Human Anatomy and Physiology in Health and Disease

THIRD EDITION

Shirley R. Burke, R. N.

Instructor
St. Francis Medical Center
School of Respiratory Care
Pittsburgh, Pennsylvania

DELMAR PUBLISHERS INC.

Cover design by John DeSieno.
Cover illustration by Bruce Kaiser.

Delmar staff:
Associate Editor: Marion Waldman
Project Editor: Judith Boyd Nelson
Production Coordinator: Teresa Luterbach
Design Coordinator: Karen Kunz Kemp
Art Supervisor: John Lent

For information, address Delmar Publishers Inc.
2 Computer Drive, West, Box 15-015
Albany, NY 12212-9985

Printed in the United States of America
Published simultaneously in Canada
by Nelson Canada,
a division of the Thomson Corporation

10 9 8 7 6 5 4 3 2 1

Library of Congress Cataloging-in-Publication Data:

Burke, Shirley R.
    Human anatomy and physiology in health and disease / Shirley R. Burke.—3rd ed.
        p.   cm.
    Rev. ed. of: Human anatomy and physiology in the health sciences. 2nd ed. ©1985.
    Includes index.
    ISBN 0-8273-4853-3 (textbook).—ISBN 0-8273-4854-1 (instructor's guide)
        1. Pathology.   2. Human anatomy.   3. Human physiology.   I. Burke, Shirley R. Human anatomy and physiology in the health sciences.   II. Title.
        [DNLM: 1. Anatomy. 2. Pathology. 3. Physiology. QS 4 B959h]
RB111.B87   1992
612—dc20
DNLM/DLC
for Library of Congress   91-15095
                                                                      CIP

Contributors

Wayne C. Anderson, R.R.T., B.A.
Director of Didactic Education
St. Francis Medical Center
School of Respiratory Care
Pittsburgh, Pennsylvania

Patricia A. Bohachick, R.N., Ph.D.
Associate Professor of Nursing
School of Nursing
University of Pittsburgh
Pittsburgh, Pennsylvania

Judith A. DePalma, R.N., M.S.N.
Chairman for Clinical Services
Undergraduate Program
School of Nursing
Duquesne University
Pittsburgh, Pennsylvania

Colleen Jane Dunwoody, R.N., M.S., O.N.C.
Clinical Instructor
Nursing Staff Development Department
Presbyterian University Hospital
Pittsburgh, Pennsylvania

Kathleen B. Gaberson, R.N., Ph.D.
Assistant Professor, Graduate Nursing Program
Duquesne University
Pittsburgh, Pennsylvania

Linda M. Goodfellow, R.N., M.N.Ed.
Instructor, School of Nursing
Duquesne University
Pittsburgh, Pennsylvania

Jo Anne S. Maehling, R.N., M.S.N.
Instructor, School of Nursing
The Pennsylvania State University
University Park, Pennsylvania

Judy Wulf, CNRN, M.S.N.
Clinical Nurse Specialist
Department of Neurosurgery
University of Minnesota
Minneapolis, Minnesota

Preface

The basic philosophy underlying the earlier editions of this text is continued in this edition. This text is intended for students in the health professions whose formal academic program is one or two years in length and whose goal is an understanding of the human body and the consequences of a disruption of body processes.

The first two chapters introduce some aspects of chemistry and microbiology related to health care. Although emphasis is not placed on chemical or cellular physiology and pathology, some concepts from these disciplines are discussed throughout the text.

The major part of the text is arranged in alternating chapters; first the anatomy and physiology of a system is discussed and then common pathologic conditions of that system. This approach is particularly useful since it helps reinforce the student's knowledge of the normal while introducing important clinical considerations.

The subject of human anatomy and physiology is not like a marble statue that is carved out and allowed to stand and be admired for all time. The knowledge in these fields is increasing at an astonishing rate, as is the application and uses to which we put this knowledge. For this reason, major changes have been made in the presentations of normal physiology and the clinical chapters have been extensively revised. Also, at the beginning of each chapter, the student will find a list of objectives that indicate important sections of the chapter and will help direct the study of that chapter.

In planning this revision, it quickly became obvious that what was needed was more than an updating and a cosmetic overhaul. As we in the health professions become more and more specialized, it is important that our students have access to material prepared by specialists in their fields. For this reason, the clinical chapters have been written by contributors who are knowledgeable in each particular area.

It is not surprising to find that, in this rapidly changing world, the needs of teachers and students are varied and changing. In our courses, the sequence of study of the various body systems should depend primarily on the way one course relates to another and on the time needed for the study of each system. In using this text, you will find no difficulty in adopting any systems sequence that is appropriate for your situation. When students who have little background in medical terminology encounter a word in the text that has not yet been defined, they can quickly find it in the glossary.

I hope that this book will be helpful to students as they begin their studies of the wonders of the human body and prepare for exciting careers in the health professions.

Shirley R. Burke

To the Student

You will probably find anatomy and physiology to be one of the most interesting courses you will ever take. It is about you, your family, and your friends. Most important, it is about those you desire to help, your patients and members of the health team with whom you will work. This course forms the foundation upon which your professional skills and judgment will be built.

Scientific information is dynamic and subject to modifications on the basis of new research. For this reason it is important that you keep your store of information up to date. Instead of preparing a bibliography that will quickly be outdated, a list of journals has been provided, which you will find in Appendix D. Reading some of these journals will help keep you up to date. The disease chapters in this text were written by individuals who are specialists and currently involved in the area of health care they write about.

The key terms at the end of each chapter represent important words and phrases covered in the chapter. These words appear in color so that you can find them easily. You should learn the spelling and definition of these terms. Some of the more difficult terms are followed by pronunciations. Vowels and consonants have their usual English sounds. A vowel followed by a consonant in the same syllable is pronounced short, as *dom* in abdominal (ab-dom'inal), and a vowel not followed by a consonant is pronounced long, as *do* in abdomen (ab-do'men).

The objectives at the beginning of each chapter should fix in your mind exactly what you should accomplish in your study of the chapter. Keep these objectives in mind while you are studying and, at the conclusion of your review, assess how well you have accomplished your objectives. Having goals in mind when you study will make the learning process more efficient. The process becomes self-accelerating: as you increase your store of information, you increase your capabilities of meeting your own needs as well as the needs of those you intend to serve.

Chapters 1 and 2 introduce some concepts from chemistry and microbiology that are applicable to your study of the human body. Following this introduction, Chapter 3 presents some of the causes of disease and a discussion of symptoms that are common to most disease processes. Chapter 4 discusses the general organization of the body. This chapter is particularly important since you will learn the proper way to describe different parts of the body. Pay particular attention to how regions of the body are named. Later, you will find that bones, muscles, nerves, and blood vessels are often named after the region in which they are located. The subsequent chapters present first the anatomy and physiology of a body system and then the common procedures used to diagnose disorders of that system, common disorders of the system, and the usual treatment.

At the conclusion of each chapter, you will find a list of questions. If you can answer these questions, you have mastered the essential content of the chapter. These questions are not necessarily sequenced in the order in which the material was discussed in the chapter since, in your clinical experience, you will find you need this information in ways other than those presented in your text. Likewise, your teacher may sequence the systems in your course differently than they are sequenced in the text. The course sequence is that which will best meet your needs. Even though a systems approach is used to describe the structure and function of the body, you should keep in mind that the body functions as a whole, not as individual parts or systems. This concept explains why, when you have a head cold, you may "ache all over." It is this interdependency of the different organ systems that helps the body compensate for specific disabilities. This concept of the interdependency of body systems will become more obvious to you as your studies progress.

If you have had little previous experience with medical terminology, you will find the glossary helpful. You will also find in the Appendixes common medical prefixes and suffixes, medical abbreviations, and weights, measures, and equivalents used in medical practice.

In previous educational experiences, you may have been required to memorize many facts. In this course, you are encouraged, for the most part, to discard this habit. It is better for you to understand one generalization and, thereby, predict three out of five facts correctly than it is to remember all five facts but not understand them and, therefore, not be able to apply your knowledge. By understanding general concepts, you will be able to deal with unpredictable situations. In your profession, you are going to meet many situations that are completely unexpected. This is one of the reasons why the health professions are so exciting.

A clear exposition of the purpose of this text will assist you in the learning process. For this reason, you should at the outset consider the following statements of purpose. Following your study of a body system and the conditions related to this system, use these to help assess your progress. If there are gaps, you will be able to identify them quickly and know precisely the areas that need more attention.

The study of this text will enable you to:

1. Know the names of the structures in each of the organ systems.

2. Be able to describe the locations of the parts of the body.

3. Know some of the parts of the various organs.

4. Know the functions of the organs.

5. Understand how the particular organ functions are accomplished.

6. Be able to predict many of the symptoms that result from malfunction of a particular organ or system.

7. Become familiar with common diagnostic procedures and how patients are prepared for examinations.

8. Gain a knowledge of how the human body attempts to compensate in the presence of disease.

9. Therapeutically support some of the normal body defense mechanisms.

10. Become a skillful observer and an accurate reporter of your observations.

Shirley R. Burke

Contents

1.
An Introduction to Chemistry 1

2.
Microscopic Life 17

3.
The Fundamental Processes of Disease 29

4.
Body Organization 55

5.
Tissues and Membranes 71

6.
Diseases of the Skin 79

7.
The Musculoskeletal System 91

8.
Disorders of the Musculoskeletal System 143

9.
The Nervous System 161

10.
Diseases of the Nervous System 197

11.
Sense Organs 223

12.
Disorders of the Sense Organs 237

13
The Cardiovascular System 249

14.
Diseases of the Cardiovascular System 287

15.
The Respiratory System 309

16.
Diseases of the Respiratory System 325

17.
The Gastrointestinal System 347

18.
Diseases of the Gastrointestinal System 367

19.
The Urinary System 387

20.
Diseases of the Urinary System 395

21.
The Reproductive Systems 411

22.
Diseases of the Reproductive Systems 433

23.
The Endocrine System 457

24.
Diseases of the Endocrine System 475

25.
Aging 489

Appendix A.
Common Medical Prefixes and Suffixes 499

Appendix B.
Medical Abbreviations 501

Appendix C.
Weights, Measures, and Equivalents 503

Appendix D.
Suggested Readings 505

Glossary
507

Index
535

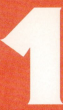

An Introduction to Chemistry

OBJECTIVES

On completion of this chapter, you will be able to:

1. Identify the major chemical elements found in the body.
2. Give examples of both organic and inorganic compounds involved in life processes.
3. Discuss factors influencing the speed of the chemical reactions in the body.
4. Give examples of the clinical uses of radioactivity.
5. Explain how to protect living cells from the harmful effects of radiation.
6. Explain how pH influences body functions.

OVERVIEW

I. THE STRUCTURE OF ATOMS
II. THE ROLE OF ELECTRONS IN CHEMICAL REACTIONS
III. ELECTROLYTES
IV. ATOMS, MOLECULES, ELEMENTS, COMPOUNDS, AND MIXTURES
V. CHEMICAL SUBSTANCES IN THE BODY
   A. Acids, Bases, and Salts
   B. Acidity and Alkalinity
VI. CHEMICAL REACTIONS
   A. Speed of Reaction
      1. Temperature
      2. Catalysis
      3. Concentration
VII. MEASUREMENT
VIII. NUCLEAR CHEMISTRY
   A. Radioactivity
   B. Radioactive Isotopes
   C. Radiation Damage
      1. Somatic Damage
      2. Germ Cell Mutation
   D. Protection from Radiation

Chemistry is the study of matter. This, of course, includes living substances as well as nonliving materials such as salt and sugar. In our study of biology to prepare for careers in the health professions, we will be concerned with matter and changes in matter. These changes may be physical or chemical.

A physical change alters the form but not the composition of matter. For example, water is composed of hydrogen and oxygen. When we boil water to sterilize surgical instruments, some of the water changes form, becoming steam, but it is still hydrogen and oxygen.

Chemical changes alter the composition of matter. The digestion of food is an example of a chemical change taking place in our bodies. The movement of oxygen and carbon dioxide through our bloodstream involves chemical reactions. Chemical reactions also take place within our muscles and nervous system when we move about. These are but a few examples of the importance of chemistry in the study of the human body.

THE STRUCTURE OF ATOMS

Matter is made up of atoms. Although an atom is extremely small, it is the arrangement and behavior of the particles that make up the atom that determine the characteristics or properties of the particular atom. Within the **nucleus** (nu'kle-us) of an atom, there are positively charged particles called **protons** and other particles that have no charge called **neutrons**. The protons and neutrons are made of more basic particles—quarks, muons, gluons and neutrinos. The weight of the atom is determined by the number of protons and neutrons. The protons determine the atomic number. All atoms of an element have the same atomic number.

Revolving around the nucleus are negatively charged particles called **electrons**. There are the same number of electrons surrounding the nucleus as there are protons inside the nucleus. Therefore, the atom is electrically neutral. It is the electrons that determine the behavior of the atom.

The electrons are located in shells or energy levels. Each level has the ability to hold a specific number of electrons. The level nearest the nucleus contains no more than 2 electrons, the next level no more than 8, the third no more than

18, the fourth no more than 32, and so on. It is important to know, however, that the outermost shell of an atom, regardless of the number of shells, can contain no more than 8 electrons.

THE ROLE OF ELECTRONS IN CHEMICAL REACTIONS

When an atom contains the full eight electrons in its outer shell, the atom is chemically stable. That is, it does not readily combine with other atoms. Atoms with less than eight electrons in the outer shell either can give off electrons to a nearby atom or can accept electrons to complete the outer shell. The activity of an atom tends to move it toward stability. Atoms with less than four electrons in the outer shell usually give off electrons to a nearby atom; those with more than four can accept electrons. Figure 1-1 illustrates the combining of sodium and chlorine atoms to form sodium chloride. The sodium atom has only one electron in its outer shell, and the chlorine has seven. The sodium will give up one electron, and the chlorine will accept this electron. If an atom gives up electrons to become stable as the sodium did, it will have a positive charge. If it takes on electrons, it acquires a negative charge. The process of gaining or losing electrons is called **ionization** (i-on-i-za'shun), and the resulting particles are called ions. Specifically, the negatively charged ions are **anions** (an'i-ons), and the positively charged ions are **cations** (kat'i-ons).

In addition to gaining or losing electrons in order to complete the outer shells, atoms can also share one, two, or three electron pairs. This type of chemical bonding is more common in organisms than is ionization. Figure 1-1 illustrates the sharing of electrons in the formation of water.

ELECTROLYTES

Substances, such as sodium chloride, that ionize in solution are called **electrolytes** (e-lek'tro-lits). Electrolytes can conduct an electric current. Since electrolytes are present in the body, their ability to conduct electric current is utilized in several diagnostic procedures. For example, the electrocardiogram (e-lek-tro-kar'de-o-gram), or ECG, gives a graphic tracing of the electrical impulses involved in the contraction and relaxation of the heart.

ATOMS, MOLECULES, ELEMENTS, COMPOUNDS, AND MIXTURES

The structure of an atom or, more specifically, the arrangement of the electrons, determines the behavior or properties of the atom. When two or more atoms combine, they form a molecule. A molecule composed of like atoms is called an element. A molecule that is a combination of different types of atoms is called a compound.

An element cannot be changed into another element by ordinary physical or chemical means. It can be separated into its individual atoms, and the resulting atoms will have the same properties as the molecule. When atoms of different elements combine, forming compounds, a chemical reaction occurs.

Compounds possess properties that differ significantly from those of their constituent elements. For example, water is a compound made of two hydrogen atoms and one oxygen atom. Under ordinary conditions, both hydrogen and oxygen are gases, nothing like the clear, colorless liquid water.

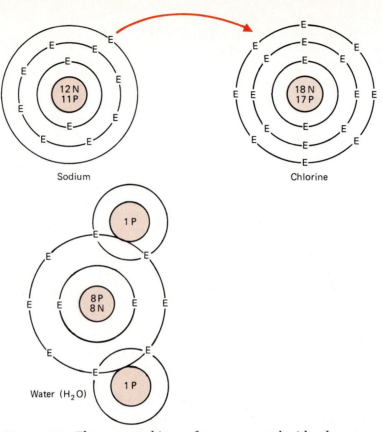

Sodium

Chlorine

Water (H_2O)

Figure 1-1. *Elements combine to form compounds either by transferring electrons or by sharing electrons. This is illustrated above with sodium and chlorine combining to form sodium chloride. One electron on the outer shell of the sodium atom is being transferred to the outer shell of the chlorine atom. This transfer makes the outer shell of both ions complete with eight electrons, and the elements are bonded together. Sharing of electrons is illustrated with the formation of water. Oxygen, with six electrons on the outer shell, will combine with two hydrogen atoms, each having one electron on its outer shell. The three atoms share the electrons so the outer shell of each atom has its complete number of electrons, eight for oxygen and two for each of the hydrogens. Symbols: **P**, proton; **N**, neutron; **E**, electron.*

A mixture contains two or more compounds, such as salt and water. A mixture can be made in various proportions, but the proportions of the molecules combining to form a compound are fixed. If water is to be formed, for example, the proportions must be two hydrogens to each oxygen. In salt water, however, a teaspoon of sodium chloride (table salt) in a cup of water or in a liter is still a mixture, and we still call it salt water.

CHEMICAL SUBSTANCES IN THE BODY

The hundred or so elements found in nature combine to make an almost unlimited number of compounds. Relatively few elements are found in the body in large quantities. Carbon, hydrogen, oxygen, and nitrogen make up more than 96% of the body weight. The major mineral elements in the body are calcium, phosphorus, potassium, sulfur, sodium, chlorine, and magnesium. There are also trace amounts of several other elements such as iron, iodine, copper, and zinc found in the body.

The relative amount of a particular element does not necessarily reflect the importance of the element in the body. All are important in the healthy structure and function of the human body.

The organic compounds (those containing carbon) are also found in the body. Those that we are mainly concerned with are carbohydrates, lipids, and proteins.

Carbohydrates are sugars and starches. For example, blood sugar or glucose is a simple sugar. Another type of sugar (deoxyribose) is a building block for the molecules that carry hereditary information. Glycogen is a more complex carbohydrate or starch. It is a reserve form of fuel that, when needed, can be broken down to usable glucose.

Lipids (fat-like substances) represent the body's most concentrated source of fuel. Although they provide more than twice as many calories (a form of energy) as carbohydrates, they are much less efficient as fuels.

Proteins are much more complex in structure than the carbohydrates or lipids. Antibodies are proteins that help provide our defenses against invading bacteria. Enzymes are proteins that act as **catalysts** (kat′ah-lists), substances that affect the speed of body chemical reactions. The contractile portion of muscle tissue is protein.

Nucleic acids, DNA and RNA, are organic compounds that contain hereditary materials and help regulate protein synthesis in the body. These important compounds will be discussed in more detail in Chapter 4.

Another organic compound, **adenosine triphosphate** (ah-den″o-sin tri-fos′fate), or ATP, is a form of stored energy found in all living cells. The breakdown of this compound provides the energy for the cell's functions. Closely related to ATP is an important organic compound, cyclic AMP, which is necessary for the proper functioning of hormones.

ACIDS, BASES, AND SALTS

The inorganic compounds with which we will be concerned are acids, bases, and salts. When an acid ionizes it will yield a hydrogen ion ($H+$). The ionization of hydrochloric acid will illustrate this.

$$HCl \rightarrow H^+ + Cl^-$$

Normally hydrochloric acid is present in the stomach, where it not only helps in the process of digestion but provides an acid medium that is not favorable for the growth of bacteria.

Although digestion in the stomach is favored by an acid medium, the digestive processes in the intestine require an alkaline medium. Bases (alkali) yield a hydroxyl ion (OH-) when in solution. This is illustrated by the ionization of sodium hydroxide.

$$NaOH \rightarrow Na^+ + OH^-$$

The combination of an acid and a base will produce a salt and water. If hydrochloric acid and sodium hydroxide are combined, the result will be sodium chloride and water.

$$HCl + NaOH \rightarrow NaCl + H_2O$$

Salts are compounds that yield neither a hydrogen nor hydroxyl ion when they dissociate. The ionization of sodium chloride will illustrate this.

$$NaCl \rightarrow Na^+ + Cl^-$$

ACIDITY AND ALKALINITY

The strength of an acid or base is expressed by the symbol pH. The values for pH range from 0 to 14, with 7 as the neutral point. A pH of 7 shows that the compound contains the same concentration of H^+ ions as of OH^- ions. Acid solutions have greater concentrations of hydrogen ions, while basic or alkaline solutions contain more hydroxyl ions.

A number on the pH scale is obtained by dividing 1 by the common logarithm (log) of the reciprocal of the hydrogen ion concentration $(H+)$ in a liter of the solution.

$$pH = \log\frac{1}{(H+)}$$

The result is that the greater the concentration of hydrogen ions (meaning the stronger the acidity), the lower the number on the pH scale. Each number on the scale represents a tenfold increase in the concentration of the acid from 7 down to 1. On the other side of the neutral point of 7, the alkalinity increases in the same manner; a base with a pH of 9 is ten times stronger than a pH of 8.

In the human body, pH is of concern to us in understanding normal functions as well as disease processes. All chemical reactions in the body are pH sensitive. The pH of different body fluids is specific for particular chemical reactions occurring within these fluids. For example, urine has a pH of about 5 or 6, secretions in the stomach are normally acid with a reaction of about 1 to 4, the intestinal secretions are alkaline with a pH of about 8 to 10.

Acid Range	*Alkaline Range*

0.0 1.0 2.0 3.0 4.0 5.0 6.0 7.0 8.0 9.0 10.0 11.0 12.0 13.0

       stomach   urine   intestine

H^+ ←neutral→ OH^-

The pH of normal blood is about 7.4. This does not vary much from a pH of 7.3 to 7.5 without manifestations of disease. Values above 8 or below 7 are not compatible with life for a prolonged period of time. When the blood pH is above 7.5, the patient is said to be in alkalosis, and values below 7.3 are evidence of acidosis. You will recall that a pH of 7 is neutral so that when we talk about acidosis we mean the blood pH is lower than the normal of 7.4 but not really below the neutral point of 7.

Since the hydrogen ion acts as a depressant, a person in acidosis will be drowsy and, in severe acidosis, may be unconscious. The patient complains of weakness and headache. There is usually dehydration. This condition can be caused by a variety of problems such as diseased kidneys that cannot eliminate acid waste products properly. Severe diarrhea with excess loss of base can also cause acidosis. Patients with chronic respiratory diseases often cannot eliminate carbon dioxide. The retained carbon dioxide combines with body water and forms carbonic acid that will cause a respiratory acidosis.

Regardless of the cause of the acidosis, the kidney will attempt to compensate by eliminating more hydrogen and retaining more bicarbonate. Respirations will increase, thereby eliminating more carbon dioxide and preventing the formation of carbonic acid.

Any condition that either increases the base content of the body or causes excessive loss of acid will produce alkalosis. The patient in alkalosis is anxious, nervous, and perspires excessively. To compensate, there will be a slowing of respiration with a retention of carbon dioxide in order to increase the formation of carbonic acid, and the kidneys will increase their excretion of bicarbonate and retain increased amounts of hydrogen.

Buffers

Since our blood must maintain such a narrow range of pH, there are mechanisms that help neutralize excess acids or bases until they can be eliminated from the body. **Buffers** are one of the mechanisms that help regulate the blood pH. Buffers are pairs of chemicals, one of which dominates if the medium is too acid and one of which dominates if the medium becomes too alkaline. There are four sets of blood buffers: alkaline and acid phosphate, proteins, bicarbonate-carbonic acid, and hemoglobin. When there is either excess acid or excess base in the blood, these buffers will help neutralize the excess acid or base until it can be eliminated by the respiratory or urinary systems. For a detailed discussion of acidosis and alkalosis see Chapters 15 and 19.

CHEMICAL REACTIONS

A chemical reaction occurs when two or more substances react with one another to form a new substance. These chemical reactions involve energy. Most chemical reactions release energy in the form of heat. The type of chemical reaction in which heat is released is called exothermic (ek'so-thur'mik). The release of energy in an exothermic reaction may occur slowly as it does in reactions in our body, or the energy release can be explosive, as it is in a blast of dynamite. There are some reactions, however, in which energy must be supplied in the form of heat, light, or electricity. These are called endothermic (en'do-thur'mik) reactions.

SPEED OF REACTION

There are many factors that influence the speed of a chemical reaction. Obviously, this is of practical importance to a chemist in a laboratory, but it is also of considerable importance to us. For example, disinfectants and antiseptics destroy bacteria by chemical reactions. We need to know how much time is required for a reaction to accomplish the desired effect.

Temperature

Chemical reactions occur more rapidly when the temperature is increased. Refrigeration helps preserve our food because it retards the chemical reactions in food. Our body temperature helps to regulate the speed of chemical reactions in our bodies.

A fever is evidence of an increase in the chemical reactions taking place in the body, and these reactions consume energy. This is one of the reasons why you are so tired when you are sick, even though you are at rest in bed.

Depending on the functions being done in different parts of the body, there are slight differences in the body temperatures. The temperature is highest in the liver where many chemical reactions are taking place. Perhaps you have wondered why oxygen combines with hemoglobin (he-mo-glo'bin) in the red blood cells in the vessels within the lungs, and seconds later the oxygen dissociates from the hemoglobin. This is partly because of temperature differences. The temperature in the lungs is somewhat lower than elsewhere in the body where there are active muscles.

Catalysis

As mentioned earlier, a catalyst is an agent that influences the speed of a chemical reaction. As a result of the action of a catalyst, the speed of a chemical reaction may be increased or retarded, but the catalyst itself remains unchanged.

Hydrogen peroxide is an effective cleansing agent because it liberates oxygen. When you apply hydrogen peroxide to a wound, you will see it bubble; this is the oxygen being liberated and cleansing the wound. To prevent the decomposition of hydrogen peroxide in the bottle, the manufacturer adds a little acetanilid (as-e-tan′i-lid) to the solution. This acetanilid is a catalyst.

Digestive enzymes are catalysts. Bread cannot be utilized by our bodies until it is broken down to a very simple chemical form. The speed of this process is enhanced by digestive enzymes.

Not only is the chemistry of digestion accomplished by enzymes, but all chemical reactions in the body are influenced by specific enzymes, the biological catalysts. Since internal body temperature must remain relatively stable, the speed of these chemical reactions is chiefly dependent on enzymes.

Concentration

The speed of a chemical reaction is directly proportional to the concentration of the reacting substances. If we use the example of an antiseptic, we might assume that the stronger the antiseptic, the more rapidly the bacteria are destroyed. Although this may be true, there are other important considerations. If we are using the antiseptic on the skin, we must be sure that a strong concentration will not harm the skin. A lower concentration may take longer to destroy the bacteria but be safer for use on the skin.

MEASUREMENT

In science, we need to know how to make precise measurements and how to communicate them. For this reason, the measuring devices used must be accurate, and a consistent system of units must be used. The metric system has worldwide use among scientists. If you are not familiar with this system, refer to Appendix C.

NUCLEAR CHEMISTRY

We have seen that ordinary chemical reactions occur because the electrons of atoms are not as stable as they might be. In some of the heavier chemical elements, nuclear reactions are possible because the nuclear particles of these elements are not stable. Over 99% of the energy of an atom is found in the nucleus. If four grams of hydrogen are burned in the presence of oxygen, the result is the production of 120,000 calories. Four grams of hydrogen undergoing a nuclear reaction produce 592 billion calories. This tremendous nuclear energy results when radioactive atoms attempt to achieve stability by throwing off nuclear particles. The change in the composition of the nucleus results in transmutation, the formation of an entirely different element.

Radioactive decay, arising from the instability of the nucleus of radioactive elements, is measured in terms of **half-life**. Half-life is the time it takes for an initial quantity of radioactive material to decay to one half the original amount. The half-lives of different radioactive materials vary from billions of years (uranium, U^{238}, has a half-life of 5 billion years) to a matter of hours (bromine, Br^{82}, has a half-life of 36 hours). Some of the more recently discovered radioactive materials have half-lives of only a few seconds.

RADIOACTIVITY

Rays are emitted in the process of decay. The naturally occurring rays are alpha rays, beta rays, and gamma rays. X-rays are man-made gamma rays. The penetrating ability of the alpha, beta, and gamma rays varies considerably. This fact is of importance not only because of the medical usefulness of the rays but also because of the necessity for protecting vulnerable tissues from the harmful effects of the rays.

Alpha rays are two protons and two neutrons that move with a velocity equal to light. These rays are particles. Alpha rays cannot penetrate the epidermis, the outer layer of the skin, which is nonliving tissue. These rays can be stopped with cardboard. If alpha rays are ingested (swallowed or inhaled), they can penetrate up to a depth of five living cells. Uranium that is naturally radioactive is an alpha emitter. When uranium decays, it becomes thorium and radium, which emit beta and gamma rays.

Beta rays are also particles. Electrons released within the nucleus are thrown out and a neutron becomes a proton. Beta rays are much smaller than alpha rays and are more penetrating. They can "burn" the skin but cannot reach the internal organs from outside.

Gamma rays are not particles but are electromagnetic radiation. Gamma rays as well as the manmade X-rays are very penetrating. Because early workers with X-rays did not realize the danger, many physicists, doctors, and radiologists died over the years from excessive exposure to X-rays.

The three atomic radiations and X-rays are all ionizing radiations that convert atoms of matter through which they pass to ions. This procedure is not the orderly sort of ionizing that takes place when a sodium atom interacts with a chlorine atom. Rather, it is a ruthless, indiscriminate knocking of electrons away from atoms and molecules. Although this type of behavior makes radiation dangerous to human tissues, at the same time, radiation can be useful as a diagnostic tool and also in the treatment of diseases, particularly cancer.

Neutrons are very penetrating and do not need oxygen as much as do gamma and X-rays. For this reason, neutrons may be more effective in the treatment of cancer since, frequently, the growth is surrounded by **necrotic** (ne-kro'tic) tissue. There is no oxygen in this dead tissue. Therefore, it shields the cancer from penetration by gamma or X-rays, whereas neutrons can usually penetrate this shield.

RADIOACTIVE ISOTOPES

Radioactive materials may be either radioactive elements, such as uranium, or an **isotope** (i'sotop) of an element that is normally stable. Isotopes are forms of the same element, having identical chemical properties but differing in weight.

Chemical properties are a function of the electrons whereas physical properties, such as weight, are a function of the nucleus. For example, the stable element iodine has an atomic weight of 127. There is a radioactive isotope of iodine with an atomic weight of 131. Both forms of iodine have the same number of electrons, 53, and therefore the same chemical properties. However, the radioactive form is heavier because there are more neutrons in the nucleus. This radioactive isotope of iodine, called I^{131}, does not occur in nature but is manufactured by bombardment of the stable iodine with neutrons.

Since isotopes have the same chemical behavior as the stable form of the element, some isotopes can be used for tracers, that is, for diagnostic studies. For example, iodine tends to concentrate in the thyroid gland. Therefore, 24 hours after the oral administration of I^{131}, its presence in the thyroid can be detected and graphed on a film showing the size and shape of the thyroid. Instruments used for this recording are called scanners. An imaging device known as a gamma camera can also be used.

Radioactive isotopes can be used to measure the volume of blood in the body. A sample of human red blood cells containing a measured amount of radioactive chromium is injected into a vein, and time is allowed for the sample to thoroughly mix with the circulating blood. Fol-

lowing this, a sample of blood is withdrawn and the amount of radioactivity it contains is measured. The ratio between the total radioactivity injected and the small fraction recovered in the blood sample allows the circulating volume of red blood cells to be calculated. A similar procedure can be used to measure the liquid portion of circulating blood.

Radioactive isotopes can be utilized for a variety of diagnostic and therapeutic purposes. Table 1-1 lists some radioisotopes commonly used in medical practice. When the half-life of an isotope is short, the material may be left perma-

Table 1-1. Commonly Used Radioisotopes

Isotope	Type of Ray	Uses Related to Disease
Iodine (I^{131})	beta, gamma	Evaluation of thyroid, liver, kidney function; pulmonary circulation; localization of brain tumors; treatment of some thyroid diseases and thyroid cancer
Technetium (Tc^{99})	gamma	Studies of blood circulation; scanning of liver, bone marrow, and spleen; localization of brain tumors
Iron (Fe^{59})	beta, gamma	Iron turnover study, measurements of iron in blood, utilization of red blood cells
Chromium (Cr^{51})	gamma	Detection of gastrointestinal bleeding, diagnosis of certain blood diseases, determination of the red blood cell survival time
Strontium (Sr^{85})	beta	Bone scan
Phosphorus (P^{32})	beta	Localization of tumors, treatment of certain leukemias and other blood diseases, treatment of cancer of the prostate, pleura, and peritoneum
Cobalt (Co^{60})	beta, gamma	Cancer treatment
Gold (Au^{198})	beta, gamma	Cancer treatment
Iridium (Ir^{92})	beta, gamma	Cancer treatment
Yttrium (Y^{90})	beta	Cancer treatment
Radium (Ra^{226})	alpha, beta, gamma	Cancer treatment
Radon (Rn^{222})	alpha, beta, gamma	Cancer treatment

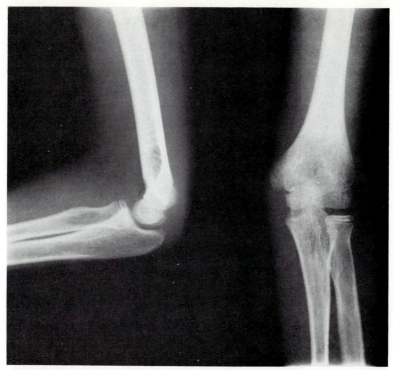

Figure 1-2. X-ray views of an elbow. X-rays can penetrate the human body; they are stopped to a great extent by dense tissues and by elements that have a high atomic number. Bone is denser than muscle and contains calcium, which has a high atomic number. The film is blackest where the X-rays pass easily through the soft tissue.

nently in the body. When a radioactive substance with a very long half-life is used for therapy, the substance is placed in or near a tumor and removed after the desired dose of radiation has been received.

In addition to the internal use of radiation, machines that use radiation can also be employed. Conventional diagnostic X-ray films enable an examiner to discover problems not otherwise detectable. Radiation treatments can be administered by machines that deliver X-rays or gamma rays to lesions in or on the patient's body (see Figs. 1-2 and 1-3).

Although radioactive iodine is used in the diagnosis of thyroid diseases, it is also used in the treatment of cancer of the thyroid and also of an overactive thyroid. Most therapeutic uses of radiation are for cancer. This treatment is based on the ability of ionizing radiation to kill cells in the sense that the cells lose their ability to divide and reproduce and thus the growth of the tumor is controlled. The radiation is not selective for the tumor cells alone and, therefore, the treatment must deliver lethal doses of radiation to the tumor while not producing too much damage to the surrounding normal tissue.

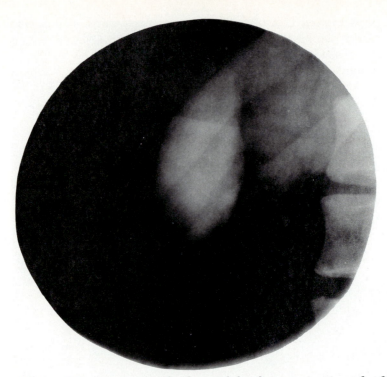

Figure 1-3. X-rays can also be used for the examination of soft tissue by administering a substance that will increase the density of the structure to be examined. In this X-ray, the gall bladder is visible because the patient was given a drug containing iodine (atomic number 53), which the gall bladder stores temporarily.

RADIATION DAMAGE

Radiation damage to living cells can be to adult cells of the present population (somatic damage) or the damage can cause germ cell mutations, in which case future generations will be affected.

Somatic Damage

Most patients receiving radiation therapy experience some degree of radiation sickness. However, with the precision of modern radiation therapy technology, these reactions are minimal. The vulnerability of living cells to radiation damage depends on the pattern of cellular division of the particular cells being radiated. The damage occurs when the cells being radiated are in the process of dividing. Since adult nerve cells do not divide, these cells are not vulnerable to this type of damage. There are other cells such as those of the bones and liver that divide only when necessary. Evidence of damage to these cells, therefore, will not be apparent for quite some time following the injury. The cells that are most vulnerable to radiation are those that divide frequently. These are the cells of the skin, those lining the gastrointestinal tract, and the blood cells. Since we know the usual life span of these cells, we can predict with some accuracy when, following a radiation injury, the symptoms of damage to these cells will appear.

If the person has received external radiation, symptoms of skin reactions occur fairly early. The skin may be unusually dry, irritated, and have the appearance of a sunburn, which is also a radiation injury. During the treatment period, the patient should not use powders, perfumes, or ointments on these areas since many of these preparations contain metallic elements that can intensify the radiation. Only mild soaps should be used, and the affected areas should be patted, not rubbed dry, after bathing. When treatments are finished, the patient may bathe and powder as he pleases.

The patient should avoid exposure to the sun as the skin subjected to radiation is more sensitive to the sun's rays. Following radiation treatments, sunburns or any skin wound will not heal as readily as it once did.

Loss of hair in the area being treated with external radiation is fairly common. The more rapidly the hair grows, the more sensitive the hair follicle is to radiation because cells that divide rapidly are most vulnerable to radiation damage. The hair may grow again, but never at its former rate or density.

Evidence of radiation damage to cells lining the gastrointestinal tract will appear in about 5 to 10 days after the radiation. The time delay is the approximate lifetime of the cells that cannot be replaced. The damaged cells cannot absorb fluids. It is important to note that all nutrients must be in fluid form in order to be utilized by the body. Compounding the problem of not being able to absorb much of the dietary intake,

the patient suffers nausea, vomiting, and diarrhea. Small, frequent meals that are high in calories, proteins, carbohydrates, and fluids but low in roughage may be helpful. Since the diet will be deficient in raw fruits and vegetables, supplementary vitamins should be taken. Fried and spicy food should be avoided.

Not only are these damaged cells unable to do their job of absorbing nutrients, they are also unable to prevent bacteria that may be present in the gastrointestinal tract from entering the bloodstream. The problems of bloodstream infections can be life threatening.

Radiation damage to the blood cells will be evident in about a month. The patient will have a decreased number of white blood cells. White blood cells normally help to protect against infection. Therefore, this patient will be particularly vulnerable to what otherwise might be considered a minor infection. Since there will be a deficiency of oxygen-carrying red blood cells, even mild activity will cause extreme fatigue. There will be bleeding tendencies because of damage to the blood platelets.

The signs and symptoms of damage in an individual who has received a lethal dose of radiation from a bomb blast or a nuclear power plant accident will be evident within four or five hours and persist for a few days before death. There will be loss of hair and nails will turn black. Lymph nodes, spleen, thymus, and bone marrow, all important in producing blood, will be seriously affected. The total amounts of red blood cells, white blood cells, and platelets will decrease markedly. If the individual survives this blood crisis, death will occur in a week to ten days from the erosion of the intestinal lining.

If a very large lethal dose is involved, death could come in 24 to 48 hours from massive trauma to the central nervous system. The individual will be quickly disoriented, lose coordination, develop convulsions, and, in a matter of hours, lapse into a coma and die.

Leukemia resulting from radiation is due to damage to bone, not to blood cells. For this reason, evidence of this sort of damage occurs much later, probably not until five years following the injury. Malignancies of the breast, lung, and thyroid caused by radiation appear later and are usually more fatal than leukemia.

Germ Cell Mutation

Somatic damage caused by radiation is due to cellular divisions without regard for the total needs of the body. Radiation to the germ cells will affect future generations. Radiation does not cause any special kinds of birth defects but, rather, increases the probability of such defects.

Pregnant women should avoid radiation. The fertilized ovum undergoes differentiation between the ninth day after conception and the sixth week of the pregnancy. It is during this time that the organs and limbs are forming. For this reason, the unborn child is most vulnerable during this period. After the sixth week of pregnancy, the baby may be perfectly formed but have cancer, low intelligence, and stunted growth.

Considering the fact that it is unlikely that any woman knows she is two or three weeks pregnant, it is important that any diagnostic X-ray tests for young women be scheduled only during the 10 day period following the start of a menstrual period.

PROTECTION FROM RADIATION

Measures for protection against radiation depend on the amount and kind of radioactivity present. They are based on the following principles: shielding around the source of radiation, distance from the source, and length of time of exposure.

Radioactive materials must be stored in lead-lined containers. The thickness of this lining is determined by the radiation physicist or safety officer. Depending on the type of radioactive material being used, special techniques may be required to shield the body secretions of the patient.

Because it follows the inverse square law—that is, if the distance from the source of radiation is doubled, exposure decreases by a factor of four—distance provides great protection from the hazards of radiation. Generally, patients who are being treated with radioactive materials should be hospitalized in a private room, and the bed should be as far from the door as possible. Many hospitals assign patients who are to receive this type of therapy to a corner room or to a room next to a linen or supply closet. Such practices provide protection for other patients by taking into account both distance and the shielding protection of the additional walls.

The length of time necessary to observe the precautions depends on the type of radioactive material being used. In some instances no unusual precautions are necessary. For example, if the half-life of the radioactive material being used is only a matter of minutes or a few hours, there is little danger to those attending these patients or to visitors.

The uses of radiation in medical practice are numerous and are constantly being revised and expanded. If you are working with radioactivity, you should constantly update your knowledge of the subject and be thoroughly familiar with proper safety measures.

Safe utilization of radiation is one of the major concerns of the International Atomic Energy Agency. The use of nuclear chemistry in medicine and in other areas, such as insect control and food preparation, is supervised in this country by the United States Atomic Energy Commission and by state agencies.

SUMMARY QUESTIONS

1. What are the four major chemical elements found in the body?
2. What are electrolytes?
3. What is the function of a blood buffer?
4. Discuss three major organic compounds needed by the body.
5. What factors influence the speed of the chemical reactions taking place in the body?
6. Give two examples of medical uses of radioactivity.
7. Discuss methods of protecting living cells from the harmful effects of radiation.
8. Discuss the symptoms of radiation sickness.
9. Compare the relative penetrating power of alpha, beta, and gamma rays.
10. How does radiation help to control the growth of cancer?
11. Compare and contrast the pH of blood, urine, gastric juice, and intestinal secretions.
12. List four sets of blood buffers.

KEY TERMS

adenosine triphosphate

anions

buffers

catalysts

cations

electrolytes

electrons

half-life

ionization

isotope

necrotic

neutrons

nucleus

protons

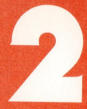

Microscopic Life

OBJECTIVES

On completion of this chapter, you will be able to:

1. List the six groups of microorganisms.
2. Explain how bacteria are classified according to their shape.
3. Discuss the environmental factors necessary for the growth and multiplication of bacteria.
4. Explain how infections are transmitted.
5. Give examples of factors that must be considered when selecting a chemical antimicrobial agent.
6. List important general rules to follow when collecting specimens that are to be examined microscopically.

OVERVIEW

I. CLASSIFICATION OF MICROBES
   A. Algae
   B. Fungi
   C. Rickettsiae
   D. Protozoa
   E. Viruses
   F. Bacteria
      1. Shape
         a. Rod-shaped—bacilli
         b. Spherical cells—cocci
         c. Curved cells—vibrio, spirillus, spirochetes
         d. Spores
      2. Distribution of Bacteria
      3. Needs of Bacteria
         a. Nutrition
         b. Moisture
         c. Temperature
         d. Reaction
         e. Oxygen
         f. Osmotic pressure
         g. Light
         h. Interrelationships
II. MICROBIAL CONTROL
   A. Transmission of Infection
   B. Antimicrobial Methods
      1. Chemical means
      2. Physical means
III. THE HANDLING OF MICROORGANISMS
   A. Collecting Specimens
   B. Identification of Organisms
IV. USE OF THE MICROSCOPE

Microbiology is the study of organisms that cannot be seen with the naked eye. Although some microorganisms (or microbes) cause disease, it is important to realize that they are generally beneficial to us. Some microbes that normally inhabit the human intestine are essential to the normal processes of the colon. Dead plants and animals are decomposed by the action of microbes and are transformed into substances that enrich the soil. Microorganisms are needed in the manufacturing of wine, cheese, antibiotics, and many other products.

The terms **pathogen** and **nonpathogen** are often used in relation to microorganisms. The implication is that pathogens cause disease and nonpathogens do not. Although this may be a useful division of these organisms for some purposes, keep in mind that the environment of the organism and the characteristics of the host influence whether a particular type of organism causes disease or not. For example, the normal, helpful bacteria that live in our intestines do not cause disease there. However, they can cause disease in other parts of the body if they reproduce in sufficient numbers. Other organisms that are normally classified as nonpathogens can cause disease in an individual who has a low resistance to infection, or if these organisms multiply excessively.

CLASSIFICATION OF MICROBES

Microorganisms can be divided into six general groups: algae (al'je), **fungi** (fun'ji), rickettsiae (rik-et'se-ah), protozoa (pro-to-zo'ah), **viruses** (vi'rus-ez), and **bacteria** (see Fig. 2-1).

ALGAE

Algae are simple plants that occur in a variety of shapes and sizes. Many are microscopic. Some of the most common forms of algae are seaweeds and those that form the green scum on ponds.

FUNGI

Fungi are plants that rarely cause disease, but there are some fairly widespread skin infections caused by fungi. Athlete's foot and ringworm are fungus diseases. Thrush, a fungus infection of the mucous membranes of the mouth, is common in infants and children.

RICKETTSIAE

Rickettsiae are parasites that live inside living cells. Rickettsial infections are transferred by lice, fleas, ticks, and mites, and thus are limited to the portion of the human population that has contact with the insect bearers. Rocky Mountain spotted fever is a severe rickettsial infection that occurs throughout North America. The disease is characterized by a widespread hemorrhagic rash and is similar to other tick-borne diseases occurring in other parts of the world.

PROTOZOA

Protozoa are the simplest organisms in the animal kingdom. There are more than 64,000 species of protozoa. Only a few of these species cause disease in humans, but those species represent serious health hazards to millions of people.

Trichomonas vaginalis (trik-om'o-nas vaj-in-a'lis) is a fairly common vaginal infection caused by a parasitic protozoa. The patient complains of itching and has a whitish vaginal discharge. Other protozoal diseases are malaria and African sleeping sickness.

VIRUSES

Viruses grow only within living cells and use the host cell's energy and biochemical machinery. They are usually not susceptible to antibiotics; however, interferon is a nonspecific antiviral agent. There are many types of viruses. They are all extremely small and grow only on living cells. The most familiar of the viral diseases is the common cold; however, measles, mumps, chickenpox, poliomyelitis, rabies, hepatitis, and influenza are also caused by viruses.

BACTERIA

Bacteria are unicellular plantlike microorganisms that are much larger than viruses. Bacteria cause the bulk of all infectious diseases. There are many different types of these organisms and their classification is complicated. For our purposes, their shape provides a simple and convenient method of grouping the different types of bacteria (see Fig. 2-1).

Shape

1. Rod-shaped bacteria are called **bacilli** (bah"sil'i). Examples of diseases caused by bacilli are tuberculosis, tetanus, whooping cough, typhoid fever, and diphtheria.
2. Spherical bacteria are called **cocci** (kok'si). These can be further divided into groups according to the way the cells are arranged. Those occurring in pairs are called **diplococci** (dip-lo-kok'si). Among the diseases caused by diplococci are gonorrhea and meningitis. **Streptococci** (strep-to-kok'si) are arranged in chains and are frequently responsible for diseases such as tonsillitis, pneumonia, boils, scarlet fever, sore throats, and skin infections. Clusters of cocci are known as **staphylococci** (staf-lo-kok'si). Boils, abscesses, wound infections, pneumonia, meningitis, urinary infections, and skin infections are a few of the diseases caused by staphylococci.
3. Some bacteria are curved. Vibrio (vib're-o) is shaped like a comma; spirillus (spir-ril'us) and **spirochete** (spi'ro-kete) are shaped like corkscrews. The most serious and wide-

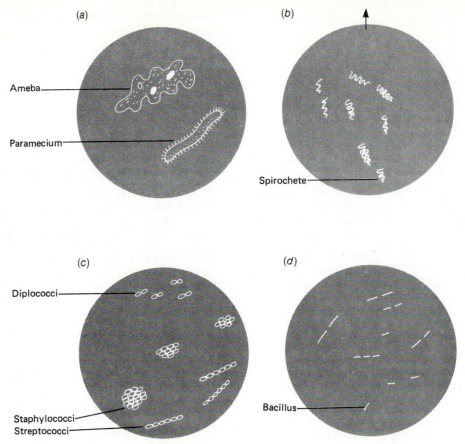

Figure 2-1. Microbes as seen with a light microscope. (a) Protozoa. (b), (c), and (d) Types of bacteria. Viruses and rickettsiae are not shown since they can only be seen with an electron microscope.

spread disease caused by curved bacteria is syphilis.

4. Certain bacilli have the ability to form round or oval resistant structures called spores. The spores are created in response to adverse factors such as high temperatures or drying. These spore-forming bacteria are much more difficult to destroy than nonspore-formers. Unless a spore is destroyed, it will germinate back into the bacterial cell.

Distribution of Bacteria

Bacteria are probably the most widely distributed of the different types of microbes since they are able to move about independently in their environment. They are in the food we eat, the water we drink, and the air we breathe. Bacteria are present on practically every article in our environment. They are on our skin and in our digestive and respiratory tracts. It is not uncommon to find large populations of streptococci and staphylococci in the throats of healthy individuals.

It should be emphasized that relatively few of the several thousand species of bacteria cause disease, and the fact that these organisms are so widespread is not, under ordinary circumstances, a matter to cause alarm or concern. In individuals whose resistance to infection is decreased, it is possible that some of these organisms may cause disease, particularly if they multiply rapidly or spread to an area of the body where they are not normally found. The significance of this fact is that wounds should be kept clean and that materials used for dressings should be sterilized.

Needs of Bacteria

Bacteria need certain environmental factors to grow and multiply. A knowledge of these factors provides a basis for techniques used to disinfect or to sterilize equipment. These needs must also be taken into consideration in the laboratory where bacteria are examined.

Nutrition. Sufficient food of the proper kind must be available. In the laboratory setting, bacteria are grown on material called culture media. Some bacteria require special nutrient media while others will grow on simple culture media.

Moisture. Water is essential for the growth and reproduction of bacteria. Some bacteria are particularly sensitive to drying or desiccation (des"ic-ca'shun) and can live for only a few hours in a dry environment, while others can resist drying for a few days. Some bacteria can surround themselves with capsules (spores) that not only make the bacteria particularly resistant to drying but also help protect them from the actions of some drugs and disinfectants.

Temperature. Each species of bacteria has a range of temperature that is best suited for its growth. Most bacteria are unable to reproduce at temperatures much below 20°C or above 45°C. Normal body temperature of 37°C is ideal for many bacteria.

Cold retards or stops bacterial growth and, therefore, refrigeration helps preserve food. Any bacteria that were present in the food before refrigeration, however, may begin to multiply when the food is removed from the refrigerator. High temperatures are much more injurious to bacteria than low temperatures, and heat is frequently used as a means of destroying bacteria.

Reaction. Bacteria require a proper degree of alkalinity or acidity. Usually the range of pH is rather narrow, not more than 8 or less than 6. Most pathogens grow best in a slightly alkaline medium.

Oxygen. Organisms that grow in the presence of atmospheric oxygen are called **aerobes** (a'er-obs), and those that cannot live in the presence of oxygen are **anaerobes** (an-a'er-obs). Although there are not many pathogenic anaerobes, the bacteria that cause tetanus and gas gangrene are anaerobic. Therefore, deep puncture wounds require particular attention. Skin heals more readily than underlying tissue and can seal these anaerobic bacteria in the wound where they can multiply.

Osmotic Pressure. The membrane of the bacteria is affected by changes in osmotic (oz-mot'ik) pressure. If exposed to solutions with a higher concentration of particles than are in the bacteria, the cell loses its water and shrinks. In a solution with a lower concentration of particles the cell will swell. The bacteria cell will not burst, however, since its membrane is stronger than the membrane of blood cells. The reactions of bacteria to changes in osmotic pressure are useful in the preparation of chemical disinfectants.

Light.   All microbes are either inhibited or killed by ultraviolet rays. Many bacteria are killed by direct sunlight within a few hours. Bright daylight is not as injurious as direct sun but does have a similar effect. Ultraviolet light can be used as a sterilization technique.

Interrelationships.   A relationship in which two organisms live together and at least one benefits from the relationship is called **symbiosis** (sim-bi-o′sis). There are three types of symbiotic relationships: mutualism, commensalism, and parasitism. In mutualism, both benefit and neither is harmed. In commensalism, only one benefits and the other neither benefits nor is harmed. In parasitism, one benefits and the other is harmed. An example of a symbiotic relationship is the rapid multiplication of both staphylococci and the influenza bacilli when the two are grown together.

Some organisms are unable to live together at all. This is called antibiosis (an-te-bi-o′sis). It is as a result of the phenomenon of antibiosis that antibiotics have been developed.

MICROBIAL CONTROL

To prevent the spread of infection, we need to be able to control the growth and reproduction of microbes. The methods used will depend on how the particular infection is transmitted as well as what techniques are effective for the destruction of the specific organisms.

TRANSMISSION OF INFECTION

Microbes are transmitted from their host either directly or indirectly. Direct transmission is made either by direct body contact or by droplet infection (the spread of organisms by coughing, sneezing, or laughing). Indirect transmission means the spread of infection by water, food, soil, contaminated objects, or other carriers such as insects.

A knowledge of the method of transmission and the route through which the pathogen enters and leaves the body is of considerable importance in the control of specific infections. For example, if the pathogen is spread by means of droplet infection, then a physical barrier such as a mask may be effective in preventing the spread of the infection. However, microbes thrive in a moist environment, and if the mask is slightly damp from expired air, it may not serve the purpose for which it is intended. Indeed, it may incubate the bacteria, increase their numbers, and spread them. If a person with an infection covers his mouth and nose with a tissue when coughing or sneezing, the danger of transmission by droplets is greatly reduced. Droplets leaving the mouth during the process of ordinary speech do not travel more than three feet, and under these circumstances, a little distance can serve as a barrier.

ANTIMICROBIAL METHODS

The inhibition and destruction of microorganisms can be accomplished by either chemical or physical means. Both are based on a knowledge of the biological needs of microbes as well as methods of transmission.

Chemical Means
Disinfectants and antiseptics are chemicals that inhibit the growth and reproduction of microbes. No chemical antimicrobial agent is best for all purposes. Following are some of the factors to be considered in the selection of such an agent.

1. *Nature of the material to be cleaned.* A chemical agent used to disinfect contaminated instruments might be totally unsatisfactory for the skin since it might seriously injure these sensitive cells.

2. *Type of organisms.* Not all organisms are equally sensitive to the inhibiting actions of specific chemicals. For example, spores are more resistant than most other microbes. The agent selected must be effective against the type of microorganism to be destroyed.

3. *Environmental conditions.* The factors discussed above under Needs of Bacteria (nutrition, moisture, temperature, reaction, oxygen, osmotic pressure, light, and interrelationships) may all have effects on the rate and efficiency of the chemical agent.

Before any chemical antimicrobial agent is used, any obvious soil, such as pus or blood, should be removed by thorough washing. The effectiveness of chemical agents depends on their strength and the length of time they are in contact with the microorganism.

Antibiotics are examples of chemicals that are fairly specific for the destruction of organisms that have caused a human infection. The antibiotic to be used for a particular infection is determined by doing a culture and sensitivity test. This procedure is done by growing the infection-causing organism on a medium that has been treated with a variety of antibiotics. After this culture medium has incubated (kept at a temperature of 37°C for 48 hours), it is observed for microbial growth. The areas on the culture medium that have been treated with the antibiotic most effective in destroying the pathogen will have the least amount of microbial growth.

Physical Means

Exposure to sunlight destroys microbes both by the effects of ultraviolet light and by drying. The value of this method is limited primarily because it may be difficult or impossible to expose all the surfaces that harbor microbes.

Since microbes cannot withstand high temperatures, heat is used in a variety of sterilization methods. Sterilization is a term used to indicate a method by which all microbes are destroyed, while disinfection refers to the destruction of most pathogens and inhibition of microbial growth in general. Antiseptics are usually not as strong as disinfectants, and therefore are more appropriate for use on the skin.

Dry heat at 170°C for two hours is an effective method of sterilization for instruments or glassware. Articles that will not be damaged by boiling can be boiled for 30 minutes. This method will destroy pathogens and most, but not all, other microbes. Boiling does not destroy spores, however; therefore, it is not an entirely reliable method of sterilization. In hospitals, most sterilization is done in an **autoclave** (au′to-klav), which is a technique of using steam under pressure. Most articles are sterile after 15 minutes at 120°C with 15 pounds of pressure.

Pasteurization is the disinfection of milk and other substances by heating. One method, called the holding method, is to heat the milk at 62°C for 30 minutes. In the flash method, the milk is heated to 71°C for 15 seconds, and then immediately cooled and bottled. Some microbes are still present in the milk, but these are harmless.

The value of washing with soap and water as a means of controlling microbes cannot be overemphasized. The soap functions chemically to limit bacterial growth; the friction of the washing and rinsing action is useful in removing the microbes and in eliminating materials that otherwise might serve as nutrition for the microbes.

With the increasing incidence of blood-borne infections, many hospitals and health agencies have developed policies to protect their employees and clients. These policies are often called "Universal Precautions" and usually require that workers and students observe some of the following procedures.

1. Gloves should be worn for contact with blood or blood-containing fluids and for procedures that involve exposure to blood.
2. For procedures that may involve spilling or splattering of blood or blood-contaminated body fluids, gloves, gowns, masks, and some form of eye protection should be worn.
3. Handwashing after patient contact should be routine.

THE HANDLING OF MICROORGANISMS

COLLECTING SPECIMENS

Specimens of pus or secretions from various parts of the body that might be infected may need to be examined microscopically. Microbes from such specimens are placed on culture media and grown until there is sufficient multiplication of the microbes so that they can be examined microscopically.

The exact method used to obtain the specimen and to prepare the culture will vary from one laboratory to another. However, there are some general rules that should be observed.

1. Use sterile equipment to collect the specimen and put it in a sterile container.
2. Label the container with the patient's name, source of the specimen, and any other identification required by the particular laboratory, such as the patient's social security number.
3. Collect the specimen from the exact site. For example, a specimen from the throat should not be unduly contaminated with secretions from the mouth.

4. Adequate amounts of material must be collected. If swabs are used, it will be necessary to have several swabs of the material.
5. No preservative or antiseptic should be added to the specimen, and the collection should be made before the patient has received any antimicrobial treatment. If treatment has been started, notation should be made of this.
6. Collect the specimen in such a manner as not to endanger others. For example, the outside of the container must not be soiled with materials likely to contain microbes.
7. Since most microbes cannot resist drying, care must be taken that the specimen is delivered to the laboratory when it is fresh. Specimens on cotton swabs dry very rapidly.
8. The culture media used to grow the microbes for examination must meet the nutritional and moisture needs of the organism.
9. The temperature and length of time required for the growth of the culture should be appropriate for the multiplication of the microbes. This is usually about 48 hours at 37°C.
10. If for some reason the specimen cannot be put on the culture media when it is delivered to the laboratory, it should be refrigerated.

IDENTIFICATION OF ORGANISMS

There are so many different kinds of bacteria that it is necessary to use a number of procedures for identifying the organisms. Some of the laboratory techniques involve the following.

1. Growing the bacteria on different types of media that will cause bacteria to grow in some characteristic fashion.
2. Counting the bacteria in a given specimen.

3. Inoculating animals with the organisms and observing the reactions to the inoculation.

4. Growing the organisms in air and in carbon dioxide to determine their aerobic or anaerobic characteristics.

5. Staining.

One of the most common stains used to identify bacteria is a Gram stain. A thin smear of microbial growth is allowed to dry on a glass slide and is then stained with a dye called crystal violet. The slide is then washed with water and covered with Gram's iodine for about one minute before it is washed again with water. Ninety-five percent alcohol is then applied to the slide until no color leaves the slide. Finally, the smear is covered with Safranine and washed with water. After the slide is dry, it can be examined with a microscope. Gram-positive organisms will have a blue stain and gram-negative organisms will stain red.

Acid-fast bacteria retain their stain even though the slide is washed with acid-alcohol. The prepared smear is first covered with carbolfuchsin and gently heated for five minutes. The slide is then washed with water and decolorized with acid-alcohol. After the slide has dried, the smear is counterstained with methylene blue, washed with water, and allowed to dry. The acid-fast organisms will be red and the others blue.

USE OF THE MICROSCOPE

The light or optical microscope is used to examine microorganisms. This instrument is a tube with a lens system at the bottom called the objective and a lens at the top called the eyepiece. It is called a compound microscope because it incorporates two or more lens systems so that the magnification of one system is increased by the other. Study the picture of the microscope shown in Figure 2-2.

There is a mirror to direct a beam of light through the object on the stage and an iris diaphragm to regulate the amount of light entering the condenser. The image is viewed through the eyepiece. The most commonly used eyepiece or ocular magnifies ten times.

Most compound microscopes have three objectives: low power ($10 \times$, meaning it magnifies ten times), high power (43, 44, or $45 \times$), and oil immersion (95 or $97 \times$). The total amount of magnification depends on the power of both the objective and the ocular; therefore, if you are using an objective designated $45 \times$ and an ocular that magnifies ten times, you have magnification of 450 ($10 \times 45 = 450$).

The specimen to be examined is put on a slide and covered with a coverslip. Place the slide on the microscope stage with the specimen centered over the condenser. The low-power objective should be positioned approximately 5 mm from the slide. Adjust the light and the mirror so that the field is uniformly bright. If the specimen is heavily stained, you will want a strong light; for a slide with little stain, close the iris diaphragm so there is less light entering the field.

While looking through the ocular of the microscope, turn the coarse adjustment slowly toward you until the specimen comes into focus. If the specimen does not come into focus by the time the tip of the objective is about 2 cm from the slide, either you have turned the coarse adjustment too rapidly, thereby missing the proper focus, or you have not centered the specimen accurately. Correct the problem and begin again.

Once the object is clearly focused on low power, make sure it is directly in the center of the field. Turn the high-power objective into position, and bring the object into focus by turning the fine adjustment slowly back and forth. It

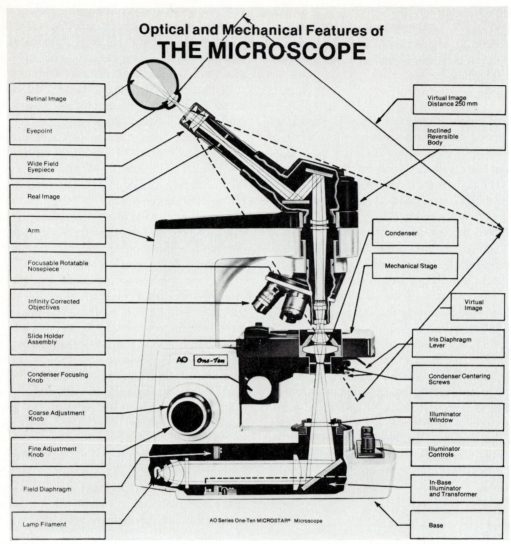

Figure 2-2. *A light or optical microscope. (Courtesy of A.O. Reichert Scientific Instruments)*

may be necessary to readjust the amount of light for the higher magnification.

You can use the oil-immersion objective once the specimen is clearly focused and centered with high power. Rotate the objective so you can put a drop of immersion oil on a slide and bring the oil-immersion objective into place. The tip of the objective will be in the oil nearly touching the slide. It will be necessary to use the fine adjustment to focus.

Keep the microscope clean and handle all parts with care. Lens paper should be used to clean the glass parts of the microscope. To remove oil from the glass parts, wipe with lens paper moistened with xylol. The microscope should be stored with the low power objective in working position. This precaution ensures that the least expensive objective will be injured should the optical system be jammed down accidentally. Keep the microscope covered when not in use.

SUMMARY QUESTIONS

1. List three types of bacteria.
2. Explain how bacteria are classified according to their shape.
3. Discuss chemical and physical means of microbial control.
4. Describe a favorable environment for the growth of bacteria.
5. List some important rules to be observed when collecting specimens for microscopic examination.
6. What is the difference between direct and indirect transmission of microbes?
7. What factors need to be considered in selecting a chemical disinfectant?

KEY TERMS

aerobes
anaerobes
autoclave
bacilli
bacteria
cocci
diplococci
fungi

nonpathogen
pathogen
spirochete
staphylococci
streptococci
symbiosis
viruses

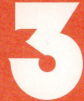

The Fundamental Processes of Disease

OBJECTIVES

On completion of this chapter, you will be able to:

1. Identify some of the major predisposing causes of disease.
2. List three ways in which cancer spreads to other parts of the body.
3. Differentiate between heat exhaustion and heat stroke.
4. Discuss two methods of estimating the severity of a burn.
5. List five major body defenses against invading bacteria.
6. Explain how immunity is acquired.
7. Explain how normal body temperature is maintained.
8. Explain how the body compensates for hypovolemic shock.
9. Discuss emergency treatment of shock.
10. List five harmful consequences of immobility and tell what measures can be taken to prevent these.

OVERVIEW

I. ETIOLOGY OF DISEASE
  A. Predisposing Causes
  B. Direct Causes
    1. Poisons
    2. Biochemical Alterations
    3. Oxygen Lack
    4. Disturbances in Immunity
      a. Allergy and hypersensitivity
      b. Immunologic depression
      c. Autoimmune diseases
    5. Neoplasms
    6. Bacterial or Viral Invasion
    7. Trauma
      a. Cold trauma
      b. Heat exhaustion and heat stroke
      c. Burns
      d. Radiation injury
      e. Wounds of bones and soft tissue
      f. Wound healing

II. NORMAL BODY DEFENSES
  A. Intact Skin
  B. Hairs in the Nares
  C. Mucous Membranes
  D. Saliva and Tears
  E. Acid Urine
  F. Gastric Juice
  G. The Reticuloendothelial System
  H. Interferon
  I. Immunity

III. TEMPERATURE CONTROL AND FEVER

IV. SHOCK

V. PAIN
  A. Anesthesia and Analgesics
  B. Electrical Stimulators
  C. Neurosurgical Procedures
  D. Biofeedback

VI. IMMOBILITY

In this chapter, the general causes or etiology of disease and the body's usual responses to specific health problems will be discussed. Some of the physiologic responses are protective. Some help minimize the cellular damage and are a part of nature's defense. These concepts are important because part of the role of workers in the health professions is to support the normal body defenses.

After considering some causes of disease and local body defenses, some common general factors, such as fever and pain, which are likely to be obvious aspects of any illness will be discussed. It is important to keep in mind that although we divide the body into systems and we study one system at a time, the body usually responds as a whole. Examples of total body responses to disease are evidenced in common manifestations such as fever, shock, pain, and immobility. To some degree, these are likely to be a part of any disease process.

Later, as each body system is presented, some of the specific system responses to disease will be discussed. As you progress in your study of human biology, you will develop an increasing awareness not only of the interdependency of the body systems but also of the interdependency of the healthy individual and his surroundings.

Pathology (pah-thol′o-je) is the study of changes that take place in the body as a result of disease. These may be gross changes in structure, such as **atrophy** (at′ro-fe) or **hypertrophy** (hi-per′tro-fe) of an organ. In the case of atrophy, the part becomes visibly smaller than normal. In hypertrophy, the size is increased. These structural changes may also be accompanied by microscopic changes. The study of the cell, which is the structural and functional unit of the body, is called **cytology** (si-tol′o-je). The microscopic study of tissues is called **histology** (his-tol′o-je). In many instances, structural changes result in alterations in the physiology or functions of the organs involved. Occasionally there are functional changes without any apparent structural change, and the disease is said to be functional rather than organic.

Subjective information about disease is called symptoms. Pain and anxiety are symptoms. Objective information, such as a blood pressure reading, is a sign. A combination of signs and symptoms that occur frequently together is a **syndrome** (sin′drom). The prognosis (progno′sis) is the ultimate outcome. Acute and chronic are terms frequently used to describe the duration of a disease. Acute is generally used to describe diseases with rapid onsets and severe consequences. Chronic is generally applied to long-term illnesses.

ETIOLOGY OF DISEASE

PREDISPOSING CAUSES

There are many predisposing causes of illness. Most are a result of a decreased body resistance. This decreased resistance can be the consequence of many different factors or a combination of factors.

Our abilities and limitations are also a combination of many different factors, one of which is our heredity. That there are inherited predispositions to certain diseases has been known by scientists for many years. However, in recent years great advances have been made in the field of genetics and genetic counseling. In Chapter 21, we shall discuss in greater detail some of the mechanisms of genetic transmission of both normal and pathological traits.

Improper diet, either in quantity or quality, can predispose to disease. Dietary deficiencies and the consequences of poor dietary practices are discussed in detail in Chapter 18. We shall point out here that the food we eat is the fuel used to accomplish the metabolic processes necessary to maintain health.

Inadequate protection obviously predisposes one to illness. Some of the obvious offenders in this area are improper or inadequate clothing and improper sanitation. In addition, every year many people die or are injured because of dangerous cars, power tools, faulty heaters, wiring, or ventilation.

In recent years we have turned our attention to environmental factors that affect our health and that of future generations. We are becoming increasingly aware of the devastating effects of overcrowding and noise. Pollution of our air and waterways is becoming a serious threat to our health.

Chlorofluorocarbons are used widely in many spray cans, foam products, and refrigerants. Over the years these chemicals have been destroying the protective ozone layer in the upper atmosphere, allowing increased amounts of ultraviolet radiation to reach the earth's surface. This is likely to cause an increased incidence of skin cancer.

It is well established that a combination of environmental and hereditary factors can cause some very serious diseases. Although at this time there are relatively few major U.S. corporations using genetic testing to spot employees who are likely to react adversely to toxic substances in the work environment, there is reason to believe this practice may become more common in the next few years. It is not only blue collar workers who are involved, but also up-and-coming executives in high-pressure businesses could be passed over for promotion if identified by genetic screening as being likely to have a heart attack at an early age.

One of the most tragic predisposing causes of disease is the lack of information or, worse still, inaccurate information. Health teaching is an important role for all members of the health professions. A well-informed person is better equipped to prevent disease and, if disease is present, to help the professionals in their role of correcting the problem.

Many things that were once considered helpful, or at least harmless, are indeed injurious to our health. One of the most dramatic and tragic examples of how inaccurate information can prove disastrous occurred in early attempts to treat morphine addicts. During the Civil War, and for some time thereafter, morphine was widely used for relieving pain. Not only was it given freely to those in acute pain, but it was also administered long into convalescence. Many people became addicted to morphine as a result of this practice. It was finally recognized that although morphine may be necessary to control severe pain, it is not without serious harmful effects when used over prolonged periods. A new drug was then discovered to be quite effective in curing the morphine addiction. The name of the drug was heroin!

Before discussing some specific causes of disease, we need to consider one other very important predisposing cause—unhappiness. It may have been this relationship between a person's outlook on life and his health that the Biblical psalmist recognized when he wrote, "That which I feared has come upon me." There is a great deal of empirical evidence that unhappy people are unusually disease- and accident-prone. In a hospital setting, of course, patients are likely to be unhappy. However, we are not talking about that sort of unhappiness. Consider instead your acquaintances or associates who are generally unhappy or who seem to derive little pleasure from their occupations and everyday activities. It is this group of people who seem to be afflicted with all sorts of ailments with greater frequency and greater severity than are those of us who are more satisfied and op-

timistic about our lives. There are people with serious disabilities who are essentially optimistic. Happy people are much better able to cope with their unfortunate situations than are their unhappy counterparts.

Think about this idea the next time you have had a very frustrating day at work or school. It seemed like nothing would go your way. Perhaps you are angry with your boss but, of course, it is inappropriate to display this anger. Better get yourself in a better frame of mind before you get behind the wheel of your car to go home. An angry, frustrated person is not a very safe driver.

DIRECT CAUSES

Many different types of agents can directly cause structural and/or functional changes in the body. When the cause of the disease can be identified, the management of the problem is generally directed toward removing this cause. If the etiology is unknown or if we have no means of counteracting its cause, the treatment is more difficult and can usually only be of a **palliative** (pal′e-a-tiv) nature. The treatment then involves minimizing the symptoms, supporting the normal body defenses, and helping to retard or limit the progression of the disease.

Poisons

Although poison will be discussed more thoroughly in Chapter 18, these toxins are mentioned here because they are important agents in the etiology of disease. If ingested or inhaled, many can seriously damage the lining of the gastrointestinal or respiratory tracts. Others can cause lethal damage to the kidneys, liver, or other vital organs.

Biochemical Alterations

Biochemical problems that can cause disease are mainly the result of pathology of the endocrine glands. These glands, together with the nervous system, control many important metabolic activities of the body. Clearly, any pathology of these glands can seriously impair normal body functions. In Chapter 24 we shall explore this complex matter in greater depth.

Oxygen Lack

Whether a deficiency of oxygen is the result of an inability of the respiratory tract to oxygenate the blood properly or whether the circulatory system is unable to deliver adequate amounts of oxygen to the tissue cells, disease will result. **Dyspnea** (disp-ne′ah), or labored breathing, may be subjective as in fear, or it may be due to **anoxia** (an-ok′se-ah), or the lack of oxygen. **Ischemia** (is-ke′me-ah) is the lack of adequate amounts of oxygen in the tissue cells because of a greatly reduced blood supply. If the ischemia is severe, necrosis, or tissue death, will result.

Disturbances in Immunity

Allergy and Hypersensitivity. Allergy is a result of altered reactions of the tissues in certain individuals on exposure to agents that are innocuous to most other people. Sensitivity is a term closely related to allergy; often the two may be indistinguishable. There is both an immediate and a delayed type of sensitivity. A delayed reaction appears from 24 to 48 hours after exposure. In this type, there are no circulating antibodies (specific immune substances). Delayed sensitivity can be transferred only with whole cells. A positive tuberculin reaction is an example of delayed sensitivity.

Immediate sensitivity can be life threatening. In this type of sensitivity, there are circulating antibodies in the serum, the fluid portion of the blood. The treatment of the allergic reaction is primarily symptomatic. The patient's symptoms may be relieved by an **antihistamine** (an″te-his′tah-min) drug. For example, pyribenzamine (pir-e-ben′zah-men) or, in the case of asthma, a drug such as theophylline (the″o-fel′in) will cause bronchial dilatation and relieve the respiratory distress. Antihistamines are of no value in the treatment of cell-mediated (delayed) hypersensitivity, but steroid hormones seem to be of some value.

In the process of developing a hypersensitivity, a susceptible person is exposed to the allergen (allergy-provoking agent) and develops an antibody to this allergen. Upon a later exposure to the allergen to which the person has been sensitized, the allergic signs and symptoms will develop.

The treatment of allergy is complex. Possibly the individual can be desensitized by taking small, periodic doses of the allergen. In some forms of allergy, this can be accomplished only with great difficulty, and the allergic individual may have to avoid exposure to the allergen completely.

The types of substances that may cause allergic reactions in sensitive individuals include dust, molds, and animal dander. Certain foods or drugs may also be a source of an allergic reaction. Some people are sensitive to weeds, particularly poison ivy, which come into contact with their skin. Insect bites or stings can also cause allergic reactions.

Immunologic Depression. Antimetabolic (an″te-meh-tab′o-lik) drugs and alkylating (al″kah-la′ting) agents are used in the treatment of certain cancers. These chemicals interfere with cell division and thereby stop the rapidly growing neoplasm. However, they affect all cells adversely and so can suppress the normal immune response, in much the same way irradiation used for cancer treatment can cause immunologic depression.

Immunologic depression can reduce the normal protection provided by the immune response to infection. Normal wound healing may also be impaired.

Massive doses of steroid drugs, such as cortisone, are sometimes given to suppress the immune response in patients who have had an organ transplant. The purpose of the medicine is to prevent rejection of the transplant, but the drug cannot selectively suppress only one aspect of the immune reaction, and the transplant patient becomes unusually vulnerable to infections.

Autoimmune Diseases.   Normally, the human body is able to recognize its "self" proteins and only produces antibodies when "foreign" (nonself) proteins invade. Autoimmune diseases, however, are conditions in which the body fails to recognize its own proteins and produces antibodies against them. Cells are damaged by antibodies or aggressive lymphocytes. In most of these conditions, autoantibodies can be detected in the patient's blood. Some apparently healthy people, particularly those of advanced years also have autoantibodies in their blood.

Examples of conditions in which autoimmune phenomena are conspicuous include rheumatoid arthritis, thyroid disease, diabetes mellitus, Addison's disease, colitis, lupus erythematosus, and pernicious anemia. These diseases are described elsewhere in the text.

Neoplasms

At present there is not a great deal known about the causes of **neoplasms** (ne'o-plasmz), or tumors. Some tumors are caused by certain viruses and others may be caused by chemical or mechanical irritation. Some neoplasms are benign (be-nine'), others are malignant (mah-lig'nant). Malignant tumors spread to other parts of the body by means of direct extension, by way of the bloodstream, or by way of the lymphatic system. Because malignant tumors undergo more rapid cellular division than do other cells of the body, they demand a large blood supply. The inability of the body to provide adequate blood supply can result in necrosis of the surrounding tissues. Because both benign and malignant tumors may become quite large, some of the symptoms produced are a result of pressure on surrounding structures.

Benign tumors are usually encapsulated and freely movable, whereas malignant tumors attach themselves to the surrounding normal soft tissues and so are not very movable. At these points of attachment there is dimpling in the overlying skin, particularly if the tumor is near the surface.

In the case of benign tumors that do not spread or metastasize (me-tas'tah-siz) to other parts of the body, surgery is usually the treatment of choice. Surgery is also used for treatment of malignant tumors, but in this case the surgical procedure is usually much more radical. Malignant tumors also are sometimes treated with radiation or with antineoplastic drugs. These drugs retard cellular division and decrease the growth of the tumor. Often the tumor is radiated first in an attempt to reduce its size, and then surgery is performed. Radiation therapy following surgery may be continued for a prolonged period of time in the hope of destroying any malignant cells not removed at surgery.

Immunotherapy for the treatment of cancer seems to have a great deal of promise. Immunotherapy is based on the theory that the patient with cancer has a defect in his immune system. Normally our phagocytic (fag"o-si'tik) cells recognize abnormal cells such as bacteria or tumor cells and destroy them. In a defective immune system these cells are allowed to multiply.

In general, immunotherapy is directed toward improving the cancer patient's immune system. Currently, there are three major approaches used in immunotherapy. One is nonspecific in that the intent is to improve the general immune capacity of the patient. BCG vaccine has been used for malignant melanoma, soft tissue sarcoma, and leukemia. A second type of immunotherapy is specific in that the substances are antigenically related to the tumor or its products. They may be killed tumor cells or an antigen substance extracted from the tumor cells. The third type of immunotherapy transfers lymphocytes from one tumor patient to another or uses molecules of immune RNA and transfer factor which have been recovered by lymphoid cells.

Leukemia is a form of cancer. There are several types of leukemia. All are serious diseases of the bone marrow in which there is a tremendous increase or decrease in the number of white blood cells and a decrease in red blood cells and platelets. The white blood cells produced in leukemia are immature cells not capable of fighting infection. For this reason, what otherwise might be a relatively mild infection may prove fatal to someone with leukemia. As the number of white cells increases, there is often a marked decrease in the production of platelets resulting in a tendency for abnormal bleeding.

Leukemia is treated with chemotherapy and the effect of the chemotherapy is to destroy the cells of the bone marrow resulting in leukopenia, thrombocytopenia, and anemia. The goal of chemotherapy is to achieve a remission of the disease process. Bone marrow transplantation is a relatively new treatment that is being researched for its effectiveness.

The procedure for a bone marrow transplant involves finding a suitable donor who has the same tissue type as the patient. About 25 ml of the donor's marrow is treated with soybean lic-

tin, which causes the T cells responsible for rejection to form a heavy clump and sink to the bottom of the tube. The remaining cells at the top are almost entirely free of T cells but they are given a second purification with sheep red blood cells that capture any remaining T cells.

Bacterial or Viral Invasion

Certain types of microorganisms can cause disease when body resistance is decreased, when they invade parts of the body that they do not normally inhabit, or when their numbers or **virulence** (vir'u-lens) is increased. Several factors influence the severity of the diseases caused by microorganisms.

Microorganisms normally inhabit many parts of the body. When they are in their usual habitat they usually do not cause disease. If, however, they invade other parts of the body, they will very likely cause disease. Infections caused by these resident bacteria are not communicable.

Communicable infections are caused by nonresident organisms that are transmitted either directly or indirectly from one host to another. Contagious diseases are also caused by nonresident organisms; however, in this instance direct contact is necessary. These nonresident organisms enter the body through some portal. Most organisms cannot invade the intact skin; however, they can enter the body through the respiratory tract, the gastrointestinal tract, or the genitourinary tract.

An infection is said to be local when it is confined to a certain area, a boil, for example, and systemic when it involves the whole body, such as influenza. Often, however, a local manifestation is merely the beginning of a systemic involvement, in which case it is referred to as a focal infection.

As the number of microorganisms increases, the likelihood of an infection and the severity of that infection increases. The strength, or virulence, of the organism is also a factor in determining the extent of the infection. Virulence usually increases by rapid transfer of the organism through a series of susceptible individuals.

A final important factor in determining the extent of the infection is the defensive powers of the host. These powers include anatomical and chemical barriers, immunity, and the ability of the phagocytic cells to destroy the invaders. Normal body defenses will be discussed in detail later in this chapter.

Trauma

Injury, or trauma, is one of the more obvious causes of disease. There are many different types of traumatic agents. All result in varying degrees of damage to the cells and consequent disturbances in body structure and function. We shall discuss briefly a few general types of trauma. Later chapters describe more fully the results of trauma to the various organ systems.

Cold Trauma. Extreme changes in environmental temperature can result in serious cellular damage. Injury owing to cold is much more severe if the cold is moist and if the exposure occurred during prolonged periods of inactivity. If the patient also has some preexisting condition that interferes with normal blood flow to the part involved or if the blood circulation is diminished by tight clothing, the trauma is likely to be more serious than it would be otherwise. The very young and the aged are especially vulnerable to cellular damage from cold.

If frostbite, for example, is superficial, the frozen part is soft, and white skin does not redden with pressure. Dark skin will have a dull ashen color. **Edema** (e-de′mah), or excess tissue fluid, is likely to develop and there may be blisters. Heat should not be applied, but the part may be immersed in warm water. The frozen part should never be rubbed with snow as this will increase the injury.

With deep frostbite, the frozen tissue will be hard. It is important to decrease the oxygen needs of the involved tissues and increase the blood supply to the part. Any necrotic tissue will have to be removed before healing can take place.

There are three main aspects to the treatment of cold trauma. First, maintain a relatively low environmental temperature to reduce metabolism to the tissues involved so that the available blood supply may be adequate to prevent tissue death. Second, maximum circulation must be maintained. Vessels in the traumatized area are likely to go into spasm, further impairing circulation and favoring blood clot formation, which may completely occlude (obstruct) circulation to the part. The **vasospasms** (va′so-spasms) may be relieved by keeping the uninvolved parts of the body warm and thereby producing a reflex **vasodilation** (vas-o-di-la′shun). Medications that favor vasodilation, such as papaverine (pah-pav′er-in), may be helpful. To reduce the tendency toward clot formation, it may be necessary to give some **anticoagulant** (an″te-ko-ag′u-lant), such as heparin (hep′ah-rin). Finally, every effort must be made to prevent the wound from becoming infected by using soft, nonirritating, sterile dressings and by applications of antiseptics. If infection does occur, specific antibiotic therapy will be needed.

Hypothermia, like radiation sickness, was unheard of 70 years ago. Now it is estimated that 25,000 people, mostly elderly, die of hypothermia every year in the United States. Although it is recognized that the person is ill, the nature of the illness is not recognized because most clinical thermometers do not register below 94°F or 35°C.

As recently as 25 years ago most people regarded drowning as the only hazard to life in the water. In the case of the Titanic, about one-third of the passengers and crew got on lifeboats safely. Most of these were saved when a nearby ship, the Carpathia, arrived and rescued them. None of the 1,489 people who had on good life jackets were saved. They probably had been in 32°F water for about two hours. The official report listed the cause of death of these people as drowning. There was little mention of immersion hypothermia.

Heat Exhaustion and Heat Stroke. Heat exhaustion is characterized by circulatory disturbances with resulting inability of the body to supply the peripheral vessels with enough fluid to produce perspiration needed for cooling. The patient is pale and feels dizzy and faint. Temperature is usually normal or below normal. The treatment is to hydrate the person.

Heat stroke (sunstroke) is a very serious condition in which the body's heat-regulatory center in the brain is not functioning properly and the body temperature increases greatly. The skin is hot, dry, and flushed. The victim becomes confused, dizzy, and faint. He is likely to lose consciousness. Without treatment it is very likely that the patient will die. If the fever remains around 40.5°C (105°F) for very long, permanent brain damage can occur. The aim of treatment, therefore, is to reduce the body temperature to a safe range as rapidly as possible since brain damage can be a function of body temperature and time. Cold, moist applications and a fan will help. Treatment must continue until the temperature has been lowered to at least 39°C (102°F) and the temperature must be checked frequently for the next several hours. Patients who have experienced heat stroke often have faulty heat regulation for several days and a lowered tolerance to heat for years or perhaps for the rest of their lives.

Burns. In the case of trauma owing to thermal burns, the severity of the damage depends on several factors, mainly the depth of the burn and the extent of the surface area involved. Generally speaking, burns that involve only superficial tissues are not serious. However, when large areas of the body are superficially burned, as in the case of sunburn, severe disruption of body physiology can occur.

In estimating the severity of a burn with respect to the depth of tissues involved, the severity is described as being first, second, or third degree. In first degree burns the skin is reddened; there are no blisters, but there may be some edema. A first degree burn usually peels or **desquamates** (des′kwah-mates) in three to six days and heals without scarring. Second degree burns are characterized by blisters that contain fluid having a composition similar to that of blood plasma. Most of the outermost layer of the skin, but not the deeper layers, are involved. The deepest layers contain the nerve endings. (See Chapter 5 for a more complete discussion of the anatomy and physiology of the skin.) For this reason, second degree burns are very painful. Second degree burns heal without scar formation in 10 to 14 days if they do not become infected. In third degree burns the entire skin and subcutaneous tissues in the burned area are involved. These burns develop massive edema within a very short time following the burn. There will be necrosis of the involved tissues. This type of burn heals with scar formation. The length of time required for healing depends on the size of the area involved; however, it will be more than three weeks.

The extent of the surface area involved in a burn is also used to estimate the severity of the trauma. The "Rule of Nines" is used to determine the percentage of surface area involved (see Figs. 3-1 and 3-2). Severe first and second degree sunburns that involve as much as 70 to 75% of the body surface cause more disturbances in body function than does a third degree burn of the fingertip. When 40% of the surface area is involved, regardless of the depth of the

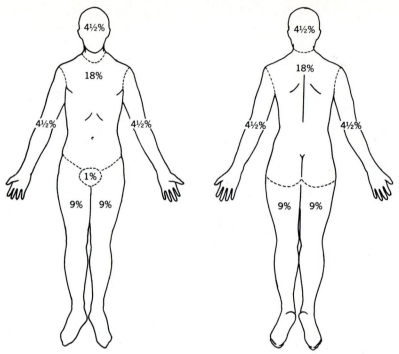

Figure 3-1. *Anterior and posterior views of the body divided into areas—9% or multiples thereof—for the purposes of quickly estimating amounts of burned surface. The "Rule of Nines" is usually attributed to Pulaski and Tennison.*

burn, there is cause for concern; if burns happen to be mostly third degree, the trauma may be fatal. People rarely survive burns involving 80% of the body surface, particularly if the burns are mostly second and third degree burns.

In the case of electrical burns, the skin first turns white and then black. These burns are usually severe and may involve not only the skin but also blood vessels, muscles, tendons, and even bones. As a result of the electrical shock, the strong skeletal muscles may have such severe contractions that they cause fractures of bones. Patients may die from heart failure before any first aid is available. The first concern with electrical burns is to maintain cardiopulmonary function and, second, to attend to the burns.

Chemical burns from either acid or alkali solutions can be very injurious. In some instances, the chemical not only burns the skin but is absorbed into the body, in which case the injury will be very serious even though a small area is involved. There are also some chemicals that will continue burning even after a thorough washing. This effect will become apparent a day or two later unless suitable early treatment has been carried out.

Regardless of the cause, burns may so severely disrupt the whole body physiology that patients with preexisting health problems, such as kidney disease, lung disease, or heart disease, can have serious trouble with what otherwise would be a relatively mild burn trauma. Again, the

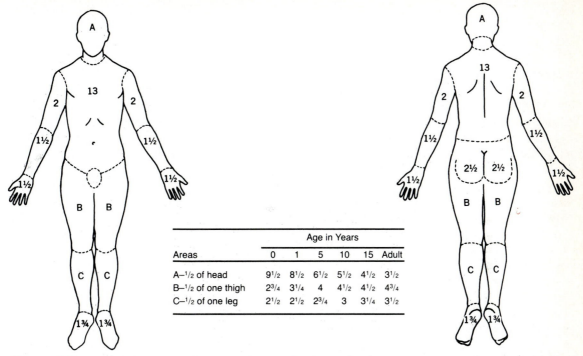

| | Age in Years | | | | | |
Areas	0	1	5	10	15	Adult
A–$\frac{1}{2}$ of head	$9\frac{1}{2}$	$8\frac{1}{2}$	$6\frac{1}{2}$	$5\frac{1}{2}$	$4\frac{1}{2}$	$3\frac{1}{2}$
B–$\frac{1}{2}$ of one thigh	$2\frac{3}{4}$	$3\frac{1}{4}$	4	$4\frac{1}{2}$	$4\frac{1}{2}$	$4\frac{3}{4}$
C–$\frac{1}{2}$ of one leg	$2\frac{1}{2}$	$2\frac{1}{2}$	$2\frac{3}{4}$	3	$3\frac{1}{4}$	$3\frac{1}{2}$

Figure 3-2. *Body proportions change with growth. Shown here, in percentage, is the relationship of body area to whole body surface at various ages. This method of determining the extent of the burned area is attributed to Lund and Browder.*

very young and the elderly are especially vulnerable to burns.

The current practice of first aid for a burn victim is to cover the area, ideally, with a moist, sterile covering. No two body surfaces should be in contact with each other while the patient is being transported to a treatment center. No ointments or salves should be applied. Although such lotions may temporarily help relieve the pain by sealing off the burned area from the air, they may be a source of infection and will have to be scrubbed off when hospital treatment is instituted. This procedure may cause additional tissue damage.

Radiation Injury. Radioactive substances give off alpha, beta, and gamma rays that can cause tissue damage. X-rays are manmade gamma rays. Although the damage caused by gamma and X-rays is much more severe than that caused by the alpha and beta rays, all are potentially hazardous. The duration of the exposure to the rays and the distance between the exposed individual and the source of the radiation are important factors in determining the degree of radiation damage.

The cells most vulnerable to radiation injury are those that most frequently undergo cell division, such as those of the skin, those lining the gastrointestinal tract, blood cells, and germ cells of the ovaries and testes. To protect from radiation injury, it is necessary to limit the time of exposure, to maintain as much distance from the source of radiation as possible, and to shield the body from the rays.

Wounds of Bones and Soft Tissue.   Injury to bones will be discussed in detail in Chapter 8. However, we shall point out here that fractures of bones can be caused not only by a direct blow but also by diseases of the bone that interfere with their ability to provide adequate structural support. A compound fracture is one in which there are fragments of broken bone protruding through the skin. A simple fracture is one in which there may be some damage to the nearby soft tissue, but no bone protrudes through the skin. A comminuted (kom'in-uted) fracture is one in which there is a shattering of the bone in the fracture area. Fragments of bone may be imbedded in the surrounding soft tissue. A greenstick fracture, which occurs almost exclusively in young children, is an incomplete break in the bone.

The following terms are used to describe trauma to soft tissue. An abrasion (ah-bra'sion) is a superficial lesion that results from the scraping or rubbing off of skin. Although this type of trauma is usually not serious, it is quite painful. Abrasions should be cleansed with soap and water. If bits of dirt or debris have entered the wound, they can best be removed by application of hydrogen peroxide. Stronger antiseptics such as iodine (particularly if the solution is not fresh and has become concentrated) may actually cause additional damage to the delicate, abraded tissues. A scab will form on the abrasion, usually within a day. This scab provides protection to the wounded tissues while healing is occurring and therefore should not be removed unless infection occurs. If the wound becomes infected, remove the scab so the wound will drain.

A laceration (las-er-a'shun) is a wound made by tearing. Again, the most important aspect of the care of the wound is cleanliness. Bleeding is not usually a problem of any major proportions if pressure is applied directly to the wound. If there is considerable bleeding, it can usually be controlled by elevation of the part or by applying ice for a short time. Venous bleeding (bleeding from veins) is usually easily controlled, because venous blood pressure is low and veins are thin walled and collapse when they are opened. Since artery walls are much thicker and do not collapse when cut, arterial bleeding is another matter. This blood is bright red and spurts from the wound. In this case, in addition to the pressure over the wound, pressure must be applied at the nearest pressure point. These sites are illustrated in Figure 3-3. As a last resort, a tourniquet can be applied proximal to the laceration. If the bleeding has not stopped within ten minutes, the wound will have to have surgical attention.

Because a laceration is due to tearing, the edges of the wound are likely to be irregular. It may therefore have to be sutured if a scar is cosmetically undesirable or if the wound is extensive. If the wound is a minor laceration on a part of the body where appearance is not an important consideration, the edges of the wound can be brought closely together and taped securely in place with a Band-aid adhesive bandage. When adhesive tape is removed from the dressing of any wound, it should always be pulled toward the wound, first from one side and then from the other. Because children frequently fear the dressing change, the tape can be moistened first with a little mineral oil to allow it to be removed without undue pulling of the skin. If the dressing must be reapplied, the skin must be thoroughly cleansed to remove all of the oil before a new dressing can be applied. For people who are sensitive to adhesive tape, it may be helpful first to paint the skin where the tape is to be applied with tincture of benzoin, which will protect the skin. Tincture of benzoin will also make the tape more adherent.

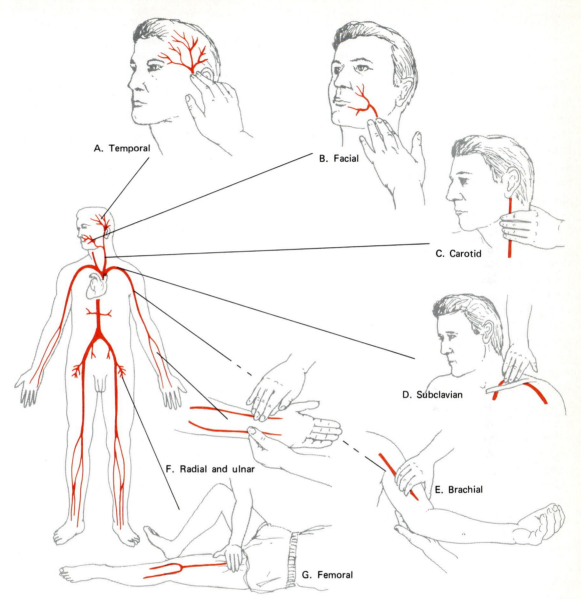

Figure 3-3. *Pressure applied at the locations illustrated can help control arterial bleeding distal to the pressure point.*

A bruise, or **ecchymosis** (ek-e-mo′sis), is due to the rupture of small superficial blood vessels in the wounded area. If there is a large amount of bleeding from these ruptured vessels, a **he"matoma** (he″mah-to′mah) may be formed. A hematoma is a swelling caused by blood in the tissues.

Penetrating wounds that damage only a small area of skin but extend deep into the body tissues can be especially dangerous. Skin heals rapidly, but the underlying tissues heal far more slowly. If the wound becomes infected, it may have to be reopened to allow drainage. In the case of any wound that may be contaminated, the person should be given protection against tetanus.

Wound Healing.   Wound healing differs very little from one type of tissue to another. It is generally independent of the type of injury. Let us consider some of the events involved in the healing of a wound. First, blood flows into the wound and fills the space with clots that help to unite the edges of the wound by retracting. Clot retraction usually begins about one half hour after the wound is incurred. In several hours, the clot loses fluid and forms a hard protective scab.

After the clot has formed, the injured and dying tissues produce necrosin (nek′ro-sin), a substance that causes nearby blood vessels to become more permeable; serum containing albumin, globulin, and antibodies leaks out of the vessels. These substances may be able to attack any microorganisms that are in the wound. The fluid also provides a sustaining environment for the white blood cells that will appear about six hours later. This fluid causes swelling and pain in the injured area. The neutrophils (nu′tro-fils), the first white blood cells to arrive, push a bit of their cytoplasm between the cells of the blood vessel wall and squeeze out. They may be able to ingest the organisms and digest most of the

remains. If no bacteria are in the wound, the neutrophils rupture and release enzymes to attack the cellular debris so that it can be removed more easily. These white blood cells are attracted to the area because the injured tissues produce a substance called leukotaxin (lu-ko-tak′sin).

About 12 hours later, monocytes (mon′o-sits) arrive. These white blood cells have great phagocytic abilities (the ability to engulf cells and foreign matter). They can also produce enzymes that digest the fatty protective coverings of some bacteria. Heat is produced by the activity of the working cells and by extensive localized vasodilatation. This heat may destroy or at least injure some bacteria. The vasodilatation also causes redness in the inflamed tissues.

Toward the end of the inflammatory period, fibroblasts (fi′bro-blasts) appear and produce collagen, a protein that will become scar tissue. During the time that the collagen is being formed, an increasing number of capillaries migrate into the wound so that the area is supplied with oxygen and the raw materials for protein synthesis. In the case of skin wounds, the final scar resembles the original tissue, except that it is denser; hair follicles, sweat glands, and sebaceous glands are usually absent. The amount of scar tissue formed depends mainly on how much stress the wound received and whether the wound was infected.

NORMAL BODY DEFENSES

INTACT SKIN

The body's first line of defense against penetration by foreign materials, including pathogenic microorganisms, is the skin. It provides an efficient physical barrier to harmful agents and environmental forces such as cold, heat, and trauma.

Most organisms cannot invade the intact skin. Fresh sweat, sebaceous (se-ba′shus) secretions, and cerumen (se-ru′men), a waxlike secretion in the outer ear canal, further discourage the growth of microorganisms. If these secretions are not fresh, not only are they unesthetic, but on decomposition they lose their antibacterial properties and actually provide nutrient media for a growing bacterial population.

Normal skin flora are toxic to the underlying tissues. Therefore, keeping their numbers at a minimum is obviously advantageous in the event that the skin is cut or abraded. The thickening of the epidermis at sites of friction, such as the palms of the hands and soles of the feet, is also a normal protective mechanism.

HAIRS IN THE NARES

The hairs in the nasal cavities also provide protection. They trap dust and other inhaled particles so that the particles cannot go farther down the respiratory tract to sites where the tissues are more sensitive.

MUCOUS MEMBRANES

Body orifices (or′i-fises), or openings, are protected by mucous membranes that produce an antibacterial protective mucus. Organisms invading the respiratory, genitourinary, or gastrointestinal tracts stimulate an increased production of this mucus, which is usually observable before other signs of infection, such as an increased body temperature.

Localized swelling of the mucous membrane in response to irritation helps to prevent the irritant from penetrating into deeper, more vulnerable tissues. Heat is also produced in response to the irritant. Increased temperature may accelerate phagocytosis and the production of immune bodies.

In the respiratory tract the mucous membrane is ciliated (cilium means lashlike process). The microscopic cilia are very powerful; when stimulated by some irritant, they wave it toward the outside of the body.

The mucous membrane of the female vagina during the childbearing years of life is particularly effective in protecting against irritation and infection. During this period, the acid secretions of the vaginal mucosa are **bacteriostatic** (bakter″e-o-stat′ik) (halting the growth of bacteria), and the mucosa is thick and resistant to irritation.

SALIVA AND TEARS

Saliva contains enzymes that are bacteriostatic. In the presence of fever, the dry mouth predisposes patients to infections of the salivary glands. Tears, saliva, mucus, skin secretions, and many internal fluids of the body contain **lysozyme** (li′so-zim), a bacteriostatic enzyme. Tears constantly bathe the outer exposed surface of the eyes. This function provides important protection since these are living cells that are exposed. (The cells of the outer layer of the skin are not living cells.) The eyelids and lashes also provide protection for the eyes.

ACID URINE

The normal acidity of the urine not only is antibacterial but also helps to keep the calcium salts in solution and prevents the formation of **calculi** (kal′ku-li), or stones. Foods that favor increased acidity of the urine are meats, cereals, and cranberry juice. Most other fruits favor alkalinity of the urine, as do most vegetables.

GASTRIC JUICE

The hydrochloric acid of the gastric juice is very effective in destroying most bacteria. However, even with **achlorhydria** (ah-klor-hi′dre-ah), a lack of hydrochloric acid, ingested bacteria can usually be phagocytized by Kupffer's (koop′ferz) cells in the liver. Kupffer's cells are a part of the **reticuloendothelial** (re-tik″u-lo-en-do-the′le-al) **system**, which is very effective in destroying invading organisms.

Newborns have relatively low gastric acidity and, as their other defense mechanisms are not well developed, special care should be taken in feeding and handling babies to prevent exposure to pathogens by the oral route.

THE RETICULOENDOTHELIAL SYSTEM

In addition to Kupffer's cells in the liver, the reticuloendothelial system also includes cells in a variety of tissues such as the spleen, bone marrow, lymph nodes, and other lymphatic tissue. All of these structures are important in the normal body defenses. Bone marrow and lymph nodes produce white blood cells to phagocytize bacteria. The lymph nodes also function to filter any bacteria or foreign material in the tissue fluid before it is returned to the bloodstream.

Histocytes (his′to-sits) are located in almost all body tissues. The histocytes in infected tissues become monocytes that have great phagocytic properties. Circulating lymphocytes are probably spent cells that have already done their part in combating infection when they were in the lymph nodes. Recent evidence suggests that lymphocytes in the bloodstream can become histocytes, which in turn become monocytes. The lymphocytes in the bloodstream may also become plasma cells to help produce immunity. Circulating lymphocytes may become fibroblasts, which can make collagen (a protein) and build scar tissue.

INTERFERON

Interferon is a protein produced by certain virally infected cells. This protein is released into the extracellular environment and, when taken up by uninfected tissues, it can protect them from viral multiplication. While viruses seem to be the main inducers of interferon production, other microorganisms such as those that cause malaria, rickettsial diseases, and tularemia can also stimulate its synthesis. This interferon mediated protection lasts for only about 24 hours.

IMMUNITY

The body defenses discussed above provide us with a nonspecific immunity and serve as a barrier excluding or destroying invading agents. In addition to these protectors we have some protectors that are more specific for particular invading organisms. Some of these protectors are hereditary. This process is called natural immunity and may be at the species, racial, or individual level. Humans, for example, are not affected by the distemper virus that is so deadly to dogs and cats. Black people are much more resistant to malaria than are white people. We have all known people who are more resistant than others to certain infections and, although this may be because of the defenses we have identified as nonspecific immunity, more likely it is traceable to their parents.

Acquired immunity is a specific defense that the body has been able to develop. **Antigens** are toxins or chemical factors produced by microorganisms that stimulate the reticuloendothelial system to produce antibodies, specific immune substances in the blood. A specific antigen provokes a specific antibody. The important thing is that this antibody will destroy or neutralize the microbe or its toxin that caused it to be formed.

This type of acquired immunity is called active. We can acquire an active immunity either by having the infection, as is the case with measles, or we can be immunized and develop an acquired active immunity without having had the infection. Artificial active immunization was first demonstrated by Jenner against smallpox in 1795. This type of protection represents a great medical discovery.

Immunization can also be accomplished by injecting the antibodies developed by one person into another. This process is called passive acquired immunity and, as you might suspect, this type does not last as long as does the active immunity. In some instances, once stimulated, the reticuloendothelial system continues to produce antibodies throughout life, whereas the injected antibodies start to disappear from the blood in a few days.

Passive immunity can also be acquired naturally. It is natural when antibodies from the mother's blood diffuse across the placenta into the circulation of the unborn child. Thus, for a short while the newborn is protected by passive immunity it acquired before it was born. In 1983 the results of research on protecting newborns by means of immunizing their mothers near the end of pregnancy were published. These results indicate that the infant may be protected for as long as one year from some of the immunizations given to the mother.

TEMPERATURE CONTROL AND FEVER

The remarkable stability of body temperature in the healthy adult, regardless of activity and environment, gives us a convenient and reasonably reliable measure of the relative health of the individual. The control center for the regulation of body temperature is located in the **hypothalamus** (hi-po-thal′ah-mus) in the brain. The temperature of the blood circulating through the hypothalamus causes this center to set into operation mechanisms either to conserve heat or to dissipate excess heat.

If the temperature of the blood circulating through the hypothalamus is lower than it should be, the following changes will take place to conserve heat and to increase heat production: **Vasoconstriction** (vas-o-kon-strik′shin) in the skin decreases heat loss by radiation and conduction. The adrenal glands increase their production of **epinephrine** (ep-i-nef′rin) and norepinephrine to cause further vasoconstriction and to increase metabolism and, therefore, heat production. Shivering also increases the production of heat as does an increased production of thyroxin (thi-rok′sin) by the thyroid gland.

If a patient who has a fever is pale (vasoconstriction is present) and feels cold (heat production is not sufficient to satisfy the temperature control center in the hypothalamus), the fever is increasing. On the other hand, once the compensatory mechanisms have conserved and produced sufficient heat to increase the temperature of the blood above the requirements of the temperature control center, the patient becomes flushed (vasodilatation is occurring), the skin feels warm, and there is increased perspiration (all helping to eliminate the excess heat). You can be certain that the temperature is now decreasing.

Some authorities believe that an elevated temperature may enhance the inflammatory process and thus may be helpful in eliminating the cause of fever. Fever may provide an unfavorable environment for the survival and reproduction of organisms causing disease. There are, however, several detrimental effects of fever, particularly if it continues over a prolonged period of time; for example, weight loss from the increased metabolism, increased heart work, and the loss of valuable body water and salts. If the fever is very high for a long period of time, brain damage may occur.

Although the reason is obscure, aspirin, an **antipyretic** (an″ti-pi-ret′ik), is usually effective in reducing fever. Aspirin, however, does not lower the body temperature in an individual who does not have a fever. For very high fevers, cold sponge baths and ice packs may be necessary to reduce the fever.

The normal oral temperature of an adult is 37°C (98.6°F). Upon arising in the morning, the healthy adult usually has an oral temperature of around 36°C because of the reduced metabolism during sleep. Babies and young children who are ill usually will have much higher temperatures than do feverish young adults. From middle age on, fevers of 38.5°C are usually indicative of much more serious illnesses than would be the case for a young child.

SHOCK

Shock may be caused either by loss of vascular volume or by an excessive vasodilatation that may greatly increase the size of the vascular bed. Hypovolemic shock is caused by the loss of vascular volume that may be the result of hemorrhage (see Fig 3-4), inadequate intake of fluids with excess losses of fluids from perspiration,

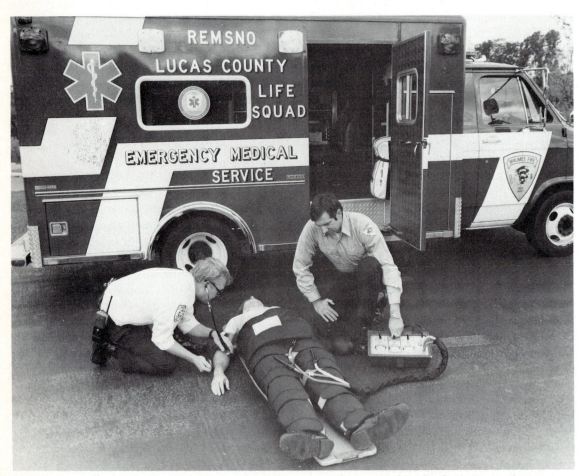

Figure 3-4. Paramedics sometimes use inflatable pants shown on this shock victim to compress the large veins in the legs. This procedure will improve circulation to the heart and brain. (Courtesy of Jobst Institute, Inc., Toledo, OH)

gastrointestinal loss of fluids as in severe diarrhea, or plasma loss as occurs with burn edema. Surgical shock can occur even though there has been no significant bleeding during the surgery. In this case, the stress of the surgery has caused the capillaries to become excessively permeable, and vascular fluid has been lost to the interstitial tissue spaces. In addition to this loss of vascular fluid, the injured cells release potassium into the bloodstream that will decrease the efficiency of the heart.

Cardiogenic shock is the result of ventricular failure. Although blood volume is adequate, there is inadequate perfusion.

Neurogenic shock or vasogenic shock occurs as a result of widespread vasodilatation. This is often associated with an allergic reaction. However, it also can occur following severe cerebral trauma or hepatic failure.

Septic shock is associated with bacterial infections. The toxins produced cause vasodilatation resulting in a relative hypovolemia. Toxic shock is a type of septic shock. The bacteria multiply in the tampon and produce a toxin that is absorbed, causing high fever and diarrhea. This leads to hypovolemia and possibly renal failure.

Regardless of the cause of shock, the normal body compensatory mechanisms are the same. These compensatory mechanisms can compensate for up to a 40% loss of vascular volume. Vasoconstrictor substances are produced to decrease the size of the vascular bed so that vital centers, the heart and brain, are supplied while the less important structures receive only minimal supplies of blood. As a result of this compensatory mechanism, there is decreased metabolism in the peripheral tissues so the patient in shock appears pale and the skin is cool.

The low blood pressure characteristic of shock causes less fluid to be filtered out of the capillaries and thereby conserves vascular volume. Actually, if the blood pressure is very low, the capillaries will increase the return of tissue fluid to the vascular compartment and thereby increase the vascular volume but cause some dehydration to the peripheral tissues. In this case, the patient will be thirsty.

With a significant decrease in the vascular volume, the heart must increase its rate in order to maintain an adequate supply of oxygen to the tissues. In addition to the pulse being rapid, it is also weak as the relative quantity of blood being ejected with each contraction is reduced.

The kidneys also help compensate for the decreased vascular volume. Less urine will be produced, so that water can be saved for the vascular compartment.

With such effective compensatory mechanisms, you might wonder why shock sometimes leads to deeper and deeper shock and becomes irreversible even with vigorous treatment. The smooth muscles of the blood vessel walls may themselves be too ischemic to contract and, therefore, cannot constrict the vessels. The blood flow becomes sluggish in these vessels and tends to clot. Clotting can entirely obstruct the blood flow in a local area and can also decrease the cardiac output of blood, further increasing the severity of the shock.

The aged individual, whose blood vessel walls have lost much of their elasticity, is much more dependent on the pumping action of the heart to perfuse blood through the circulatory system. These patients are much more likely to suffer irreversible shock with blood pressure levels that would not be particularly dangerous to a younger patient.

Measures must be taken to treat the cause of the shock. In addition to specific therapy, simple first aid measures can be lifesaving. The patient should be kept flat with both legs elevated. Although light blankets may be used to decrease chilling, no excessive heat should be applied. Heat will cause vasodilatation and increase the metabolism of the peripheral tissues, both of which will oppose the normal body compensatory mechanisms. If the patient is conscious, oral fluids should be given liberally. If the shock is severe, intravenous fluids must be given. Drugs that cause vasoconstriction and elevate the blood pressure are sometimes prescribed. Some doctors, however, believe that such drugs should not be used to treat shock because they may significantly decrease blood supply to vital organs.

PAIN

Pain is a major protective mechanism. It gives us warning that something is wrong so that we can take measures to help correct the difficulty. Diseases, such as cancer, which are not evidenced by pain until the process is well advanced, are more difficult to manage than is a disease such as acute appendicitis, which gives pain warning early in the disease process.

Perhaps it is impossible to define pain because it is largely subjective. There is probably an emotion of pain as well as the sensation of pain and both are whatever the person experiencing the pain says it is. Factors influencing the meaning of pain are many and varied. Age, sex, cultural background, psychosocial factors, and many other factors influence how we experience pain. The setting in which the pain occurs may be important. For example, an athlete who has been injured during an important sports event may view this pain in quite a different manner than the pain of a headache.

Pain threshold refers to the intensity of the stimulus necessary for the person to perceive pain. This threshold is approximately the same for all individuals. Pain tolerance refers to the length of time or intensity of the stimulus that the person will allow before making an overt response to the pain. Pain tolerance is lowered by persistent pain such as that of advanced cancer. A weak, debilitated person usually tolerates pain less well than a strong, healthy individual. Fatigue, anger, worry, and fear will also decrease one's ability to tolerate pain. Tolerance of pain is increased by some drugs, alcohol, warmth, rubbing, and companionship. Strong religious beliefs also increase tolerance of pain. Generally speaking, most people can tolerate pain better during the daytime hours than they can at night.

Cutaneous pain is mediated mostly by superficial pain nerve endings. If these superficial nerves are destroyed, the pain is not as severe. Abrasions are often more painful than deep cuts.

There are visceral pain receptors in the blood vessel walls, the outer covering of the brain and spinal cord, the periosteum covering the bones, and parietal (pah-ri'e-tal) membranes (membranes that are nearest the body wall). Visceral sensation is not well localized because there are so few visceral nerve fibers. For pain to be felt, a large area of the organ must be stimulated. Visceral sensation may take either of two pathways to the brain, where the sensation is interpreted. It may go over the parietal pathway, in which case the sensation will be felt in the skin covering the organ involved. Or, if the nerve impulse travels over a visceral pathway, it enters the spinal cord a few segments above the organ involved; therefore, the pain will be experienced higher than the actual location of the stimulus.

Several types of stimuli may cause visceral pain. Although cutting the skin will cause pain, an incision into viscera does not result in pain. Ischemia is probably the most important stimulus that causes visceral pain. This type of pain is provoked by movement and relieved by rest. In the case of a stomach ulcer, the pain is caused by a chemical irritant. This pain may be decreased by the ingestion of food, particularly milk or some bland food. Stretching of the viscera also produces pain. This type of pain is similar to the pain of ischemia because the blood vessels in the distended viscera are compressed. Spasm also causes compression of blood vessels and decreases blood supply. The increased activity of the organ in spasm increases the need for blood supply and causes an increased production of acid metabolites that cannot be readily removed because of the diminished blood supply.

Visceral pain may sometimes result in the sensation being experienced in cutaneous areas somewhat remote from the stimulus. This is called referred pain and can be of considerable diagnostic significance. For example, the pain of a heart attack is not uncommonly felt in the left shoulder and down the left arm instead of in the area of the heart. Figure 3-5 shows the usual areas involved in referred pain.

ANESTHESIA AND ANALGESICS

For pain to be perceived, the brain must be functioning, the pathway to the brain must be intact,

and the pain receptors must respond to the stimulus. Each of these three factors is important in the different types of conventional anesthesia. In general anesthesia, the brain cannot perceive the pain. When a nerve is blocked, the pathway to the brain is interrupted. A local injection of procaine renders the pain receptors insensitive to the pain stimulus.

Medications for pain, **analgesics** (an-al-je'ziks), may be effective if they relieve the cause of the pain. For example, atropine is a drug that causes relaxation of smooth muscles and so may diminish the pain caused by spasms of smooth muscles. If the pain is caused by constriction of blood vessels, drugs such as nitroglycerin that dilate blood vessels may be helpful.

Other types of drugs used to treat pain alter a person's attitude to the pain rather than relieve the pain. The patient feels the pain, but is indifferent to it. Narcotics, tranquilizers, and sedatives function in this manner. It is important to realize that under the influence of this

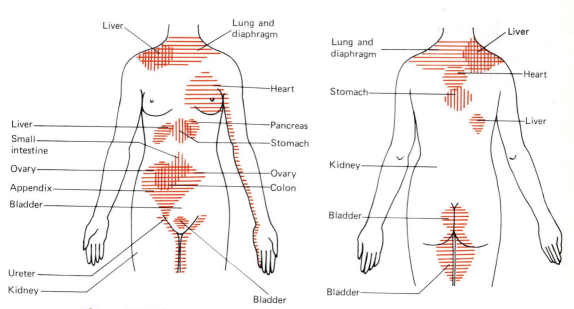

Figure 3-5. *The cutaneous areas where internal pain may be referred*

type of medication, judgment and attitudes about things other than pain will also be influenced.

ELECTRICAL STIMULATORS

Electrical stimulators are a great help to some people who suffer chronic pain. A transcutaneous electrical stimulator is a battery-powered stimulator about the size of a small transistor radio. Two or more electrodes attached to the battery box are applied to the skin on or near the site of the pain. The patient can produce electrical signals that counteract the pain either by inhibiting the responses within the brain or by blocking the pathway of the pain impulse. It is possible that the electrical signal may also

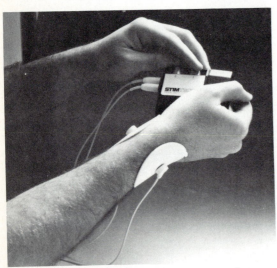

Figure 3-6. *An electrical stimulator can be useful in controlling chronic pain. The sponge electrodes shown on the right wrist are glued to the skin over the painful area. The patient can adjust the level of the impulses with the controls on the small battery pack shown. The stimulator battery pack can be carried in the patient's pocket. (Courtesy of Stimtech, Inc., 9440 Science Center Drive, Minneapolis, MN)*

cause the release of **endorphins** (en-dor′finz), chemicals produced by the brain that alleviate pain. Endorphins are normally produced in response to severe and acute pain. One type of transcutaneous electrical stimulator is shown in Figure 3-6.

Since the transcutaneous stimulator is noninvasive in its application, it is particularly useful for a person who cannot tolerate more extensive surgical procedures. The only contraindication to the use of this device is the presence of certain types of cardiac pacemakers.

A dorsal column stimulator is similar to the transcutaneous stimulator except that the electrode is surgically implanted in the spinal column. Since this surgical procedure is considered major surgery, candidates for it are usually selected only after their success with a transcutaneous stimulator has been demonstrated. There is a newer system that is a less intrusive approach to spinal cord stimulation. The leads are inserted through the skin into the space surrounding the cord. Only local anesthesia is required for this procedure.

NEUROSURGICAL PROCEDURES

Constant, unrelenting pain that cannot be controlled by any of the above measures may be reduced or abolished by various neurosurgical procedures. A cordotomy involves the surgical interruption of the pain-conducting pathway in the spinal cord. Since this pathway also conducts impulses concerned with temperature, the patient will have neither sensations of heat or cold nor pain below the level that is severed. As this deprives the patient of some very important sensory input, it is usually only done for patients in the terminal stages of their illness.

BIOFEEDBACK

Biofeedback is a technique that can be utilized by some patients for the relief of their pain. With this method, the patient is taught to control the tenseness of his muscles by visualizing relaxing experiences. Although the outcome of such biofeedback training varies with age, motivation, and ability to think abstractly, the overall success rate is good. A distinct advantage of this method for the relief of pain is that there are few known risks or side effects.

IMMOBILITY

Immobility can be caused by paralysis, pain, trauma, limited joint action, or restriction of activity for either medical or psychiatric reasons. Regardless of the cause of the inactivity, it has devastating effects on all of the organ systems if it is prolonged. Immobility alters the total biopsychosocial responses of the person, and the limits placed on activity cause physiological and psychological interference with basic needs and with normal development. This patient's helper, therefore, must keep this in mind and realize that the immobilized patient may not react to everyday events in the same way that other people do.

With prolonged immobility, a desalting of the bones and a weakening of the structural supports can result, particularly if there is a deficiency of estrogen, as in women past menopause. Calcium is withdrawn from the bone and excreted by the kidney. An increase in the dietary calcium or supplemental calcium is contraindicated in postmenopausal women because without estrogen the bones cannot use it. Any excess calcium may cause kidney stones to form, particularly if the urine is more alkaline than normal. The excess calcium may also be deposited in muscle and cause myositis ossificans (mi-o-si′tis os-if′′i-cans). It may also be deposited in joints and cause **osteoarthropathy** (os′′te-o-ar-throp′ah-the).

About 45% of the body weight is muscle. Thus, it is not surprising that weakness owing to immobility comprises a major factor in any illness. We lose about 5% of our muscle strength each day of immobility. In addition to inactivity causing muscle weakness, the muscles also atrophy. As little as one or two months of immobility can reduce muscle mass by as much as 50%. With prolonged immobility of about a year, the muscle fibers may become infiltrated with fat and fibrous tissue. Atrophy of skeletal muscles decreases muscle size, functional movement, and strength of contraction and causes impaired coordination.

Contractures can develop as a result of prolonged immobility. Atrophy and shortening of the muscles may involve the joints. Flexors and adductors are the strongest muscles. Therefore, the deformed extremity will be in a flexed and adducted position unless careful attention is given to positioning that favors the extensors and abductors, and unless the part is frequently exercised in as full a range of motions as possible. It is not uncommon for a person who has been on bed rest for a prolonged period of time to develop foot drop unless measures are taken to keep the feet in a neutral position for a more normal walking position. This procedure can be done by positioning the soles of the feet against a foot board and allowing this board to support the weight of the bed clothes.

Lessened muscle activity decreases the circulation to the skin and other soft tissues. Prolonged pressure also decreases blood supply and nerve impulses. Under these circumstances, **decubital** (de-ku′be-tal) **ulcers** (bed sores) may develop, particularly over bony prominences like the base of the spine. Prevention of this complication depends on positioning and massage to improve circulation. Once the ulcer has occurred, treatment is difficult because all wound healing depends on a good blood supply to the affected part.

The effects of immobility on the cardiopulmonary system can also be serious. Even after a few days of bed rest, some loss of muscle tone occurs. Upon arising for the first time following a period of bed rest, the patient is likely to have **orthostatic** (or′tho-stat-ik) **hypotension**, decreased blood pressure owing to an increase in the diameter of the blood vessels and to the fact that when the patient gets out of bed, the nervous system may not be able to adjust rapidly enough to regulate vascular diameters properly. Thus, the patient may become light-headed and may faint.

With prolonged bed rest, there is a decreased venous return of blood to the heart that, in turn, favors clot formation. The most likely place for the **thrombus** (throm′bus), or clot, to form is in the large veins of the legs. If the thrombus begins to move, it becomes an **embolus** (em′bo-lus) and may be fatal when it reaches the vessels of the lungs.

In addition to the decreased venous return, there will also be a poor return of tissue fluids via the lymphatics, as this fluid return depends greatly on active skeletal muscles. Under these circumstances, the patient will very likely have edema, particularly if the person sits for long hours in a chair.

Decreased respirations while a patient is immobile not only decrease venous return to the heart but also decrease chest expansion. These conditions can lead to complications such as hypostatic pneumonia and retained mucus that may also favor respiratory infections.

With immobility, tissue **catabolism** (kah-tab′o-lizm), or tissue breakdown, increases and **anabolism** (ah-nab′o-lizm), or tissue buildup, decreases. Both of these conditions can cause **anorexia** (an-o-rek′se-ah) (loss of appetite) and malnutrition. Gastric and intestinal distention with constipation is also a common complication of immobility. If the constipation is severe enough, fecal impaction can lead to bowel obstruction.

In the urinary system, prolonged immobility can lead to **stasis** (sta′sis) of urine and urine retention. As mentioned earlier, the kidneys may not be able to eliminate bone minerals and stone formation may occur, particularly if the urine is alkaline and dehydration with decreased urine volume exists.

Many psychological problems are also associated with prolonged periods of immobility. Motor function constitutes one of the most important aspects of human behavior. Even much of our thought processes are concerned with planning some action. Immobility and isolation decrease motivation, problem-solving ability, and learning.

Three major types of behavioral changes may occur in the immobilized patient. The patient's inability to manipulate himself or the environment can result in frustration, anger, and fear. Perceptual changes also occur when the person has a reduction in both the quantity and the quality of information available to him. This type of sensory deprivation can cause stressful interpersonal relationships. The third type of psychological problem occurring with prolonged immobility is that of role change. Our society highly values both youth and activity. Whether or not there is actually a decrease in a person's social status is not relevant. Relevant is the fact that the patient feels that his status has deteriorated and that those contributions he can make to his family and society are of little value. Perhaps the magnitude of this aspect of the problem is best illustrated by our "getting acquainted" conversations. One of the first things we ask a new acquaintance is "What do you do?" The implication is that we are what we *do*. These three problems are very difficult for both the patient and the helpers. If a patient can be helped through the stage of frustration and anger into a stage of accepting the disability and focusing attention on what can be done rather than on what cannot be accomplished, great progress toward a full and rich life can be made in spite of serious disability.

SUMMARY QUESTIONS

1. How does cancer spread from one part of the body to another?
2. Discuss two ways to estimate the severity of a burn.
3. Differentiate between heat exhaustion and heat stroke.
4. Discuss the treatment of heat stroke.
5. Discuss four major predisposing causes of disease.
6. Discuss four ways in which the body protects itself from bacterial invasion.
7. What signs would you look for to tell whether a person's fever is going down?
8. Explain how the body compensates for shock.
9. What people are most vulnerable to shock?
10. What are the appropriate first aid measures in the treatment of shock?
11. List five complications of immobility.
12. With immobility what can be done to prevent contractures?
13. Discuss how immunity is acquired.

KEY TERMS

achlorhydria
anabolism
analgesics
anorexia
anoxia
anticoagulant
antigens
antihistamine
antipyretic
atrophy
bacteriostatic
calculi
catabolism
cytology
decubital ulcers
desquamates
dyspnea
ecchymosis
edema
embolus
endorphins

epinephrine
hematoma
histology
hypertrophy
hypothalamus
ischemia
lysozyme
neoplasms
orthostatic hypotension
osteoarthropathy
palliative
pathology
reticuloendothelial system
stasis
syndrome
thrombus
vasoconstriction
vasodilation
vasospasms
virulence

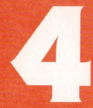

4

Body Organization

OBJECTIVES

On completion of this chapter, you will be able to:

1. Describe the locations of all of the internal organs of the human body.
2. Differentiate between skeletal, visceral, and cardiac muscle.
3. Describe the structure of a living cell.
4. List the functions of five cellular organelles.
5. Describe how substances enter and leave living cells.
6. Explain what happens when living cells are put in hypotonic, isotonic, and hypertonic solutions.
7. Give examples of where in the body three different types of epithelial tissues are located.
8. List six types of connective tissue and tell where each is located in the body.
9. Differentiate between tissues and membranes.
10. Demonstrate on your body the anatomical regions.
11. Give examples of how you use the terms proximal and distal.

OVERVIEW

I. THE ANATOMICAL POSITION
   A. Planes of the Body
   B. Regions of the Body
II. INTERNAL BODY ORGANIZATION
   A. Body Cavities
   B. Systems
III. CELLS
   A. Nucleus
      1. Deoxyribonucleic Acid
      2. Mitosis
      3. Meiosis
   B. Cytoplasm and Organelles
   C. Cell Membrane
      1. Diffusion
      2. Osmosis
      3. Filtration
      4. Active Transport
      5. Phagocytosis, Pinocytosis, and
         Exocytosis
IV. TISSUES
   A. Epithelial Tissue
   B. Connective Tissue
   C. Muscle Tissue
   D. Nerve Tissue
V. MEMBRANES

Anatomy is the study of structure and physiology is the study of function. Structure and function are interdependent and, in many instances, it is the function that determines the structure.

In this chapter, we shall first consider the gross external appearance of the body and learn a few terms used to describe the position of a body part. Then we will consider the internal body organization, and finally we shall explore the structural and functional unit of all living matter, the cell.

THE ANATOMICAL POSITION

In order to describe the position of a structure or locate one structure in relation to another, we must assume that the body is in a specific position. We call this position the anatomical position. The person in this position is standing erect, facing the viewer, hands at sides with palms forward. Terms we use to describe the relationship of one body part to another are lateral, medial, superior, inferior, proximal, distal, anterior or ventral, and posterior or dorsal. Medial means toward the midline; lateral means toward the side. For example, when you are in the anatomical position your thumb is on the lateral side of your hand. Superior means above and inferior means below. Anterior or ventral means in front and dorsal or posterior means in back. Proximal means closest to the point of attachment or origin; distal means farther away. The elbow is proximal to the hand and the hand is distal to the elbow.

PLANES OF THE BODY

The body as a whole, as well as individual organs, can be divided into different planes. Figure 4-1 illustrates the sagittal, coronal or frontal, and transverse or horizontal planes of the body.

REGIONS OF THE BODY

Figures 4-2 and 4-3 show the regions of the body. You should learn these regions of the body, as this knowledge will be essential in understanding medical reports. For example, when someone wants to report where a particular wound or pain is located, they will do so using the terms of position discussed above and those terms describing the regions of the body. This information will also be a great help to you in learning subsequent lessons. For example, the

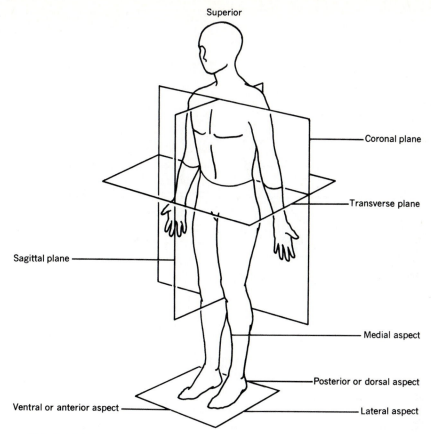

Figure 4-1. Planes of the body and terms of location and position

pectoral (pek′to-ral) muscle is located in the pectoral region. The brachial (bra′ke-al) artery, vein, and nerve are located in the brachial region.

INTERNAL BODY ORGANIZATION

BODY CAVITIES

The thoracic cavity is protected by the rib cage. The floor of the thoracic cavity is the diaphragm.

This cavity contains the heart, lungs, bronchi, great blood vessels, thymus gland, esophagus, and lymphatic ducts.

The abdominal cavity is inferior to the diaphragm and contains the organs of digestion, spleen, kidneys, adrenal glands, liver, gall bladder, and pancreas. The abdominal aorta, the largest abdominal artery, sends branching blood vessels to supply these structures with blood. The inferior vena cava and large portal vein receive the venous blood from these organs.

The pelvic cavity is inferior to the abdominal cavity. This cavity contains the empty urinary

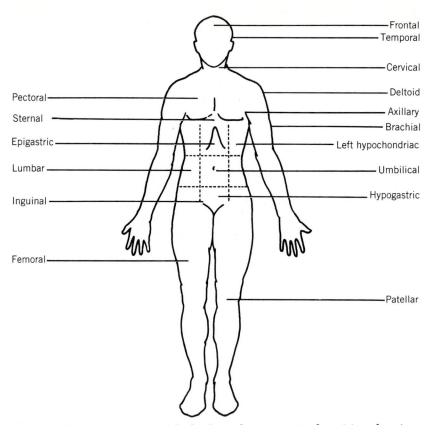

Figure 4-2. Anterior view of the body in the anatomical position showing the regions. Sometimes the regions of the abdomen are designated as the right and left upper quadrants and the right and left lower quadrants.

bladder, some of the organs of reproduction, and the distal part of the gastrointestinal tract.

The dorsal cavity contains the brain and spinal cord as well as the spinal nerve roots. These vital structures are well protected by the bones of the skull and vertebral column.

SYSTEMS

A body system is a group of organs that performs related functions or different stages of some complex function. Each of the body systems performs a specific function. However, all of the body systems are greatly dependent on the proper functioning of each of the other systems. For this reason, disease processes of one system may well be evidenced by malfunctioning of some of the other systems. For example, patients with certain types of heart disease may have great difficulty breathing. We shall discuss briefly each of the body systems and the major functions of each system.

The respiratory system is primarily concerned with the exchange of gases between the bloodstream and the microscopic **alveoli** (al-ve'o-li)

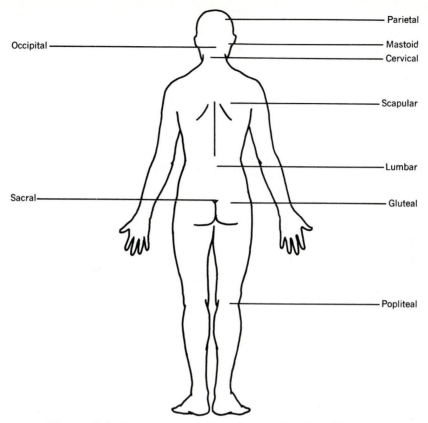

Figure 4-3. *Posterior view of the human body and regions*

of the lungs. The most important gases exchanged are oxygen and carbon dioxide.

The circulatory system has two divisions: lymphatic and blood. The lymphatic division is composed of lymph vessels, lymph nodes, and other lymphatic tissue. Its chief functions are to return tissue fluid to the bloodstream and to filter this fluid, removing the foreign material and bacteria before they can enter the bloodstream. The blood circulation depends on the pumping action of the heart, which sends blood containing nutrients and oxygen into the arteries and capillaries where these products are deliv-

ered to the tissue cells. The capillaries return the products of cellular metabolism to the veins and back to the heart. If the products of cellular metabolism are waste products, they will be carried to the organs of excretion, chiefly the kidneys and lungs. If the products of cellular metabolism are substances such as enzymes and hormones needed for proper functioning of other cells, the circulatory system will deliver these products to the cells where they are needed.

The skeletal system is composed of bones and joints. The chief functions of the skeletal system are to provide a supporting framework for the body and a place for the attachment of muscles and ligaments. The skeletal system also provides protection for many delicate internal organs such as the brain. Many blood cells are produced in the bones.

There are three different types of muscle: skeletal, visceral, and cardiac muscle. Skeletal muscles are voluntary; they provide locomotion and support of the body. Visceral muscles, which are involuntary, are found in many of the organs of digestion where they move the products of digestion through the gastrointestinal tract at the proper speed. Visceral muscles are also found in blood vessels whose diameter they regulate. Cardiac muscle is also involuntary and is located only in the heart.

The gastrointestinal system processes the foods we eat and renders them into an absorbable form so that they can enter the bloodstream and be distributed to the cells that need them. The gastrointestinal tract also aids in eliminating waste products.

The urinary system is composed of the kidneys, ureters (u-re′ters), urinary bladder, and urethra. This system, which brings about the elimination of soluble waste products, is very important in maintaining the acid-base balance of the body. This balance is critical to health and will be discussed in Chapter 19.

The brain, spinal cord, and peripheral nerves (nerves extending to and from the brain and cord) make up the nervous system. This system is concerned with our thought processes and also regulates both voluntary and involuntary actions of muscles and glands.

The endocrine system works with the nervous system in controlling and integrating all the normal biochemical processes of the body. The pituitary gland, thyroid gland, parathyroids, pancreas, adrenals, gonads, pineal (pin′e-al), and thymus (thi′mus) are some of the major components of the endocrine system.

The reproductive system functions to continue the species. Organs of the male and female reproductive systems differ both in their structures and locations.

CELLS

The structural and functional unit of all living matter is the cell (see Fig. 4-4). Most cells can be seen only with a microscope. Cells are made up of protoplasm (pro′to-plazm), which is mainly water containing various organic and inorganic substances as well as several important organelles (or-ga-nel′ez) or "little organs." The cell is surrounded by a membrane that determines to some extent which substances will enter the cell from the liquid cellular environment.

The chemical composition of protoplasm is very complex. About 99% of the substance of the protoplasm is carbon, hydrogen, oxygen, and nitrogen. The remaining 1% is sodium, chlorine, potassium, phosphorus, sulfur, magnesium, and calcium. Iron, copper, iodine, fluorine, and several other elements are present in trace amounts.

NUCLEUS

The activities of the cell are directed by the nucleus, which is located near the center of the cell. Chromosomes (kro′mo-somz) within the nucleus are made up of thousands of genes. A human gene is a segment of a deoxyribonucleic (de-ok′se-ri′bo-nu′kle″ic) acid (DNA) molecule, the hereditary material.

Deoxyribonucleic Acid

Each of the 46 chromosomes of the normal human cell contains DNA, which is shaped like a long spiral ladder. The rungs of the ladder are paired bases. Adenine (A), guanine (G), cytosine

CELL

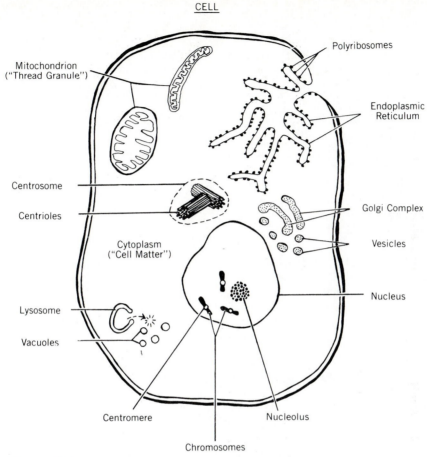

Mitochondrion
("Thread Granule")

Polyribosomes

Endoplasmic
Reticulum

Centrosome

Centrioles

Golgi Complex

Vesicles

Cytoplasm
("Cell Matter")

Nucleus

Lysosome

Vacuoles

Centromere

Nucleolus

Chromosomes

Figure 4-4. *Diagram of a typical cell illustrating some of the major cellular structures visible with an electron microscope (From Layman, D.,* The Terminology of Anatomy and Physiology: A Programmed Approach. *New York: John Wiley & Sons, Inc., 1983. Used with permission.)*

(C), and thymine (T) are the most common bases. The pairing of the bases is such that A will only fit with T and G will only fit with C; therefore, the sequence of the bases on one side of the ladder determines the sequence along the other side. The sides of the ladder are sugar-phosphate chains twisted into a double helix as shown in Figure 4-5. In this illustration, you see two new DNA molecules being formed from a parent DNA. With each nuclear division, exact duplicate DNA molecules are formed and, ultimately, two identical daughter cells.

Mitosis
Body growth, replacement of cells that have a short life span, and repair of injured tissues depend on the reproduction of cells. The most common form of cell division is **mitosis** (mi-to'sis). The different stages of mitosis are shown in Figure 4-6.

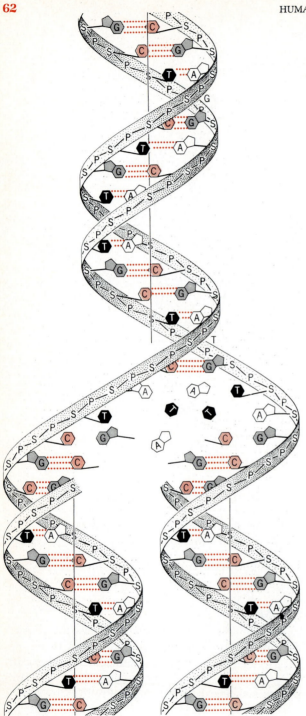

Figure 4-5. A schematic representation of DNA. As the strands separate, two new DNA molecules are formed. DNA contains the hereditary material and is located in the nucleus of every cell.

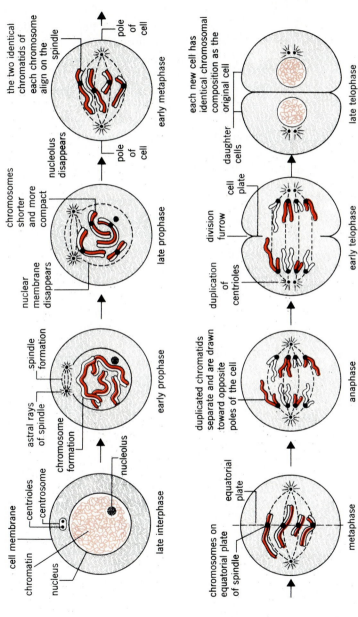

Figure 4-6. *The major events in mitosis or cellular division resulting in two daughter cells with the same number of chromosomes and containing the same hereditary code as the parent cell*

Interphase. This is the stage or period when cells are not undergoing division. During this period, the duplication of DNA takes place.

Prophase. The centrioles (sen′tre-olz″) separate and begin to move to opposite sides of the cell. Chromosome threads become more tightly coiled and the two halves called chromatids can be seen.

Metaphase. The nuclear membrane dissolves, and fine tubules are seen extending toward the midline of the cell. The chromosomes form a line in the middle of the cell attaching themselves to the tubules.

Anaphase. The two chromatids of each chromosome are completely separated from each other and can be considered chromosomes. The tubules pull them to their respective sides of the cell.

Telephase. The cell membrane constricts at the midpoint, the chromosomes begin to uncoil, and the nuclear membranes of the daughter cells are formed. Finally, mitosis is complete with two new cells formed, each with 46 chromosomes containing the hereditary code of the cell.

Meiosis

The sex cells, the female ovum and male sperm, are formed not by mitosis but by **meiosis** (mi-o′sis), or a process called **reduction division**, because during division the number of chromosomes is reduced. Each mature sex cell formed in this process has half the number of chromosomes of the parent cell. Thus, when the ovum with 23 chromosomes is fertilized by a sperm with 23 chromosomes, the cell produced will have the proper number of 46.

CYTOPLASM AND ORGANELLES

The nucleus is surrounded by **cytoplasm** (ci′to-plazm). Within the cytoplasm are organelles that carry out the many functions of the cell. These functions are determined by DNA, and the instructions are carried into the cytoplasm by RNA, ribonucleic (ri″bo-nu-kla′ic) acid.

The most important organelles are the **ribosomes** (ri′bo-somz), **endoplasmic reticulum** (en′do-plas′mik re-tik′u-lum), **mitochondria** (mi′to-kon′dre-ah), **lysosomes** (li′so-somz), centrioles, **Golgi** (gol′je) **complex**, **microtubules** (mi″kro-tub′ulz), and **microfilaments** (mi″kro-fil′a-ments). We shall consider briefly the functions of each of these organelles.

Protein synthesis takes place in the ribosomes, which are attached to the endoplasmic reticulum (ER). Some of the endoplasmic reticula have no ribosomes, and these synthesize lipids. Both types of endoplasmic reticula have fluid-filled channels that appear to connect all parts of the cytoplasm. This suggests that the ER may function as a transportation system within the cell.

The mitochondria are frequently called the "powerhouses" of the cell because they contain the enzymes and other molecules that carry out the energy-producing reactions of the cell. This energy results from the breakdown of a high-energy phosphate compound, ATP, adenosine triphosphate. The ATP is resynthesized from the utilization of foodstuffs, chiefly carbohydrates.

The lysosomes contain powerful enzymes and are considered the digestive organs of the cell. These organelles also function to remove damaged cells or damaged portions of cells. Rupture of the lysosomes will result in the death of the cell.

The centrioles play a major role in cellular division. These organelles are located close to the nucleus of the cell and become active during cellular division, or mitosis.

Enzymes and hormones that have been manufactured by the cell are transported through the cell membrane by the Golgi complex. Once outside the cell, they enter the bloodstream where they can be taken where needed in the body.

Microtubules and microfilaments are believed to be involved, directly or indirectly, in attainment and maintenance of cell shapes. These organelles also probably contribute to the motility of the cell.

In addition to the organelles found in the cytoplasm are ribonucleic acid, some DNA, glycogen, lipids, proteins, and inorganic substances. Some cells—such as muscle and nerve cells—also contain fibrils, microscopic threadlike structures.

CELL MEMBRANE

The membrane of the cell, or plasma membrane, is a meshwork of protein threads with a **matrix** (ma′triks) of fat and other organic compounds. The membrane separates the protoplasm of the cell from the liquid cellular environment and plays an important role in the movement of food, wastes, and the products of cellular metabolism in and out of the cell.

Diffusion

Diffusion is a process by which particles are moved from an area of higher concentration to an area of lower concentration. For example, if you put a drop of dye in a glass of water, you will see the dye spread through the water by a process of diffusion (see Fig. 4-7). The pores in the cell membrane permit the diffusion of water, oxygen, carbon dioxide, and a few **crystalloid** (kris′tal-oid) particles in and out of the cell. Most of the small crystalloid particles diffusing through a cell membrane are probably food particles needed by the cell.

Fat-soluble substances that are too large to get

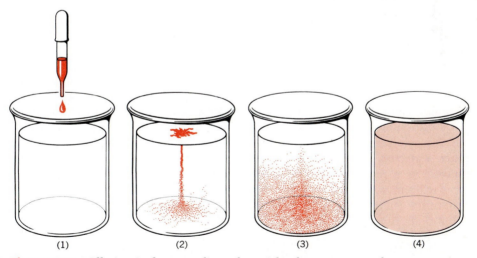

Figure 4-7. Diffusion is the spreading of particles from an area of greater concentration to areas of lesser concentration. Here some dye has been put into a beaker of water and the color is gradually spreading throughout the water by diffusion.

through the pores of the cell membrane may travel in and out of the cell by dissolving in the fat of the membrane.

Osmosis

Water can move in and out of the cell by diffusion; however, water can also pass through the cell membrane by a process of **osmosis** (os-mo′sis). The direction the water will be pulled by osmosis depends on the concentration of particles in the fluids on either side of the cell membrane.

Normally, the fluid surrounding the cell is **isotonic** (i″so-ton′ik). This means that the concentration of the fluid (or the number of particles within the fluid) is the same as the concentration within the cells. Under these circumstances, water moves freely in the same quantities in and out of the cell. Because the same quantity of water is simultaneously moving in and out of the cell, for all practical purposes the concentration on both sides of the membrane stays the same. Clinically, isotonic solutions are used for intravenous feedings. An example of an isotonic solution is normal saline which is 0.85% sodium chloride. Because glucose does not ionize and sodium chloride does ionize, a 5% solution of glucose is also isotonic to human cells.

A **hypertonic** solution is one that has a greater concentration of particles than that inside the cell. If a cell is surrounded by a hypertonic solution, water will be pulled out of the cell by osmosis. As a result of the cell losing water, the cell will shrink. How much water will be pulled out of the cell depends on the concentration of the fluid surrounding the cell. The quantity of water moved by osmosis is directly proportional to the difference in concentration on either side of the membrane. Since cells can be damaged by hypertonic solutions, these so-lutions are only used for intravenous injections in special circumstances.

A **hypotonic** solution is one that has a lower concentration of particles than is present inside the cell. If a cell is surrounded by a hypotonic solution, for example distilled water, it will swell with water, which is being pulled in by osmosis. If enough water enters the cell in this manner, the cell membrane will burst.

Filtration

Filtration is a process by which materials are forced through a membrane from an area of higher pressure to an area of lower pressure. In the laboratory, you have probably seen a solution poured through a filter paper in a funnel. In this instance, it is the weight of the solution that forces fluid through the paper. In our bodies, the blood pressure forces water and very small particles through the capillary membrane. The blood pressure in the capillary is higher than the pressure of the fluid outside the capillary. Therefore, the direction of movement is from the capillary into the fluid around the tissue cells (intercellular space).

Active Transport

Diffusion and osmosis are passive modes of moving substances through cell membranes. These methods of transport depend completely on the concentration gradient. In active transport, the mitochondria of the cell provide energy (from the breakdown of ATP) to move materials across the cell membrane regardless of the concentration factors. For example, on the one hand, potassium is in greater concentrations inside the cell than it is in the intercellular space. Under these circumstances, potassium cannot diffuse into the cell, and indeed intracellular potassium should diffuse into the intercellular space until the concentrations of potassium are equal on both sides of the cell membrane. Sodium, on the other hand, is needed in greater concentrations outside the cell than inside. With active transport, these ions are moved back and forth across the cell membrane, maintaining the proper physiological balance without regard for concentration differences.

Phagocytosis, Pinocytosis, and Exocytosis

Phagocytosis (fag″o-si-to′sis) is a process in which the cell membrane develops a small sac and slowly envelops a particle, bringing it inside the cell. **Pinocytosis** (pi″no-si-to′sis) is a similar process except that, instead of a solid particle, a liquid is brought into the cell. **Exocytosis** is the discharge from the cell of particles that are too large to diffuse through the cell membrane.

TISSUES

Several different types of cells exist, and each has a specialized function and a characteristic appearance. Cells of the same type combine to make tissues. In the human body, there are four primary tissues: epithelial (ep″i-the′le-al), connective, muscular, and nervous tissue. Each of these primary tissues may be subdivided into various types with each type specialized for a particular function.

EPITHELIAL TISSUE

Simple squamous (skwa′mus) **epithelial tissue** is made of a single layer of thin, flat cells. This type of tissue is found in the lungs where it facilitates the exchange of gases between the air sacs and the capillaries. This tissue also provides a smooth lining for the blood vessels and lymphatics and facilitates the exchange of gases, nutrients, and products of cellular metabolism between the capillaries and other body cells. In the blood vessels, this tissue is also called **endothelium** (en″do-the′le-um).

Stratified squamous epithelium is made of several layers of cells and is found in areas of the body needing protection against friction. For example, it lines the nose and mouth and is part of the epidermis (ep″i-der′mis), the outer layer of the skin.

Simple cuboidal epithelium is found in certain glands, for example the thyroid, and on the surface of the ovary. Cuboidal cells secrete glandular products.

Columnar epithelial tissue is made of cells that resemble columns. There are four types of columnar cells. The simple columnar cells that line the gastrointestinal tract facilitate the absorption of nutrients. Ciliated columnar cells have processes on their free surfaces that help to move substances toward the outside of the body. These cells are found in the respiratory tract and in parts of the reproductive system. Goblet columnar cells, which are found in the top layer of mucous (mu′kus) membrane, secrete mucus to keep the membrane moist. The end organs of certain nerve fibers, such as the taste buds and the rods and cones of the eye, are a special type of columnar cell.

Glandular epithelium is found in both the endocrine (en′do-krin) and the exocrine glands of the body. These cells secrete substances such as digestive juices, hormones, and perspiration.

CONNECTIVE TISSUE

Connective tissue is primarily a supporting and binding type of tissue. Connective tissue can readily repair itself if injured and it also helps to repair damage to other types of tissue.

Areolar connective tissue, the most common

of all connective tissues, is thin and glistening. It connects the skin and other membranes to their underlying structures and exists as packing around blood vessels and organs.

Adipose (ad'i-poz) tissue cells have the ability to take up fat and store it. They help to insulate and to protect as well as to provide a reserve food supply.

White fibrous connective tissue or dense connective tissue is very strong and flexible. Tendons and ligaments are made of this type of connective tissue.

There are three types of cartilaginous connective tissue. Hyaline (hi'ah-lin) cartilage, which is found at the ends of bones in freely movable joints, is glossy and bluish white. It forms the preliminary skeleton of the embryo. The intervertebral discs and the pubic symphysis (sim'fi-sis) contain fibrous cartilage. Elastic cartilage is found in the external ear.

Osseous (os'e-us) connective tissue is bone. Deposits of calcium and phosphate salts cause the intercellular material of osseous tissue to be hard.

Blood is liquid connective tissue. All cells are dependent on blood to receive their nutrients and to transport the products of cellular metabolism.

MUSCLE TISSUE

There are three types of muscle tissue. Skeletal muscle is voluntary (controlled by the mind) and is attached to the skeleton. This muscle tissue is also called striated because, when viewed microscopically, fine striations are evident. Visceral (vis'er-el) muscle or smooth muscle is not under voluntary control (involuntary) and is found in the walls of blood vessels and in many of the organs of digestion. Cardiac muscle is found only in the heart. It is also involuntary.

NERVE TISSUE

Nerve tissue is highly specialized with properties of irritability and conductivity. This tissue transmits nerve impulses which assist in the integration of all physiological functions.

MEMBRANES

Membranes are composed of combinations of epithelial and connective tissue.

Mucous membrane lines cavities that open to the outside of the body, such as the respiratory and gastrointestinal tracts. Serous membrane lines closed cavities and secretes a slippery serous fluid for protection from friction. The pleura (ploor'ah), which covers the lungs, and the peritoneum (per"i-to-ne-'um), which covers the organs of the abdominal cavity, are examples of serous membranes. **Synovial membrane** is tough because of the presence of much fibrous tissue. Synovial membranes line the cavities of freely movable joints. Dense fibrous membrane is tough and opaque. It is primarily a protective membrane and covers the brain and bones. It also makes up the **sclera** (skle'rah), the outer coat of the eye.

The cutaneous (cu-ta'-ne-us) membrane is the skin. Its principal functions are as follows: It protects the underlying structures from injury and bacterial invasion; it helps regulate body temperature; it is a sense organ, keeping us aware of our environment; it helps to some extent in the excretion of some body water and soluble wastes. Although the skin is classified as a membrane, it is also the largest organ of our body.

Tissues and membranes will be discussed in more detail in Chapter 5.

SUMMARY QUESTIONS

1. What organs are located in the abdominal cavity? pelvic cavity? thoracic cavity? dorsal cavity?
2. In what region of the body is the liver located? spleen? empty urinary bladder? heart?
3. Give examples of where in the body you will find three different types of epithelial tissues.
4. Where in the body will you find osseous connective tissue?
5. What type of tissue is found in ligaments and tendons?
6. How does a tissue differ from a membrane?
7. List the functions of five different cellular organelles.
8. Explain three ways in which substances pass through the cell membrane.
9. Explain what happens when living cells are put in hypotonic, isotonic, and hypertonic solutions.
10. Differentiate between skeletal, visceral, and cardiac muscle.
11. Where are mucous membranes located?
12. What kind of membrane is the pleura?
13. Where is hyaline cartilage located?
14. What is the region between the shoulder and the elbow?
15. Where is the hypochondriac region?
16. Where is the hypogastric region?
17. Give two examples of how you would use the terms proximal and distal.

KEY TERMS

alveoli
crystalloid
cytoplasm
endoplasmic reticulum
endothelium
epithelial tissue
exocytosis
filtration
Golgi complex
hypertonic
hypotonic
isotonic
lysosomes

matrix
meiosis
microfilaments
microtubules
mitochondria
mitosis
osmosis
phagocytosis
pinocytosis
reduction division
ribosomes
sclera
synovial membrane

5

Tissues and Membranes

OBJECTIVES

On completion of this chapter, you will be able to:

1. Name the five different types of epithelial tissue and tell where each is located in the body.
2. Describe six kinds of connective tissue.
3. Give examples of the specific functions of each of the different types of epithelial and connective tissues.
4. Differentiate between the three types of muscle tissue.
5. Describe the characteristics of nerve tissue.
6. Discuss the characteristics and locations of three different types of membranes.
7. Describe the structure of the skin.
8. Discuss the functions of the skin.

OVERVIEW

I. TISSUES
    A. Epithelial Tissues
        1. Simple Squamous Epithelium
        2. Cuboidal Epithelium
        3. Columnar Epithelium
        4. Stratified Epithelium
        5. Glandular Epithelium
    B. Connective Tissues
        1. Areolar Connective Tissue
        2. Adipose Tissue
        3. Dense Fibrous Connective Tissue
        4. Cartilage
        5. Osseous Connective Tissue
        6. Liquid Connective Tissue
    C. Muscle Tissue
    D. Nerve Tissue
II. MEMBRANES
    A. Mucous Membrane
    B. Serous Membrane
    C. Synovial Membrane
    D. Fibrous Membrane
III. THE SKIN OR CUTANEOUS MEMBRANE

Tissues and membranes are composed of cells, which are the structural and functional units of all living organisms. The study of cells is called **cytology** (si-tol′o-je). There are several different types of cells in the human body. Although all cells are composed of protoplasm surrounded by the cell membrane, the characteristics and structures of cells vary depending on their specialized functions.

Cytological examinations can help in the diagnosis of a **neoplasm** (ne′o-plasm) or new growth. The cells of a benign tumor resemble those of the parent tissue. They are regular in size and uniform in shape. Malignant cells are not uniform in shape or size. Normal cells are destroyed, and there is evidence of excessive mitosis.

Cells respond to signals causing them to start or stop some process. This concept is not really very different from a switch you might turn to activate some equipment. What the switch is wired to determines whether a light will go on or the radio will start playing. Most equipment is rather specific; a TV is not a garbage disposal. Body cells are also specific in their functions. The switches to activate most cells are called receptors. For nerve cells, the signaling is done by transmitters.

A hormone affects cells that have the particular type of receptor for that hormone. Drugs, like hormones, affect every cell capable of responding to them. If only one type of cell responds, the drug action is quite specific. Most drugs affect many different kinds of cells. This is one of the reasons most drugs have so many untoward side effects.

The activated cell can change shape, as is the case when a muscle contracts. An activated nerve cell sends an electrical impulse. Some of our cells, when activated, store supplies such as fat, or they may manufacture hormones or enzymes.

Cancer cells lose their receptors and, therefore, their ability to perform their normal function. They are insensitive to signals that should start or stop their growth.

TISSUES

Tissues are made of cells that are similar to one another in structure and in intercellular substance. Each type of tissue is specialized for the performance of specific functions. One can observe the structural differences with an ordinary light microscope. Figure 5-1 shows the micro-

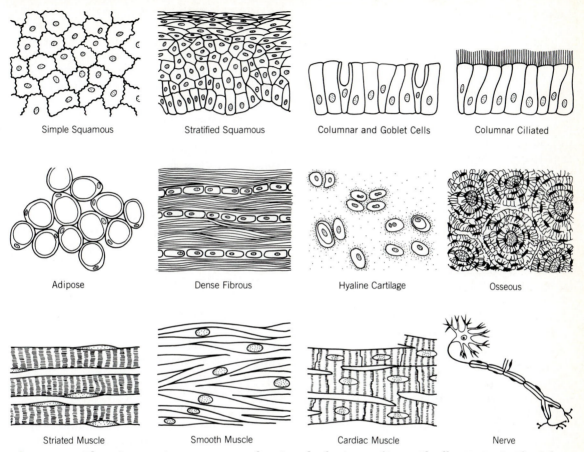

Simple Squamous   Stratified Squamous   Columnar and Goblet Cells   Columnar Ciliated

Adipose   Dense Fibrous   Hyaline Cartilage   Osseous

Striated Muscle   Smooth Muscle   Cardiac Muscle   Nerve

Figure 5-1. The microscopic appearance of various body tissues (From Chaffee, E., Basic Physiology and Anatomy Laboratory Manual, *3rd ed. Philadelphia: J.B. Lippincott, Co., 1974. Used with permission.)*

scopic appearance of various tissues found in the body.

EPITHELIAL TISSUES

In general, epithelial tissues cover the body surface and line the body cavities. These tissues primarily protect the underlying structures, secrete fluids, and absorb substances needed by the body.

Epithelial tissues form thin sheets and are not very strong. The cells are packed closely together

so there is not much true intercellular substance. They have no blood vessels of their own but depend on capillaries in the underlying connective tissues for their supplies and for the removal of the products of their metabolism.

Simple Squamous Epithelium

Simple squamous epithelial tissue consists of a single layer of smooth, flat, platelike cells that are fitted closely together. Simple squamous epithelium lines the blood and lymph vessels as well as the air spaces in the lungs. It provides for the exchange of nutrients, gases, and the products of cellular metabolism between the bloodstream and the other cells of the body.

Cuboidal Epithelium

The cells of cuboidal epithelial tissue are shaped like cubes. This type of tissue is found in the thyroid gland, on the surface of the ovary, and in parts of the kidney.

Columnar Epithelium

Cells of columnar epithelium are tall and narrow. One area in which this type of tissue is found is the lining of the small intestine, where the cells are specialized for the absorption of the products of digestion. Some columnar cells, called goblet columnar cells, produce a protective and lubricating mucus. Other columnar cells have cilia (hairlike processes) on their free surfaces; the cilia move particles and secretions across the surface of the tissue. Some of the columnar cells of the epithelial lining of the respiratory tract are ciliated.

Stratified Epithelium

Stratified epithelium consists of more than one layer of cells, but the outer layer is always made of flattened (squamous) cells. As the surface cells are brushed off by friction, new cells are pushed to the surface by the deeper layers of the tissue. The outer layer of our skin is stratified squamous epithelium. This type of tissue is also found lining the mouth.

Glandular Epithelium

Glandular epithelium is specialized to secrete a variety of different substances. Exocrine glands secrete substances through ducts onto the surface of the body (for example, sweat) or into hollow organs such as the stomach. Endocrine glands pour their secretions directly into the bloodstream.

CONNECTIVE TISSUES

Connective tissues support, protect, and bind together other tissues. The particular function of the connective tissue can depend on the cells of the tissue or the characteristics of the substance found between the connective tissue cells. All connective tissues have more intercellular substance than do epithelial tissues; however, the amount as well as the nature of the intercellular substance differs greatly among the varieties of connective tissue.

Areolar Connective Tissue

Areolar or loose connective tissue is widely distributed throughout the body. It is thin and glistening and is not as strong as most of the other connective tissues. It lies beneath most of the epithelial tissues and serves as packing around blood vessels and nerves.

Adipose Tissue

Adipose tissue has the ability to store fat droplets. It is found beneath the skin; around the kidneys, where it provides support and protection; in joints, where it serves as padding; and in the yellow marrow of long bones. Adipose tissue is a reserve food supply, supports and protects various organs, and provides insulation against heat loss.

Dense Fibrous Connective Tissue

Tendons and ligaments are dense fibrous tissue. This very strong tissue is particularly suited to connect bones together or to connect muscles to bones. Dense fibrous tissue is also found covering muscles.

Cartilage

The intercellular material of cartilage is a firm, jellylike substance. There are three types of cartilage: elastic, hyaline, and fibrous. Elastic cartilage, which is flexible, is found in the external ear. Hyaline cartilage is found at the ends of bones in freely movable joints and in part of the nasal septum. This type of cartilage connects the ribs to the sternum, or breast bone. The skeleton of the embryo is formed from hyaline cartilage. Fibrous cartilage, which is not as firm as hyaline cartilage but is very strong, is found in the discs between the vertebrae and in some other partly movable joints.

Osseous Connective Tissue

Osseous tissue is bone. The intercellular substance of osseous tissue in an adult is mostly calcium phosphate salts. In a young child, there is relatively less of the mineral salts and more protein in the bone. For this reason, the bones of children are somewhat more flexible than those of adults. Osseous tissue provides a supporting framework for the body and provides bony protection for some organs, such as the brain. Bone also serves as a calcium depot. If the blood calcium level gets too low, calcium is withdrawn from the bone so that a normal level of calcium can be maintained in the blood.

Liquid Connective Tissue

Blood is liquid connective tissue. The intercellular material of this tissue is fluid. Blood serves as a vital transport system for distributing nutrients, gases, and the products of cellular metabolism throughout the body. For a detailed discussion of the composition of blood, see Chapter 13.

MUSCLE TISSUE

As discussed in Chapter 4, there are three types of muscle tissue: skeletal, visceral, and cardiac. Skeletal muscle is voluntary and must have a nerve supply in order to contract. Visceral and cardiac muscles are involuntary and, under ordinary circumstances, we cannot control the contractions of these muscles. In subsequent chapters, we shall present a more detailed discussion of muscle tissue.

NERVE TISSUE

Nerves are composed of nerve cells or neurons and supporting cells called **neuroglia** (nu-rog′le-ah). These neurons are highly specialized and serve to transmit impulses to and from various parts of the body. Sensory impulses originate in the periphery and go to the brain for interpretation to keep us advised of conditions in our environment. Motor impulses originate in the central nervous system, brain and cord, and result in muscle or glandular activity.

MEMBRANES

Membranes are combinations of tissues. The membranes that are of particular importance to your understanding of the human body are mucous, serous, synovial, fibrous, and cutaneous.

MUCOUS MEMBRANE

Mucous membrane is a combination of epithelial and connective tissues. Mucous membranes line the body cavities that open to the outside of the body: the respiratory tract, the gastrointestinal tract, and the genitourinary tract. All mucous membranes contain some goblet cells that secrete mucus for lubrication and protection.

SEROUS MEMBRANE

Connective and epithelial tissues make up the serous membranes that line closed cavities of the body. Examples are the **pleura** (ploor′ah), which covers the lungs and lines the thorax, and the **peritoneum** (per″i-to-ne′um), which is found in the abdominal cavity. Serous membrane secretes a slippery fluid that protects against friction.

SYNOVIAL MEMBRANE

Freely movable joint cavities are lined with synovial (si-no′ve-al) membrane. The cells in the surface layer secrete synovial fluid to provide lubrication.

FIBROUS MEMBRANE

Fibrous membranes are strong, protective membranes composed entirely of connective tissues. Examples of this type of membrane are the **dura mater** (du′rah ma′ter) covering the brain, the **periosteum** (par″e-os′te-um) covering the bones, and most of the outer covering of the eye, which is called the **sclera** (skle′rah).

THE SKIN OR CUTANEOUS MEMBRANE

The skin, or **integument** (in-teg′u-ment), is a more complex combination of tissues than is found in the membranes previously described. It is subjected to many more insults, and its structure varies accordingly. Although technically a membrane, it is also considered an organ. In fact, it is the largest organ of our bodies.

The skin is almost entirely waterproof and provides a protective barrier for the more delicate underlying tissues. Although the outer layer of skin has no blood vessels, the total skin receives about one-third of all blood circulating through the body.

The outer layer of the skin is stratified squamous epithelium called the epidermis (ep″e-der′mis). The inner layer, or **dermis**, is connective tissue. Although these two layers are firmly attached to each other, they are quite different in their characteristics (see Fig. 5-2).

The epidermis has no blood vessels. The outermost layer of the epidermis is composed of dead cells, which are constantly being worn away and replaced by the living cells in the deeper layer of the epidermis. The deep layer of the epidermis produces **melanin** (mel′ah-nin), which is responsible for the skin color. Exposure to sunlight increases the production of melanin and therefore causes "sun tan." Freckles are irregular patches of melanin. Exposure to sunlight also causes the skin to produce vitamin D, which is important in the absorption of dietary calcium.

The dermis is the inner layer of skin. Conelike elevations, or **papillae** (pah-pil′e), on the surface of the dermis are the structures responsible for fingerprints.

Elastic fibers in the dermis allow for extensibility and elasticity of the skin. There are considerably more elastic fibers in the dermis of a young person than that of an elderly person. This fact and the disappearance of fat from the subcutaneous tissue result in the characteristic wrinkled appearance of the skin in elderly people.

Certain cutaneous glands deserve special mention because they produce secretions important to the functions of the skin. **Sebaceous** (se-ba′shus) **glands** are found almost everywhere on the surface of the body except on the palms of the hands and the soles of the feet. Sebaceous glands produce **sebum** (se′bum), an oily secretion that helps to keep the skin soft and prevents the hair from becoming dry and brittle.

Sweat glands in the dermis pour their secretions onto the surface of the skin through ducts that pass through the epidermis. The evaporation of perspiration is one mechanism by which the body is able to maintain a stable internal temperature in the presence of high external temperatures. In a person who is acclimated to the heat, sweat does not accumulate in droplets and roll from the skin as it does when a person is not accustomed to the heat. Droplets that do not evaporate do not cool the body, and they waste water and salts.

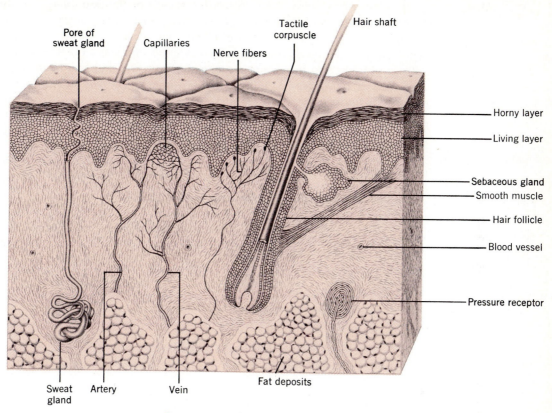

Figure 5-2. *Skin, three-dimensional view*

Sweat glands are most abundant on the palms and soles. However, although sweating in response to high temperatures is general, it is not marked on the palms of the hands and soles of the feet. Psychologically produced sweat, on the other hand, predominates on the palms and soles. Many different kinds of emotions can cause the production of this type of sweat. In muscular exercise, the sweating is both thermal and emotional.

Ceruminous (se-ru′mi-nus) glands are found in the skin of the passages leading into the ear. These glands secrete **cerumen** (se-ru′men), a waxy substance that helps to protect the ear-

drum. If the amount of cerumen is excessive, it can interfere with hearing.

Hair is present on most of the skin surfaces. However, it is most abundant on the scalp. The hair grows from a follicle deep in the dermis. Because the hair that we see is not living tissue, cutting or shaving has no effect on its growth.

Fingernails and toenails protect the distal parts of our fingers and toes. The nails are most firmly attached at the base of the nail. This crescent-shaped area is called the lunula (lu′nu-lah).

In summary, the function of the skin is to protect the underlying structures from bacterial invasion and from drying out. It serves as a sense organ because it contains nerve endings that respond to touch, pain, and changes in temperature. The skin helps to regulate body temperature by the evaporation of perspiration and by the vasoconstriction or dilatation of blood vessels in the skin. If the internal body temperature increases, the vessels of the skin dilate and the warm blood flows more freely near the cooler surface of the body where the heat can be dissipated by radiation and conduction. Although not a major function, the skin also helps in the elimination of some of the body wastes.

SUMMARY QUESTIONS

1. Name the types of cartilaginous tissues and tell where each is located.
2. Of what type of tissue is bone composed?
3. Where are mucous membranes located?
4. Name the glands of the skin and discuss the functions of each.
5. What type of membrane lines the closed cavities of the body?
6. What is the function of adipose tissue?
7. Where is dense fibrous connective tissue found in the body?
8. What is the function of stratified epithelium and where is it found in the body?
9. Name the various types of muscle tissue and discuss the functions of each type.
10. What are the functions of the cutaneous membrane?
11. Give some examples of fibrous membranes.
12. What are the unique characteristics of nerve tissue?
13. How does a membrane differ from a tissue?

KEY TERMS

cerumen
cytology
dermis
dura mater
integument
melanin
neoplasm
neuroglia

papillae
periosteum
peritoneum
pleura
sclera
sebaceous glands
sebum

Diseases of the Skin

OBJECTIVES

On completion of this chapter, you will be able to:

1. Describe three common diagnostic procedures used for patients with skin lesions.
2. Describe six types of skin lesions.
3. Describe three common therapeutic measures used to relieve skin lesions.
4. List four common skin irritants and give suggestions on how to avoid these irritants.

OVERVIEW

I. DIAGNOSTIC PROCEDURES
   A. Direct Examination
   B. Biopsy
   C. Sensitivity Tests
II. SKIN LESIONS
III. THERAPEUTIC MEASURES
IV. INTEGUMENTARY DISORDERS
   A. Acne
   B. Seborrheic Dermatitis (Dandruff)
   C. Eczema
   D. Urticaria (Hives)
   E. Contact Dermatitis
   F. Psoriasis
   G. Impetigo
   H. Warts
   I. Herpes Simplex (Cold Sores)
   J. Herpes Zoster (Shingles)
   K. Furuncles and Carbuncles
   L. Paronychia
   M. Sebaceous Cysts
   N. Miliaria (Prickly Heat)
   O. Diaper Rash
   P. Dermatophytosis (Athlete's Foot)
   Q. Corns and Calluses
   R. Infestations and Bites
   S. Lupus Erythematosus
   T. Scleroderma
   U. Pilonidal Sinus

The appearance of our skin is important to all of us. It reflects something about our way of life, age, the climate in which we live, our general health, and even a bit about our personality in the way the skin is groomed. It is our largest organ and is complex not only in its normal structure but in its pathology. It is not surprising, therefore, that a very large percentage of the people seeking medical help come to the doctor because of problems related to the skin.

The constant exposure of the skin to the environment is a factor that may contribute to the incidence of skin diseases as well as to some of the difficulties in dealing with such illnesses and frequently to their recurrence.

There are a variety of diseases of the skin with which you should be familiar. Many of these diseases are of unknown etiology and, as a result, treatment is usually directed toward relief of the signs and symptoms. Fortunately, although skin diseases cause discomfort, most are self-limiting.

DIAGNOSTIC PROCEDURES

Considering the enormous number of diagnostic tests, imaging techniques, and laboratory procedures that are used today, there are relatively few parameters employed in the diagnosis of skin disorders.

DIRECT EXAMINATION

In order to properly examine the skin, good lighting is essential. It is important to note the distribution of any skin lesions. If a rash is localized, it may indicate that the cause is local; for example, a rash only on the feet may be related to footwear. The rashes of some diseases are more pronounced on the trunk, whereas other rashes are more noticeable on the distal body parts. Notice particularly areas where body parts come into contact with each other. It is helpful to know whether the lesions are more bothersome after bathing. Determine whether there seems to be any relationship between the onset of the problem and some significant change in the patient's way of living.

Microscopic examinations of scales taken from the lesions may reveal fungi. A Wood's light is used to examine the scalp for ringworms.

Such an examination is done in a dark room. An ultraviolet light and a Wood's filter produce a fluorescence in hair infested with human or animal fungus.

BIOPSY

A small section of the skin can be removed surgically with a dermal punch. This instrument is an electrical punch that can penetrate the skin to a desired depth. The skin is first cleansed with an antiseptic solution and a local anesthetic is injected into the area. The specimen obtained will be examined by a histologist (his-tol'o-gist), who specializes in the study of tissues.

SENSITIVITY TESTS

A Patch test is used to identify substances to which the patient is sensitive. A gauze pad is saturated with the test material in a concentration not likely to cause irritation and applied to uninjured skin. The area is covered with a piece of protective material such as cellophane. Unless marked irritation appears, the patch is usually left on for 24 to 48 hours. Twenty minutes after the patch is removed, a reading is made. There will be erythema or blisters if the reaction is positive. The area should be observed for two or three days since there may be a delayed reaction.

If more than one test material is used, each area is numbered and a record made of which material was used where. There are ready-made patches available.

Percutaneous and intradermal tests are useful for testing sensitivities to various foods and pollens. These tests are particularly helpful in identifying the causes of eczema.

Percutaneous tests are done by making a scratch about 1/2 inch long through the epidermis without causing bleeding. The foreign material is placed on the scratch with a toothpick. The scratch is usually made on some covered part of the body such as the anterior surface of the thigh or the lower back. The material is left on the scratch for 15 minutes and then the skin is rinsed and dried. If there is a positive reaction, edematous elevations will develop at the site. If a positive reaction does not appear, the patient is instructed to observe the area for another 24 hours because delayed reactions can occur.

If the patient does have a positive reaction to the percutaneous test, the suspected material should be eliminated from the patient's environment. If this is not possible, sometimes the patient can be desensitized to the material by administering small, repeated doses of the **allergen** (al'er-jen).

A small amount (0.2 ml) of a prepared solution can be injected intradermally into the anterior surface of the forearm. Readings are made after 30 minutes and then daily for one week. A positive reading (an edematous, reddened area) does not necessarily mean that the patient is presently sensitive since such a reaction also may represent a past sensitivity. When these sensitivity tests are positive, there may also be systemic symptoms such as nausea, chills, flushing, and shortness of breath. For this reason, epinephrine should always be readily available when these tests are done. Epinephrine is an emergency drug useful in treating a severe allergy.

SKIN LESIONS

Skin lesions vary in size, color, and shape. It is important that you learn the correct terms used to describe the patient's lesions. The following are some common primary lesions:

1. Bullae (bul'i) (blebs, blisters) are large elevations that contain serous fluid.
2. Desquamation (des"kwah-ma'shun) is a peeling of the skin.

3. Macule (mak'u-le) are level, circumscribed areas on the skin.

4. Nodules (nod'yulz), or tubercles are large, circumscribed solid elevations.

5. Papules (pap'ulz) are smaller, circumscribed solid elevations. They do not contain fluid. The largest papules are no larger than a pea.

6. Pustules (pus'tulz) are small elevations that contain pus.

7. Tumors are soft or firm masses that may either be freely movable or fixed.

8. Vesicles (ves'i-k'ls) are small blisters, the largest of which are no larger than a pea.

9. Wheals are edematous elevations. There usually is itching accompanying the wheals.

Secondary lesions are the results of some primary lesion. Excoriation (eks-kor'e-a'shun) is used to describe the appearance of skin that has shallow ulcers, which may be due to scratching. A **fissure** (fish'ur) is a linear break in the skin.

Exudate (eks'u-dat) is drainage. If the drainage is watery, it is called serous exudate. If it has pus in it, it is said to be purulent (pu'roolent). A sanguineous (sang-gwin'e-us) exudate is a bloody drainage.

THERAPEUTIC MEASURES

One of the most common symptoms associated with diseases of the skin is itching or **pruritus** (proo-ri'tus). Excessive warmth, rough prickly fabrics, and emotional stress aggravate itching. Frequently, it is more noticeable at night, probably because the patient's attention is not occupied elsewhere. Scratching will only relieve an itch if it removes the irritant, which it rarely does. More likely the scratching will increase the severity of the itch by spreading the irritant or even denude the skin and make the patient more

susceptible to infection. Antipruritic lotions such as calamine are helpful. Starch baths (one pound of corn starch in a tub of warm water) may also help relieve itching. The patient should be instructed not to use soap when taking the starch bath and to pat the skin with a soft towel rather than to rub it when drying.

Although pruritis is frequently the first symptom of a relatively minor skin disorder, it may also be an early indication of a more serious disease such as leukemia or Hodgkin's disease. Other causes of pruritis include sensitivity to various drugs, chemicals, soaps, and pollens. Physical changes in the skin, such as dryness from excessive bathing or chafing and irritation from various fabrics, can cause pruritis.

Crust and scales that accumulate on the skin must be removed. The ideal technique for this procedure is wet dressings. They are not only helpful in the gentle removal of these sorts of skin debris but are also beneficial in cleansing wounds, softening the skin, promoting drainage, and soothing inflamed skin.

Either warm or cold water can be used for these dressings. Cold, wet dressings produce vasoconstriction and reduce metabolism in the area. Warm, wet dressings cause vasodilatation, which will facilitate phagocytosis. Medicated solutions can also be used.

Wet dressings must be kept wet. If the dressing becomes dry, it will very likely become a source of irritation, particularly if someone attempts to remove a dry dressing that has adhered to the skin.

Baths have the same effect as wet dressings and are more practical if the skin problem being treated is generalized or if the area is one that is difficult to dress.

Cryosurgery (krio-ser'jer-e) can be used to remove small skin lesions. Liquid nitrogen is a cold, liquefied gas that can be applied directly to a benign or precancerous lesion. The lesion will first become swollen and red and a blister may form. Next, a scab forms and falls off in one to three weeks. The skin lesion will be sloughed along with the scab. Growth of new skin follows.

A chemical face peel utilizes a cauterant to the skin to cause a controlled burn. This procedure results in superficial destruction of the upper layers of the skin and a tightening of the deep layers. The most common indications for a chemical peel include pigmentation problems, skin damage due to radiation, removal of freckles, and superficial acne scarring. Following the treatment, there is moderate swelling and crusting for a week. Redness persists for six to eight weeks. Once the healing is completed, the skin will have a more youthful appearance.

Good general hygienic measures are important for healthful living, and this is particularly true for the patient with skin problems. The patient should be given instructions for a balanced diet with adequate roughage. Exercise and rest are also important aspects of good health. It is advisable that the patient with skin problems avoid exercise that causes excessive perspiring as this will stimulate the skin to produce more sebum, which may be a problem, particularly if the nature of the skin problem is an infection.

INTEGUMENTARY DISORDERS

ACNE

Acne characteristically occurs during adolescence. It is usually self-limiting and will disappear in the late teens or early twenties. However, eight or ten years is a long time for a young person who longs to be attractive and popular to endure the pimples and blackheads of acne (see Fig. 6-1).

Frequent, thorough washing of the affected areas with a mild soap is helpful because it

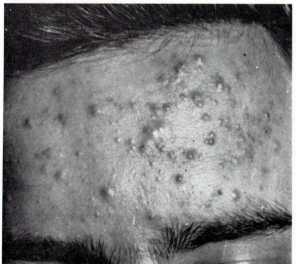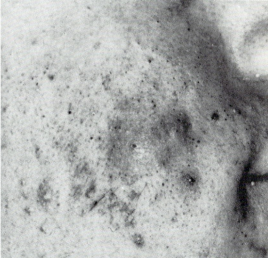

Figure 6-1. Acne. Note the papular pustules. (From Stewart, W.D., Danto, J.L., and Maddin, S., Dermatology, 4th ed. St. Louis: The C.V. Mosby Co., 1978. Used with permission.)

helps to reduce the oiliness and at least temporarily reduces the number of bacteria causing the infection on the skin. The blackheads and pimples or pustules should not be picked at or squeezed because unskilled manipulation of these lesions can result in secondary infections and perhaps permanent scarring.

The doctor may order steroid (ste′roid) creams to be applied to the affected areas. Before applying any medication, the patient's hands and the affected area should be washed thoroughly. Short treatments with ultraviolet light, under the direction of a doctor, may be beneficial because this treatment will lessen the oiliness and reduce the number of infection-causing bacteria. Excessive use of ultraviolet light can be harmful.

Recently, a new medication, Accutanen (isotretinoin), has been used for acne with a great deal of success. Unfortunately, it is known to cause birth defects and, therefore, young women are cautioned against using this drug. Recall that the fetus is most vulnerable during the time that the cells are differentiating (from the tenth day following conception through the sixth week).

Certain foods are thought to aggravate acne. It may be helpful, therefore, to avoid chocolates, nuts, and fatty foods. Some doctors completely restrict dietary caffeine. If caffeine is restricted, the patient should be informed that caffeine is found not only in coffee but also in many soft drinks.

If the acne has caused scarring, this condition can be made less conspicuous by a chemical face peel or by dermabrasion. Under anesthesia, the outermost layers of the skin are removed by sandpaper or a rotating wire brush. Following dermabrasion, the skin feels raw and sore. Some serous exudate and crusting will take place, but the patient should not wash the area for five or six days and avoid picking or touching it until sufficient healing has occurred.

SEBORRHEIC DERMATITIS (DANDRUFF)

Dandruff frequently occurs with acne; however, it is not limited to the adolescent period of life. The symptoms are an oily scalp, itching, irritation, and the formation of greasy scales. Severe or prolonged seborrheic (seb-o-re′ik) dermatitis can cause the premature loss of hair.

Dandruff usually responds well to frequent shampooing (two or three times a week) with tincture of green soap, brushing the hair, and massaging the scalp. Although the condition improves with treatment, the symptoms frequently return if the regimen of treatment is interrupted.

ECZEMA

Eczema (ek′za-mah) is characterized by vesicles on reddened skin. The blisters burst and weep; crusts form later from the dried fluid. Because the condition is usually aggravated by emotional stress, tranquilizers may be ordered. Antihistamines and steroids are also helpful in the treatment of eczema. Wet dressings and starch baths may relieve some of the symptoms. Infantile eczema is shown in Figure 6-2.

URTICARIA (HIVES)

Urticaria (ur″ti-ka′re-ah) is usually the result of an allergy, but the condition is sometimes related to emotional stress. The most familiar example of urticaria is a mosquito bite. In severe cases, there will be wheals or rounded, white elevations and itching of the entire body. Steroids and antihistamines are used to treat urticaria.

CONTACT DERMATITIS

The most common causes of contact dermatitis are contact with poison ivy, poison sumac, or poison oak. Prompt cleansing of the exposed

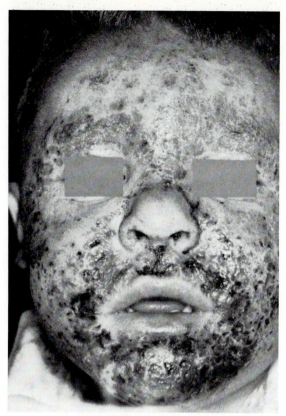

Figure 6-2. Infantile eczema (From Stewart, W.D., Danto, J.L., and Maddin, S., Dermatology, 4th ed. St. Louis: The C.V. Mosby Co., 1978. Used with permission.)

the patient to the allergen by giving repeated small doses of the substance.

PSORIASIS

Psoriasis (so-ri′ah-sis) is characterized by patchy erythema and scales. It most frequently occurs in young adults and middle-aged people. Its cause is unknown. Ointments can be used to soften the scales; sometimes, ultraviolet light treatments are helpful. Low-fat diets are usually recommended. Steroids, antihistamines, and tranquilizers may also be used, as they are for many other skin diseases.

IMPETIGO

Impetigo (im″pe-ti′go) usually is the result of infection by streptococci or staphylococci. It is more common in infants and children than in adults. Because this condition, unlike most other skin diseases, is contagious, care must be taken in treating and handling the lesions.

The symptoms of impetigo are erythema and vesicles that rupture and cover the skin with a sticky yellow crust. The crust must be removed with soap and water or mineral oil before antibiotic ointments are applied. The condition can usually be cured in a few days. However, if it is severe in the newborn infant, it can be fatal.

skin with soap and water followed by application of alcohol may prevent or lessen the reaction to these allergens. The symptoms include redness, itching, blisters, and edema. Scratching spreads the lesions. Antipruritis lotions and cold, wet dressings help to relieve the symptoms.

Many people are allergic to cleansing agents, cosmetics, other chemicals, and certain metals. In such cases, it is well to avoid the particular allergen. The doctor may be able to desensitize

WARTS

Warts are caused by a virus. Susceptibility to warts varies considerably from one person to another. Sometimes warts disappear spontaneously. If they do not, nitric or sulfuric acid can be applied deep into the root of the wart after the thick, horny outer tissue has been pared away. Although most warts are not painful, plantar warts that occur on the soles of the feet can cause considerable discomfort.

HERPES SIMPLEX (COLD SORES)

Herpes (her'pez) **simplex** is also caused by a virus. Many healthy people harbor this virus and under such circumstances as emotional stress or respiratory infections the herpes simplex can appear (see Fig. 6-3).

The condition is characterized by blisters on inflamed skin, usually around the mouth. Although there is no specific treatment and the lesions subside in about a week, topical applications of tincture of benzoin can help to relieve the pain and burning. The patient should be told that when the benzoin is first applied the burning will be more severe but that subsequent applications will not be painful.

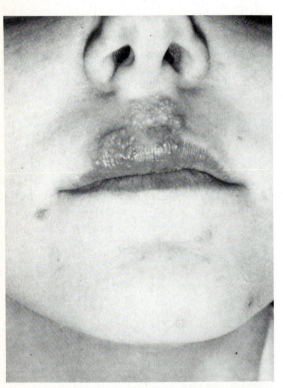

Figure 6-3. Herpes simplex (From Stewart, W.D., Danto, J.L., and Maddin, S., Dermatology, 4th ed. St. Louis: The C.V. Mosby Co., 1978. Used with permission.)

HERPES ZOSTER (SHINGLES)

The cause of herpes zoster is a viral infection. Patients have fever and **malaise** (ma-laz'). After a few days, erythema and vesicles appear along the course of a nerve. Although there is no specific treatment for this painful condition and it can last for months, analgesics and calamine lotion can be used for symptomatic treatment.

FURUNCLES AND CARBUNCLES

A furuncle (fu'rung-kul) is a boil. A carbuncle is a large, swollen erythematous lesion, often on the back of the neck. The carbuncle is very painful and has several openings through which pus drains. Both conditions are usually the result of staphylococcal or streptococcal infections.

Hot, moist compresses help to localize the infection and to promote drainage. It may be necessary to incise and drain the lesions surgically. Antibiotics are usually ordered.

Because furuncles and carbuncles frequently occur in patients who have diabetes mellitus, the patient should have blood and urine examinations to rule out this endocrine disease. If diabetes is present, it must also be treated.

PARONYCHIA

A **paronychia** (par"o-nik'e-ah) is an infected hangnail. Often, the patient needs only to soak the finger frequently in warm water. If this treatment is not successful, the base of the nail will have to be surgically removed. Painful as such a procedure might seem, it usually is not. The nail will grow back in about three to four months.

SEBACEOUS CYSTS

Sebaceous cysts are the result of the blockage of a duct of a sebaceous gland. Usually, the swelling is small, and a doctor can simply incise and drain the cyst in the office. Occasionally, the cyst becomes very large and unsightly. In such cases, it will have to be removed in a hospital operating room. The doctor usually will discharge the patient immediately after the surgery with instructions to return to the office in four or five days to have the dressing changed. If a drain was placed in the wound, it is removed at this time.

MILIARIA (PRICKLY HEAT)

Miliaria (mil″e-a′re-ah) is a condition in which there is an obstruction of the ducts of the sweat glands and the sweat escapes into the epidermis, producing a red pruritic rash. The discomfort of the condition may be relieved by cool baths using mild soap. The patient should apply a light coating of corn starch powder. Too much powder will cause caking, particularly in folds of skin, and will further aggravate the condition. Lightweight clothing and absorbent underwear should be worn.

DIAPER RASH

The most common skin problem in infancy is diaper rash. It is more frequent during hot weather. The skin under the diaper is irritated and erythematous from the organic acids in the stool or from ammonia produced by bacterial decomposition of urine.

Exposing the area to the air will help to dry the rash. Antibacterial creams and topical vitamin creams may be prescribed. The area should be cleansed with mineral oil. Prompt diaper changes are important. The use of rubber or plastic pants should be discouraged.

DERMATOPHYTOSIS (ATHLETE'S FOOT)

Athlete's foot is a fungus infection. Susceptibility to the infection varies considerably from one person to another. Usually, it first affects the skin between the toes; the skin is red, cracked, and sore. It can spread to other parts of the feet,

the hands, axillae, and the groin. Because it is an infectious condition, care must be taken to avoid transmission from one person to another by means of contaminated towels and toilet articles. People with the infection should avoid going barefoot in dormitory bathrooms and gym locker rooms.

Antifungal agents such as Desenex powder or ointment are usually effective in treatment of dermatophytosis (der″mah-to-fi-to′sis). The patient must take particular care to dry between the toes and should avoid footwear that causes the feet to perspire. Frequent changes of shoes and socks may be helpful.

CORNS AND CALLUSES

Corns and calluses are usually the result of friction caused by poorly fitted shoes. Corns are hard, raised areas that are often painful. Calluses are flat, thickened patches. The only effective treatment is to relieve the pressure or friction. Keratolytic (ker″ah-to-lit′ik) agents such as salicylic acid help to remove the thickened hard skin. Rubbing cream can also soften the calluses.

INFESTATIONS AND BITES

Pediculosis (pe-dik″u-lo′sis) is caused by lice. Lice can infest scalp hair, body hair, or pubic hair. Symptoms are itching and irritation of the skin. Scratching denudes the skin and makes it more susceptible to infection. A variety of ointments, powders, and lotions containing benzyl benzoate or benzine hexachloride are effective in the treatment of pediculosis. If the patient continues to have close contact with others who harbor the parasites, the condition will recur.

Scabies is caused by a mite that burrows deep into the skin. The itching of this condition is intense. Scabies can be readily transmitted from one person to another by close personal contact. The treatment of scabies is thorough bathing followed by the application of ointments or lotions that contain benzine hexachloride or benzyl benzoate. After the treatment, the patient should completely change his clothing.

LUPUS ERYTHEMATOSUS

Lupus (lu'pus) erythematosus (er-e-them"ah-to'sis) is a rare condition characterized by erythematous macular lesions. These itchy lesions frequently appear on the face in a butterfly pattern. In addition to skin lesions, many patients with lupus have dysfunction of the kidneys, joints, lungs, and heart.

Although there is no specific treatment for lupus, steroids help to relieve the symptoms and salicylates such as aspirin relieve joint pains and reduce fever. There are remissions and **exacerbations** (eg-zas"er-ba'shunz) of this disease. Prognosis is guarded and ultimately the disease can be fatal.

SCLERODERMA

Scleroderma (skle"re-der'mah) is a systemic disease involving not only the skin but also the muscles, bones, heart, and lungs. The skin becomes smooth, hard, and tight. Although the disease is progressive, there are periods of remissions and exacerbations. In severe cases, the disease is usually fatal.

There is no specific treatment for scleroderma. However, symptomatic treatment with ointments, massage, and heat may help relieve the stiffness and inelasticity of the skin. Steroids can provide temporary relief.

PILONIDAL SINUS

A **pilonidal** (pi"lo-ni'dal) cyst is a sac in the sacral region that often contains hair. The cyst usually does not cause any problems until it becomes infected and a draining sinus develops. In such a case, the sinus can be very painful. People whose occupations require long hours of sitting are predisposed to pilonidal sinuses. The lesion should be treated several times a day with warm water compresses or sitz baths. With this treatment, the lesion will probably heal in a matter of a few days to a week. Unfortunately, the sinus frequently recurs.

The surgical treatment of a pilonidal sinus is usually quite extensive, considering the fact that the visible lesion is so small. The tract is laid open with a deep and wide V-shaped incision and packed with gauze to keep it open so it will heal from the bottom up. It will take two or three weeks for the incision to heal.

SUMMARY QUESTIONS

1. Describe how a patient is examined for a skin disease.
2. How are sensitivity tests done?
3. List and define six primary skin lesions.
4. What measures would you recommend to relieve the symptoms of eczema?
5. What should you do if you come into contact with poison ivy?
6. How would you instruct a patient who has pruritus?
7. What measures can you recommend to someone who suffers from acne?

KEY TERMS

allergen
cryosurgery
eczema
exacerbations
exudate
fissure
herpes simplex
impetigo

malaise
paronychia
pediculosis
pilonidal
pruritus
psoriasis
scleroderma
urticaria

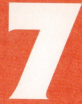

The Musculoskeletal System

OBJECTIVES

On completion of this chapter, you will be able to:

1. Explain how bones are formed.
2. Describe the functions of the three types of bone cells.
3. List 7 of the 13 major bone markings.
4. Identify the bones of the appendicular skeleton.
5. Identify the bones of the axial skeleton.
6. List the sinuses of the skull.
7. Give examples of where each type of cartilage is located.
8. Give examples of the three different types of joints.
9. Demonstrate the different types of movements in diarthrotic joints.
10. Explain what is meant by oxygen debt.
11. Describe the chemical changes that take place during muscle contraction.
12. Explain the All or None Law as it applies to muscle.
13. List the functions of all of the major prime movers.

OVERVIEW

I. COMPOSITION OF BONE

II. GROSS STRUCTURE OF BONE
  A. Classification of Bones According to Shape
  B. Bone Markings
  C. Bone Marrow
  D. Blood Supply

III. BONE FORMATION

IV. THE SKELETON AS A WHOLE
  A. The Appendicular Skeleton
    1. The Shoulder Girdle
    2. Arm and Hand
    3. Pelvic Girdle
    4. Lower Extremities
  B. The Axial Skeleton
    1. Bones of the Skull
      a. Cranium
      b. Bones of the Face
      c. Sinuses
      d. Sutures
      e. Fontanels
    2. Vertebral Column
    3. Thorax

V. CARTILAGE

VI. ARTICULATIONS OR JOINTS

VII. BURSAE

VIII. ORGANS OF LOCOMOTION
  A. Types of Muscle Tissue
  B. Physiology of Contraction
    1. Energy Sources
    2. Contractility
      a. Chemical Changes
      b. Electrical Changes
    3. Muscle Tone
    4. Excitability
  C. Naming of Muscles

IX. PRIME MOVERS AND ANTAGONISTS

Bones, which are composed mainly of osseous connective tissue, have many important functions. They provide a supporting framework for the body, protect the viscera (organs), and provide a place for attachment of muscles. Bones store minerals, mainly calcium salts, that can be used to increase the blood calcium level in circumstances that deplete the blood calcium. Some bones contain red bone marrow which forms red blood cells and some white blood cells. This marrow also aids in the destruction of old, worn-out red blood cells. Together with other organs, the red marrow plays an important role in the body's immune process.

COMPOSITION OF BONE

The chief organic constituent of bone is **collagen** (kol'ah-jen), which is a protein. About two-thirds of the adult bone is inorganic calcium salts, notably calcium phosphate and calcium carbonate. The source of the protein and the inorganic salts is the food we eat. Because calcium phosphate is the primary ingredient for proper bone density, we shall consider some of the factors involved in the metabolism of this inorganic salt.

Vitamin D is essential for the absorption of these minerals into the blood vessels of the intestine. Although it can be synthesized by the skin on exposure to sunlight, the best and safest sources of vitamin D are fish-liver oils, eggs, milk, and butter. Because it is a fat-soluble vitamin, the action of vitamin D is dependent on proper fat metabolism. The action of vitamin D is opposed by cortisone and other glucocorticoids (hormones from the adrenal gland). For this reason, patients on long-term steroid therapy (cortisone treatment) may have decreased bone density and are predisposed to pathological fractures. The sex hormones, estrogen and testosterone, favor the deposition of calcium in the bones. Postmenopausal women who have low levels of estrogen may have diminished bone density.

The enzyme alkaline phosphatase is the catalyst needed for the regulation of bone and blood levels of calcium. Hormones from the thyroid and parathyroid glands are also important in the regulation of bone and blood levels of calcium. Thyrocalcitonin favors the deposition of calcium into the bone, and parathormone favors the withdrawal of calcium from the bone, thereby increasing the calcium blood level.

Mechanical stress also favors bone formation, whereas inactivity favors the desalting of bones. Patients with fractures of the weight-bearing bones are frequently put in traction until they can be mobilized. The traction supplies the mechanical stress that will favor bone healing while the patient is inactive. Traction also helps keep the bone fragments in correct alignment. Without traction, the strong leg muscles may go into spasm and cause overriding (overlapping) of the fractured ends of the bone (see Fig. 7-1).

Bone, like other tissues, consists of living cells and nonliving intercellular substance. The intercellular material or **matrix** (ma′trix) predominates. **Osteoblasts** (os′te-o-blasts) are bone building and bone-repairing cells. In healthy adult bone, these cells are located in the deep layer of the periosteum, the dense fibrous membrane that covers the bone. The periosteum also contains many small blood vessels that send branches into the bone. Because of these blood vessels and the osteoblasts, the periosteum is essential for bone cell survival and bone formation, a process that continues throughout life.

Beneath the periosteum is compact bone. This type of osseous tissue, as its name implies, is very dense. Microscopically, compact bone is made up of **haversian** (ha-ver′se-an) **systems** (see Fig. 7-2). The structures that make up each haversian system include lamellae (la-mel′eh),

which are concentric, cylinder-shaped calcified structures, lacunae (la-kun′e) or small lakes containing tissue fluid, **osteocytes** (os′te-o-sits), another type of bone cell, and canaliculi (kan″ah-lik′u-le), which are canals connecting all of the lacunae together and to a larger canal, the haversian canal. These canals carry nutrients to the osteocytes and also carry away the products of their metabolism. It is the osteocytes that facilitate the exchange of calcium between bone and blood.

Cancellous bone is light and spongy. This type of bone is found in areas that are not subjected to great mechanical stress and where the weight of the compact bone would be a problem. Cancellous bone has no haversian systems. It is a weblike arrangement of marrow-filled spaces separated by thin processes of bone.

GROSS STRUCTURE OF BONE

CLASSIFICATION OF BONES ACCORDING TO SHAPE

Bones can be classified according to their shape. Long bones are located in the extremities. The two ends of the long bones are called **epiphyses** (e-pif′is-ez). Each epiphysis is covered with hyaline cartilage that supplies a smooth surface for the articulating bones. There is cancellous bone in the epiphysis. The shaft of the bone, or **diaphysis** (di-af′is-is), is compact bone and covered with periosteum.

The center of the bone is the medullary cavity, which contains yellow bone marrow that consists largely of adipose tissue (see Fig. 7-3). **Osteoclasts** (os′te-o-klasts) are cells found at the medullary cavity. These cells are concerned with the absorption and removal of bone. By increasing the diameter of the medullary cavity, these cells cause the bone to grow in diameter. At the

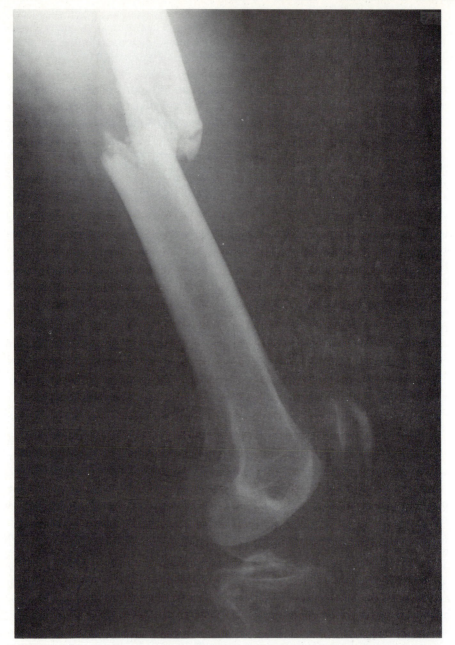

Figure 7-1. X-ray showing a fractured femur with overriding caused by contraction of the thigh muscles surrounding the broken bone. Traction will correct the overriding and favor the action of the bone-building osteoblasts.

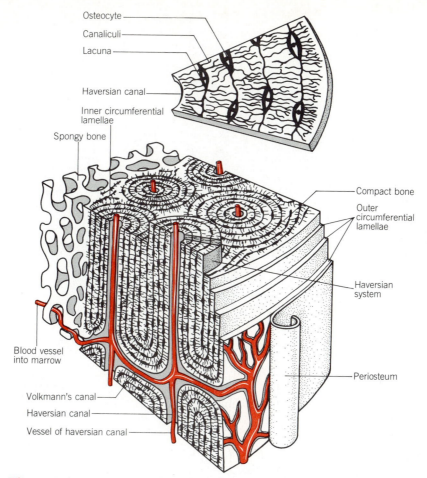

Osteocyte
Canaliculi
Lacuna
Haversian canal
Inner circumferential lamellae
Spongy bone
Blood vessel into marrow
Volkmann's canal
Haversian canal
Vessel of haversian canal
Compact bone
Outer circumferential lamellae
Haversian system
Periosteum

Figure 7-2. *Microscopically, the osseous tissue in compact bone is honeycombed with canaliculi (tiny canals) and lacunae (lakes) containing osteocytes. The haversian system is the anatomical unit of compact bone. (From Chaffee, E. E., Lytle, I. M., Basic Physiology and Anatomy, 4th ed. Philadelphia: J.B. Lippincott, Co., 1980. Used with permission.)*

same time, the osteoblasts from the periosteum are building new bone around the outside of the bone. This process goes on throughout our lives. In early adulthood and middle-age, the two processes, bone formation or **ossification** (os″i-fi-ka′shun) and bone destruction occur at the

same rate so that the bones neither grow nor shrink. During childhood and adolescence, ossification goes on at a faster rate than does bone destruction. Sometime after the age of 35, bone loss exceeds bone gain.

It is not the length of the bone that determines

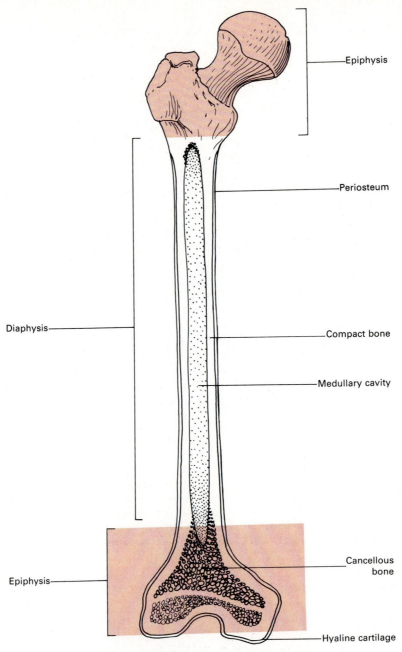

Epiphysis

Periosteum

Diaphysis

Compact bone

Medullary cavity

Epiphysis

Cancellous bone

Hyaline cartilage

Figure 7-3. Transverse section of a long bone

if a bone is to be classified as a long bone. Long bones have medullary cavities whereas the other bones do not. The bones of the phalanges in the fingers and toes have medullary cavities and are classified as long bones.

Short, flat, and irregular bones have an inner portion of cancellous bone covered over on the outside with compact bone. Short bones, found in the wrists and ankles, are the carpals and tarsals. Flat bones are the bones that form the outside of the cranium, the ribs, scapula, sternum, and patella. The rest of the bones are classified as irregular bones. Sesamoid (ses'ah-moid) bones are extra bones found in certain tendons. The kneecap, or patella, is a sesamoid bone. Excluding the sesamoid bones, except for the patella, there are 206 bones in the human body.

BONE MARKINGS

The surfaces of bones have characteristic markings. These markings serve many purposes: They join one bone to another, provide a surface for the attachment of muscles, or create an opening for the passage of blood vessels or nerves. These markings can also be used as landmarks. Table 7-1 lists some of the more common terms used in reference to these markings.

BONE MARROW

Yellow bone marrow is located in the medullary cavity of long bones. Primarily composed of adipose tissue, it serves as an area of fat storage.

Red bone marrow is found in all cancellous bone of children. In adults, it is located only in the cancellous bone of the vertebrae, hips, sternum, ribs, cranial bones, and the proximal ends of the femur and humerus. Red bone marrow is composed of many cells supported by a highly vascular, delicate connective tissue. The red bone marrow forms red blood cells, platelets, and some white blood cells. It also destroys old red blood cells and some foreign materials.

Because of the important role of red bone marrow in the manufacture of blood, the analysis of specimens of bone marrow is often helpful in the diagnosis of diseases of the blood. This marrow not only functions as blood-building, or **hemopoietic** (he"mo-poi-et'ik), tissue, but it is also involved in the body's immune response.

Table 7-1. Bone Markings

Process	a bony prominence or projection
Condyle (kon'dil)	a rounded knuckle-like prominence usually at a point of articulation
Head	a rounded articulating process at the end of a bone
Spine	a sharp slender projection
Tubercle (tu'ber-kl)	a small rounded process
Tuberosity (tu-beros'i-te)	a large rounded process
Trochanter (tro-kan'ter)	a large process for muscle attachment
Fossa (fos'ah)	a depression or hollow
Foramen (fo-ra'men)	a hole
Crest	a ridge
Line	a less prominent ridge of a bone than a crest
Meatus (me-a'tus)	a tubelike passage
Sinus or antrum	a cavity within a bone

Bone marrow transplants have proven to be life-saving measures for patients with defective immune systems.

BLOOD SUPPLY

Unlike active muscles and many other organs of the body, bone is a quiet organ that does not require wide variations in its blood supply. Its normal needs for blood are minimal and relatively constant. All bones have microscopic periosteal arteries. The long bones also have nutrient or medullary arteries. These arteries enter the medullary cavity through a tunnel in the shaft of the bone.

BONE FORMATION

By three months after fertilization of the ovum, the skeletal system has been formed, although not of bone. The bones of the skull begin as fibrous membrane and the rest of the bones of the body are formed from hyaline cartilage.

In membranous bone formation, the fibrous membrane already has the shape of the bone to be formed. There is an ossification center in the middle of the membrane, and ossification (laying down of the inorganic salts) begins in the center and radiates toward the periphery. The ossification process is not complete at the time of birth. The fibrous membrane that has not been ossified at the time of birth forms the **fontanels** (fon-tah-nelz′), or soft spots, of the infant's head. These fontanels allow for molding of the skull and an easier passage through the birth canal. The fontanels and the open joints between the cranial bones also allow for growth of the skull. Although the skull does grow, the relative head size decreases from one-fourth to one-eighth of the body's total height.

The cartilaginous bone of the embryo is formed from hyaline cartilage. Slightly different patterns of ossification exist in the different types of bones. Short bones have one ossification center in the middle of the forming bone and ossification proceeds toward the periphery. Long bones usually have three centers of ossification: one at each end of the forming bone and one in the center of the shaft. In these bones, the inorganic salts are being deposited from the center toward each end and from each end toward the center.

As the bone develops, the cartilage cells degenerate and osteoblasts move in, causing the deposition of the calcium salts. Until this process is completed, there will be a strip of cartilage at each epiphysis. Finally, at about age 18 or 20, most of the bones are completely ossified, and the epiphyseal cartilages are no longer visible on the X-ray film. As discussed above, long bones grow in circumference by the combined activities of the osteoblasts in the periosteum and the osteoclasts in the medullary cavity.

An X-ray film of the long bones of an infant's hand will show the presence of the epiphyseal cartilages where bone growth is still incomplete. The cartilage appears as a dark line on the relatively white bone, since cartilage has less density than the ossified bone (see Fig. 7-4).

From this discussion of the ossification of bones you can see that mature bones are more brittle than young bones since they contain relatively more inorganic salts than the more flexible organic collagen. This is one of the reasons that, as a result of a simple fall, fractures are more common in adults than in children.

After the osteoblasts have completed their initial function of bone formation, some will be-

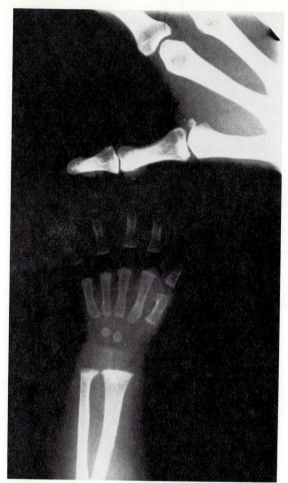

Figure 7-4. *X-ray of the hand of a 5-month-old infant showing epiphyseal cartilages (dark area) near the ends of the bone where growth is incomplete. Compare this with the appearance of a portion of an adult hand at the top of the picture.*

come maintenance cells or osteocytes. The osteocytes help in the exchange of calcium salts between bone and blood. In the fully grown adult, there are still functioning osteoblasts in the deep layer of the periosteum.

THE SKELETON AS A WHOLE

The skeleton is divided into two main parts, the appendicular skeleton and the axial skeleton (see Figs. 7-5 and 7-6). The appendicular skeleton is made up of the bones of the shoulder, upper extremities, hips, and lower extremities. The name appendicular identifies these parts as appendages (or extensions) of the axis or axial skeleton. The bones of the skull, thorax, and vertebral column comprise the axial skeleton.

THE APPENDICULAR SKELETON

There are 126 bones in the appendicular skeleton. These bones as well as some of their important markings are illustrated in Figures 7-5 through 7-26.

The Shoulder Girdle

The shoulder girdle includes the clavicle (klav′e-kel) (Fig.7-7). The glenoid (gle′noid) cavity, an indentation in the scapula (Fig. 7-8), receives the head of the humerus (hu′mer-us). The spinous process is on the posterior of the scapula and the lateral end of this process is called the acromion (ak-ro′me-on). The clavical articulates (joins) with the sternum (ster′num), or breast bone, and extends laterally to the acromion.

Arm and Hand

The humerus is the bone in the brachial region (see Fig. 7-9). The head of the humerus articulates with the glenoid cavity. On the posterior, the distal end of the humerus is the olecranon fossa (o-lek′ra-non fos′ah), which receives the olecranon process of the ulna (ul′nah) of the forearm. The ulna is on the medial aspect of the forearm, and on the lateral aspect is the radius (ra′de-us) (see Fig. 7-10).

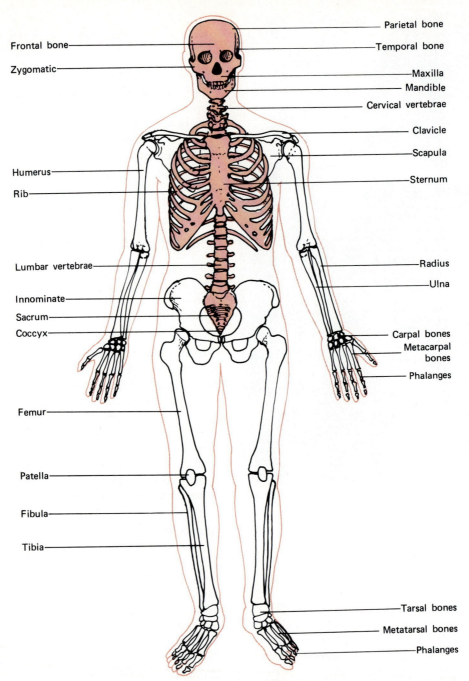

Figure 7-5. *Anterior view of the skeleton. The shaded portion is the axial skeleton.*

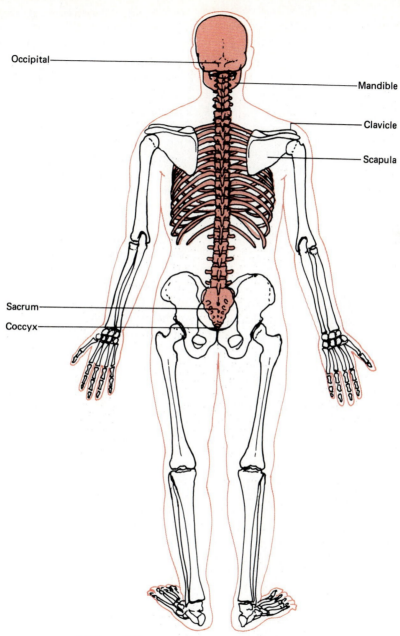

Figure 7-6. *Posterior view of the skeleton*

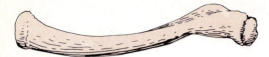

Figure 7-7. *Left clavicle*

There are eight carpal (kar′pal) bones in each wrist. The palm of the hand has five metacarpal bones; there are 14 phalanges (fa-lan′jez) in the fingers, two in the thumb, and three in the other fingers (see Fig. 7-11). This combination of so many small bones in the hands provides a structure that is capable of a greater variety of motions than is possible in other parts of the body.

Pelvic Girdle

The pelvic girdle is made up of two innominate (in-om′i-nat) bones (hip bones), the sacrum (sa′krum) and coccyx (kok′siks) (see Figs. 7-12, 7-13, and 7-14). (Note: the sacrum and coccyx are a part of the vertebral column.) The sacrum is a fusion of five vertebrae and the coccyx is a fusion of four or five vertebrae. The pelvic girdle protects the urinary bladder, some reproductive organs, the lower colon, and the rectum. In the female, it is broad and roomy with a large outlet, whereas in the male it is narrow and funnel-shaped. The pubic arch in the male is narrower than a right angle, whereas in the female it is broader than a right angle (see Fig. 7-15).

The innominate bone begins as three separate bones that fuse by adulthood into one. The ilium (il′e-um) is the upper flared portion of this hip bone; the ischium (is′ke-um) is the lower, strongest part; the pubis (pu′bis) is the anterior part. The large opening in this bone is the obturator (ob′tu-ra″tor) foramen. The two innominate bones unite anteriorly to form the **symphysis** (sim′fi-sis) **pubis**. On the lateral aspect of the innominate bone is the acetabulum (as″e-tab′u-lum), the socket that holds the head of the femur.

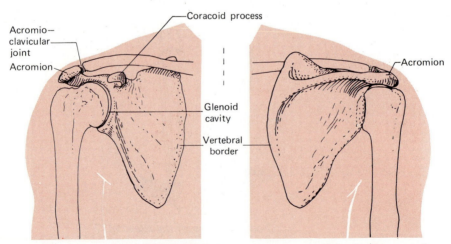

Figure 7-8. *Anterior view (left) and posterior view (right) of right scapula*

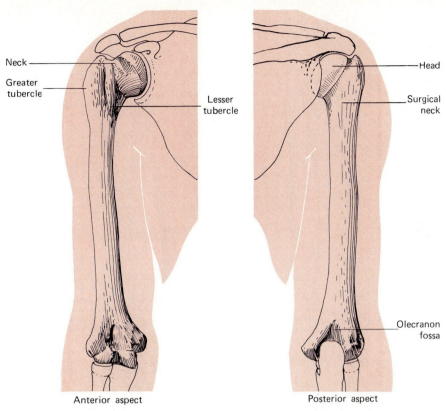

Neck

Greater
tubercle

Lesser
tubercle

Head

Surgical
neck

Olecranon
fossa

Anterior aspect

Posterior aspect

Figure 7-9. *Anterior view (left) and posterior view (right) of right humerus*

Lower Extremities

The femur (thigh bone) is the largest and heaviest bone of the lower extremity (see Fig. 7-16). At the proximal end of the femur are two large processes called **trochanters** (tro-kan′terz) for the attachment of the leg muscles. The greater trochanter is on the lateral aspect and the lesser trochanter is on the medial aspect. On the posterior, there is a sharp ridge called the linea aspera (lin′e-ah as′per-ah). There are two bones in the lower leg. The tibia (tib′e-ah) is the larger of the two and is on the medial aspect. On the anterior surface of the proximal end of the tibia is a small, rounded protrusion called a **tuberosity** (tu″ber-os′it-e) and at the distal end on the medial aspect is the medial malleolus (mal-e′o-lus). The fibula (fib′u-lah) is a slender bone on the lateral aspect of the leg (see Fig. 7-17). There are seven tarsal (tar′sal) bones in the ankle. The calcaneus (kal-ka′ne-us), which is the largest tarsal bone, forms the heel. The talus (tal′us) is the tarsal bone that articulates with

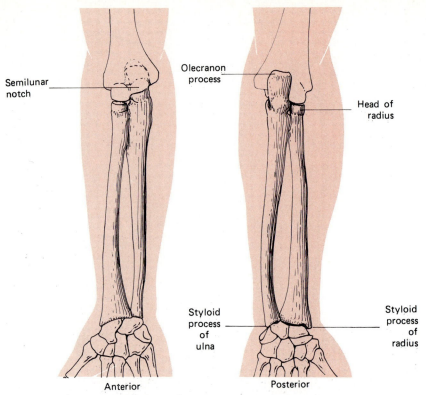

Figure 7-10. *Anterior view (left) and posterior view (right) of left ulna and radius*

the tibia and fibula. Five metatarsal bones form the arch and ball of the foot and there are 14 phalanges in the toes (see Fig. 7-18).

THE AXIAL SKELETON

There are 80 bones in the axial skeleton. These are the bones of the skull, vertebral column, and thorax. This number includes six small bones (malleus, incus, and stapes) of the middle ears, which are concerned with transmission of sound waves.

There is a single hyoid (hi'oid) bone, which

is unique since it has no articulations. This bone is U-shaped and lies in the anterior part of the neck just below the chin. It serves for the attachment of certain muscles that move the tongue and aid in speaking and swallowing.

Bones of the Skull

The skull is made up of 28 bones. With the exception of the small bones of the middle ear and the lower jaw bone, these bones unite together to form immovable joints and provide an excellent protection for the brain, eyes, and inner

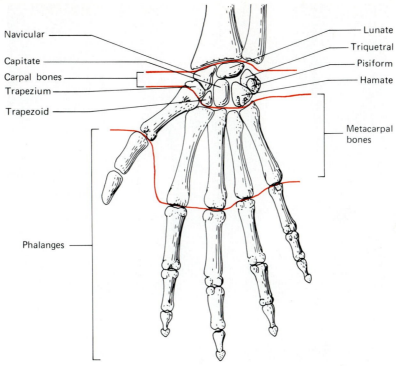

Figure 7-11. *Bones of the right hand and wrist, anterior view*

Navicular
Capitate
Carpal bones
Trapezium
Trapezoid
Phalanges
Lunate
Triquetral
Pisiform
Hamate
Metacarpal bones

ears. To facilitate study, the bones of the skull will be divided into the bones of the cranium and of the face.

Cranium   The cranium is formed by eight bones (see Fig. 7-19). The frontal bone in the frontal region forms the forehead and the roof of the orbits of the eyes. This bone contains the frontal sinuses, which are air spaces lined with mucous membrane. Secretions from these sinuses drain into the nose. The two parietal bones form the roof and sides of the head (see Fig. 7-20). The occipital bone is the base of the skull. The foramen magnum is an opening in the oc-

cipital bone through which the spinal cord communicates with the brain. On each side of the foramen magnum are condyles for articulation with the first cervical vertebra, the atlas (see Fig. 7-21). The two temporal bones are located in the temporal region. The petrous (pet′rus) portion of the temporal bone is a wedge-shaped mass of bone that houses structures concerned with equilibrium and hearing. The mastoid process of the temporal bone contains the mastoid sinus, which drains into the middle ear.

The ethmoid (eth′moid) bone is a small bone, part of which forms the upper part of the bony nasal septum. The roof of the nasal cavity is

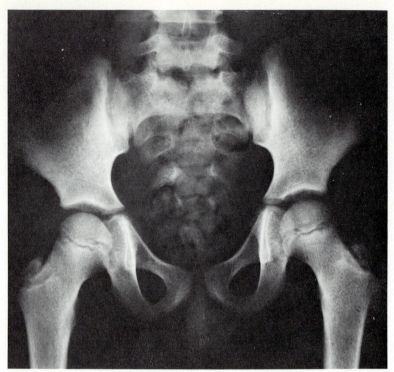

Figure 7-12. X-ray view of the pelvis of a 6-year-old boy. Notice the incomplete bone growth as evidenced by the dark line at the hip joint as well as the thinner dark line at the head of the femur.

formed by the horizontal plate of the ethmoid. This horizontal plate has foramen for the passage of the nerves of smell from the nasal cavity to the brain. The superior and middle **conchae** (kong′ke) are located on the lateral walls of the nasal cavity. The ethmoid also contains sinuses that drain into the nose.

Just posterior to the ethmoid is the sphenoid (sfe′noid) bone. The sphenoid articulates with all of the other cranial bones. The middle portion of this bone is called the body and contains the sphenoid sinus, which opens into the posterior part of the nasal cavity. On the upper surface of the sphenoid is a saddle-shaped depression called the sella turcica (sel′ah tur-si-kah), or Turkish saddle (see Fig. 7-22). The pituitary gland lies in this depression. Extending laterally from the body are the great wings of the sphenoid and above them are the small wings.

Bones of the Face   Two nasal bones form the bridge of the nose. On the medial wall of the socket of the eye are the lacrimal (lak′re-mal) bones. These lacrimal bones contain the lacrimal ducts through which tears from the eye drain into the nasal cavity. Two inferior con-

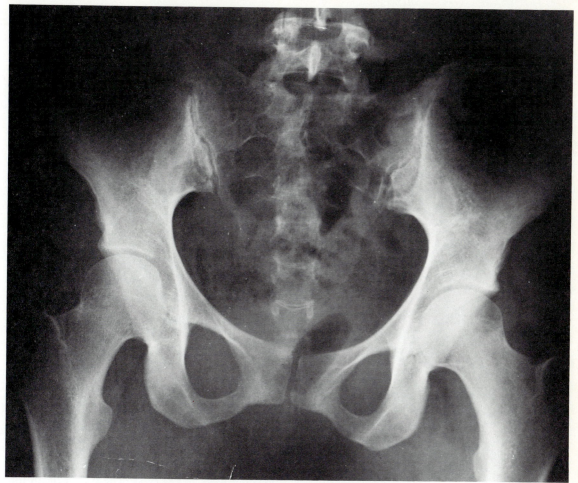

Figure 7-13. *X-ray view of adult female pelvis*

chae, or turbinates (tur′bi-natz), are scroll-like bony projections that extend from the lateral walls of the nasal cavity. These structures, together with the middle and superior conchae of the ethmoid bone, greatly increase the inner surface area of the nose. Inhaled air will be warmed and moistened by the mucous membrane covering the conchae. The vomer (vo′mer) forms the posterior and lower part of the bony nasal septum.

Two palatine (pal′ah-tin) bones form the posterior part of the roof of the mouth. The anterior part of the roof of the mouth is a part of the maxillary (mak′se-ler-e) bone. The maxilla (mak-sil′ah) has alveolar (al-ve′o-lar) processes, or sockets, that support the upper teeth. The

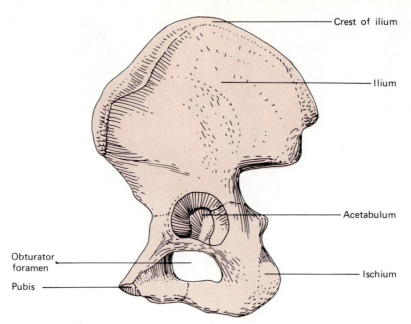

Crest of ilium

Ilium

Acetabulum

Obturator foramen

Ischium

Pubis

Figure 7-14. Left innominate bone, lateral view

maxillary bone also contains a pair of sinuses that drain into the nasal cavity. The maxillary sinus is sometimes called the antrum of Highmore. The maxilla is actually a fusion of two bones that join during fetal life. Faulty union of these bones can result in a cleft palate. Infants with this congenital defect have difficulty in nursing since their mouths communicate with the nasal cavity. The zygomatic (zi″go-mat′ik) bone is located at the upper and lateral part of the face. These bones are the prominent bones of the cheek.

The mandible (man′di-bl) is the lower jaw bone. Place your finger just in front of the opening of the external ear, and you will feel the sliding movement of the condyle of the mandible as it articulates (joins) with the temporal bone. The hyoid bone is a horseshoe-shaped

bone fastened by muscles in the neck below the mandible.

Sinuses   The air spaces, or sinuses, in the bones of the skull help to give resonance to the voice and lightness to the skull. Those that drain into the nose are called paranasal sinuses (see Fig. 7-23). The mucous membrane lining of these paranasal sinuses is contiguous with that of the nose and throat so it is not unusual for the sinuses to be involved in upper respiratory infections. These sinuses are named for the bones in which they are located: frontal, ethmoid, sphenoid, and maxillary.

Sutures   The joints of the skull are called sutures. There are a few of these with which you

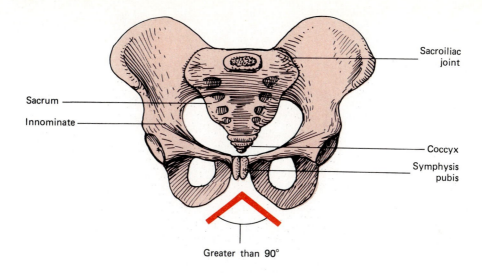

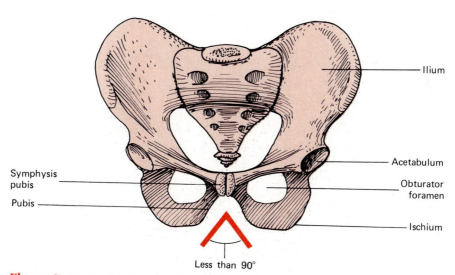

Figure 7-15. *In the female, the angle at the pubic arch is 90 or broader. In the male, it is narrower than a right angle.*

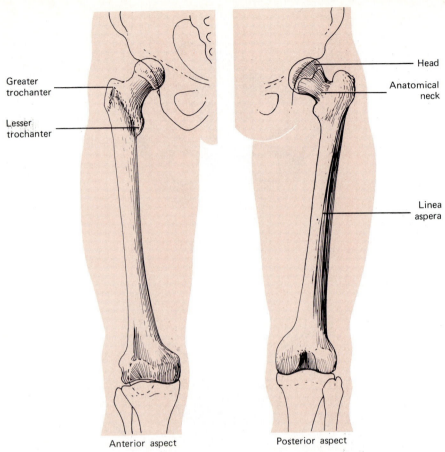

Greater
trochanter

Lesser
trochanter

Head

Anatomical
neck

Linea
aspera

Anterior aspect   Posterior aspect

Figure 7-16. *Anterior view (left) and posterior view (right) of right femur*

should be familiar. The coronal suture is located between the frontal and parietal bones. Recall that a coronal plane divides the body into front and back parts. The sagittal suture is between the two parietal bones. The temporal bone joins the parietal and sphenoid bones at the squamosal (skwa′mo-sal) suture. The lambdoidal (lam-doi′dal) suture is just posterior to the parietal bones and the temporal bones.

Fontanels   As mentioned earlier, the fontanels are composed of fibrous membrane in which ossification is incomplete at the time of birth. The anterior fontanel, which is the largest, is located at the junction of the sagittal and coronal sutures. The posterior fontanel lies between the sagittal and lambdoidal sutures. The anterolateral fontanels are located at the junction of the frontal, parietal, sphenoid, and temporal

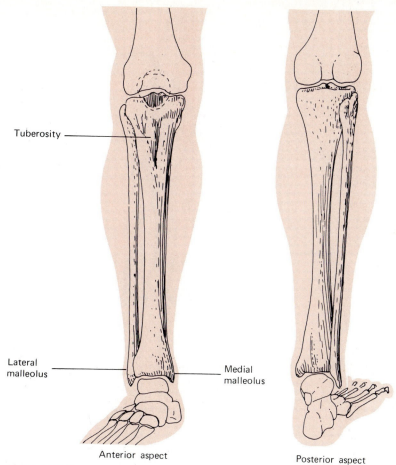

Tuberosity

Lateral malleolus

Medial malleolus

Anterior aspect

Posterior aspect

Figure 7-17. Anterior view (left) and posterior view (right) of right tibia and fibula

bones. The posterolateral fontanels are located at the junctions of the parietal, occipital, and temporal bones (see Fig. 7-24).

Within a few months after birth, only the anterior fontanel remains palpable (feels soft to the touch). This fontanel usually closes after about 16 months of age.

Vertebral Column

The vertebral column supports the head and trunk and provides protection to the spinal cord and nerve roots (see Fig. 7-25). In the adult, there are 26 bones in the vertebral column. In the child, however, there are 33 vertebrae since those of the sacrum and coccyx have not fused.

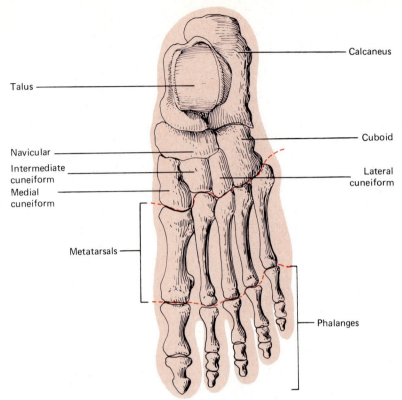

Talus

Navicular

Intermediate
cuneiform

Medial
cuneiform

Metatarsals

Calcaneus

Cuboid

Lateral
cuneiform

Phalanges

Figure 7-18. Bones of the left foot and ankle

Between each pair of vertebrae there is an intervertebral disc of fibrous cartilage that functions as a cushion or shock absorber. The different types of vertebrae are named for the regions in which they are located: cervical, thoracic, lumbar, sacral, and coccygeal. Although there are regional variations in the different vertebrae, there are some markings that all have in common.

With the exception of the first two cervical vertebrae, all have drum-shaped bodies that are just anterior to the vertebral foramen. There are

two short projections that extend posteriorly from the body; these are called pedicles (ped′e-kelz). From the pedicles, the laminae (lam′i-ne) extend posteriorly and unite to form the **spinous process**. Between the pedicle and the lamina is the transverse process (see Fig. 7-26).

There are seven cervical vertebrae. The first cervical vertebra is the atlas, or C1, which articulates with the condyles of the occipital bone of the skull. The second is the axis, or C2, from which arises the odontoid (o-don′toid) process to articulate with the atlas. The cervical verte-

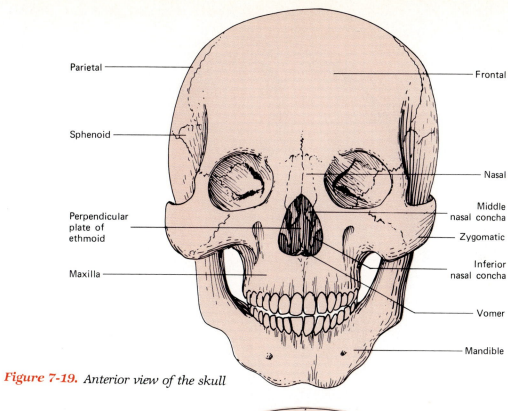

Figure 7-19. *Anterior view of the skull*

Parietal

Sphenoid

Perpendicular plate of ethmoid

Maxilla

Frontal

Nasal

Middle nasal concha

Zygomatic

Inferior nasal concha

Vomer

Mandible

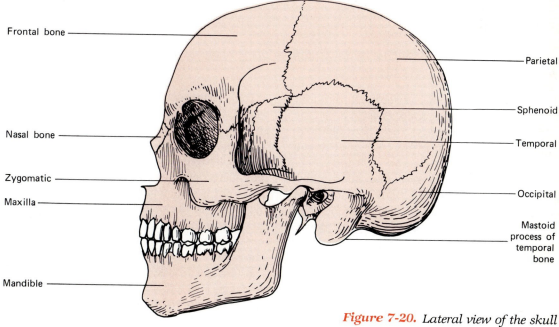

Frontal bone

Nasal bone

Zygomatic

Maxilla

Mandible

Parietal

Sphenoid

Temporal

Occipital

Mastoid process of temporal bone

Figure 7-20. *Lateral view of the skull*

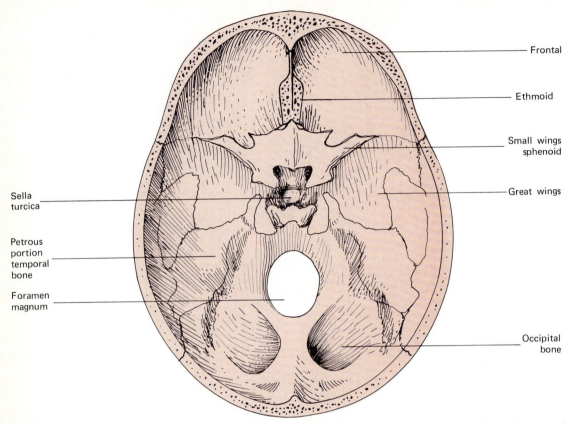

Frontal

Ethmoid

Small wings
sphenoid

Great wings

Sella
turcica

Petrous
portion
temporal
bone

Foramen
magnum

Occipital
bone

Figure 7-21. A view of the base of the skull from above showing the internal surface of some of the cranial bones

brae differ from the other vertebrae in that they are smaller and have transverse foramen on their transverse processes. These foramen provide a passageway for the vertebral blood vessels.

There are 12 thoracic vertebrae, all of which have facets for articulation with the ribs. They are larger than the cervical vertebrae and their spinous processes are longer and point downward more than do the spinous processes of any of the other vertebrae.

The five lumbar vertebrae are the heaviest of the vertebrae. The processes of these vertebrae are short and thick.

The sacrum consists of five fused sacral vertebrae. It forms the posterior part of the pelvic girdle.

A fusion of four or five vertebrae forms the coccyx. Between the sacrum and the coccyx is the sacrococcygeal (sa'kro-kok-sij'e-al) joint. This joint is somewhat more movable in the female than in the male, an adaptation for pregnancy and childbirth.

Thorax

The thorax is made up of a cage of bones and cartilage, covered with muscles and skin. The floor of the thorax is the diaphragm. The chief

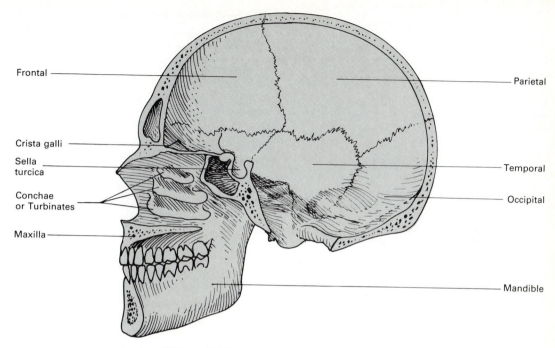

Frontal

Crista galli

Sella turcica

Conchae or Turbinates

Maxilla

Parietal

Temporal

Occipital

Mandible

Figure 7-22. *Sagittal section of the skull*

function of this bony cage is to protect the thoracic viscera.

The sternum, which is approximately six inches long, is located in the anterior midline of the thorax. It consists of a fusion of three parts: the manubrium (man-u'bre-um), the body or middle portion, and the xiphoid (zif'oid), which is the inferior portion (see Fig 7-27). These three parts are the last bones to fuse. This fusion usually does not occur until after the age of 30.

There are 12 ribs on each side of the thorax; they are all attached to the thoracic vertebrae. The first seven pairs, called the true ribs, are attached directly to the sternum by separate costal cartilages. Each of the next three pairs, called the false ribs, is attached to the cartilage of the rib above it and thence to the sternum. Because

they have no anterior attachment, the last two pairs of ribs are called the floating ribs.

CARTILAGE

Cartilage, like bone, has more intercellular substance than cells. The intercellular substance of cartilage, however, is a firm gel. The cells of cartilage are also located in lacunae, but there are no canals or blood vessels in the matrix of cartilage. Cartilage is avascular. Nutrients and oxygen reach these scattered cartilaginous cells

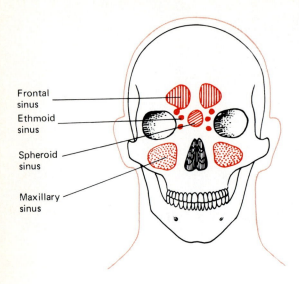

Frontal
sinus

Ethmoid
sinus

Spheroid
sinus

Maxillary
sinus

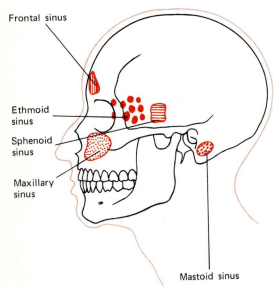

Frontal sinus

Ethmoid
sinus

Sphenoid
sinus

Maxillary
sinus

Mastoid sinus

Figure 7-23. Cranial sinuses

only by diffusion from the capillaries in the fibrous covering of the cartilage or from the synovial fluid in the case of articular cartilage.

There are three types of cartilage: hyaline, fibrous, and elastic. These types differ structurally primarily in the makeup of the intercellular substances. Hyaline cartilage is the most common type. It resembles milk glass and, indeed, its name is derived from the Greek word meaning glassy. Fibrous cartilage is very strong and functions as a cushion in some of the joints with limited motion. Elastic cartilage has elastic fibers in it so that it has some elasticity as well as some firmness.

ARTICULATIONS OR JOINTS

Joints can be classified according to the amount of motion they permit (see Fig. 7-28). The joints of the skull are immovable and are called **synarthrotic** (sin″ar-thro′tic) **joints**

Amphiarthrotic (am″fe-ar-thro′tic) **joints** have limited motion. The bones that form most of these joints are united by fibrous cartilage. Examples of amphiarthrotic joints are the symphysis pubis, vertebral joints, and the sacroiliac (sak″ro-il′e-ak) joints.

Diarthrotic (di″ar-thro′tic) **joints** are freely movable. The articulating ends of the bones that meet at these joints are covered with hyaline cartilage, and a strong fibrous capsule surrounds the joint and is firmly attached to both bones. The capsule is lined with synovial membrane. This membrane secretes a slippery synovial fluid for lubrication. Several types of movement can be accomplished at diarthrotic joints. These motions are described in Table 7-2 and Figure 7-29.

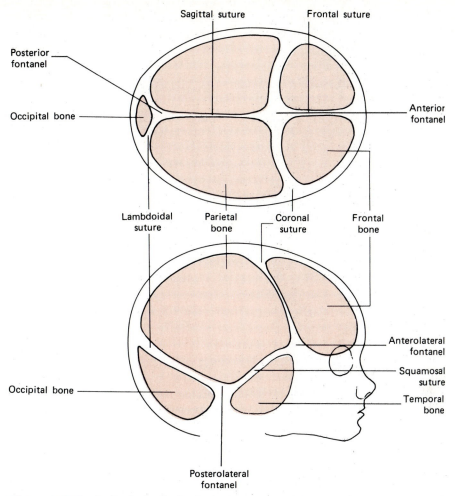

Figure 7-24. *A fetal skull showing fontanels and sutures, superior aspect (above), lateral aspect (below)*

BURSAE

Bursae (bur'se) are little sacs that function as slippery cushions in areas where pressure is exerted during movement of the body parts, for example, between bones and the overlying mus-

cle, tendons, or skin. The bursae are lined with synovial membrane and lubricated with synovial fluid. The bursae are named according to their location. The most important are the acromial (ah-kro'me-al), olecranon (o-lek'rah-non), prepatellar, subdeltoid, and subscapular.

Injury to bursae can result in inflammation or

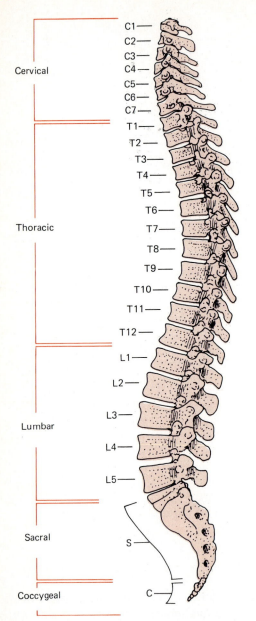

Figure 7-25. *Lateral view of the adult vertebral column.*

Table 7-2. Motion in Diarthrotic Joints

Action	Description
Flexion	Decreases the angle at a joint
Extension	Increases the angle at a joint
Hyperextension	Increases the angle beyond the anatomical position
Circumduction	The distal end of an extremity inscribes a circle while the shaft inscribes a cone
Adduction	Moves a body part toward the midline
Abduction	Moves a body part away from the midline
Rotation	Revolves a part about the longitudinal axis
Internal	Moves toward the midline or medially
External	Moves away from the midline or laterally
Supination	Turns the palm upward
Pronation	Turns the palm downward
Inversion	Turns the plantar surface toward the midline
Eversion	Turns the plantar surface away from the midline
Plantar flexion (extension)	Moves the sole of the foot downward as in standing on the toes
Dorsiflexion	Moves the sole of the foot upward

bursitis. Movement of the affected part can be very painful. The prepatellar bursa is most commonly affected. Working for prolonged periods of time in a kneeling position predisposes this area to trauma and inflammation. The condition is sometimes called housemaid's knee. A bunion is a swelling of a bursa of the foot, particularly at the metatarsophangeal joint of the great toe.

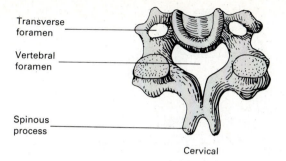

Transverse
foramen

Vertebral
foramen

Spinous
process

Cervical

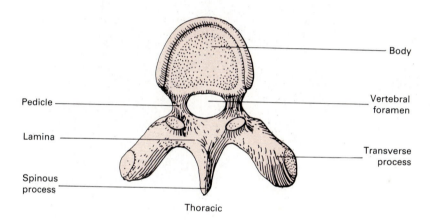

Pedicle

Lamina

Spinous
process

Body

Vertebral
foramen

Transverse
process

Thoracic

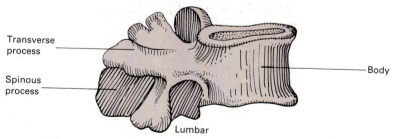

Transverse
process

Spinous
process

Body

Lumbar

Figure 7-26. *Cervical, thoracic, and lumbar vertebrae.*

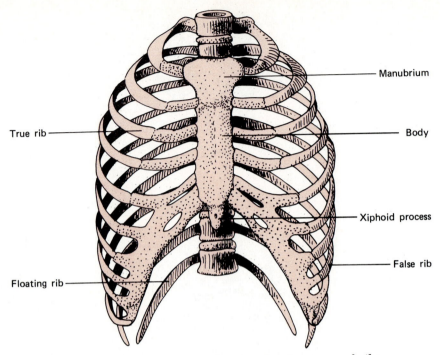

Figure 7-27. *Bony thorax showing the sternum and ribs.*

ORGANS OF LOCOMOTION

There are over 600 individual muscles in the human body. Muscle tissue comprises about 45% of the total body weight of an adult.

In addition to the property of contractility (the ability to exert force), muscles also have other important properties. Excitability is the ability to respond to a stimulus. Elasticity is the ability of the muscle to return to its original shape after it has contracted or stretched. Extensibility is the ability of muscle to stretch.

Muscles produce heat when they contract. After strenuous exercise you may feel hot, which is the result of the heat produced by your active muscles. Contractions of muscles are a major factor in maintaining body temperature.

TYPES OF MUSCLE TISSUE

There are three different types of muscle tissue. Skeletal muscle, which is attached to the skeleton, exerts force across joints. These muscles are under our voluntary control, and for this reason, they are sometimes called voluntary muscles. When seen through a microscope, this type of tissue has lines through it; thus, skeletal muscle is also called striated muscle.

Visceral muscles, which are involuntary, are located in the walls of organs and blood vessels.

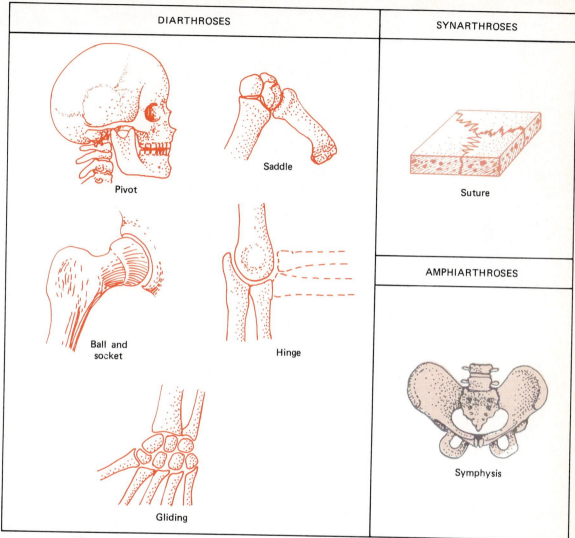

Figure 7-28. Joints classified according to the degree of movement permitted.

Microscopically, these cells appear smooth and spindle shaped. Visceral muscle is also called smooth muscle.

Cardiac muscle, also involuntary, and striated, is located only in the heart. Figure 5-1 illustrates diagrammatically the microscopic appearance of each of these types of muscle tissue.

Skeletal muscle is capable of contracting rapidly and powerfully for short periods of time.

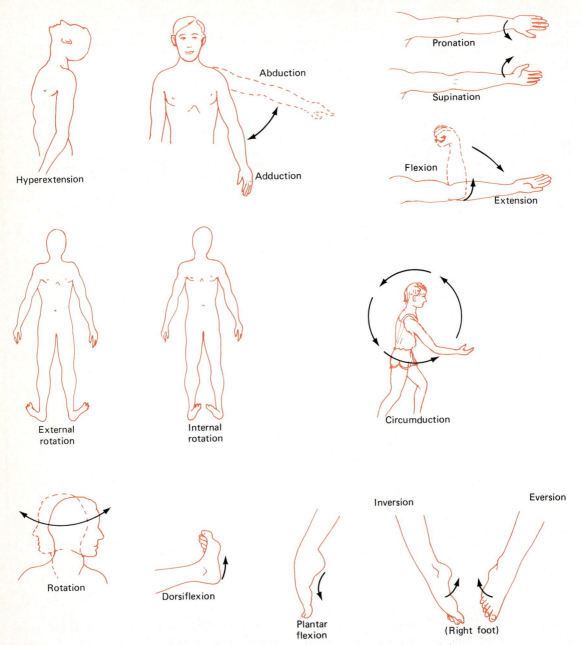

Figure 7-29. *Types of movement permitted at diarthrotic joints.*

There must be nerve impulses to bring about contraction of skeletal muscles. Efferent nerve fibers from the brain and spinal cord send impulses for contraction and afferent fibers from the muscles to the central nervous system inform the brain of the degree of contraction taking place.

Visceral and cardiac muscles also have efferent and afferent nerve fibers. In the case of visceral muscle, the efferent or motor nerves are less important than in skeletal muscle because visceral muscle has automaticity, that is, the ability to contract without nerve supply. In the case of cardiac muscle, which also has automaticity, the efferent nerve impulses control the rate of contraction according to the needs of the body. In both visceral and cardiac muscle, the afferent impulses are concerned with sensations of pain, spasm, and stretch.

PHYSIOLOGY OF CONTRACTION

When a muscle is contracting the muscle cells become shorter and thicker. The contraction causes the part to move.

Energy Sources

Recall that cellular energy is the result of chemical processes taking place in the mitochondria. The immediate energy for muscle contraction comes from the breakdown of adenosine triphosphate (ATP), an energy-rich phosphate compound. When a muscle cell is stimulated, an enzyme causes one of the phosphates to split from ATP, releasing energy and forming adenosine diphosphate:

$$ATP \rightarrow ADP + PO_4 + \Delta$$

The resynthesis of ATP occurs almost immediately when ADP reacts with phosphocreatine, another high-energy compound found in the cell. Therefore, the reaction is reversible:

$$ATP \leftrightarrows ADP + PO_4 + \Delta$$

The energy for the resynthesis of the phosphocreatine comes from the breakdown of carbohydrates, specifically glycogen or glucose, found within the cell. As the carbohydrate is broken down, pyruvic acid is formed. Following the formation of pyruvic acid there is a complex series of chemical reactions with the results depending on the amount of oxygen available. There are two possibilities: (1) In moderate activity, with adequate amounts of oxygen, some of the pyruvic acid is converted to carbon dioxide, water, and energy. (2) With strenuous activity, when one cannot breathe oxygen rapidly enough to deal with large amounts of pyruvic acid being formed, the pyruvic acid becomes lactic acid. This condition is called oxygen debt. The person will be out of breath until the debt is paid. Rapid breathing will supply the oxygen needed to convert the lactic acid back to pyruvic acid.

Eighty percent of the lactic acid will be recycled back to carbohydrates for reuse. Twenty percent will be oxidized to provide energy for the production of more phosphocreatine. The waste products of this metabolic activity are carbon dioxide and water.

Contractility

The actual contraction or shortening of a skeletal muscle cell involves protein filaments, actin (ak′tin) and myosin (mi′o-sin), located in the muscle cytoplasm or sarcoplasm (sar′ko-plazm). The arrangement of the actin and myosin filaments gives skeletal muscle its striated appearance. Each muscle fiber consists of smaller muscle fibrils that have alternating light and dark bands, as shown in Figure 7-30. These bands are the thin filaments of actin and thicker myosin filaments arranged longitudinally in the middle of a relaxed sarcomere (sar′ko-mer), or contractile unit. The actin filament is composed of two spiral strands of actin. Wound around these actin strands are two

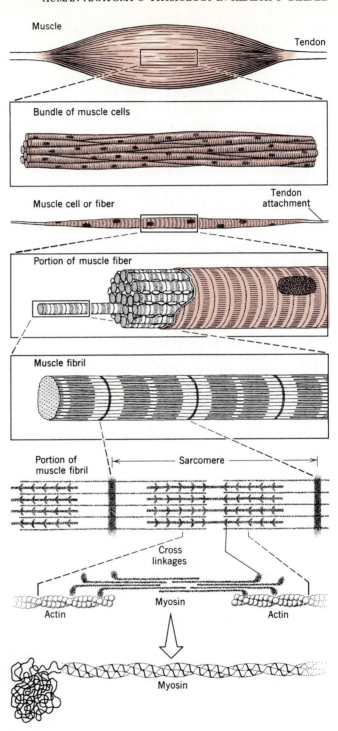

Figure 7-30. *Muscles contain bundles of muscle cells or fibers. A single fiber is composed of fibrils that contain actin and myosin filaments. During contraction, the actin and myosin filaments move close together, shortening the muscle.*

strands of tropomyosin. Attached periodically along the tropomyosin strands is a third protein, troponin, which has a great affinity for calcium ions. A thick myosin filament is composed of approximately 200 myosin molecules.

Chemical Changes   At the junction between the nerve and muscle cell, the stimulating nerve releases **acetylcholine** (as″et-ul-ko′lin), which alters the muscle cell membrane or sarcolemma (sar′ko-lem-a) so that sodium enters the cell. Once the sodium is in the muscle cell, the acetylcholine is destroyed by cholinesterase (ko-lin-es′ter-as) and the sarcolemma will not allow large amounts of sodium to enter the cell. The sodium causes the sarcoplasmic reticulum to release calcium which combines with the troponin (tro′po-nin) on the actin. As soon as the actin filaments are activated by calcium, they are pulled toward the myosin. This process decreases the overall length of the sarcomere and results in contraction of the total muscle. The energy for this contraction comes from the breakdown of ATP.

As long as the calcium remains combined with troponin, contraction continues. Relaxation of the muscle is not a passive process. Relaxation requires energy from the breakdown of ATP to actively transport the calcium back into the sarcoplasmic reticulum.

The contractile process of smooth muscle is essentially the same as that of skeletal muscle except that smooth muscle uses less ATP and both the contraction and relaxation phases are slower. Cardiac muscle cells have the same arrangement of actin and myosin with the same mechanism of contraction; however, the manner of excitation is different from that of skeletal muscle.

Electrical Changes   In addition to chemical changes, electrical changes also take place during muscle contraction. Electrical changes have considerable clinical significance because they can be measured and recorded and can provide valuable diagnostic information. In the case of cardiac contraction, electrical changes are measured by an electrocardiograph, or ECG. Electromyography (EMG) measures the electrical changes taking place during the contraction of skeletal muscles. The electrical impulses liberated are conducted to the body surface by electrolytes in the body fluids.

All muscle cells abide by the All or None Law. Each muscle cell, when stimulated, gives a total response or it does not contract at all. The strength of the contraction of the entire muscle depends on the number of cells stimulated and the condition of the muscle.

Muscle Tone

Muscle tone is a steady, partial contraction that is probably present at all times in healthy muscles. Muscle tone is lowest when we are asleep or ill. When a person has been ill and has had even a relatively short period of bed rest, the muscle tone can be markedly diminished. Because the patient is generally unaware of this condition, assistance should be available when the patient gets out of bed.

Excitability

The ability of a muscle to respond to a stimulus is called excitability. Nerve tissue most often supplies the stimulus. Cardiac and smooth muscle tissues, however, have automaticity and will contract without nerve impulses. The stimulus for visceral muscle contraction can be distention, temperature changes, hormones, and the composition of the body fluids surrounding the muscle. Visceral muscle, as well as skeletal and cardiac muscles, will contract in response to electrical stimulation. During contraction, the muscle gets shorter and thicker and pulls the body parts into action. For example, with your left elbow in extension, place your right hand on the anterior aspect of the brachial region, feeling your biceps brachii. Flex your elbow and you will feel the biceps thicken as it pulls the forearm upward. Now extend your elbow while you feel the biceps relax and lengthen.

Although there are variations in the duration and strength of contraction of different skeletal muscles, we can make some generalizations about the features of skeletal muscle contraction as opposed to visceral and cardiac muscle contractions. Skeletal muscle responds to a stimulus quickly with a forceful contraction and then relaxes promptly. Visceral muscle responds slowly, maintaining the contraction over a

longer period of time. Cardiac muscle response is somewhat quicker than visceral, and the contraction is stronger but of shorter duration. This concept is illustrated in Figure 7-31.

NAMING OF MUSCLES

Skeletal muscles are sometimes named according to their action, such as flexors or extensors. They also may be named according to their location, the direction of their fibers, the gross shape of the muscle, or the number of divisions that the specific muscle has.

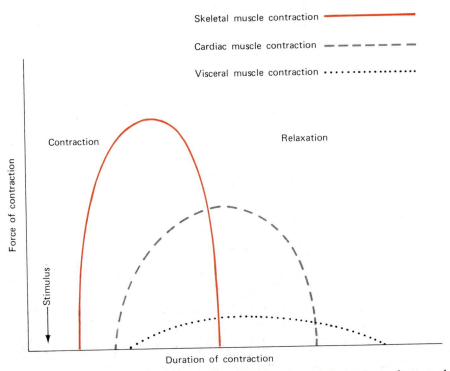

Figure 7-31. *Comparison of the force and duration of skeletal, cardiac, and visceral muscle contractions. Note the latent period, the time from the application of the stimulus and the muscle response, varies in the different muscle tissues.*

PRIME MOVERS AND ANTAGONISTS

The muscles with which we will be concerned are called prime movers. When a prime mover contracts, its antagonist must relax (see Fig. 7-32). The antagonist, therefore, does the opposite of the prime mover. For example, when the elbow is flexed, the biceps is the prime mover and the antagonist, the triceps, must relax. In order to extend the elbow, the triceps becomes the prime mover, and the biceps must relax. Muscles that assist a prime mover are called synergists (sin'er-jists). Clinically, synergists become increasingly important when there is a loss of muscle strength.

There are over 600 muscles that are under our conscious control. The functions and locations

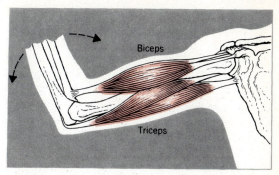

Figure 7-32. *Antagonist muscles. During elbow flexion, the triceps relaxes while the biceps contracts. For extension, the biceps relax while the triceps contract.*

of some of the more important of these muscles are listed in Table 7-3. Figures 7-33 through 7-48 will help you visualize these skeletal muscles and their actions.

Table 7-3. Skeletal Muscles

Muscle	Location	Function
Muscles of Facial Expression		
Orbicularis oculi	Circles eyelids	Closes eyelid
Levator palpebrae superior	Posterior part of eye orbits and eyelids	Opens eyelid
Oculi recti (4)	Superior part of orbits	Rolls eye upward
	Inferior part of orbits	Rolls eye downward
	Lateral and medial parts of orbits	Turn eye side to side
	Superior lateral side of eyeball	Turns eyeball downward and laterally
Oculi obliques (2)	Inferior lateral side of eyeball	Turns eyeball upward and laterally
Orbicularis oris	Circles the mouth	Purses lips
Masseter	From zygomatic bone to mandible	Closes jaw
External pterygoid	From sphenoid to mandible	Opens mouth
Movement of the Head		
Sternocleidomastoids	From sternum and clavicle to the temporal bone	Flex and rotate head
Semispinalis capitus	From thoracic vertebrae to occipital bone	Extends head

Table 7-3. (continued)

Muscle	Location	Function
Movement of the Shoulder		
Trapezius	From occipital bone to scapulae	Raises and pulls shoulders back
Pectoralis minor	From shoulder girdle to ribs	Depresses shoulder forward
Movement of the Upper Extremity		
Pectoralis major	Pectoral region	Flexes and adducts anteriorly
Latissimus dorsi	Lateral aspect of the back	Extend and adduct posteriorly
Deltoid	Deltoid region	Abducts arm
Biceps brachii	Anterior aspect of brachial region	Flex forearm and supinate hand
Triceps brachii	Posterior aspect of brachial region	Extend forearm
Anterior forearm muscles	Anterior aspect of the forearm	Flex wrist and pronate hand
Posterior forearm muscles	Posterior aspect of the forearm	Extend wrist and supinate hand
Muscles of Inspiration		
Diaphragm	Floor of thoracic cavity	Increases vertical diameter of thorax
Muscles of the Abdominal Wall		
External obliques	Superficial layer of abdominal muscles	Compress viscera and aid in forced expiration. Flex and rotate vertebral column
Internal obliques	Beneath external obliques	Same action as the external obliques
Transversus	Beneath internal obliques	Compresses viscera and aids in forced expiration
Rectus abdominus	From symphysis pubis to sternum	Depresses thorax, flexes and rotates vertebral column
Muscles of the Back		
Sacrospinalis	From sacrum to occipit	Extends vertebrae
Muscles of the Pelvic Floor		
Levator ani	Pelvic floor	Support pelvic viscera
Coccygeus	Pelvic floor	Supports pelvic viscera
Rectal sphincter	Surrounds anus	Keeps anus closed
Movement of the Lower Extremities		
Gluteal group	Gluteal region	Some muscles of this group extend the thigh and rotate thigh outward. Others abduct and internally rotate the thigh
Adductor group	Anterior and medial aspect of the thigh	Adduct the thigh
Hamstrings	Posterior aspect of the thigh	Flex lower leg
Quadriceps femoris	Anterior aspect of femoral region	Extends lower leg
Anterior tibial	Anterior aspect of lower leg	Dorsiflexes and inverts the foot
Posterior tibial	Posterior aspect of the tibia	Inverts and plantar flexes
Gastrocnemius	Prominent muscle of the calf	Adducts and inverts the foot, plantar flexes

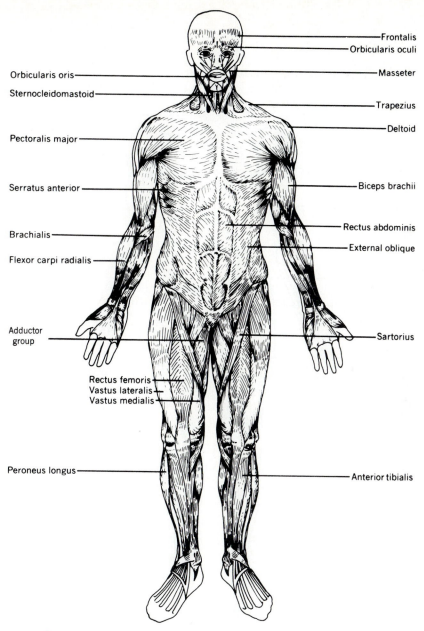

Frontalis
Orbicularis oculi
Orbicularis oris
Masseter
Sternocleidomastoid
Trapezius
Deltoid
Pectoralis major
Serratus anterior
Biceps brachii
Brachialis
Rectus abdominis
Flexor carpi radialis
External oblique
Adductor group
Sartorius
Rectus femoris
Vastus lateralis
Vastus medialis
Peroneus longus
Anterior tibialis

Figure 7-33. *Superficial muscles of the body, anterior view.*

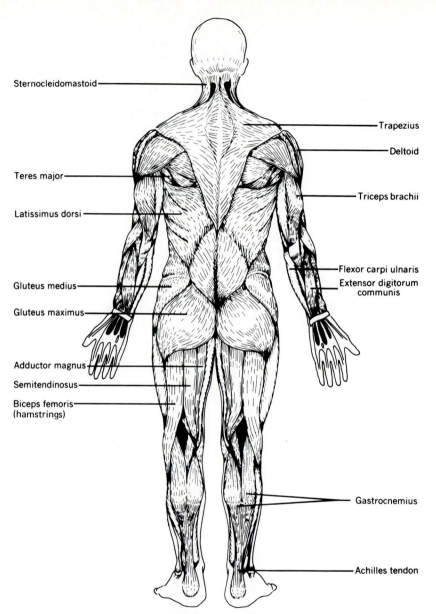

Figure 7-34. *Superficial muscles, posterior view.*

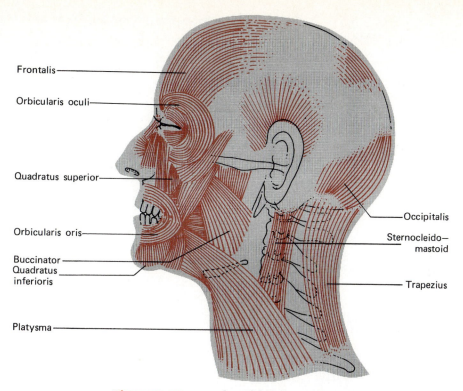

Frontalis

Orbicularis oculi

Quadratus superior

Orbicularis oris

Buccinator

Quadratus inferioris

Platysma

Occipitalis

Sternocleido—mastoid

Trapezius

Figure 7-35. Muscles of facial expression.

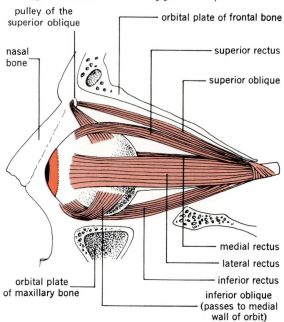

pulley of the superior oblique

nasal bone

orbital plate of frontal bone

superior rectus

superior oblique

medial rectus

lateral rectus

inferior rectus

inferior oblique (passes to medial wall of orbit)

orbital plate of maxillary bone

Figure 7-36. Extrinsic muscles of the left eye, lateral view.

131

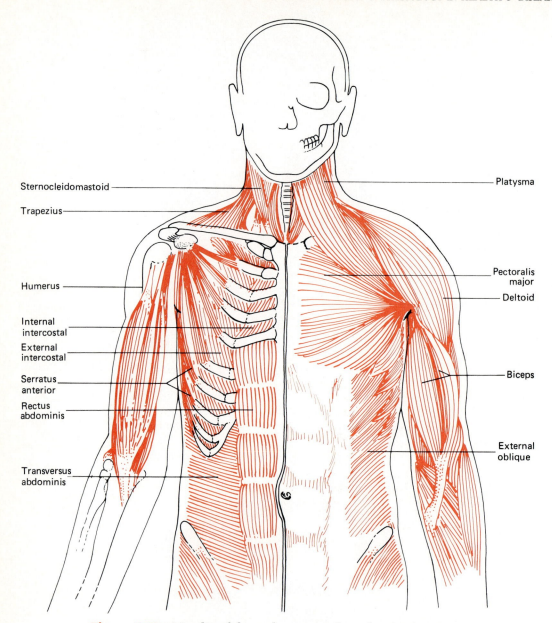

Figure 7-37. *Muscles of the neck, arm, and trunk, anterior view.*

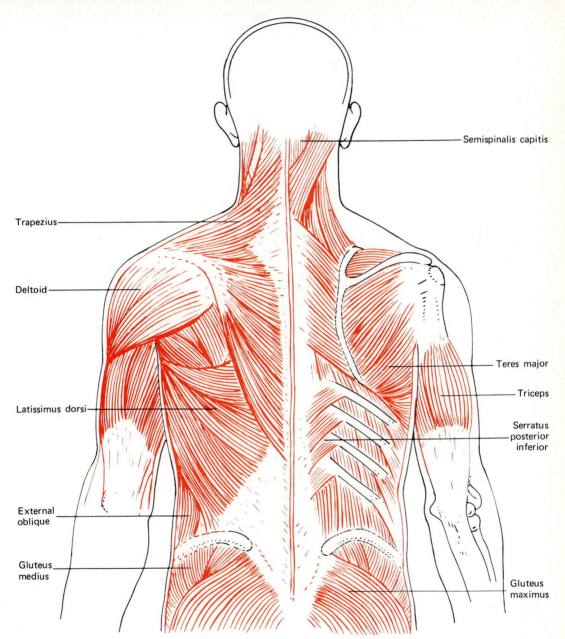

Figure 7-38. *Muscles of the neck, arm, and trunk, posterior view.*

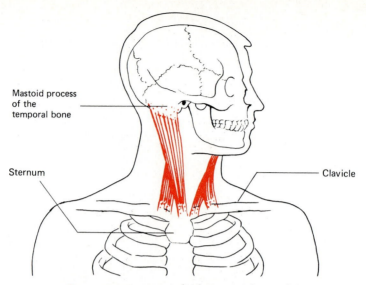

Mastoid process
of the
temporal bone

Sternum

Clavicle

Figure 7-39. *Sternocleidomastoid muscles.*

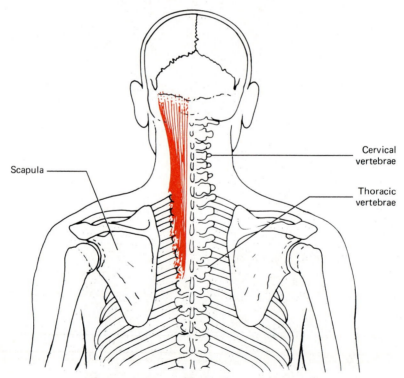

Scapula

Cervical
vertebrae

Thoracic
vertebrae

Figure 7-40. *Semispinalis capitis muscle.*

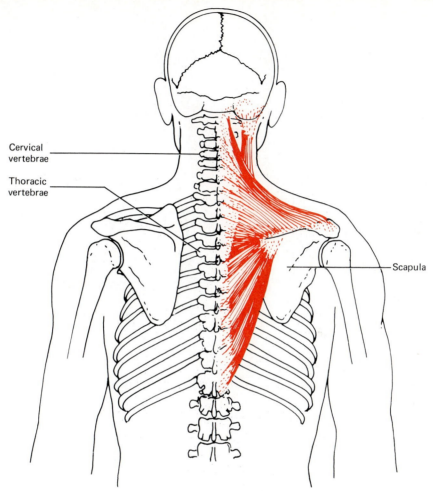

Cervical
vertebrae

Thoracic
vertebrae

Scapula

Figure 7-41. *Trapezius muscle.*

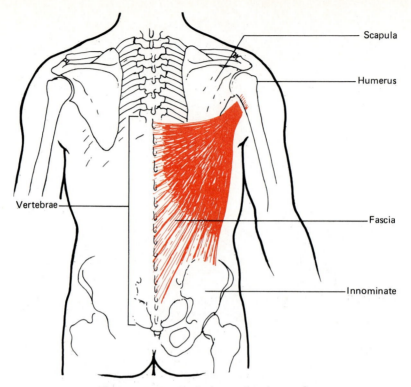

Figure 7-42. *Latissimus dorsi muscle.*

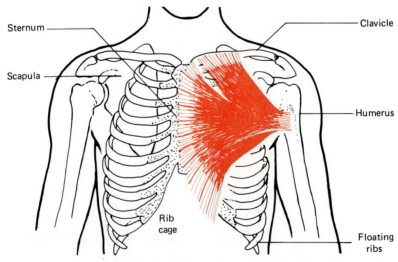

Figure 7-43. *Pectoralis major muscle.*

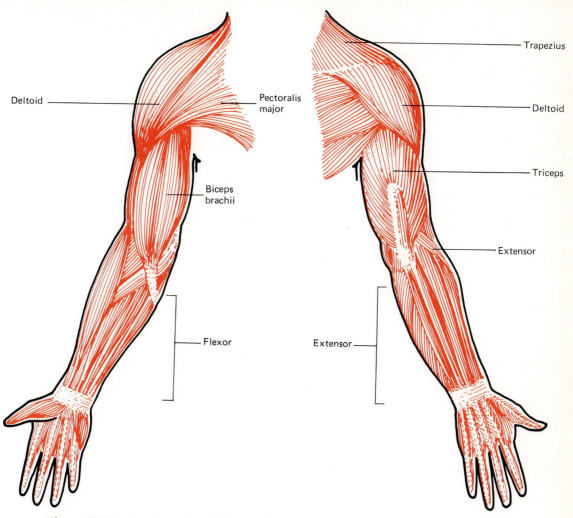

Figure 7-44. *Anterior view (left) and posterior view (right) of the right arm muscles.*

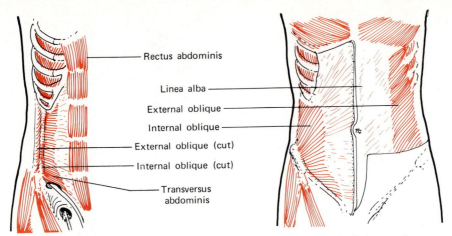

Rectus abdominis

Linea alba

External oblique

Internal oblique

External oblique (cut)

Internal oblique (cut)

Transversus abdominis

Figure 7-45. *Deep abdominal muscles (left) and superficial abdominal muscles (right) of the abdominal wall.*

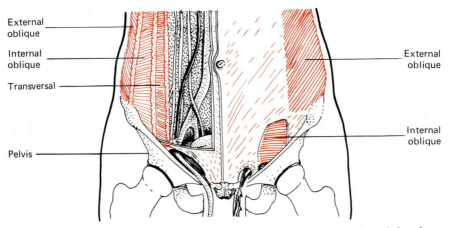

External oblique

Internal oblique

Transversal

Pelvis

External oblique

Internal oblique

Figure 7-46. *Abdominal wall muscles are intact (right). Each of the three layers of muscles is cut (left).*

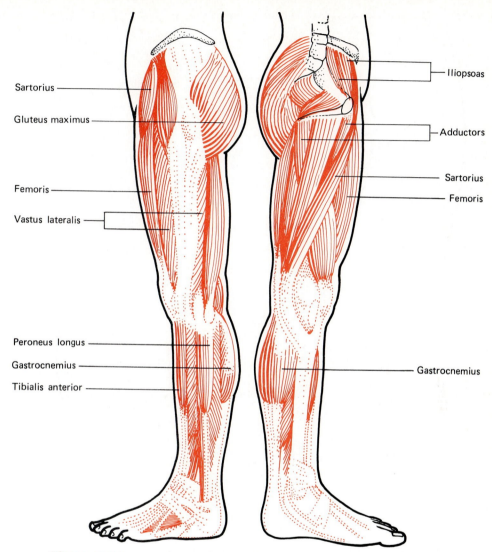

Sartorius

Gluteus maximus

Femoris

Vastus lateralis

Peroneus longus

Gastrocnemius

Tibialis anterior

Iliopsoas

Adductors

Sartorius

Femoris

Gastrocnemius

Figure 7-47. *Lateral view (left) and medial view (right) of leg muscles.*

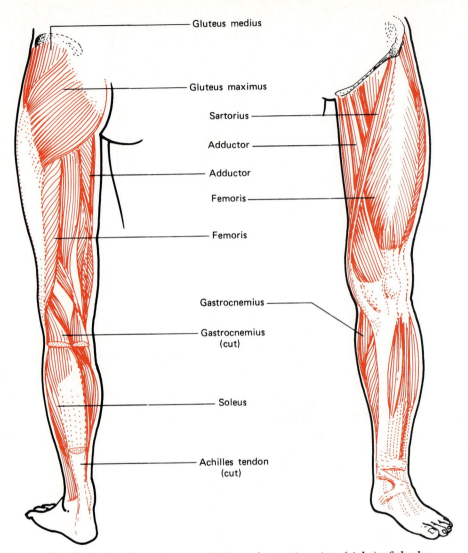

Gluteus medius

Gluteus maximus

Sartorius

Adductor

Adductor

Femoris

Femoris

Gastrocnemius

Gastrocnemius
(cut)

Soleus

Achilles tendon
(cut)

Figure 7-48. *Posterior view (left) and anterior view (right) of the leg.*

SUMMARY QUESTIONS

1. What factors favor the deposition of calcium into bone?
2. How are the bones of the skull formed?
3. How are the bones of the appendicular skeleton formed?
4. What are the bone-building cells called?
5. How do the functions of osteocytes differ from those of osteoclasts?
6. List the cranial sinuses and describe their functions.
7. How does a condyle differ from a fossa?
8. What is a tuberosity?
9. What is a foramen?
10. What bone is located in the brachial region?
11. Where is the femur located?
12. Where is the acetabulum?
13. Name the bone at the base of the skull.
14. Name the bone in the temporal region.
15. Name the bones that make up the roof of the mouth.
16. Name the first and second cervical vertebrae.
17. What are the three bony parts of the innominate bone?
18. Classify joints according to the amount of motion they permit.
19. What is the difference between abduction and adduction?
20. What is dorsiflexion?
21. Differentiate between the three types of muscle tissue.
22. What is the All or None Law as it applies to muscle?
23. Discuss sources of energy used for muscle contraction.
24. Explain what is meant by oxygen debt.
25. How is ATP resynthesized?
26. Describe three types of cartilage and explain where each is located.

KEY TERMS

acetylcholine
amphiarthrotic joints
collagen
conchae
diaphysis
diarthrotic joints
epiphyses
fontanels
haversian systems
hemopoietic

matrix
ossification
osteoblasts
osteoclasts
osteocytes
spinous process
symphysis pubis
synarthrotic joints
trochanters
tuberosity

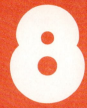

Disorders of the Musculoskeletal System

OBJECTIVES

On completion of this chapter, you will be able to:

1. State the difference between a simple fracture and a compound fracture.
2. Identify the type of fracture that is likely to become infected.
3. List first aid measures to be taken prior to transporting a fracture victim.
4. Differentiate between open and closed reduction of fractures.
5. Define osteomyelitis.
6. Identify the type of patient most likely to develop an incisional hernia.
7. Name the most common primary bone cancer.
8. List three types of hernias and discuss the treatment of each.
9. Discuss complications of hernias.
10. Contrast rheumatoid arthritis and osteoarthritis.

OVERVIEW

I. FRACTURES
   A. Types of Fractures
   B. First Aid
   C. Fracture Treatment
      1. Reduction of Fractures
      2. Casting and Cast Care
      3. Traction
   D. Complications of Fractures
      1. Failed Union
      2. Fat Emboli
      3. Infection
      4. Compartment Syndrome
   E. Crutch Walking
II. DISLOCATIONS AND SUBLUXATIONS
III. SPRAINS AND STRAINS
IV. EPICONDYLITIS
V. ARTHRITIS
   A. Rheumatoid Arthritis
   B. Osteoarthritis (Osteoarthrosis)
VI. OSTEOPOROSIS
VII. LOW BACK PAIN
VIII. DEFORMITIES OF THE BACK
IX. OSTEOMYELITIS
X. HERNIAS
XI. CANCER

Major functions of the musculoskeletal system include making movement possible, protecting vital organs, storing calcium and other minerals, and providing the site for blood cell production. Injury and pathology in this system frequently limit mobility and cause pain, instability, and deformity. In this chapter, we shall consider some of the more common disorders of the musculoskeletal system and examples of how these might be treated.

This chapter was written by Colleen Dunwoody.

FRACTURES

One of the most common disorders of the musculoskeletal system is that of broken bones. Frequently, the cause of a fracture is trauma resulting from a fall or motor vehicle accident. Another cause may be disease that weakens the structure of the bones making them unable to bear the stresses produced by normal activity. Such fractures are called pathological and may be caused by metastatic lesions (cancer), chronic inflammation or infection, and osteoporosis (porous, brittle bones).

TYPES OF FRACTURES

Fractures are classified as follows (see Fig. 8-1):

1. Undisplaced fracture: The fracture line goes all the way through the bone with fragments remaining in anatomical position.

2. Displaced fracture: The fracture line goes all the way through the bone with fragments out of anatomical position and separated.

3. Incomplete fracture: The fracture line does not extend through the bone or disrupt the entire thickness of the bone.

4. Complete fracture: The fracture line goes all the way through the bone (can be undisplaced or displaced).

5. Comminuted fracture: The bone is broken in several places and splinters of bone can be embedded in surrounding tissue.

6. Segmental fracture: The shaft of the bone is broken into several large fragments.

7. Butterfly fracture: The bone is broken in two places with the resulting fracture resembling the wing of a butterfly (triangular).

8. Spiral fracture: The bone has been twisted apart and the fracture line is oblique to the shaft of the bone.

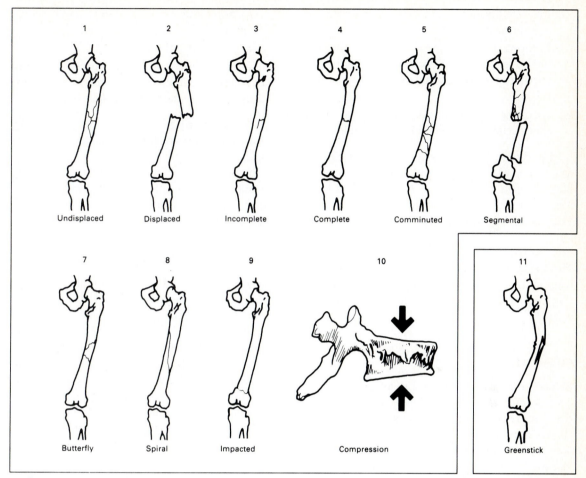

Figure 8-1. Types of fractures (1–10 Courtesy of Presbyterian University Hospital, Pittsburgh, PA)

9. Impacted fracture: The broken ends of bone are jammed into each other.

10. Compression fracture: The bone collapses due to disruption of bone tissue, usually occurring in a short bone such as a vertebral bone.

11. Greenstick fracture: An incomplete break that occurs almost exclusively in children.

In addition, fractures are classified as simple or compound. A simple fracture does not produce an open wound whereas a compound fracture causes disruption of skin and soft tissue. The wound is caused when a fragment of bone punctures the skin. Even when bone is not observed protruding through the skin, it is necessary to inspect the skin carefully since the bone fragment could be imbedded in the soft tissue. Compound fractures are likely to be complicated by infection.

FIRST AID

Before transporting an accident victim with limb fractures (or dislocations), it is important to evaluate the neurovascular status of the involved extremity. This process includes checking sensation, temperature, color, pulses, and the victim's ability to move fingers or toes.

Prevention of movement of bone fragments at the fracture site prior to transporting the victim is of utmost importance. Further damage to soft tissues, the vascular system, and nerves could result from improper or inadequate immobilization. Splints are used to protect the fracture and are applied before the victim is moved, including the joints above and below the fracture site.

Types of splints include:

1. Soft splint: a nonrigid splint such as a pillow or blanket.

2. Hard splint: a rigid splint with a hard surface such as a board or plaster (such a splint must be padded to protect soft tissues).

3. Air splint: an inflatable splint.

4. Traction splint: a splint that uses traction to decrease angulation and reduce pain (examples: Hare and Thomas splints).

It is important to apply the splint carefully and most injuries are splinted "as they lie." Two people should apply the splint, one supporting the injured part, the other applying the padding and splint. The splint should be held in place with straps or unstretchable gauze. Elastic bandages should never be used since the elasticity may allow too much mobility in the injured part. Air splints may be open at both ends to allow adequate neurovascular assessment.

When multiple injuries are apparent, always suspect spinal trauma. Cervical spine injuries should be immobilized with a cervical collar and victims of thoracic and lumbar spinal trauma should be transported on a backboard.

Bleeding may be a problem when the victim has compound fractures. Cover open wounds with sterile dressings and apply direct pressure if arterial bleeding is suspected. Care givers must use Universal Precautions when the potential for contamination with blood or body fluids exists. Protective gloves are worn by the care giver to prevent such contamination, and all blood and body fluids are considered to be infected. Severe injuries may cause shock and, when it is present, treatment of shock has priority over treatment of fractures. Be alert for signs of occult bleeding that may occur in pelvic and femoral fractures. A tape measure should be used to measure the girth of the affected part to detect any enlargement suggesting internal bleeding.

Pain caused by muscle spasm around the fracture site may be alleviated by splinting and applying gentle traction. When long bones such as the femur are fractured, muscles around the fracture contract and may cause the bone ends to override (overlap) and cause the extremity to be shortened. Traction may be applied manually by gentle, steady pulling of the intact part distal to the fracture. If trained medical personnel are not available to apply a traction splint, manual traction must be maintained during transport to a hospital.

FRACTURE TREATMENT

Reduction of Fractures

X-rays are used to confirm the presence of a fracture. Computed tomography (CT) uses X-rays to provide a clear, cross-sectional image and is especially useful when pelvic fracture is suspected. Computer reconstruction of the radiation levels absorbed by various tissues identifies the injured bone and surrounding tissues. CT is used to provide two-dimensional and

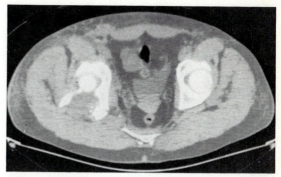

Figure 8-3. Computed tomography of the pelvis, two-dimensional (Courtesy of Central Imaging Services, Inc., University of Pittsburgh Medical Center)

three-dimensional images (see Figs. 8-2, 8-3, 8-4, and 8-5).

Magnetic resonance imaging (MRI), also called nuclear magnetic resonance (NMR), utilizes a magnetic field and radio waves to create a computer image (see Fig. 8-6). The word nuclear refers to the nucleus or center of each cell in the body. The cells of the body release energy that form images that can be scanned by using

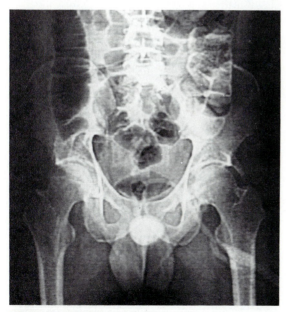

Figure 8-2. Flat plate of the pelvis (Courtesy of Central Imaging Services, Inc., University of Pittsburgh Medical Center)

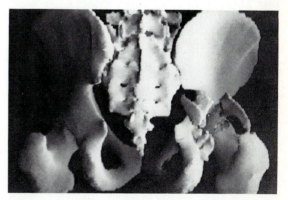

Figure 8-4. Computed tomography of the pelvis, three-dimensional, posterior view (Courtesy of Central Imaging Services, Inc., University of Pittsburgh Medical Center)

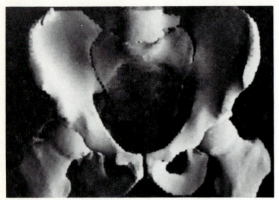

Figure 8-5. Computed tomography of the pelvis, three-dimensional, anterior view (Courtesy of Central Imaging Services, Inc., University of Pittsburgh Medical Center)

magnetic forces. This information is collected by the computer and transformed into an image that can be read by the radiologist.

When X-rays have confirmed the diagnosis of a fracture, reduction (manipulation) may be necessary to restore correct anatomical position of the fractured parts. When a fracture is simple and undisplaced, manipulation is not necessary prior to immobilization with a cast or splint.

A closed reduction is performed by manipulating the bone back into its normal position. Local or general anesthesia may be used. Following reduction, the part is immobilized by some type of external fixation such as a cast or splint until evidence of healing is apparent on an X-ray.

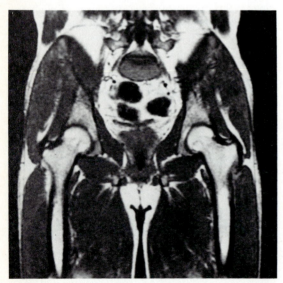

Figure 8-6. Magnetic resonance image of the pelvis (Courtesy of Central Imaging Services, Inc., University of Pittsburgh Medical Center)

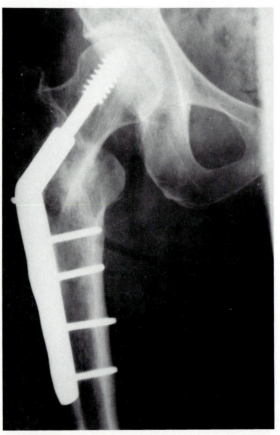

Figure 8-7. Internal fixation of a right hip fracture (Courtesy of Harold E. Swensen M.D.)

An open reduction is performed through a surgical incision to expose the fracture site. Bone fragments are realigned and maintained in position with internal fixation such as rods, plates, and screws (see Fig. 8-7). Following an open reduction with internal fixation, immobilization with a cast or splint may or may not be necessary, depending on the fracture and the type of internal fixation used.

External fixation is a method of fracture immobilization in which a system of percutaneous pins or wires are connected to a rigid external frame (see Fig. 8-8). External fixation is highly versatile, may be constructed in many different configurations, and permits three-plane correction of deformities. Meticulous care is required at the pin-skin interface to prevent infection while the external fixator is in place. When fracture healing is complete and the external fixator is removed, a cast or splint may be necessary.

The Ilisarov (il-is'arov) external fixation device is used to lengthen bones (see Fig. 8-9). This can be used to treat dwarfs or someone who has one leg shorter than the other. It is also used for a badly comminuted fracture when bone has been lost and the defect must be filled.

Casting and Cast Care

The most common type of casting material in use today is made from gauze bandages impregnated with plaster of Paris. To prepare the roll for application, it is dipped in tepid water on its end so bubbles can escape and water can penetrate the roll. When the bubbling stops, the roll is removed and gently squeezed to remove excess water. The orthopedic surgeon then wraps the involved part, starting at the distal end and wrapping uniformly to above the fracture site. Following cast application, X-rays are

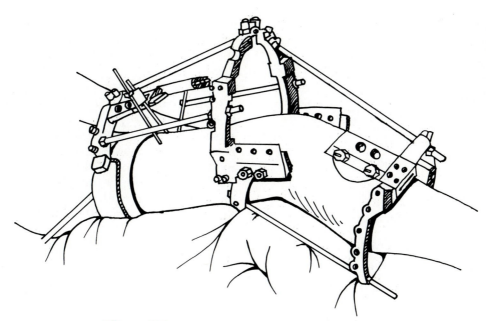

Figure 8-8. Patient with external fixation therapy

lighter and, if they become wet, they still maintain their stability.

Regardless of what casting material is used, protection of skin under the cast is an absolute necessity. Prior to cast application, the involved part is wrapped with a special cotton padding or stockinette. Wrinkles must be carefully prevented in whatever padding material is used, especially over bony prominences.

As a plaster of Paris cast hardens, it feels hot, then cold. Patients should be told to expect a short period of heat followed by a cool, damp sensation under the cast. The cast should be left uncovered during the drying period, which may last as long as 24 hours depending on the size of the cast. When a wet cast is moved, it must be handled carefully with the palms of the hands, since finger or thumb imprints could result in pressure necrosis to skin under the cast. If possible, the casted part should be elevated above heart level to prevent swelling.

The padding under the cast should always extend beyond the edges of the casting material. It may be necessary to secure the padding and provide additional protection to cast edges by applying adhesive tape or moleskin around the edges.

Plaster of Paris casts can be cleaned by using a small amount of white cleanser on a damp cloth. Soaking the cast with water must be avoided as this will soften the plaster. Casts can be decorated as long as water soluble paints or marking pens are used. Oil-based paints occlude (plug up) the pores in the plaster and do not allow it to breathe and, thus, can cause maceration (excessive softening) of the skin under the cast.

During the time the extremity is casted, the fingers or toes should be observed regularly to assess neurovascular status. Any swelling, change in color, decreased sensation, or abnormal temperature that is unrelieved by elevation

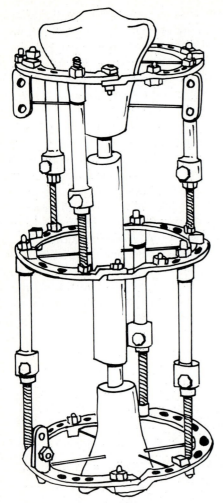

Figure 8-9. *The Ilisarov device*

repeated to assure correct alignment at the fracture site.

Several lightweight synthetic casting materials are also currently available. These materials are more expensive because they require special equipment for application. The advantage of using these materials is that they are

should be promptly reported to the physician. Such symptoms may indicate impairment to vital structures (nerves or blood vessels) beneath the cast. A localized area of pain under the cast may indicate a blister or pressure area that can result in serious tissue destruction.

Cast removal is performed by splitting the cast with a cast saw. Since the blade on the cast saw oscillates rather than rotates, it is unlikely to damage skin beneath the padded cast. The patient should be warned that the cast saw is noisy. After the cast is removed, the patient will notice dry, flaky skin that has accumulated under the cast. This can be removed over several days with normal bathing and application of moisturizing lotions. The patient should also be instructed to expect that joints that have been enclosed in a cast will be stiff and perhaps sore following cast removal. Muscle atrophy can also be apparent. The patient who has had a leg cast and has been ambulating without the use of a cane or crutches may require them after cast removal to protect the weakened extremity from injury. Exercises may be prescribed to strengthen weakened muscles and return joints to full range of motion. It is important that the patient understands the importance of carrying out the exercise program so that full muscle strength and joint range of motion will be regained.

Traction

Traction is sometimes used, particularly for fractures of the femur. The traction is applied to a pin which is inserted through the distal bone fragment and the pulling force helps return the overriding bone fragments to normal anatomical position. It may be used until healing takes place or until internal fixation can be performed. When a pin is used, the traction weight must never be removed, otherwise fracture fragments might return to the overriding position, causing pain and muscle spasm and disrupting the healing process. The weight at the foot of the bed of a patient with a femur fracture may reach as much as 40 pounds. This much weight is likely to cause the patient to slide down in the bed; therefore, counter traction is used. This type of traction is accomplished by elevating the foot of the bed by placing an electrical bed in shock position or placing blocks under the wheels at the foot. Weights must always be hanging free at the ends of the bed. A firm mattress should always be used for a patient in traction; a bed board may be necessary to provide comfort and support. Since the patient in traction may be on bedrest for an extended period of time, exercise will be necessary to regain muscle strength. Supervision and instruction from the physical therapist for ambulation with assistive devices (cane, crutches, walker) may be required.

COMPLICATIONS OF FRACTURES

Failed Union

Inadequate immobilization, either external (casts, splints) or internal (screws, plates, rods), can result in failure of the fracture healing process. Failed unions are classified as follows:

1. Delayed union: failure of the fracture to consolidate (heal) within the time usually required
2. Malunion: healing of the fracture occurs but with an increased degree of angulation or deformity at the fracture site
3. Nonunion: failure of a fracture to heal and produce a complete, firm, stable union. It is characterized by motion at the fracture site

Fat Emboli

Although fat embolus is not a common complication, it does occur and can be life-threatening.

Fat embolism is probably the result of fat droplets being released from the bone marrow into the venous bloodstream and ultimately lodging in the vessels of the pulmonary circuit. This condition usually occurs within the first 24 hours following severe fractures of the long bones, although it can occur as much as 72 hours after the accident. Symptoms of fat embolism include apprehension, sweating, fever, rapid pulse, shortness of breath, and pallor. The most distinctive sign is a petechial rash over the chest and shoulders. The presence of fat emboli is an emergency since the patient's ability to breathe properly is affected and mechanical ventilation may be necessary.

Infection

Infection can be a serious complication and is especially prevalent following compound fractures. Signs of infection include pain, fever, redness, and yellow, foul-smelling drainage. When crepitation (krep'i-ta-shun), a crackling sound and sensation produced when the area is palpated, is felt, it may be due to gas bubbles formed by the gas-gangrene bacillus. Wound drainage is cultured to identify the organism causing the infection and tested to determine the antibiotic to which the organism is sensitive. The antibiotics are then given intravenously. Surgical removal of the infected tissue may also be necessary.

Compartment Syndrome

Compartment syndrome is a complication of fractures that occurs when pressure, either from internal or external forces, causes compression of vital structures in the upper or lower extremity, which affects blood supply and nerve function. The signs and symptoms are specific to the nerve, artery, and muscle involved. It is, therefore, important to check the exposed fingers and toes carefully for sensation, temperature, color, pulses, and movement. Permanent damage and deformity can result if changes are not detected early in the course of compartment syndrome.

CRUTCH WALKING

The patient must have correctly fitting crutches and must be instructed in their proper use. Improperly fitted crutches can contribute to an unstable, unsafe gait. Crutches that are too long can exert pressure on the brachial nerve plexus in the axilla and cause nerve damage more disabling than the fracture. The patient must be alerted not to lean on the crutches which will place weight on the axilla, as nerve palsy can result from this maneuver even when crutches are properly fitted.

The patient should usually perform exercises to strengthen muscles in the upper extremities in preparation for crutch walking. Doing push-ups and lifting weights while lying in bed are good exercises for these patients.

Several types of gaits are used by patients who must walk on crutches. The physician prescribes what gait the physical therapist should teach the patient and specifies how much weight can be borne on the affected extremity.

A single crutch should never be used because it stresses the injured side by shifting the center of gravity. If support is needed on one side only, a cane should be used. The cane is always used on the unaffected side.

To assist in ambulation, you should walk on the unaffected side and slightly behind the disabled person. It is preferable for patients to wear trousers or pajama bottoms when ambulating. This type of clothing gives the assistant a place at the waist to support the patient. When assisting on a stairway, you should walk behind the patient going up the stairs and in front when going down the stairs.

DISLOCATIONS AND SUBLUXATIONS

Dislocations and subluxations can occur at the joints of the shoulder, elbow, wrist, finger joints, hips, knees, ankles, and toes. When a dislocation occurs, the bones are displaced so that the articulating surfaces totally lose contact. When a joint is subluxated, the articulating surfaces partially lose contact. These problems are frequently the result of trauma but may also occur due to disease that weakens the supporting structures around the joint. The patient experiences pain, loss of function of the joint, and malposition (the joint is not in the normal position). Both are treated by manipulation until the parts are in their normal position. Immobilization with a cast, splint, or elastic bandages for several weeks will allow the joint capsule and surrounding ligaments to heal.

SPRAINS AND STRAINS

A sprain is an injury causing tearing of the supporting ligaments surrounding a joint and usually follows a sharp twisting motion. A strain is an injury to a muscle or its tendon attachment. With each injury, there is swelling, pain, and loss of motion to the affected joint. There may be a bluish discoloration, or **ecchymosis** (ek"e-mo'sis), in the area due to bleeding under the skin. The part should be X-rayed to rule out the possibility of a fracture. Treatment consists of controlling pain and swelling and immobilization of the affected area to promote healing. An immobilized sprain usually heals in two to three weeks; usually, a strain does not take as long to heal as a sprain.

EPICONDYLITIS

Epicondylitis (ep"e-kon-dil-i'tis) (tennis elbow, epitrochlear bursitis), is inflammation of the forearm extensor supinator tendon fibers at their attachment to the lateral humeral epicondyle. It is common in tennis players whose activities require a forceful grasp, wrist extension against resistance, or frequent rotation of the forearm. Grasping an object or twisting the elbow causes elbow pain, often radiating to the forearm and back of the hand. Treatment includes local injections of corticosteroid and local anesthetic, as well as some systemic antiinflammatory drug. Aspirin is often helpful. An immobilizing splint may be necessary as well as muscle strengthening exercises. In some cases, avoiding the type of activity that caused the inflammation for a few weeks may be all that is necessary to resolve the problem.

ARTHRITIS

RHEUMATOID ARTHRITIS

Rheumatoid arthritis is a chronic, systemic, inflammatory disease that primarily attacks peripheral joints and surrounding muscles, tendons, ligaments, and blood vessels. The disease is characterized by spontaneous remissions and unpredictable exacerbations (flare-ups), though the onset may be insidious. The disease affects females three times more frequently than it does males and may be due to a genetic defect in the body's autoimmune system. Besides joint discomfort, patients often have a fever, feel general malaise, and are intolerant of weather changes. Exacerbations often follow some stressful situation. Diagnosis is made by X-ray, blood studies,

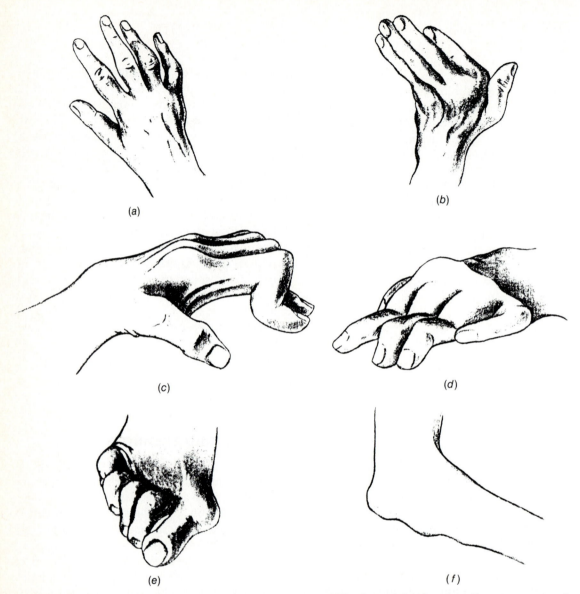

Figure 8-10. *Rheumatoid arthritis deformities. (a) Spindle-shaped fusiform swelling in proximal interphalangeal joints. (b) Ulnar deviation of metacarpophalangeal joints. (c) Boutonniere deformity, flexion of proximal interphalangeal joints and hyperextension of distal interphalangeal joints. (d) Swan neck deformity, flexion of the metacarpophalangeal joints with hyperextension of the proximal interphalangeal joints and flexion of the distal interphalangeal joints. (e) Hallux valgus (bunion) with claw toe deformity. (f) Rheumatoid nodules near the elbow. (Courtesy of Cready and White, Western Pennsylvania Arthritis Project, St. Margaret Memorial Hospital, Pittsburgh, PA)*

and synovial fluid analysis. Common deformities found in rheumatoid arthritis are pictured in Figure 8-10.

Drug therapy is used to decrease the inflammation and relieve joint pain. The first drug prescribed is usually aspirin, a salicylate. Nonsteroidal antiinflammatory drugs and steroids may also be prescribed. Because these drugs are often irritating to the mucosal lining of the stomach, patients are encouraged to take them with food or milk. They should be instructed to watch for evidence of gastrointestinal bleeding such as black, tarry stools. Side effects of prolonged steroid therapy include fluid retention, peptic ulcers, poor wound healing, adrenal atrophy, and emotional problems such as euphoria.

Supportive measures include getting enough rest at night as well as rest periods during the day. Splinting can be used to rest inflamed joints. Frequent range of motion exercises and individualized therapeutic exercises help to maintain joint motion. Heat is used to relax muscles, relieve pain, and decrease inflammation.

Extensive damage to the affected joints may require surgical repair, which often includes a total joint replacement (see Figs. 8-11, 8-12).

OSTEOARTHRITIS (OSTEOARTHROSIS)

The most common form of arthritis is **osteoarthritis.** It is a chronic, progressive disease that causes deterioration of the joint cartilage and formation of reactive new bone at the margins and subchondral parts of the joints. It may be due to a genetic defect. Symptoms usually appear during middle-age with one or several joints involved. Little swelling occurs but the joints are painful and stiff, especially during weather changes and after activity at the end of the day.

The diagnosis is confirmed by X-rays, which characteristically show narrowed joint space,

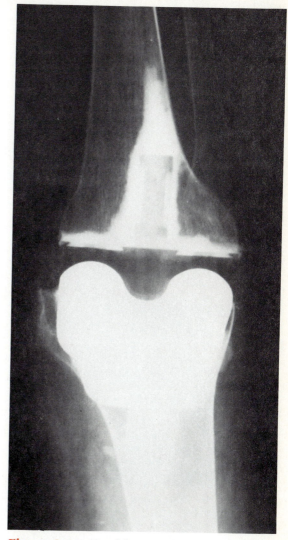

Figure 8-11. Total knee replacement, anterior-posterior view

cystlike bony deposits in the joint space and margins, joint deformity (bow legs, knock knees), and bony growths on weight-bearing areas (knees, hips).

Analgesics are used to relieve pain and antiin-

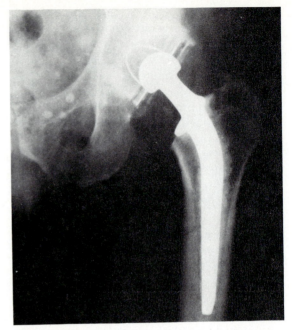

Figure 8-13. Total hip replacement

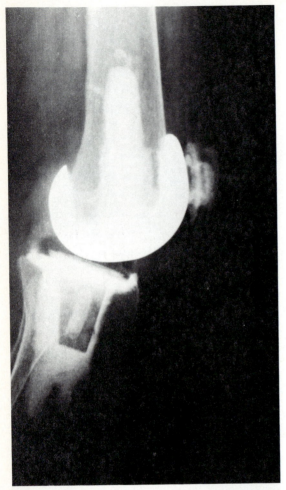

Figure 8-12. Total knee replacement, lateral view

flammatory agents can also provide relief. Local heat to the joint and rest are also helpful. Assistive devices such as a cane, crutches, or walker can reduce stress on affected joints. The affected joints may be injected with a steroid preparation. This form of steroid therapy does not have side effects as severe as those of the steroid preparations that are taken orally. Surgical intervention that may be necessary includes total hip and total knee replacement (see Fig. 8-13).

OSTEOPOROSIS

Osteoporosis is a disease where there is a loss of bone mass due to acceleration in the rate of bone resorption and a slowing down in the rate of bone formation. Calcium and phosphorus salts are lost in bones affected by this disease. They become porous, brittle, and at risk for fractures. The cause is unknown in primary osteoporosis. Secondary osteoporosis may be due to prolonged steroid therapy, prolonged immobilization, alcoholism, malnutrition, hyperthyroidism, or a deficiency of osteoblastic hormones such as estrogen and testosterone. The disease is usually discovered when an elderly person suffers a fracture and X-rays confirm the diagnosis. Treatment is symptomatic and aimed at preventing additional fractures and controlling pain.

LOW BACK PAIN

Low back pain is a common complaint and a major cause of time lost from work. It can be a source of much aggravation to both the sufferer and those who are trying to help. Because the real cause of the problem is frequently hard to identify, the ailment is difficult to treat. The pain may be due to real disease such as metastatic cancer, urological or gynecological problems, or orthopedic problems, but may also be related to emotional problems. The most frequent orthopedic causes of low back pain are osteoarthritis, lumbosacral strain, or a herniated intervertebral disc.

Acute lumbosacral strain is characterized by pain in the lumbar area that does not radiate to the buttocks or legs. It is often accompanied by muscle spasm and is relieved by bedrest, muscle relaxants, local heat, and analgesics. Exercises to strengthen abdominal and paravertebral muscles are often prescribed. A brace or lumbosacral corset may help to provide immobilization while soft tissue healing takes place.

A herniated intervertebral disc (slipped disc) causes severe pain that radiates down one leg (sciatica). The pain becomes particularly severe when the patient strains, coughs, sneezes, or lifts (even a light object) using poor body mechanics. The pain is caused by pressure on the spinal nerves, most often at the fourth or fifth lumbar disc space or the fifth lumbar and first sacral disc space. The spongy center called the nucleus pulposus (nu'kle-us pul-po'sus) of the disc herniates through the fibrous covering and can cause the pressure on the sensory nerve roots at that level (see Fig. 8-14).

About 90% of patients with a herniated intervertebral disc can be treated conservatively with bed rest on a firm mattress and analgesics. Occasionally, if conservative measures are unsuccessful, surgery may be necessary. A laminectomy and discectomy may be done, which involves the removal of the posterior arch of the vertebra and the herniated disc.

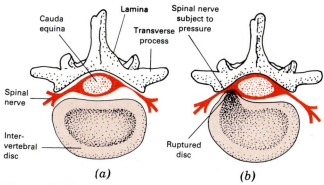

(a)   *(b)*

Figure 8-14. (a) Normal relations of the intervertebral disc and lumbar vertebra to the spinal cord and nerve branches. (b) A ruptured disc protruding into the vertebral canal where it exerts pressure on a spinal nerve root.

Sometimes a spinal fusion is necessary to provide stability to the spinal column. In this type of surgery, bone is taken from another area such as the iliac crest and grafted onto the vertebrae. Two or more vertebrae are united by means of this graft. Although mobility of the joint is permanently lost, the patient becomes accustomed to this area of stiffness.

DEFORMITIES OF THE BACK

Scoliosis (sko"le-o'sis) is an abnormal curvature of the spine, usually a lateral curvature. The cause is usually **idiopathic** (id"e-o-path'ik) (unknown), but it may be due to neuromuscular disease, vertebral anomalies, or paralysis. Postural (functional) scoliosis results from poor posture or a discrepancy in leg lengths and is not a fixed deformity.

The most common spinal segment involved is the thoracic region, with convexity to the right. Compensatory curves to the left will be found in the cervical and lumbar regions. These compensatory curves develop to maintain body balance.

When symptoms occur, they are likely to include backache, fatigue, and dyspnea. Untreated scoliosis can result in pulmonary insufficiency (due to decreased lung capacity), back pain, degenerative arthritis of the spine, disc disease, and sciatica.

Treatment is determined by the severity of the deformity and the age of the patient. It may include close observation, exercise, a brace, or a surgical spinal fusion.

Kyphosis (ki-fo'sis) is an anteroposterior curving of the spine (humpback) that causes a bowing of the back, usually in the thoracic region. Lordosis (lor-do'sis) is a curvature in the lumbar region causing a swayback appearance.

OSTEOMYELITIS

Osteomyelitis is a pyogenic (producing pus) bone infection that may be acute or chronic. Although it can result from an infected compound fracture, it is more frequently a blood-borne infection starting from a focus of infection elsewhere in the body. The most common organism causing osteomyelitis is Staphylococcus aureus; others include Streptococcus pyogens, pneumococcus, pseudomonas aeruginosa, Escherichia coli, and proteus vulgaris.

The patient has sudden, severe pain in the affected bone, with tenderness, heat, swelling, and restricted movement in adjacent parts. Systemic symptoms may include fever, malaise, rapid pulse, and nausea. Prompt treatment is necessary with appropriate antibiotics and surgical drainage of pus. There is serious danger that osteomyelitis may become chronic. Following surgical drainage, the wound is left open and packed with sterile, antibiotic-soaked dressings. The affected part can be immobilized in a cast or splint for comfort. Rest and good nutrition will facilitate healing by increasing the patient's resistance.

HERNIAS

Hernias are probably the most common type of muscle disorder. Hernias result from weakened muscles of the abdominal wall allowing the underlying viscera to protrude. The most common hernias are those that occur in the normally weak places of the abdominal wall—inguinal ring, femoral ring, umbilicus—and in the diaphragm where the esophagus enters the stomach.

With the exception of the diaphragmatic hernia, surgery is usually the treatment of choice. Trusses are usually not recommended because the uncorrected hernia is vulnerable to serious complications. An incarcerated hernia cannot be reduced (the protruding viscera cannot be pushed back into the abdominal cavity). Edema of the protruding structures and constriction of the opening through which the bowel has emerged make it impossible for them to return to the abdominal cavity.

Strangulation of a loop of bowel can occur if the incarcerated hernia has not received prompt surgical attention and the opening through which the viscera is protruding obstructs the blood supply to that part of the bowel. This condition can lead to necrosis of the trapped loop of bowel and will necessitate a bowel resection (surgical removal of the loop of bowel).

A diaphragmatic, or hiatus, hernia is the protrusion of a part of the stomach through a defect in the diaphragm at the point where the esophagus passes through the diaphragm. Patients with this type of hernia have heartburn, belching, and epigastric pressure after eating. It may help to relieve their distress if they eat frequent small meals and avoid any food for about three hours before retiring. They might also sleep in a semisitting position and avoid bending over. If the patient is obese, a weight reduction diet should be recommended. A patient with a chronic cough must be treated because coughing puts additional strain on the weakened area.

Surgical treatment of a hiatus hernia involves thoracic surgery to replace the stomach protruding from the abdominal cavity and to repair the defect in the diaphragm. Such surgery is more major than that required for other uncomplicated hernias.

Occasionally, incisional hernias occur following abdominal surgery. Obese or elderly patients and those who suffer malnutrition are more prone to developing incisional hernias than are other surgical patients. Surgical incisions that have been infected and in which wound healing has been impaired are also prone to developing an incisional hernia.

CANCER

Malignancy in the musculoskeletal system may be the result of a primary tumor originating in musculoskeletal tissue or secondary tumors that have metastasized from another site. Primary cancers likely to spread to the musculoskeletal system include breast, lung, prostate, kidney, and thyroid cancer.

The most common primary bone cancer is osteogenic sarcoma, which arises from the bone-forming mesenchyme in the long-bone metaphysis. The less common parosteal sarcoma originates in parosteal osteoblastic cells on the outer surface of the periosteum. Chondrosarcoma is a malignant cartilage-forming tumor that may arise spontaneously or from a preexisting benign lesion. Fibrosarcoma arises from nerve-sheath connective tissue. Leiomyosarcoma and rhabdomyosarcoma are myogenic tumors. Ewing's sarcoma usually arises from primitive bone marrow cells in the medullary cavity of long bones.

Most etiologies are unknown but radiation-induced sarcomas have been identified. Trauma may draw attention to an already existing lesion but is unlikely to cause musculoskeletal cancer.

Treatment includes wide surgical excision, radiation therapy, and chemotherapy. Musculoskeletal cancer may threaten the victim's life by crowding out normal tissue and spreading throughout the body.

SUMMARY QUESTIONS

1. Differentiate between a simple fracture and a compound fracture.
2. What type of fracture is most likely to become infected?
3. Discuss first aid measures that are appropriate to use for a patient who has a spinal fracture.
4. What observations are needed for a person who has had a cast applied to an extremity?
5. What is the difference between internal and external fixation of a fracture?
6. How does rheumatoid arthritis differ from osteoarthritis?
7. Define osteomyelitis.
8. What are the common types of hernias?
9. What type of patient is most likely to develop an incisional hernia?
10. Discuss complication of hernias.
11. What conservative measures can be taken to relieve the distress of a hiatus hernia?
12. List three treatments for cancer of the musculoskeletal system.

KEY TERMS

crepitation
ecchymosis
epicondylitis
idiopathic

osteoarthritis
osteomyelitis
rheumatoid arthritis

9

The Nervous System

OBJECTIVES

On completion of this chapter, you will be able to:

1. Differentiate between the central and peripheral nervous systems.
2. Describe the structures that protect the central nervous system.
3. Describe the functions of the autonomic nervous system.
4. Describe neurons and their supporting tissue.
5. Describe the nature of the nerve impulse over nerve fibers and across synapses in the central and peripheral nervous systems.
6. Give examples of first-, second-, and third-level reflexes.
7. List the factors that influence reaction time.
8. List the most important nerve emerging from each nerve plexus.
9. Discuss the various functions in each part of the brain stem.
10. List nine functions of the diencephalon.
11. Discuss the role of the reticular formation.
12. Describe the structure and functions of the cerebrum.
13. Trace the pathway of the cerebrospinal fluid from the time of its formation until it is returned to the bloodstream.
14. List the 12 cranial nerves and the principal functions of each.

OVERVIEW

I. DIVISIONS OF THE NERVOUS SYSTEM
II. NERVE TISSUE
III. CLASSIFICATION OF NEURONS
IV. NERVE CONDUCTION
    A. Electrical Transmission
    B. Chemical Transmission
V. REFLEXES
VI. REACTION TIME
VII. SPINAL CORD
VIII. SPINAL NERVE ORIGINS AND DISTRIBUTION
IX. CONNECTIONS OF THE CORD WITH THE BRAIN
X. BRAIN OR ENCEPHALON
    A. Brain Stem
        1. Medulla Oblongata
        2. Pons
        3. Midbrain
        4. Cerebellum
    B. The Interbrain
    C. The Reticular Formation
    D. The Cerebrum
XI. MENINGES
XII. CEREBROSPINAL FLUID
XIII. CRANIAL NERVES
XIV. THE AUTONOMIC NERVOUS SYSTEM
    A. Sympathetic Division
    B. Parasympathetic Division

The nervous system, together with the endocrine system, aids in the control and coordination of the other systems of the body. It provides the tools by which we reason, learn, remember, and indulge in activities that are distinctly human. It assists us in making choices. The freedom to choose is a valuable freedom that carries with it tremendous responsibilities. Frequently, the choices we make determine what future choices might be available to us.

DIVISIONS OF THE NERVOUS SYSTEM

The central nervous system (CNS) is made up of the brain and spinal cord. The brain is the largest and most complex mass of nerve tissue and is well protected by the bones of the skull. The spinal cord is well protected by the bones of the vertebrae. This bony protection of the nerve tissue of the central nervous system is particularly important because nerve tissue in the central nervous system will not regenerate if it is injured.

The peripheral nervous system (PNS) is composed of nerves that connect the central nervous system with the rest of the body. There are 12 pairs of cranial nerves and 31 pairs of spinal nerves in the peripheral nervous system. The autonomic nervous system (meaning self-governing) is made of nerve fibers that lie within the spinal nerves and some of the cranial nerves. This autonomic nervous system is concerned with visceral activities that are not usually under our conscious control.

NERVE TISSUE

Nerve tissue, one of the primary tissues of the body, is composed of neurons, which are the nerve cells with a variety of supporting cells called neuroglia (nu-rog'le-ah) which means glue. In addition to supporting the neurons, neuroglia also can function as phagocytes and are a part of the blood-brain barrier that restricts certain substances from the brain.

Neurons have special properties of irritability and conductivity. An individual nerve cell has a central mass called the cell body from which there are varying numbers of extensions or

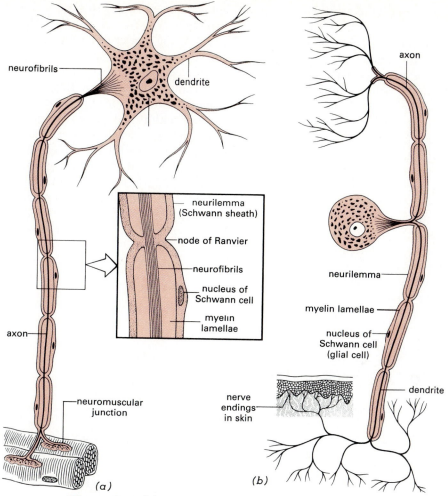

Figure 9-1. (a) Motor neuron and (b) sensory neuron

processes called **axons** (ak'sonz) and **dendrites** (den'dritz). Figure 9-1 shows a typical neuron. The dendrites (meaning tree-like) carry impulses toward the cell body and the axons transmit the impulses away from the cell body.

Within the cell body is a spherical nucleus. Neurofibrils (nu-ro-fi'brils) cross through the cytoplasm of the nerve cell body and extend into the processes that convey impulses to and from the cell body. Also in the cytoplasm are Nissl (nis'el) bodies, which are granular masses. There are many Nissl bodies in a resting neuron but few in the working neurons, a fact that suggests these structures together with numerous free ribosomes are concerned with protein synthesis needed to replace proteins used by the neurons in their metabolic activities. Neurofibrils and Nissl bodies are unique to nerve cells.

These cells have cytoplasmic structures that are common to other types of cells such as mitochondria, Golgi apparatus, and lysosomes. However, since mature neurons do not reproduce themselves, there are no centrioles.

The cell bodies of neurons must be well protected since, if the cell body is destroyed, the whole neuron dies. Cell bodies are located only in the gray matter (unmyelinated fibers) of the brain, cord, and ganglia (gang'gle-ah). Ganglia are small modules of nerve tissue that provide for some nerve connections within the autonomic nervous system and house the sensory cell bodies of the spinal neurons.

The processes extending from the nerve cell give these cells a unique appearance. Picture in your mind a microscopic cell that has processes three feet long! This is the appearance of the fibers within the nerves supplying your feet since the cell bodies of these are located at about the level of your waist. Elsewhere, the nerve processes may be very short. In no other system of the body do we have cells that vary so greatly in appearance and yet perform essentially the same function.

The dendrites carry impulses toward the cell body. The length of the dendrites and how much they branch varies greatly in different neurons. Axons convey impulses away from the cell body. Each neuron has only one axon. However, it frequently has one or more collateral axons branching from the main axon.

Some of the cell processes have **myelin** (mi'e-lin) and **neurilemma** (nu-re-lem'ah) coverings. Myelin is a white lipoprotein substance that gives some nerve tissue a white appearance. The myelin covering is not a continuous sheath since it is interrupted at intervals by constrictions called the nodes of Ranvier. At these nodes, where the nerve fiber does not have the myelin insulation, there is an exchange of sodium and potassium into and out of the nerve fiber. This exchange of ions, according to the membrane

theory of nerve transmission, assists in the transmission of the nerve impulse. The nerve fibers in the gray matter of the brain and cord do not have the myelin covering.

All peripheral neurons have neurilemma, a thin multinucleated covering believed to be essential to the repair of nerve tissue. Nerve fibers in the central nervous system do not have neurilemma and, when destroyed, normally do not regenerate. Recently, however, there have been some successful attempts in grafting peripheral nerve tissue (with neurilemma) into damaged CNS areas. In the case of brain damage, it is not uncommon for other areas of the brain to take over some of the functions of cells that have been destroyed.

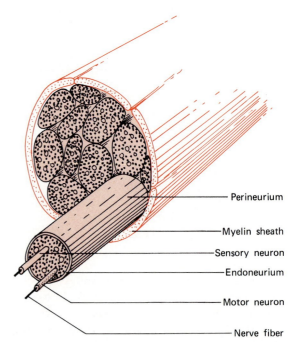

- Perineurium
- Myelin sheath
- Sensory neuron
- Endoneurium
- Motor neuron
- Nerve fiber

Figure 9-2. *Cross section of a spinal nerve. Sensory neurons carry nerve impulses toward the brain and spinal cord. Motor neurons carry impulses from the brain and cord to muscles and organs.*

Peripheral nerves are made up of many nerve fibers and the axons and dendrites of the neurons. A group of fibers is held together with endoneurium (en-do-nu're-um). Several of these groups will be held together in a bundle by a connective tissue called perineurium (per-i-nu're-um), and finally the bundles are bound together by epineurium (ep-e-nu're-um). The result looks very much like a cross section of a large electrical cable (see Fig. 9-2).

CLASSIFICATION OF NEURONS

Neurons are commonly classified according to their function. Afferent neurons are sensory and carry impulses from the periphery to the central nervous system. Their dendrites have special receptor end organs called extroceptors, interoceptors, and proprioceptors, which convert stimuli into nerve impulses. The extroceptors are located near the surface of the body and are sensitive to such stimuli as temperature, pain, or touch from the external environment. Interoceptors, found in the viscera, give rise to visceral sensation. Proprioceptors, located in muscles, joints, tendons, and the labyrinth (lab'i-rinth) of the ear, are concerned with muscle sense, position, and movement of the body in space. The interpretation of all sensation is done by the cortex of the brain.

Efferent fibers are motor and secretory. They transmit impulses from the central nervous system to muscles and glands, delivering orders for activity. Most nerves contain both motor and sensory fibers. There are a few purely sensory nerves, such as the optic nerve of the eye and the olfactory for smell, but there are no purely motor nerves because all must have afferent fibers for muscle sense. For example, nerves that are primarily motor must also carry sensory

messages to inform the brain of the degree of muscle contraction.

Connecting, or internuncial (in-ter-nun'she-al), neurons transmit impulses from one part of the brain or cord to another. These neurons do not leave the central nervous systems.

The contact between neurons is called a **synapse** (sin'apz). This is a tiny space where the impulse from the axon of one neuron is transmitted to the dendrite of another neuron. A single axon may convey impulses to a number of neurons and, conversely, a single neuron may receive impulses from the axons of several neurons.

NERVE CONDUCTION

Properties of irritability or excitability enable the nerve tissue to respond to stimuli. This property is especially well developed in the receptor endings; however, a nerve fiber may be stimulated at any point along the course. Occasionally, the receptors may lose their irritability temporarily because of prolonged stimulation. This property is called sensory adaptation. The olfactory nerves for smell become sensory adapted easily. For this reason, we quickly become unaware of unpleasant odors, such as stale cigarette smoke. If we leave a smoky room, go into fresh air for awhile, and then return, we readily notice the unpleasant odor.

Conductivity is the ability of the nerve to transmit impulses. The velocity of the impulse going to skeletal muscles is rapid. Large myelinated nerves may transmit at speeds of 100 meters per second (200 miles an hour). Small, unmyelinated fibers supplying viscera conduct at about 0.5 to 1 meter per second (about one mile an hour). Recall how slow the response of visceral muscle is to a stimulus. As the nerve impulse travels over the nerve fiber it is self-propagating. The impulse slows down a bit at the synapse where, for example, a sensory neuron gives the impulse to a connecting neuron.

Resistance at the synapses varies considerably. It is high when we are learning a new skill, but with practice the resistance is lowered and we are able to perform the skill more rapidly. When you are learning academic material, it is helpful if the information is made available to you in several different ways. For example, you can read about it, see a film concerned with the same material, have classroom discussions about it, and perhaps have it demonstrated to you in some way. In so doing, several different neural pathways are being established. When you need to reproduce the material, it is unlikely that all of these pathways will be blocked. Also, having been introduced to the material in several ways, you may be able to associate the material with something else familiar to you. Association is the basis of our long-term memory.

ELECTRICAL TRANSMISSION

For the conduction of a nerve impulse over a nerve fiber, an electrical potential must be established. This electrical potential, also called the membrane potential, results from the different concentrations of certain ions on either side of the membrane. The difference is due mainly to positively charged sodium ions that are present in greater concentrations outside the nerve fiber and to potassium ions, also positively charged, that are in greater concentrations inside the fiber. The membrane is selectively permeable, allowing potassium ions to diffuse freely but restricting the passage of sodium ions. For sodium to move across the membrane, energy is required. This energy is produced by the mitochondria of the neuron, and the process is called sodium pump. This sodium pump opens the sodium channels. Calcium is needed to close the channels. If there is a deficiency of intra-

cellular calcium the channels may remain open allowing sodium to diffuse through the membrane repeatedly, and the impulse is transmitted again and again. This is tetany. Some local anesthetics, such as procaine, decrease the membrane permeability to sodium. When the drug is in the tissue fluid around the nerve fiber sodium cannot enter the nerve, and impulses are prevented from passing through this region.

In the resting neuron, that is, one that is not transmitting, sodium ions are pumped to the outside while potassium ions are moved into the fiber. The number of sodium ions transported out is greater than the number of potassium ions that move into the fiber, and the membrane is polarized; it has a negative charge on the inside and a positive charge outside. The actual voltage of the membrane potential is about 0.085 volt.

Figure 9-3 shows the transmission of a nerve impulse. Think of the nerve impulse as moving in the direction of the arrows, one segment at a time, beginning with a stimulus applied to the nerve fiber in the upper left part of the illustration. When the nerve is stimulated, the permeability of the membrane is altered and allows sodium to enter, causing the membrane to become suddenly positive inside and negative outside. This is called depolarization because the normal polarized state (positive outside and negative inside) is reversed. The area of depolarization extends rapidly to the next segment as the membrane there becomes permeable to sodium. Sodium ions flow through the membrane in the new segment causing electrical current to spread along the fiber. This spread of the increased permeability and electrical current along the membrane is called a depolarization wave or a nerve impulse. A few ten thousandths of a second after depolarization, the membrane again becomes impermeable to sodium ions, but potassium ions can still move through the membrane. Because of the high concentrations

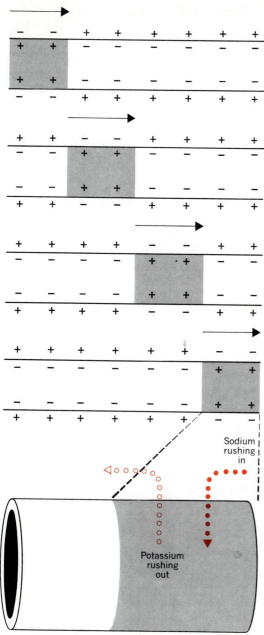

Figure 9-3. *Transmission of a nerve impulse along a neuron involves the exchange of potassium and sodium across the nerve membrane. A nerve impulse can travel from your toes to your brain and back in a fraction of a second.*

of potassium inside, many potassium ions diffuse outward carrying positive charges with them. This, once again, creates a negative charge on the inside and a positive charge outside the membrane. This process is called repolarization.

Repolarization usually begins at the same point at which the fiber was depolarized originally and spreads along the fiber as shown in Figure 9-3. The shaded area beneath each arrow is depolarization. Repolarization is represented in the segment to the left of the depolarization wave. The whole cycle of depolarization and repolarization takes place in a minute fraction of a second, and the fiber is ready to receive and transmit a new impulse. The electrical transmission of the nerve impulse continues over each segment of the nerve until, in the case of a sensory impulse, it is interpreted by the brain or, in the case of a motor impulse, muscle activity is accomplished.

The electrical changes that take place during the transmission of a nerve impulse can be observed and recorded. An electroencephalogram (e-lek″tro-en-sef′ah-lo-gram) is a graphic record of electrical changes in the brain. Such records are of diagnostic importance in the study of the brain.

During conduction of a nerve impulse, chemical and thermal changes take place. The chemical changes involve the use of glucose and oxygen by the nerve tissues. In the healthy body glucose is the only fuel that can be used by brain tissue, whereas the other tissues of the body can use other foods for fuel. While the nerve is conducting impulses, oxygen is used and carbon dioxide is produced. If the brain is deprived of the supply of either oxygen or glucose, damage occurs much sooner than in other types of tissue. Heat is also produced during the conduction of a nerve impulse but not in the quantity that it is during muscle activity. You will get quite warm when playing a fast game of tennis, but you will not get overheated from the nerve activity required for study!

Nerve, like muscle tissue, abides by the All or None Law. When stimulated, the nerve fiber will either respond completely or there will be no response. The impulse is self-propagating. That is, the depolarization of a portion of a nerve serves as the stimulus for the depolarization of the next portion of the nerve.

CHEMICAL TRANSMISSION

As we have seen, the nerve impulse as it travels rapidly over a nerve fiber is electrical. When the impulse reaches the terminal end of the axon and is to be transmitted to another neuron or muscle, the transmission becomes chemical. At the terminal ends of the axons, there are knobs or feet that contain vesicles. When stimulated by the nerve impulse, these vesicles release a transmitting substance into the gap between the neuron and the receiving structure. The transmitting substance, a chemical, causes the impulse to cross the interval (see Fig. 9-4).

Since the neural transmission at synapses is chemical, it is slower than the transmission over nerve fibers and there is a greater dependency on oxygen. The synapses, therefore, are more susceptible to fatigue than are nerve fibers.

Acetylcholine (as"e-til-ko'lin) is the chemical mediator at most synapses in the peripheral nervous system and between nerves and skeletal muscle. Once the impulse has been received, another chemical, **cholinesterase** (ko-lin-es'ter-

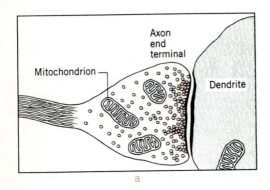

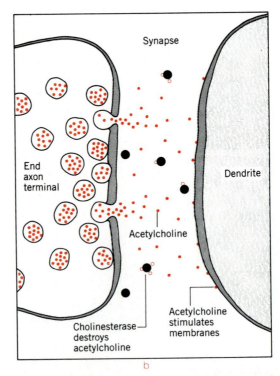

Figure 9-4. Transmission of a nerve impulse across a synapse is chemical. Acetylcholine and cholinesterase are often the chemical mediators.

as), enzymatically breaks acetylcholine into acetate and choline so that the impulse does not continue indefinitely. The acetate and choline then diffuse back to the axon vesicles where they are reunited by choline acetyltransferase and stored for future use.

In addition to acetylcholine, there are more than 40 other chemical mediators. Norepinephrine, dopamine, serotonin, histamine, glutamic acid, and aspartic amino acid all function as excitor substances while enkephalins (en-kef'a-linz), endorphins (en-dor'finz), gamma amino butyric acid, and dynorphin (di-nor'fin) are inhibitors.

Which neurotransmittor is involved not only has to do with the location of the synapse or neuroeffector but, in some instances, with the nature of the particular impulse. For example, dopamine is frequently the excitor chemical for emotional responses. Serotonin is involved in sensory perception and temperature regulation whereas the enkephalins, endorphins, and dynorphin are inhibitors when the impulse is concerned with pain. Dynorphin is 200 times as powerful as morphine.

The chemical mediators are of clinical importance because some drugs act at the synapse by influencing the action of the chemical mediators. For example, if cholinesterase is blocked, nerve impulses repeatedly stimulate the muscle, causing increased muscle contraction. With some emotional disturbances, such as depression, it may be helpful to give a drug that inhibits monamine oxidase, an enzyme that inactivates both serotonin and norepinephrine.

Facilitation refers to a lowering of synaptic resistance. Excitor substances are released lowering the postsynaptic neuron membrane potential and so the neuron becomes more excitable. The "nervous" person has such a decrease in synaptic resistance. There can also be an increase in the synaptic resistance. This is called inhibition. As a result, we do not have to respond to every stimulus in our environment since these impulses do not reach higher levels in the nervous system.

REFLEXES

Reflexes can be classified in several ways. Clinically, they are frequently classified according to the part affected. A deep tendon reflex, such as a knee jerk when the patellar tendon is tapped, is an example of a reflex classified according to the structure involved. Other examples are the corneal reflexes that cause us to blink when the cornea is touched and the pupil reflex that causes the pupil of the eye to constrict in bright light and dilate in the dark.

Testing for the presence of these reflexes and the number of reflex responses is often used for evaluating the level of consciousness of a person in a coma. Pupil reflexes are useful in assessing the severity of a head injury. Checking for the presence of a gag reflex in a patient who has had a local throat anesthetic before offering food or fluids is a reasonable safety measure. When the sole of the foot is stroked, the toes curl under. This is the plantar reflex or negative Babinski. This reflex is positive (the big toe is extended and the other toes spread out) in infants under the age of a year and a half since their corticospinal tracts (tracts carrying messages for voluntary muscle actions) are not fully developed. A positive Babinski in an older person may indicate disease or damage to these tracts.

Reflexes may also be classified according to the level of the nerve structures involved. In a first-level reflex, the sensory impulse goes only as high as the spinal cord, and a motor impulse is immediately sent from the cord to cause a muscle response. First-level reflexes are protective reflexes; the response is very rapid, easily predictable, and difficult to inhibit. An example of a first-level reflex is that of jerking your hand away from a hot stove. Quickly following the first-level reflex, second- and third-level reflexes will probably occur, but the initial protective action is the simple first-level reflex pictured in Figure 9-5.

Second-level reflexes travel as high as the brain stem. These reflexes are also protective in nature. An example of a second-level reflex is a gasp you might have when you burn your hand. Vomiting and coughing are also second level reflexes.

Third-level reflexes are learned or conditioned reflexes involving the cerebral cortex. Bladder and bowel control are third-level reflexes. The number of these reflexes is almost unlimited and examples vary considerably from one person to another. Simple job skills that a worker has performed many times become reflex acts. Although other workers can accomplish these tasks, they must give the task more conscious attention and they will not be able to do the particular task as rapidly as the experienced worker.

Regardless of how reflexes are classified, the essential structures involved are a receptor, an afferent neuron, an internuncial or connecting neuron, an efferent neuron, and an effector. Most reflex arcs involve hundreds of neurons. There are relatively few two-neuron arcs in which afferent and efferent neurons synapse directly.

In this discussion, it has been implied that a sensory impulse will always be transmitted to a connecting neuron, a motor neuron, and will result in motor activity. This is not always true. Specifically, how reflexes are inhibited is not well understood, but it is generally agreed that the site of this action is at the synapse. An example of reflex inhibition that all have experienced is the successful inhibition of a sneeze.

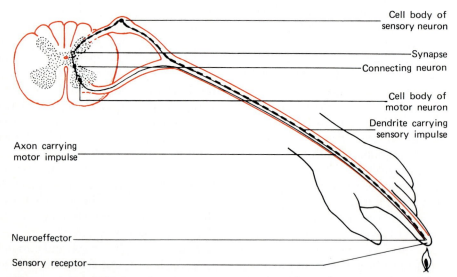

Figure 9-5. Pathway of a first-level reflex. The immediate response of this reflex is possible because the sensory impulse from the finger goes only to the spinal cord, and immediate motor impulses are sent to the muscles for action.

Synaptic resistance can also be decreased allowing a weak stimulus to evoke a strong response. How this happens is not understood, but it can be demonstrated. While pulling on your clasped hands, have someone tap your patellar tendon. The resulting knee jerk will be greatly intensified.

REACTION TIME

Reaction time is the time from the application of a stimulus to the start of the response. Reaction time is influenced by several factors: the nature and strength of the stimulus, how the situation is perceived, and the number and condition of the synapses that the impulse must cross and how many muscles must act. Removing your hand from the hot stove involves few synapses and relatively few muscles. Such a stimulus is strong enough to demand priority over most other activities. On the other hand, if you are driving a car and are alerted to a potential traffic hazard, in order to avert an accident you may have to apply the brakes, alter the direction of the car, and honk the horn to warn other motorists of the danger. Age, fatigue, and drugs, such as alcohol, can also influence reaction time. A motorist who has consumed too much alcohol, which depresses the cerebral cortex, may not be able to react fast enough to avert an accident.

SPINAL CORD

The spinal cord, located in the vertebral canal, extends from the foramen magnum to the level of the disc between the first and second lumbar vertebrae. It is thicker in the cervical and lumbar areas where the nerves supplying the extremities arise. Actually, this lumbar enlargement extends from the ninth to the twelfth thoracic vertebrae. It may seem strange that the lumbar enlargement is in the thoracic region; this is the case because the spinal cord grows at a slower rate than the vertebral column. By adulthood, the area within the vertebral column below the second lumbar vertebra contains nerves that branched from the spinal cord at higher levels. These nerves form the cauda equina (kaw'dah e-qui'na). It is called the cauda equina because it resembles a horse's tail. Thirty-one pairs of spinal nerves arise from the cord. There are eight pairs of cervical nerves, twelve pairs of thoracic, five pairs of lumbar, five pairs of sacral, and one pair of coccygeal nerves. These nerves leave the bony canal by way of the intervertebral foramen (see Fig. 9-6).

The cord is protected by the bony vertebral column and by **meninges** (me-nin'jez). The outermost meningeal covering is the **dura mater** (du'rah ma'ter) meaning tough mother. It is a fibrous membrane extending down to the level of the second sacral vertebra. The **arachnoid** (ah-rak'noid) beneath the dura is a delicate, spiderweb-like covering that also extends to the level of the second sacral vertebra. The **pia mater** (pi'ah ma'ter) or tender mother, closely covers the cord and extends only to the distal end of the cord. The pia mater is very vascular.

The spaces between the meninges are of clinical significance. The extradural space or epidural space lies above the dura. The subdural space lies between the dura and the arachnoid. Beneath the arachnoid is the subarachnoid space, that contains the cerebrospinal fluid. Analysis of this fluid, samples of which can be obtained by a lumbar puncture or spinal tap, is a valuable diagnostic aid.

Figure 9-6. *(a) In the cervical region of the cord, the spinal nerve roots penetrate the dura in the cervical region. (b) At the lower end of the cord, the nerve roots travel downward before penetrating the dura and emerging through the bony intervertebral foramen. (c) The origins of the 31 pairs of spinal nerve. (bottom) The connections of one spinal nerve to the cord.*

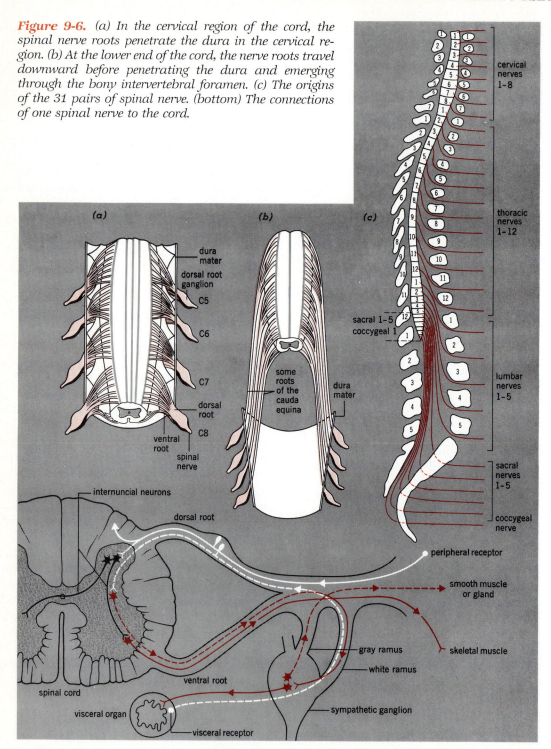

If we examine the spinal cord in cross section, we note that there are two fissures (fish'urs) or indentations. The deepest of these fissures is the anterior fissure. The gray matter of the cord contains unmyelinated nerve fibers, connecting neurons, and cell bodies. For descriptive purposes, this gray matter resembles an H and the columns of the H are designated as the right and left ventral, or anterior horns, and the dorsal or posterior horns. White matter surrounds the gray matter and the nerve fibers here are myelinated. These are the nerve fibers that transmit impulses from one segment of the cord to another and connect the brain with the rest of the body.

SPINAL NERVE ORIGINS AND DISTRIBUTION

The dorsal or sensory root ganglion contains the cell bodies of afferent or sensory nerve fibers. The ventral root contains the motor fibers. The cell bodies of the motor fibers are in the gray matter of the ventral horn. These two roots unite to form a spinal nerve just as they leave the intervertebral foramen. Thus, the spinal nerve is mixed (both motor and sensory) and, as with all peripheral nerves, it is myelinated (see Fig. 9-7).

Each spinal nerve has three main branches. The dorsal branches go to the skin and muscles of the back, the visceral branches go to the internal organs, and the ventral branches, which are the largest, go to the front of the body and to the extremities. These branches may also be called rami (ra'mi), meaning horns.

Nerve plexuses (plek'suses) are formed by the interlacing of the ventral branches of certain spinal nerves. The cervical plexus is formed by the first four cervical nerves. The most important nerves arising from this plexus are the phrenic (fren'ik) nerves, which supply the diaphragm. Specifically, the phrenic nerves have nerve fibers of the third, fourth, and fifth cervical nerves (see Figs. 9-8 and 9-9). A transection of the cord above the level of the third cervical vertebra will obviously result in a cessation of respirations and death.

The brachial plexus involves cervical nerves five through eight and the first thoracic nerve. This plexus supplies the entire upper extremity. The radial nerve is the largest from the brachial plexus. This nerve has fibers from C5 through 8 and T1. It supplies the triceps and the posterior forearm. Injury to this nerve may result in wrist drop (inability to extend the wrist). The ulnar nerve, involving nerves from C8 and T1, supplies the anterior and medial forearm and the fourth and fifth fingers. The median nerve arises from C5, 6, and 7 nerves and goes to the anterolateral forearm and to the rest of the fingers and thumb. The musculocutaneous, also from nerves C5, 6, and 7, supplies the biceps and is both motor and sensory to the skin of the lateral forearm. Improper use of crutches may cause pressure on the brachial plexus and injure the nerves of this plexus.

There is no plexus in the thoracic region. Twelve intercostal nerves arise from this level of the cord and supply the intercostal muscles, the skin in this region, and some of the abdominal muscles.

The lumbar plexus, which includes the first four lumbar nerves, supplies the lower abdominal muscles, the groin, and the external genitalia (jen-e-ta'le-ah). The femoral nerve from this plexus supplies the quadriceps and the obturator nerve supplies the adductor muscles of the thigh.

The sacral plexus arises from the fourth and fifth lumbar nerves, the first sacral nerve, and

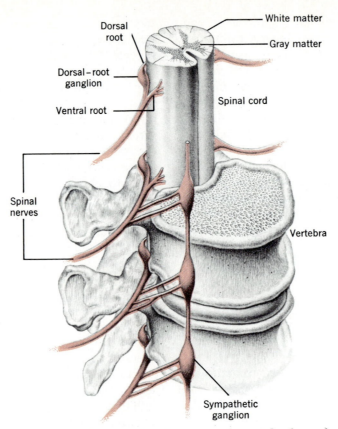

Dorsal root

White matter

Gray matter

Dorsal–root ganglion

Ventral root

Spinal cord

Spinal nerves

Vertebra

Sympathetic ganglion

Figure 9-7. The spinal cord shown in the vertebral canal. Note the mixed spinal nerves emerging through the intervertebral foramen. Sensory impulses enter through the dorsal root and motor impulses exit through the ventral root.

some of the fibers from the second and third sacral. Nerves from this plexus supply the gluteal muscles, thigh, leg, and foot. The sciatic nerve supplies the hamstrings, leg, and foot. The peroneal nerve, which arises from the lateral aspect of the sciatic nerve, supplies the lateral and anterior muscles of the lower leg. Injury to this nerve may result in foot drop. Because of the location of this nerve as it traverses through the

gluteal region, there is some danger that it might be damaged by an intramuscular injection. If the injection is made into the muscles of the upper outer quadrant of the buttock, the needle will not hit the peroneal nerve (see Fig. 9-10).

The pudendal (pu-den′dal) plexus contains fibers from sacral nerves two through four. It is a small plexus, but is of clinical significance be-

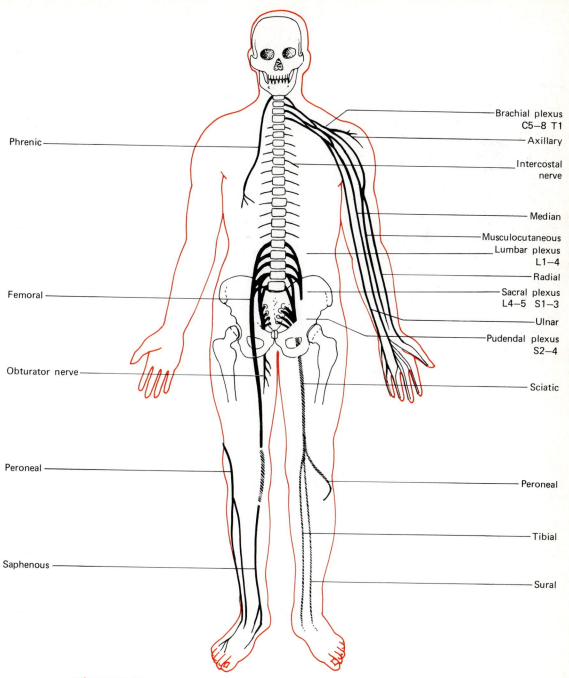

Figure 9-8. *Distribution of some major peripheral nerves, anterior view*

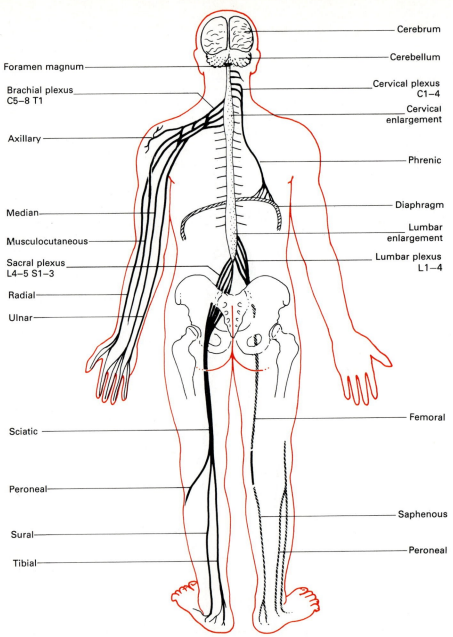

Figure 9-9. *Distribution of some major peripheral nerves, posterior view*

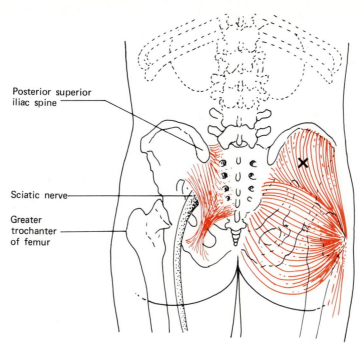

Figure 9-10. *To avoid peroneal nerve injury, it is important to consider the pathway of the sciatic nerve when giving an intramuscular injection in the gluteal region.*

Posterior superior iliac spine

Sciatic nerve

Greater trochanter of femur

cause sometimes a pudendal nerve block (saddle block) is done for anesthesia during childbirth.

The function of all of the spinal nerves is to carry impulses to and from the periphery and the spinal cord. We shall consider next how these nerve impulses ascend to the brain for higher action and from the brain to control various motor activities.

CONNECTIONS OF THE CORD WITH THE BRAIN

In the white matter of the cord there are ascending and descending tracts. The ascending tracts conduct impulses to the brain and descending tracts conduct impulses from the brain to various levels of the spinal cord. In some cases, the tracts are given names that indicate their origin and destination.

The lateral spinothalamic (from the spinal cord to the **thalamus** (thal′ah-mus) of the brain) carries impulses that are concerned with pain and temperature. The ventral spinothalamic tracts transmit impulses concerned with pressure. The spinocerebellar (spi′no-ser-e-bel′ar) tracts, which carry impulses to the cerebellum (ser-e-bel′um), play an important part in reflex adjustments of muscle tone and posture. These adjustments are not on the conscious level because the impulses do not reach the cerebral cortex and, therefore, you are unaware of them. The dorsal columns carry impulses that do reach higher centers in the brain. These impulses, which originate in proprioceptors in skeletal muscle, tendons, and joints, involve conscious muscle sense (an awareness of the movement and position of the body parts).

Descending tracts in the cord carry motor impulses from the brain. The pyramidal (pi-ram'i-dal) or corticospinal (kor"te-ko-spi'nal) tracts carry impulses for fine voluntary movement. The cell bodies of these nerve fibers are located in the motor areas of the frontal lobes of the brain; therefore, the muscle actions resulting from these nerve impulses are under conscious control. The lateral corticospinal fibers cross in the **medulla** (me-dul'ah) of the brain so that, for example, injury to motor areas in the right side of the brain will result in some degree of weakness or paralysis of the structures on the left side of the body that were controlled by the injured motor area. The smaller ventral corticospinal tracts do not cross in the medulla; some of these fibers cross at each segment of the spinal cord.

The extrapyramidal, or rubrospinal (roo-bro-spi'nal), are descending cord tracts that arise from lower levels of the brain and, therefore, are concerned with unconscious movements. Muscle coordination and reflex control or equilibrium are examples of activities resulting from nerve impulses traveling down the extrapyramidal tracts. Figure 9-11 shows the locations of the ascending and descending cord tracts.

Cord functions are by segments. In the event of a cord transection, voluntary motor activities and sensation below the level of the transection will be absent. Since visceral and cardiac muscle have automaticity, there will be no impairment of this type of motor activity. Motor functions and sensation above the level of the transection will not be impaired.

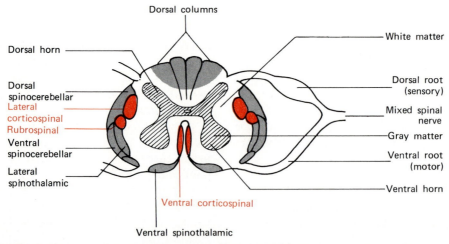

Figure 9-11. *A section of the spinal cord showing the descending motor tracts in color and the ascending sensory tracts in black*

BRAIN OR ENCEPHALON

The brain is the largest and most complex mass of nerve tissue in the body (see Fig. 9-12). The brain is well protected by the bones of the skull and by the meninges. The brain's requirement for glucose and oxygen is much more constant than that of other tissues of the body. These requirements are dependent on a rich blood supply discussed in Chapter 13.

The brain attains full physical growth in about 18 to 20 years. Although physical growth may cease, an unlimited number of neural pathways can be developed well into advanced age. Whether these pathways will be developed, regardless of age, depends on many factors, the most important of which probably is the desire to learn. How learning takes place is a very complex subject, but there is no doubt that we learn by asking questions. Language was invented to ask questions. Answers can be given by grunts or gestures, but questions must be spoken. Humankind came of age when the first question was asked. Social and intellectual stagnation result not so much from the lack of answers but from the absence of the impulse to ask questions.

BRAIN STEM

Medulla Oblongata

The medulla oblongata (ob-lon-ga′ta), or "bulb" of the brain, is an expanded continuation of the spinal cord. This vital structure is only about 3 cm (1 inch) long. It contains centers for the regulation of respirations, heartbeat, and vasomotor activities. These are called the vital centers because they are essential to life. Efferent nerve impulses originating in these centers are sent to the appropriate organs to maintain vital functions necessary for the metabolic needs of the body. For this reason, injury or disease of the medulla oblongata is serious and may be fatal.

The reflexes of coughing, vomiting, sneezing, and swallowing are mediated from the medulla. None of the functions of the medulla or other parts of the brain stem are on a conscious level. Many of the cord-brain pathways cross from one side to the other in the medulla.

Cranial nerves arising from the medulla include the acoustic, glossopharyngeal, vagus, accessory, and the hypoglossal nerves.

Pons

The pons is a bridge that contains conduction pathways between the medulla and higher brain centers. It also connects the two halves of the cerebellum. This part of the brain stem is a little smaller than the medulla. The respiratory centers of the pons include the **apneustic** (ap-nu′stik) **center,** which prolongs inspiration, and the pneumotaxic (nu-mo-tax′ik) center, which intermittently inhibits inspiratory neurons. The origins of cranial nerves V through VIII are located in the pons.

Midbrain

The midbrain connects the hindbrain with the forebrain. It extends from the pons to the lower surface of the cerebrum and is about the same size as the pons. It is a short, narrow segment that provides conduction pathways to and from higher and lower centers. Reflex centers in the midbrain include the righting, postural, and audiovisual reflexes. The righting reflexes are concerned with keeping the head right side up. Postural reflexes of the midbrain are concerned with the position of the head in relation to the trunk. The visual and auditory reflexes cause you to turn your head toward the direction of a loud sound.

The oculomotor and trochlear cranial nerves have their origins in the midbrain.

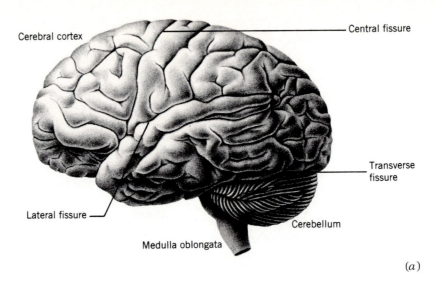

(a)

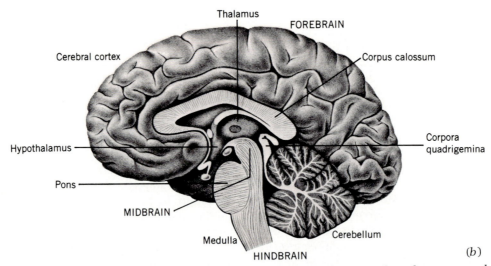

(b)

Figure 9-12. (a) Lateral external view of brain shows the cortical surface arranged in fissures or grooves and folds called convolutions. (b) Sagittal section of brain shows some principal internal structures.

Cerebellum

The cerebellum is located in the lower back part of its cranial cavity. Its functions, although not on the conscious level, are essential for coordinating muscle activity for smooth, steady movements. Reflex centers for the regulation of muscle tone, equilibrium, and posture are located in the cerebellum. The cortex of the cerebellum is gray matter. Beneath the cortex are white matter tracts that resemble the branches of a tree as they extend to all parts of the cortex. In a midsagittal section, the arrangement of white and gray matter presents a tree-like appearance that is called the arbor vitae, or tree of life.

THE INTERBRAIN

The structures of the interbrain, or **diencephalon** (di-en-sef′al-lon), are located above the midbrain and are covered by the cerebral hemispheres. Although their functions are not on the conscious level, they are essential to life.

The **hypothalamus** (hi-po-thal′-am-us) is located just posterior to the optic chiasm in the floor of the third ventricle and part of the walls of this ventricle. Some of the important functions of the hypothalamus include the manufacture of the hormones that are released from the posterior **pituitary** (pi-tu′-i-tar-e). The hypothalamus also causes the anterior pituitary to release its hormones. These hormones regulate many essential body functions and will be discussed in Chapter 23. The hypothalamus contains centers for the regulation of visceral activities, water balance, temperature control, appetite, sugar and fat metabolism, and normal waking and sleeping mechanisms. This biological clock is a very sensitive clock. If you are responsible for preparing the work schedule for the people in your department it is very important to keep this in mind. For people who must rotate shifts, it is best to move them from early shifts to later, that is, 7 to 3 AM then 3 to 11 PM and not the other way. Do not rotate them more often than every 21 days. Most mistakes are made between 3 and 5 AM. The Three Mile Island radiation accident occurred at 4 AM, when the shift people had only been on two days. These people were rotated weekly.

Neurons of the hypothalamus have extensive connections not only with our viscera but also with the cerebral cortex. It is not surprising, therefore, that our emotional state can affect visceral activity and influence our normal sleep patterns. Conversely, visceral disturbances or sleep disturbances can alter our behavioral and emotional responses.

The limbic system surrounds the hypothalamus or, according to some authorities, the hypothalamus is a part of the limbic system. Although behavior is a function of the entire nervous system, the limbic system controls the involuntary emotional aspects of behavior. Stimulation of various parts of this system will cause sensations of pain, pleasure, anger, fear, sorrow, affection, or sexual feelings.

The **thalamus** is a large mass of gray matter located in the walls of the third ventricle (see Fig. 9-13). The major portion of the diencephalon is the thalamus. All afferent or sensory impulses, except for the sensory fibers coming from the olfactory area of the nose, go first to the thalamus, where they are sorted and grouped; then they are sent on to the proper area of the cerebral cortex, where they are interpreted. The Law of Specific Nerve Energies holds that the place where a stimulus ends in the thalamus determines what sensation will be experienced. If the nerve impulse arrives in the heat area of the thalamus, the sensation will be that of heat even though the stimulus may have been something quite different.

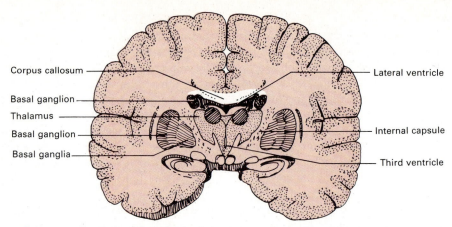

Figure 9-13. *Coronal section of the brain shows how the arrangement of fissures and convolutions increases the surface area of cortical gray matter. Note the basal ganglia are four masses of gray matter located deep within the brain.*

THE RETICULAR FORMATION

The reticular formation is composed of nerve fibers that spread through the upper portion of the spinal cord, brain stem, and diencephalon. The main function of this mass of interlacing nerve fibers is to coordinate muscle activity and to arouse the cerebral cortex via the wake center in the hypothalamus.

Stimulation of a specific motor area in the cerebral cortex will move a voluntary muscle, but the action will be jerky. It is the reticular formation that smooths and polishes the action. One theory concerning wakefulness holds that the wake center stimulates the reticular formation, which is responsible for a generalized increase in muscle tone. The proprioceptors in these muscles respond to the increased tone and send sensory impulses to the reticular formation via the thalamus. The reticular formation arouses the cerebral cortex so that the impulse can be interpreted.

The reticular formation also is concerned with inhibitory and facilitatory influences. When a stimulus needing no response reaches the reticular formation, it is prevented from going on to the cortex. This stoppage is called inhibition. Even a weak stimulus that is important will be magnified or facilitated. When one portion of the reticular formation is stimulated, a generalized increase in cerebral activity and an increase in muscle tone throughout the body take place. When you are asleep, the reticular activating system is in an almost totally dormant state. Such sensory impulses as pain or the sound of the alarm clock can activate the system and you will wake up. This impulse is called the arousal reaction. Signals from the cerebral cortex can also stimulate the reticular activating system and, thereby, increase its activity.

These functions of the reticular formation are of considerable clinical importance. Damage to the brain stem that involves parts of the reticular formation may result in prolonged coma. We know that stimulation of the cerebral cortex will not awaken the brain since it requires arousal signals from the reticular formation. The depressant actions of such drugs as tranquilizers and hypnotics are due to inhibition of the reticular formation. Since muscle coordination is a function of this system, it should be obvious that these drugs will also impair voluntary muscle action.

THE CEREBRUM

The cerebrum, the largest part of the brain, is separated into right and left hemispheres. Each hemisphere is subdivided into four lobes, which are named according to the covering cranial bones: frontal, parietal, temporal, and occipital lobes.

The cerebral cortex is a relatively thin layer of gray matter, cells, synapses, and unmyelinated fibers arranged in folds called convolutions (kon-vo-lu'shuns) or gyri (ji'ri). Between the convolutions are indentations called fissures or sulci (sul'ki). Figure 9-13 shows how these convolutions and fissures provide for a large cortical mass confined within a relatively small space.

A few of the fissures are important anatomical landmarks with which you should be familiar. The longitudinal fissure is located between the two hemispheres. This fissure extends downward to the corpus callosum (kah-lo'sum), a white matter tract connecting the two hemispheres of the cerebrum. The transverse fissure lies between the cerebrum and cerebellum; the central fissures, or fissures of Rolando, lie between the frontal and parietal lobes; and the lateral fissures, or fissures of Sylvius, lie between the temporal and frontoparietal lobes.

The cerebral cortex contains billions of neurons. The function of the cortex is to retain, to modify, and to reuse information. These quali-

ties are the bases of associative memory and the foundation of knowledge. Abstract thinking, judgment, reasoning, and moral sense use all parts of the cortex. However, it is believed that the prefrontal cortex is particularly concerned with what is called elaboration of thought. This term means simply an increase in depth and abstractness of thoughts and the ability to store information and recall it for future use. It is this ability that enables us to do such things as plan for the future, consider the consequences of our actions, delay action in response to incoming signals so that information can be weighed and the best course of action decided, and solve complicated mathematical, legal, and philosophical problems.

It has been established that certain areas of the cortex are primarily concerned with specific functions. Actually, any particular motor act or sensory interpretation probably involves the interaction of many areas of the cortex. But, in a general way, certain functions have been localized in specific cortical areas.

The general motor area of the cortex is located just anterior to the central fissure (see Fig. 9-14). Specific areas of this general motor area are concerned with movement of specific parts of the body. For example, the motor speech area, or Broca's area, located at the base of the general motor area, in the left hemisphere, is concerned with the ability to form words both in speaking and in writing. The left hemisphere does analytical and serious thinking, and the right hemisphere is artistic and emotional. For most individuals, linguistic ability is in the left hemisphere and melody is in the right hemisphere. For this reason, a person with **aphasia** (ah-fa'ze-ah), or the inability to speak, can communicate by singing.

Although the two hemispheres appear the same, some functions are not equally represented in each hemisphere. This is called cere-

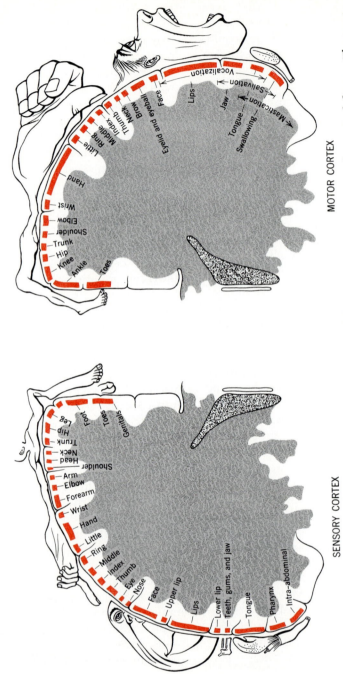

MOTOR CORTEX

SENSORY CORTEX

Figure 9-14. *The general motor and general sensory areas of the cortex are located near the central fissure. The parts of the body pictured indicate the location and relative amount of cortex required for the body part.*

bral dominance. The degree of cerebral dominance varies from one person to another and from one function to another. The superior and posterior part of the left temporal lobe is called the general interpretive area and is concerned with the interpretation of complicated meanings of different sensory experiences. Damage to this area, therefore, will leave an adult with a great intellectual void because of the inability to interpret the meanings of sensory experiences. A person without a prefrontal cortex can do a simple arithmetic computation such as 5 × 6 = 30, but without the general interpretive area the computation means nothing to the person. If the general interpretive area is destroyed in a child under the age of six years, the opposite side can usually develop to the full extent, returning the capabilities of the child essentially to normal.

Another evidence of difference in the two hemispheres of the brain is found in a person's emotional response to damage to the right or left side of the brain. Lesions in most areas of the left side result in the patient being disturbed and depressed as would be expected in response to a serious injury, while damage in much of the right hemisphere sometimes leaves the patient unconcerned about this condition.

Figure 9-15 shows how a nerve originating in the motor area descends through white matter tracts of the brain to a cord segment where it will synapse with a motor neuron that supplies the part to be moved. The motor neurons that originate in the cortex are called upper motor neurons and those that originate in the anterior part of the gray matter of the cord are called lower motor neurons. Notice that these neural pathways are funneled through a relatively narrow area called the **internal capsule.** There is a crossing of the nerve fibers so that nerves originating in one hemisphere control the skeletal muscles of the opposite side of the body.

Let us consider some clinical implications of this illustration. Damage to a motor nerve pathway can result in paralysis. If the damage is to an upper motor neuron, the muscles involved will be stiff or spastic and the deep tendon reflexes, such as the knee jerk, will be exaggerated. If the damage is to lower motor neurons, the resulting paralysis is flaccid (flak'sid). That is, the muscles will have little tone and there may be a loss of the tendon reflexes. One type of neural damage that can result in a spastic paralysis is a stroke. Because of the crossing of the fibers, the affected muscles will be in the side opposite the brain damage. The usual site of the neural damage in a stroke is the internal capsule. Peripheral nerve damage will result in flaccid paralysis on the same side as the nerve injury.

The general sensory area of the cortex is just posterior to the central fissure. In this area, true discrimination of sensations is experienced; for example, you know when your hand is touching a soft velvety surface or that you have stepped on a tack. Other sensory areas, such as those for the special senses, are located elsewhere in the cortex. The visual area is in the occipital lobe, the auditory area is in the superior part of the temporal lobe, and the olfactory and gustatory areas are in the medial aspect of the temporal lobe.

Beneath the cortex are white matter tracts. These tracts are myelinated fibers traveling in three principal directions. Commissural (kom-is'u-ral) fibers connect the right and left hemispheres of the cerebrum. Projection fibers are ascending and descending fibers such as are found in the internal capsule. Association tracts transmit impulses from front to back on the same side of the brain.

The **basal ganglia** are four masses of gray matter lying deep within the white matter of each hemisphere. These are concerned with as-

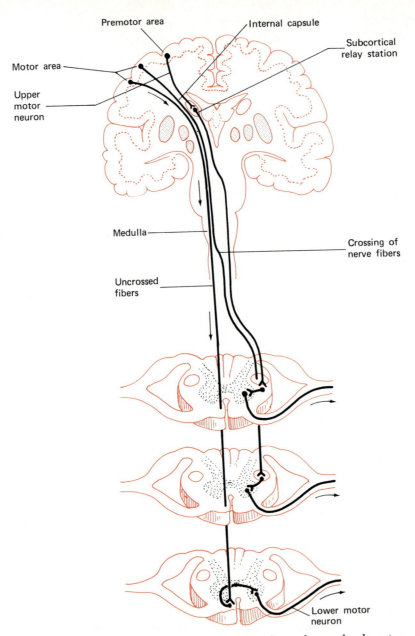

Figure 9-15. *Pathway of motor impulses from the cerebral cortex through the descending cord tracts to spinal nerves. Note that some of the fibers cross at the medulla and others cross at a lower level.*

sociative movements such as swinging your arms as you walk and unconscious facial expressions. Although obviously you can consciously alter your facial expression and determine the degree to which you will move your arms as you walk, most of the time these acts are not on the conscious level but are controlled primarily by the premotor area (located just anterior to the general motor area) and the basal ganglia. These structures, together with certain related parts of the brain stem, make up what is known as the extrapyramidal system. In general, the extrapyramidal system is concerned with muscle activities that are largely reflex in nature as opposed to fine skilled motor acts that are controlled by the pyramidal system originating in the general motor area of the cortex.

MENINGES

The **meninges** are the coverings of the brain beneath the cranial bones. The outermost covering is the dura mater, which has two layers. In most places, these layers are in contact with each other, but in other areas the internal dura sends extensions into some of the fissures of the brain while the external dura remains close to the interior of the skull. The falx cerebri (falks cer′e-bri), a fold of dura in the longitudinal fissure, forms the superior sagittal sinus. The tentorium cerebelli (ten-to′re-um ser-e-bel-i′), which lies in the transverse fissure, forms the straight sinuses in its folds. These sinuses contain venous blood that ultimately will flow into the internal jugular veins. The venous drainage of the brain is discussed in detail in Chapter 13.

The arachnoid is a delicate covering beneath the dura. The arachnoid villi are tiny projections of the arachnoid into the venous sinuses. It is through the villi that the cerebrospinal fluid is returned to the bloodstream.

The innermost covering of the brain is the pia mater. It is very vascular and dips down into the fissures of the cortex.

All of these meningeal coverings of the brain are continuous with the meningeal coverings of the cord. The spaces between the coverings are called the **subdural space** and the **subarachnoid space.** Cerebrospinal fluid is found in the subarachnoid space.

CEREBROSPINAL FLUID

The function of the cerebrospinal fluid is to provide a protective fluid cushion for the brain and cord and to aid in the exchange of nutrients and wastes between the central nervous system and bloodstream. It is a clear, colorless, watery fluid found in the ventricles of the brain and in the subarachnoid space around the brain and cord.

The blood vessels of the choroid plexus (ko′roid plek′sus) in the ventricles produce the cerebrospinal fluid. The ventricles are spaces within the brain (see Fig. 9-13). The healthy adult has about 100 to 150 ml of cerebrospinal fluid. This fluid contains about 40 to 60 mg/100 ml of glucose; however, the glucose content varies with the blood sugar level. In addition to glucose, the fluid also contains traces of protein and other nitrogenous substances as well as electrolytes such as sodium, potassium, chloride, calcium, and magnesium.

The cerebrospinal fluid is under pressure. This pressure is measured with a water manometer (see Fig. 9-16). Two pressure readings are usually recorded: the initial pressure and the

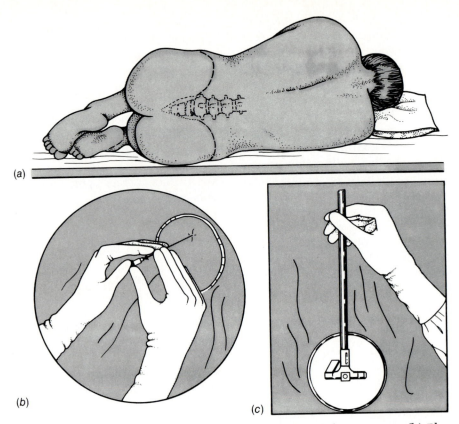

Figure 9-16. *Lumbar puncture. (a) Patient positioned for puncture. (b) Physician introducing needle and stylet. (c) Manometric determination of cerebrospinal fluid pressure. (From Barber, J.M., Stokes, L.G., and Billings, D.M.,* Adult and Child Care, *2nd ed. St. Louis: The C.V. Mosby Co., 1977)*

pressure after a small amount of fluid has been removed for chemical analysis or microscopic study. The closing pressure will be lower than the initial pressure. This pressure is clinically significant in conditions such as a head injury or brain tumor.

Cerebrospinal fluid is constantly being formed and circulated until it is returned to the blood-stream. The pathway for the circulation of the cerebrospinal fluid is as follows: lateral ventricles, foramen of Monroe, third ventricle, aqueduct of Sylvius, fourth ventricle, and then to the subarachnoid space via the foramens of Magendie and Luschka. Ultimately, it is returned by the arachnoid villi to the cranial venous sinuses (see Fig. 9-17).

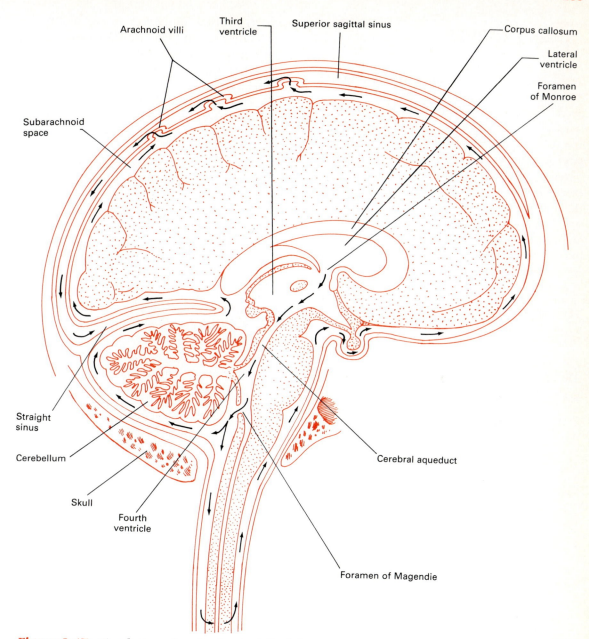

Figure 9-17. *Circulation of cerebral spinal fluid from its formation in the choroid plexus until it is returned to the blood in the cranial venous sinus*

CRANIAL NERVES

Twelve pairs of cranial nerves emerge from the underside of the brain (see Fig. 9-18). These nerves are numbered from front to back in the order in which they arise from the brain. The first, second, and eighth nerves are purely sensory; the others are both motor and sensory. There are several that are primarily motor, for example, the oculomotor and the trochlear. However, even in these nerves there must be sensory fibers for muscle sense to let us know the amount of muscle contraction needed to accomplish the movements. Table 9-1 lists the cranial nerves and the principal functions of each.

THE AUTONOMIC NERVOUS SYSTEM

The autonomic nervous system, meaning self-governing, is composed of visceral efferent nerve fibers that transmit impulses to smooth muscle, cardiac muscle, and glands. These nerve fibers lie within the cranial and spinal nerves; however, their impulses are not ordinarily under conscious control (see Fig. 9-19).

The hypothalamus integrates these impulses and makes necessary routine adjustments in the control of such vital activities as digestion and regulation of the blood pressure and heart beat. There are extensive neural connections between the hypothalamus and the cerebral cortex as well as between the hypothalamus and the viscera. For this reason, our thoughts certainly can influence visceral functions, and visceral functions (or malfunctions) can influence our conscious behavior. Expressions such as "The very thought of that makes me sick to my stomach" may indeed be very true.

As with the somatic nervous system, the motor neurons of the autonomic nervous system originate in the central nervous system. In the autonomic nervous system, however, there are two neurons between the CNS and the effector or the viscera being stimulated. This second

Table 9-1. Cranial Nerves

Nerve		Function
I	Olfactory	Smell
II	Optic	Vision
III	Oculomotor	Eye movements; regulates pupil size
IV	Trochlear	Eye movements
V	Trigeminal	Mastication; sensory to face and head
VI	Abducens	Abduction of eye
VII	Facial	Facial expression; taste; salivary secretion
VIII	Acoustic	
	Auditory branch	Hearing
	Vestibular branch	Equilibrium
IX	Glossopharyngeal	Swallowing; secretion of saliva; taste
X	Vagus	Parasympathetic fibers to viscera
XI	Accessory	Motor and sensory fibers to shoulder and head
XII	Hypoglossal	Tongue movements

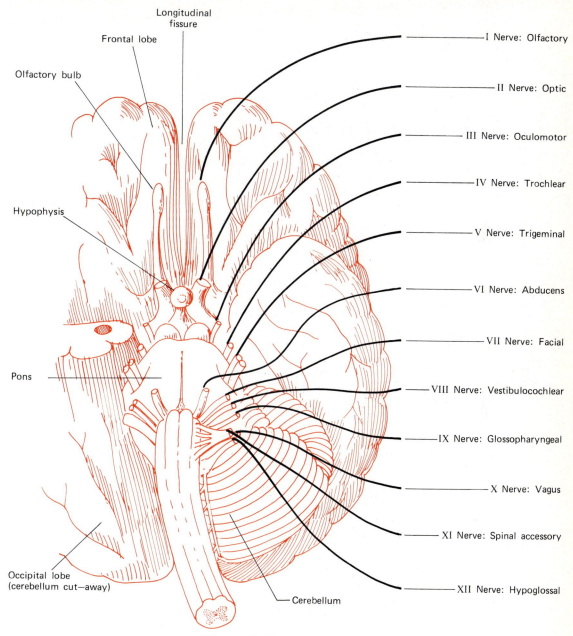

Longitudinal fissure

Frontal lobe

Olfactory bulb

Hypophysis

Pons

Occipital lobe
(cerebellum cut—away)

Cerebellum

I Nerve: Olfactory

II Nerve: Optic

III Nerve: Oculomotor

IV Nerve: Trochlear

V Nerve: Trigeminal

VI Nerve: Abducens

VII Nerve: Facial

VIII Nerve: Vestibulocochlear

IX Nerve: Glossopharyngeal

X Nerve: Vagus

XI Nerve: Spinal accessory

XII Nerve: Hypoglossal

Figure 9-18. Cranial nerves

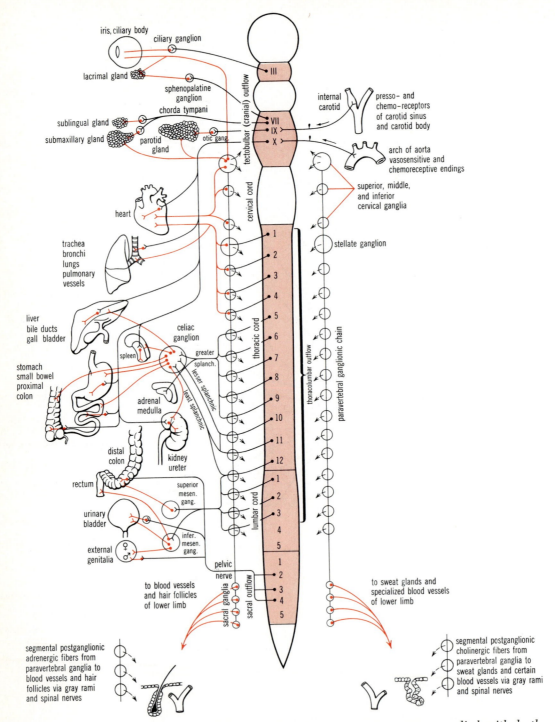

Figure 9-19. *Autonomic nervous system. Note that most organs are supplied with both sympathetic and parasympathetic fibers.*

neuron originates in autonomic ganglia. Some authorities believe that it is this additional synapse that removes the functions of the autonomic system from our conscious control. We do know, however, that with biofeedback people can learn how to control their blood pressure and many other of the autonomic functions.

There are two divisions of the autonomic nervous system and most of the viscera of the body have fibers from both divisions. The parasympathetic division, which has its origins in some of the cranial nerves and the sacral spinal nerves, calms us and conserves energy. Stimulation of this division favors digestion of food, rest, and repose. The sympathetic division, originating in the thoracic and lumbar spinal nerves, is concerned with expending energy. It is our fight and flight system. These two autonomic divisions may also be named according to their CNS origins: the parasympathetic is the craniosacral division and the sympathetic is the thoracolumbar division.

The chemical mediator at the synapse of both divisions is acetylcholine, which is inactivated by the enzyme cholinesterase. At the neuroeffectors of the sympathetic division, the chemical mediator is norepinephrine or noradrenalin, which is inactivated by monamine oxidase (MAO). At the neuroeffector of the parasympathetic division, acetylcholine is released. The parasympathetic fibers, therefore, may be called **cholinergic** fibers and the sympathetic fibers called **adrenergic** since norepinephrine is very similar to adrenalin. Cholinergic drugs stimulate the parasympathetic division and favor digestion and relaxation. Anticholinergic drugs will increase skeletal muscle tone and decrease motility and secretions of the gastrointestinal tract. MAO inhibitors facilitate the sympathetic nervous system.

Let us now consider some of the anatomical details and specific functions of each division.

SYMPATHETIC DIVISION

The ganglia of the sympathetic division are the chain or lateral ganglia and the prevertebral ganglia. The prevertebral ganglia are located in the abdomen. Here a preganglionic fiber can synapse with several postganglionic fibers. The chain ganglia are two chains located on either side of the vertebrae. One preganglionic fiber entering the chain can contact several ganglia and the branches of a single axon can synapse with thirty or more postganglionic fibers. For this reason, stimulation of the sympathetic division can quickly bring about rapid and widespread visceral activity essential for fight or flight.

The pupils of the eyes dilate, respirations increase, and the bronchioles dilate. In the circulatory system, the actions of the sympathetic division include increased heart rate and cardiac output. Blood vessels in the heart and skeletal muscles dilate and those of the skin and most viscera constrict. All digestive processes are inhibited, except the liver, which will increase the conversion of glycogen to glucose in order to meet the needs of the active skeletal muscles. There will be increased mental activity and an increased production of adrenal hormones. All of these processes will better equip you to meet the emergency.

PARASYMPATHETIC DIVISION

The general function of the parasympathetic division is to conserve energy and reverse the actions of the sympathetic division. Stimulation of this division does not bring about such widespread and rapid actions as does stimulation of the sympathetic division. Indeed, it takes some time for the parasympathetic division to erase the physiological evidences of anger or fear. The ganglia for this division are the terminal ganglia that are located within or close to the structure being innervated; therefore, in general, a parasympathetic preganglionic fiber contacts one or only a few postganglionic fibers.

The parasympathetic division favors digestive processes; peristalsis increases as does the flow of digestive secretions, and the bowel and urinary bladder sphincters relax. The physiological responses in the circulatory and respiratory systems are appropriate for rest and relaxation.

Using Figure 9-19, review the distribution of the sympathetic and parasympathetic fibers and indicate what action would occur in each of the organs as a result of stimulation of either the craniosacral or the thoracolumbar divisions of the autonomic nervous system.

SUMMARY QUESTIONS

1. Differentiate between the central nervous system and the peripheral nervous system.
2. Where are the cell bodies of neurons located?
3. What are the names of the cell processes of neurons?
4. Which nerve fibers have neurilemma and which do not?
5. Give examples of first-, second-, and third-level reflexes.
6. List several factors that influence reaction time.
7. What structures protect the spinal cord?
8. What is the most important nerve arising from the cervical plexus?
9. List four nerves that arise from the brachial plexus and tell what structures are supplied by each.
10. From what nerve plexus does the femoral nerve arise?
11. From what nerve plexus does the sciatic nerve arise and what structures does this nerve supply?
12. Where is the medulla of the brain located and what is its function?
13. What type of reflex centers are located in the cerebellum?
14. Where is the pneumotaxic center located and what is its function?
15. List several functions of the hypothalamus.
16. Where is the thalamus and what is its function?
17. What is the function of the reticular formation?
18. Where are the longitudinal, transverse, lateral, and central fissures located?
19. Where in the brain are the general motor and general sensory areas located?
20. Where is the area for motor speech?
21. Where are the basal ganglia and what is their function?
22. Trace the pathway of the cerebrospinal fluid from the place of formation until it is returned to the bloodstream.
23. Which cranial nerves are purely sensory?

24. Discuss the chemical mediators found in the brain.
25. List physiological changes that occur when the sympathetic nervous system is stimulated.
26. What is the general function of the parasympathetic nervous system?
27. Describe the structure and function of the cerebrum.
28. Describe the protection of the central nervous system.

KEY TERMS

acetylcholine   hypothalamus
adrenergic   internal capsule
aphasia   medulla
apneustic center   meninges
arachnoid   myelin
axons   neurilemma
basal ganglia   pia mater
cholinergic   pituitary
cholinesterase   subarachnoid space
dendrites   subdural space
diencephalon   synapse
dura mater   thalamus

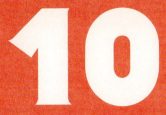

10

Diseases of the Nervous System

OBJECTIVES

On completion of this chapter, you will be able to:

1. Describe the main components of the neurological history and examination.
2. Describe the procedures for neurological diagnostic tests.
3. List the principles to consider when communicating with a confused or apprehensive patient.
4. Discuss important observations and appropriate first aid for a patient experiencing a seizure.
5. Discuss the symptoms of increased intracranial pressure and why it requires emergency treatment.
6. Describe the risk factors for CVA and identify those that can be controlled to help prevent stroke.
7. Describe measures to help prevent injuries to the head and spinal cord.
8. Discuss factors that cause hydrocephalus and tell what purpose a shunt serves.
9. Discuss the symptoms and treatment of Parkinson's disease.
10. Compare the disease processes of multiple sclerosis and Guillain-Barré syndrome.

OVERVIEW

I. NEUROLOGICAL EVALUATION
   A. Neurological History
   B. Neurological Examination
II. DIAGNOSTIC TESTS
   A. Lumbar Puncture
   B. Cisternal Puncture
   C. Computerized Tomography (CT scan)
   D. Cerebral Angiogram
   E. Electroencephalogram (EEG)
   F. Evoked Responses or Potentials
   G. Electromyogram (EMG)
   H. CT Myelogram
   I. Magnetic Resonance Imaging
III. GENERAL NEUROLOGIC PROBLEMS
   A. Behavioral Responses
   B. Delirium
   C. Seizures
   D. Increased Intracranial Pressure
   E. Coma
IV. SPECIFIC NEUROLOGIC PROBLEMS
   A. Cerebrovascular Accident
   B. Epilepsy
      1. Generalized Seizures
      2. Partial Seizures
   C. Head Injury
   D. Spinal Cord Trauma
   E. Central Nervous System Infections
   F. Poliomyelitis
   G. Hydrocephalus
   H. Muscular Dystrophy
   I. Parkinson's Disease
   J. Myasthenia Gravis
   K. Multiple Sclerosis
   L. Guillainn-Barré Syndrome

This chapter was written by Judy Wulf.

We can predict the signs and symptoms that result from nervous system diseases or injury if we know the normal functions of the various parts of the nervous system and have information concerning location of the pathology. For example, a lesion in a sensory peripheral nerve is manifested by impaired sensation in the area of the body that is served by that nerve, whereas a lesion in the motor area of the left cerebral cortex results in impaired movement on the right side. In this chapter our objective is to consider disorders of the nervous system. However, remember the nervous system functions to control and coordinate most body systems. Thus, disorders or problems in the nervous system have the potential to affect other body systems.

NEUROLOGICAL EVALUATION

NEUROLOGICAL HISTORY

During a neurological evaluation, the examiner obtains a careful history from the patient or family members. This history guides the focus of the neurological examination. The history includes a description of the main complaint, history of the present illness, past medical history, family history, review of systems, and medication history. The description of the present illness includes information about the onset, progression, frequency and duration of the problem, and other associated symptoms. It is important to identify factors that improve or aggravate the patient's symptoms. The patient's past medical history includes medical diseases or problems, surgical procedures, injuries, and allergies to foods, drugs, or medications. A brief health history of the immediate family and grandparents focuses on neurological diseases or disorders that appear to be genetic.

The review of systems focuses on questions about specific problems that the patient may have experienced. This helps detect specific symptoms of various nervous system functions the patient may not have mentioned. This includes seizures, syncope or fainting, headaches, vertigo, paralysis, paresthesias or altered sensations, and pain. It is helpful to ask if the patient has ever had problems with orientation, memory, thinking, speaking, swallowing, vision, hearing, movement, coordination, or balance. Medication history identifies the type, dose, and schedule of prescription and over-the-counter medications the patient is currently receiving.

NEUROLOGICAL EXAMINATION

Following the history, a neurological examination is usually performed. This includes screening all areas of neurological function and examining in greater detail those components where problems are suspected. Components of the neurological examination include consciousness, mental status, cranial nerves, motor and sensory function, cerebellar function, station, gait and balance, deep tendon reflexes, and superficial reflexes. Detecting signs and symptoms from the history and neurological examination help identify the location, nature, and probable cause of the pathological process. Following this, various diagnostic tests may be used to further delineate the problem and/or rule out other possible explanations for the problem. Then appropriate medical or surgical treatment can be initiated.

Tools commonly used during the neurological examination include an ophthalmoscope, Snellen eye chart or other reading material, pen light, sterile pin and wisp cotton, tongue blade, tuning fork, reflex hammer, and common objects such as pen, coin, or key. Using these tools, the examiner often looks for differences in nervous system function between the right and left side of the body, such as inequality of the pupils. This asymmetry or difference between the right and left side may be a subtle indication of a nervous system problem. The examiner needs to be sensitive to the patient responses during the examination as many tasks can be difficult if the patient is having problems. The patient's full effort and cooperation is needed so that the best responses can be obtained.

To determine the patient's consciousness, the examiner notes the responses required to maintain a wakeful or alert state in the patient. For example, the patient may need a gentle shake in order to respond to simple commands or questions. Determining the patient's mental status involves various questions that test the patient's memory and sense of time, place, person, and situation. During the history, if problems are detected in thinking or memory, the examiner may include additional questions related to general knowledge, judgment, and insight and the ability to do simple arithmetic calculations. If problems are determined with language or communication, further specific assessment of verbal, written, and gestural understanding and expression of language is completed.

Cranial nerve examination usually tests cranial nerves II through XII, unless problems in frontal function are determined. If this is the case, cranial nerve I is also included. When testing cranial nerve function, the examiner compares the right and left sides. Two groups of cranial nerves are generally tested together.

The first group includes cranial nerve III (oculomotor), cranial nerve IV (trochlear), and cranial nerve VI (abducens), which control eye movements. All nerves in this group are tested together by having the patient look at the examiner's finger through all directions of gaze.

Table 10–1. Cranial Nerve Functions and Methods of Testing

Nerves	Function	Function to Test
I. Olfactory	Smell	1. Test each nostril separately 2. Use volatile oils, tobacco, coffee, vanilla, cloves (not irritating substances that test cranial nerve V)
II. Optic	Vision	1. Test visual acuity—Snellen eye chart 2. Test visual fields by confrontation—gross screening device 3. Examine the fundus: Papilledema—blurred disc margins —hemorrhages near disc —absence of venous pulsation 4. Direct reaction 5. Consensual reaction
III. Oculomotor	1. Extraocular eye movements —inward —upward 2. Elevates eyelid 3. Constrictor of pupil (edinger-westphal nucleus) 4. Convergence, consensual reaction	1. Test consensual and direct pupil reaction 2. Observe size of pupil and ptosis 3. Test EOMs (extraocular movements) a. follow finger for EOMs b. accommodation
IV. Trochlear	Motor to superior oblique eye muscle	Test EOMs

The second group includes cranial nerve IX (glossopharyngeal), and cranial nerve X (vagus). These nerves are tested together by observing palatal movement and gag reflex. The ophthalmoscope is used during the cranial nerve examination to evaluate the optic disc. This is best accomplished by darkening the room and having the patient focus at a distant point on the ceiling. Table 10–1 lists the cranial nerves, functions, and methods of testing.

Motor system examination includes inspecting muscles for bulk or size, tone, and strength. The examiner moves the patient's extremities through various ranges of joint motion. Next, the muscle strength is evaluated between upper and lower extremities, while comparing the right and left sides among all muscle groups. An important determination is whether the patient is right or left handed as this may account for slight differences in strength between the right and left sides of the body. If weakness is found, the examiner determines the side (right or left) and the extremity and specific muscle groups involved. Muscle strength is graded on a 1–5 scale. On this scale, 5 indicates full normal strength. The number 1 indicates mild muscle twitch with no visible movement in the extremity.

Table 10–1. Cranial Nerve Functions and Methods of Testing—Cont'd

Nerves	Function	Function to Test
V. Trigeminal	1. Motor to masticatory muscles 2. Sensory to face	1. Ask to clench jaw and palpate masseters 2. Jaw jerk 3. Corneal reflex—wisp of cotton to cornea 4. Test for pinprick, touch, and temperature to face
VI. Abducens	Motor to lateral rectus of eye	Test EOMs—lateral movement
VII. Facial	1. Motor—muscles of facial expression 2. Sensory taste—anterior ⅔ tongue	1. Test facial muscles, close eyelids against resistance, smile, whistle 2. Taste—anterior ⅔ tongue
VIII. Acoustic	1. Equilibrium 2. Hearing	1. Check for nystagmus 2. Check hearing—whisper one ear and close the other
IX. Glossopharyngeal	Motor to pharynx	1. Test gag reflex 2. Taste—posterior ⅓ tongue
X. Vagus	Motor/sensory larynx, pharynx, heart, lung, bronchi	Test gag reflex
XI. Spinal accessory	Motor to SCM and trapezius	Test—push head against resistance; shrug shoulders against resistance
XII. Hypoglossal	Motor to tongue	1. Test—push tongue against cheeks 2. Check for atrophy and fasciculations 3. Look for deviation of tongue

The examiner tests the patient's sensation to pinprick and light touch using fingers or a pin and a Q-Tip cotton swab. Sometimes, sensory testing also includes sensation of vibration using a tuning fork, temperature sensation using tubes of hot and cold water, position sensation moving thumbs or great toes in an up and down fashion, and object recognition by placing an object, such as a key or coin, in the hand with the patient's eyes closed. Figure 10–1 shows the cutaneous areas served by the various spinal sensory nerves.

Cerebellar testing includes observation of gait and finger to nose testing. The patient is asked to walk a straight line placing one foot in front of the other in a heel to toe fashion. Balance is tested while the patient is standing still with feet together and eyes closed. It is helpful to be standing nearby in case the patient has problems with coordination or balance and requires assistance.

Testing reflexes is an important part of the examination. The examiner uses a reflex hammer and evaluates reflexes in the upper and lower extremities by comparing reflex responses between the right and left sides of the body and the amount of the reflex. Reflexes are graded on a 0–4 scale. On this scale, 0 indicates no re-

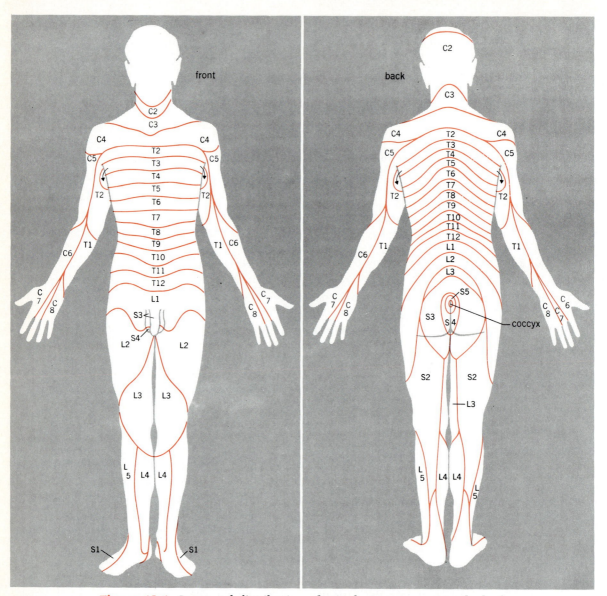

Figure 10-1. *Segmental distribution of spinal sensory nerves to the body*

sponse; 2 means a normal amount of reflex jerk; and 4 indicates an exaggerated amount of reflex. One common superficial reflex tested is the plantar reflex. This is stimulated by stroking the bottom of the foot. A normal response is to curl one's toes. If the great toe flexes upward and the other toes spread out, while this is normal for an infant, it indicates disease or damage in the cortical spinal tracts in people of other ages.

After the history and examination, the patient is informed about other diagnostic tests that may be necessary. The patient should understand the nature of the procedures, the reason for doing the tests, and any risks or complications. Some diagnostic tests require a signature of informed consent and advanced preparation before the procedure is performed.

DIAGNOSTIC TESTS

LUMBAR PUNCTURE

A **lumbar puncture** or spinal tap is a test used to obtain cerebrospinal fluid for analysis, to measure the pressure of cerebral spinal fluid, to inject substances such as contrast media, or to remove spinal fluid as a means of treatment. This procedure involves positioning the patient as shown in Figure 9–16. After positioning the patient, the area is draped and the area of skin for puncture is disinfected. A local anesthetic is given. A spinal needle is inserted between the lower lumbar vertebra until it enters the subarachnoid space containing spinal fluid. The stylet or internal part of the needle is removed and a manometer column is attached to obtain spinal fluid pressure readings. If desired, several drops of cerebrospinal fluid are placed in sterile tubes

and labeled as the first, second, or third tube collected. After all of the specimens are collected, the closing spinal fluid pressure reading is taken. Normal pressures of cerebrospinal fluid (CSF) range from 60–150 mm of water. Opening pressures are generally a little higher than closing pressures. Pressures temporarily increase if a person holds his breath or has tight muscles. Thus, a person is reminded to take slow, even breaths and to stay relaxed. Pressures ranging above 200 are considered abnormal. After the closing pressure is measured, the needle is withdrawn while gentle pressure with sterile dressing is applied to the puncture site. A Band-Aid adhesive bandage is then placed over the puncture site and is periodically checked to be certain no fluid is leaking. Because removal of spinal fluid can cause headache until the body has replenished the fluid, quiet activities and lying flat are more comfortable for the first few hours after the test.

Equipment required for this procedure includes betadine and/or alcohol for skin preparation, xylocaine or another local anesthetic, lumbar puncture tray, and sterile gloves for the physician. All equipment must be sterile.

This test is performed at the bedside or in the office. It is important to help the patient stay in the correct position and remain still during the test. Although a local anesthetic is used, there can be some discomfort during the procedure but the patient must remain still.

The CSF is examined for constituents listed in Table 10–2 or cultured for the presence and identification of microorganisms.

CISTERNAL PUNCTURE

A cisternal puncture (sis-ter′nol) is similar to the lumbar puncture except the CSF is withdrawn from the cisterna magna (just below the

Table 10-2. Composition and Characteristics of Cerebrospinal Fluid in Health and Disease

Normal Range	Conditions in Which Variations from Normal May Occur
Appearance: Clear and colorless	Hazy: with WBC count of 300–600 cells/mm^3 Turbid: with WBC count over 600 cells/mm^3 Red: fresh bleeding into the subarachnoid space, traumatic tap Xanthochromic (yellow- or amber-tinged): blood present for more than 4 hours, protein content greater than 100 mg/ 100 ml, bile pigment present
Volume: approximately 130 ml	Increased: hydrocephalus, degenerative processes in which neural tissue is decreased Decreased: temporarily following lumbar or cisternal puncture
Pressure: 60–150 mm H$_2$O	Increased: intracranial tumors, hemorrhage, hydrocephalus, meningitis, uremia Decreased: head injury, subdural hematoma, spinal tumors
Glucose: 50–80 mm/100 ml	Increased: conditions that increase blood sugar Decreased: meningitis, poliomyelitis
Protein: 20–40 mg/100 ml	Increased: meningitis, central nervous system syphilis, cerebral hemorrhage, cerebral thrombosis, paralysis agitans, dementia praecox, encephalitis, poliomyelitis

From Shirley R. Burke, *The Composition and Function of Body Fluids*, 2nd ed. (St. Louis: The C. V. Mosby Co., 1980).

occipital bone) using the aid of fluoroscopy. The same equipment is needed for this procedure as for the lumbar puncture. The examination, however, is done in the fluoroscopy room in X-ray.

COMPUTERIZED TOMOGRAPHY (CT SCAN)

Using X-ray radiation, **computerized tomography** is a cross-sectional view of tissues and structures that differentiates them by density. It is especially useful in following the progression of disease or improvement for those processes that involve blood, such as hematomas, hemorrhages, and brain tumors. It is less helpful in differentiating problems related to fractures or changes in or near the bone. Sometimes a con-

trast media is injected intravenously for better visualization. Occasionally, patients have allergic reactions to the contrast agent.

During the procedure, the patient lies on a sliding table with the head immobilized. An X-ray beam and detector are rotated around the head to measure densities in a series of cross-sectional scans about 5 mm apart. The computer averages the density for each point measured in the brain and makes a pictorial representation of the densities. On the scans, less dense structures like spinal fluid appear darker while more dense structures such as bone appear whiter. When a contrast media is injected, this increases the absorption in the areas where blood is found. Therefore, these areas appear whiter on the scan.

This test is used to scan the brain and spinal

cord and other areas of the body. There is no discomfort unless there is an IV injection of a contrast agent. A CT scan of the head takes approximately 20 minutes. Because of lack of cooperation or understanding, some patients may need sedation in order to remain motionless for the study. Figure 10-2 shows a normal CT scan of the brain and allows comparison with the abnormal scan of a patient with a tumor seen in Figure 10-3.

CEREBRAL ANGIOGRAM

During a cerebral **angiogram**, a contrast medium is injected into the carotid and/or vertebral arteries, and X-rays are taken to better

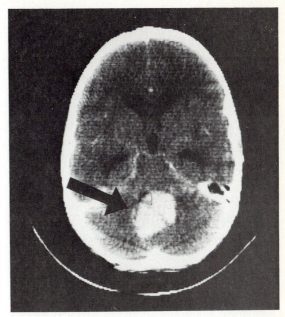

Figure 10-3. A CT scan of a patient with a tumor mass in the posterior fossa shown in the lower central portion of the film (Courtesy of Conrad S. Revak, M.D., St. Francis Hospital, Pittsburgh, PA)

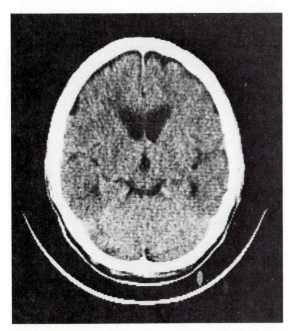

Figure 10-2. A normal CT scan of the head (Courtesy of Conrad S. Revak, M.D., St. Francis Hospital, Pittsburgh, PA)

visualize the arterial, capillary, and venous phases of the brain circulation. This helps identify problems in the cerebrovascular circulation such as arteriovenous malformation and aneurysm. Figure 14-1 shows a normal cerebral carotid angiogram or arteriogram.

This test is done in a neuroradiology suite in the hospital, takes several hours to complete, and involves specific pre- and post-procedural care. Consent is obtained by the physician.

After draping and preparation of the skin, usually the right groin, the physician punctures the femoral artery, inserting and threading the catheter through the blood vessel under fluoroscopy until it reaches the carotid artery. Occasionally the physician uses the brachial artery or a direct carotid artery puncture. When the catheter is in position, multiple injections of contrast medium are given and a rapid sequence of films are taken. When the contrast agent is injected, the patient feels hot burning sensations that quickly disappear. When all of the desired blood vessels have been studied, the catheter is removed and manual pressure is applied. This is followed by a pressure dressing on the puncture site.

After this procedure, the patient needs frequent observation and care for the first 24 hours as ordered by the physician. This usually involves neurological assessment, observation of the puncture site as well as monitoring temperature, blood pressure, pulse, and respiration. Also, the patient is monitored for any signs or symptoms of complications or allergic reactions. Usually, patients do well following this test. However, complications include hemorrhage, infection or blood clot at the puncture site, stroke, kidney failure, heart arrythmia (dysrhythmia), or high or low blood pressure.

Another method in cerebral angiography is called digital subtraction angiography. This procedure uses a similar technique but with a larger volume of contrast media injected through the veins rather than the arteries. Also, the preparation and post-procedural care differ slightly.

ELECTROENCEPHALOGRAM (EEG)

The **electroencephalogram** (e-lek″tro-en-sef a-lo-gram) or EEG is a graphic paper record of the electrical activity from the brain that is measured from the surface of the scalp. This electrical activity represents the sum of synaptic activity across large populations of neurons. The EEG is a common diagnostic test used in the management of epilepsy or seizure disorders. Also, it is used as a diagnostic test in head injury, stroke, encephalopathy, coma, psychiatric illness, and brain death determination. The study requires interpretation of the quality and characteristics of the background electrical activity and any abnormal electrical discharges that are present.

The procedure involves attaching 17 to 21 electrodes to the patient's scalp and filling them with a conductive jelly. Once the electrodes are all connected, the patient's electrical activity is transmitted to the machine for amplification, artifact filtering, and graphic display. The time needed for the test varies from 45 minutes to several hours, depending on the number of recording techniques and activation procedures used. Activation procedures may include flashing lights or photic stimulation, hyperventilation, or sleep deprivation. Once the recording is finished, all electrodes are removed and the patient should wash the hair to remove all traces of glue and gel. No risks are involved with this test. The patient should understand that the test does not read minds or deliver electrical shocks.

More sophisticated versions of EEG have evolved that combine videotape displays of the patient simultaneous with the EEG. These are usually done on patient care units or EEG recording suites. The studies last for one to several days and enable more precise differentiation of seizure activity.

EVOKED RESPONSES OR POTENTIALS

The terms **evoked response** and **evoked potential** are synonymous and indicate specific tests that measure the electrical activity in specific sensory pathways in response to external stimuli. A computer is used to average and analyze the wave forms. There are several types of evoked responses that are often referred to by their acronyms. Visual evoked responses or VERs, brainstem auditory evoked responses or BAERs, and somatosensory evoked responses or SSERs, are the main types.

Each test involves attaching several electrodes to the scalp as well as a method to deliver sensory stimuli. The sensations the patient can experience vary by study. For example, BAER involves listening to clicks through earphones; VER involves seeing a strobe light or an alternating checkerboard on a video screen; and SSER involves feeling tiny electrical currents on the forearms and shins.

These tests have no complications. However, they can be boring for the patient. Also, the patient with an altered level of consciousness or a lack of understanding may become agitated during the test and require sedation.

ELECTROMYOGRAM (EMG)

The **electromyogram** or EMG is a test that records the electrical activity associated with contraction of the skeletal muscle fibers. This test studies the muscle at rest and during voluntary muscle contraction. Another component of the EMG are nerve conduction velocities. Nerve conduction velocities measure muscle contractions evoked by electrical stimulation of a peripheral nerve. These tests help to define types of muscle disease that involve the lower motor neuron, locate nerve lesions, and quantify nerve regeneration and muscle recovery.

The procedure involves some discomfort as needle electrodes are placed into the muscles to be examined and there is a momentary prick. The study may produce dull aching in the muscle. Nerve conduction velocities are done after other recording is completed and can involve

electrical stimulation of a motor and sensory nerve. No complications are related to this test.

CT MYELOGRAM

A CT **myelogram** (mi'e-lo-gram) is used to diagnose congenital lesions affecting the vertebrae and spinal cord, spinal cord tumors, vertebral disc disease, spinal nerve root, and cord compression. The test also allows visualization of the structures surrounding the spinal cord and subarachnoid space. The technique usually involves performing a lumbar puncture and removing a small quantity of spinal fluid, injecting a contrast medium, and taking CT scans at the desired levels. Patient preparation for the test and post-procedural care differ depending on the type of contrast media used.

The oil-based contrast medium does not mix with the cerebrospinal fluid, is heavier, and can be manipulated into the study area using gravity. When the scans are completed, the substance must be removed. When an oil-based contrast is used, the patient is not permitted to eat or drink prior to the test. After the test, the patient remains flat in bed for at least 12 hours.

In comparison, if a water-based medium is used, less spinal fluid needs to be removed before the medium is injected. The contrast does not need to be removed because it is water soluble and is reabsorbed and broken down by the body. The patient is encouraged to take extra liquids both before and after the myelogram using a water-based medium. The patient remains sitting with the head of the bed elevated at least 30° for at least eight hours after the test. This position prevents the water-based medium from coming in contact with the brain, which could cause seizure activity. Headaches are less severe when a water-based contrast medium is used compared with an oil-based contrast.

The most common problem after this test is

a spinal headache, which is usually relieved by time and by drinking plenty of fluids. Mild analgesics can be used. The patient is also observed for back pain and rigidity, fever, voiding difficulties, nausea, and vomiting.

MAGNETIC RESONANCE IMAGING

Magnetic resonance imaging or MRI is a new type of imaging that does not use radiation. It is especially useful in imaging the brain and spinal cord for areas of necrotic tissue, areas of ischemia, malignancies, degenerative diseases, and problems near the bony fossae such as posterior fossa tumors. Figure 10-4 shows a coronal MRI of the head. Notice this scan differentiates the gray and white matter of the brain. Because MRI scans are safe, they are advantageous for following the progress or course of a disease in patients who require repeated scans.

During a head scan the patient lies on a sliding table with a shield placed around the neck and shoulders. The table slides into the strong magnetic field. A computer processes the measurements taken during the study and presents them in a cross-sectional picture. An MRI of the head takes about 45 minutes. Patients report that the scan is boring, that it is difficult to remain motionless throughout the study, and that they may feel claustrophobic and confined. Some patients may need sedation in order to stay motionless and tolerate the study.

No risks are involved with the study. However, patients need to be screened carefully for any contraindications to the study such as ferromagnetic objects that could be moved or affected by the strong magnetic field. Patients who have electronic devices or implants, pacemakers, metal vascular clips, metal prostheses used in joint replacements, bone pins, plates, and screws, artificial heart valves, and cerebral surgical clips are contraindicated from having the scan. Most institutions have a specific screening tool used to evaluate patients.

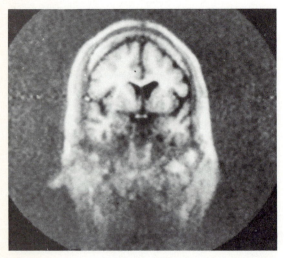

Figure 10-4. A normal magnetic resonance imaging (MRI) scan of the head

GENERAL NEUROLOGIC PROBLEMS

BEHAVIORAL RESPONSES

Many factors can affect the behavior of a person with a neurological disease or disorder. The process the patient follows from initial symptoms to examination, tests, diagnosis, and treatment may create various concerns, fears, worries, and anxieties. The person may feel helpless, overwhelmed, embarrassed, disfigured, angry, or depressed. The person may be struggling to cope with sudden changes such as paralysis and difficulty speaking and may be sensitive about other people's perceptions.

It is important to treat the person with respect and to listen to concerns. Questions should be answered honestly. If requests or questions cannot be answered, the fact that you have taken time to listen implies understanding and a caring and helpful attitude. Patients may forget instructions and may need to have instructions repeated in a simple and direct manner. It is not helpful and may actually aggravate the situation to scold, ignore, or make false statements. Although such statements may be intended to help, instead they indicate that you do not understand the situation and are of no help in dealing with the problem.

Patients who are in pain, mildly confused, or lacking adequate oxygen, may be apprehensive. The apprehension may be severe enough to cause serious problems with behavior. Clearly, the remedy for apprehension related to these problems is correcting the underlying cause. The cause of the apprehension may be difficult to identify. It is important to maintain a quiet presence, stay with the patient, and summon more experienced staff to assess the situation and provide further guidance if problems arise.

DELIRIUM

Delirium is a state of confusion and restlessness caused by various factors affecting the memory and thought processes of the brain. It may be temporary and reversible, intermittent, or permanent. The delirious patient may be disoriented as to time, place, person, or situation, and may have illusions or hallucinations. An illusion is an inaccurate interpretation of some stimuli in the environment. Hallucinations consist of hearing, seeing, or feeling things that do not exist.

The delirious patient lacks effective memory and judgment, which can produce erratic behavior and restlessness. The main concerns are to ensure safety and keep additional confusing stimuli to a minimum. Necessary instructions should come from one person and should be brief and simple. The patient may need frequent reminders of the situation, expectations, and orientation to you.

For safety, it is best to have someone with the patient at all times to observe and direct him. If this is not adequate or possible, physical restraints may be necessary. However, these may serve to increase the behavioral agitation. Judgment must be exercised by those responsible for the patient's care. Care must be used so the physical restraints do not harm the patient.

SEIZURES

Seizures result from abnormal patterns of electrical activity in the brain. There are many different causes of seizures, such as infections of the central nervous system, head injury, or epilepsy. Seizures can also result from temporary conditions, such as electrolyte imbalances, high fevers, or a sudden blow to the head. Seizure activity can be manifested through altered responses to environment, alteration in movements, and/or alteration in sensations.

Regardless of the cause, the most important aspect of care during a seizure is to stay with the patient, make careful observations, and prevent any injuries. Accurate observations are of great value to the physician in identifying the type of seizure and the underlying cause. Try to remember how the seizure first began. It may have started with a change in the patient's response to you or what was happening at the time. It may have begun with a blank stare or a loss of consciousness. If there was movement, where did it start first or did it appear to involve both sides of the body at once. Additionally, can the patient tell you anything about the seizure? Was the patient aware that a seizure had just occurred? Did the patient sense any warning prior to the seizure? What was the patient like after the seizure? After witnessing a seizure, try to remember and write down your observations in chronological order. Try to remember how it may or may not have involved responsiveness, consciousness, movements, or sensation.

Preventing injuries during a seizure requires common sense. Stay with the patient and do not panic. If the patient is not in danger of any injury, there is little you need to do. You must not attempt to restrain the movements of a patient having a seizure since it is not possible to stop a seizure. Attempting to do so could cause injuries. If the patient has stiffening or jerky movements or has fallen, help the patient to lie on the side and place something soft under the head. After the seizure, the patient should be rolled on the side with the head tipped toward the floor to allow drainage of saliva and prevent choking. If movements cause the patient to strike something, try moving the patient or the object to prevent injury. Do not place anything in the mouth because this may injure the teeth or gums. It is impossible to swallow the tongue. If swallowing or breathing is affected during the seizure, it will return to normal afterwards. As the patient starts to awaken from the seizure, let him know a seizure occurred and that everything is okay. Gradually reorient the patient to the surroundings. Share your observations with the patient or with other health care providers.

There are many different types of seizures. A seizure is classified or named according to characteristics of electrical activity in the brain together with clinical observations. Seizures may begin and end suddenly or gradually. They catch us by surprise and can appear frightening if we do not understand what is happening. Remember that the person does not have control over what happens during the seizure and that most seizures are self-limiting, ending within several minutes. If the seizure has not stopped within several minutes, stay with the patient but summon emergency help immediately.

INCREASED INTRACRANIAL PRESSURE

Since the cranial contents (brain, blood, and cerebrospinal fluid) are contained within a nonexpandable skull, any increase in the volume of one component results in an **increase in intracranial pressure**. Many different types of neurological problems (head injury, brain tumors, central nervous system infections, cerebrovascular accidents, or cerebral edema) may cause an increase in the intracranial pressure.

The signs and symptoms of increased intracranial pressure include changes in the level of consciousness. The person may become progressively more drowsy, eventually unconscious, or confused. Persistent headache and vomiting are common symptoms of increased intracranial pressure. There may be enlargement in the pupil size and a more sluggish reaction to light, affecting one or both pupils (see Figure 10–5). Changes in blood pressure, pulse, and respiration may occur if the increased intracranial pressure is not treated. Changes in blood pressure, pulse, and respiration are late signs of increased intracranial pressure and occur after other signs and symptoms have been present. Other symptoms of increased intracranial pressure may be a loss of certain gazes in the eye movements and decreases in motor strength or muscle tone.

Once increased intracranial pressure is diagnosed, it requires urgent medical and/or surgical treatment to avoid brain herniation and death.

COMA

There are many causes of coma. Coma is evident by a loss of consciousness; the patient lacks meaningful, purposeful responses to all stimuli. Comatose patients are completely dependent on health care providers. In providing any care or services to these patients, you must take on the responsibility of their special senses to protect

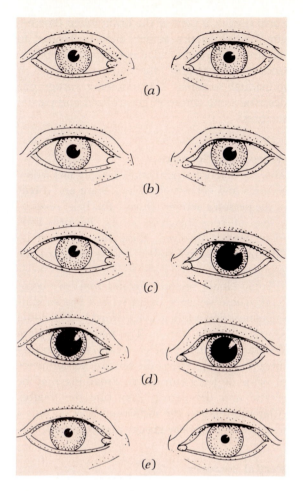

Figure 10-5. Observation of pupil size and reaction to light can indicate different types of brain damage. (a) Normal pupils. (b) Moderately dilated pupils that react sluggishly to light may indicate increased intracranial pressure. (c) When a pupil of normal size reacts normally to light and the other dilated pupil reacts sluggishly to light there is increased pressure on the left oculomotor nerve. (d) These dilated pupils are nonreactive, indicating progressive and severe damage. (e) Constricted pupils that react sluggishly or not at all may indicate damage to the pons.

them from injury and provide care. For example, they cannot sense that they are lying on a bent wrist and could injure it. The health care provider must take responsibility to prevent injury for the patient and reposition the arm.

We do not know whether comatose patients can hear or understand what is said. Therefore, never say anything in the presence of a comatose patient that would be inappropriate to say if the patient were conscious. Dignity and respect are always important, regardless of the patient's condition.

SPECIFIC NEUROLOGIC PROBLEMS

CEREBROVASCULAR ACCIDENT

A **cerebrovascular accident** or CVA (commonly termed a stroke) is caused by vascular damage within the brain as a result of a thrombus, embolus, or hemorrhage. The results of the damage depend on the cause and the area of brain that becomes affected. The patient may experience confusion, change in thinking or personality, weakness or paralysis in a part of the body (opposite side of the damaged brain area), change in vision, difficulty with speaking, understanding speech, or swallowing. A CVA may rob the person of various normal functions, which can be devastating for the patient and the family. The degree of recovery varies from patient to patient according to many factors.

Approximately one-third of CVA patients have a warning attack prior to the CVA. This is called a transient ischemic attack or TIA. This is a temporary loss of neurological function that lasts less than 24 hours. There is full recovery from this. The TIA may consist of neurological symptoms similar to CVA. A patient having a TIA must seek prompt medical attention for evaluation and treatment to help prevent a stroke. Several risk factors increase the risk of CVA, including hypertension, smoking, previous transient ischemic attack, obesity, hyperlipidemia, and a family history of CVA. Patients with atherosclerosis, diabetes mellitus, and heart disease are also at increased risk for developing CVA. Prevention of CVA involves reducing or eliminating those risk factors that we can control.

Medical treatment of CVA combines antihypertensive medications, controlling cardiac arrhythmias, anticoagulation therapy, and platelet anti-aggregation medication. Surgical treatment is used in a small number of cases. This would include carotid endarterectomy when the carotid artery is more than 70% blocked. Sometimes vascular bypass surgery is done to augment cerebral blood flow by using other blood vessels to supply blood to the damaged area.

EPILEPSY

Epilepsy is a disorder of the brain characterized by repeated seizures. For the majority of people with epilepsy, the cause is unknown. In some people, the cause may be related to a specific area of damage following head injury or CVA. While there is no treatment for the causes of epilepsy, there are anti-epileptic drugs that suppress or control the seizures. The medication must be taken daily to keep the blood level consistent so as to prevent seizures. The dosage of medication is adjusted until maximum seizure control is obtained with a minimal amount of drug side effects. Surgical treatment may be indicated for some people if treatment with anti-epileptic drugs has failed and seizures are disabling or debilitating.

Seizures are classified according to whether they are generalized or partial at the onset. Generalized seizures involve the entire brain at the onset or beginning of the seizure. Partial sei-

zures involve a part of the brain when they begin. Partial seizure activity may be limited to one area or spread to adjacent areas of the brain. Under each category, there are many types of individual seizures. The following paragraphs describe some common generalized and partial seizures.

Generalized Seizures

Absence seizures (petit mal) usually last a few seconds and consist of a blank stare and a halt in the person's activity. During this brief seizure, a loss of consciousness occurs. Because little movement is involved, these seizures may be difficult to observe unless one is aware of the problem.

Tonic clonic seizures (grand mal) are common. These seizures begin with a loss of consciousness and a fall, accompanied by a startling sound from the person. The person may have stiffening in the muscles followed by jerking muscle activity. During the seizure, incontinence of urine or feces can occur. Breathing may be erratic and the person may bite the tongue. After the seizure, the individual may go into a deep sleep or appear groggy and confused.

Partial Seizures

Simple partial seizures (jacksonian seizure) consist of a seizure that starts with movement in a part of the body and then spreads to adjacent areas. The person is usually fully conscious during this seizure but does not have control over the movements. A complex partial seizure (psychomotor or temporal lobe seizure) consists of a seizure that involves partial impairment of responsiveness. That is, the person appears conscious but does not respond appropriately to the environment. This seizure often involves automatisms or repetitive, semi-purposeful, patterned movements, such as lip smacking or picking at clothing. Although it may seem logical to shout at, shake, or restrain the person, this may cause confusion and agitation. It will not stop the seizure activity in the brain. It is better to stand by and observe. If possible harm is nearby, gently guide the person away from it.

When working with a patient who has a history of epilepsy or a seizure disorder, know what type of seizure to expect. If this information is not available, ask the patient or another health care provider for a specific description of what happens. This will aid in seizure recognition and in efforts to provide the most appropriate first aid. Again, seizures are usually self-limited, not lasting longer than several minutes. If the person's seizure lasts longer than this, seek emergency assistance.

HEAD INJURY

Seventy per cent of fatal accidents involve head injury. The causes of head injury include vehicular accidents, sports related injury, alcohol or drug ingestion and related accidents, violent acts such as shooting or knifing, and falls. The damage that results from head injury includes fractures of the skull, increased intracranial pressure, damage to delicate brain tissue and blood vessels, and swelling or edema that occurs as part of the head injury. Skull fractures may also damage cranial nerves, causing permanent loss of function. The severity of the injury depends on many factors including the type of injury, the patient's age and general health, the degree of brain damage, how quickly the person begins medical treatment, and the type of treatment.

Immediately after a head injury, a patient should be treated as though there also is a fracture in the spine until it is proven otherwise. The head, neck, and spine should be kept immobile and in a neutral position until an immobilizing support can be placed under the head and back. No other movement should be permitted until an ambulance and experienced help are available.

Scalp injuries are common to most head injuries. Scalp lacerations are likely to bleed profusely. At the scene of an accident, the wound should be covered with the cleanest material available, and bleeding controlled with pressure to the scalp. Bleeding from the nose and ears after a head injury suggests a skull fracture. A watery discharge from the nose or ears is likely to be cerebrospinal fluid and may indicate skull fracture and other more extensive damage. Wound infections are common, and most people are treated with antibiotics.

Skull fractures are associated with damage to nearby blood vessels, cranial nerves, and tissue. If the skull fracture is depressed and pressing on the brain, this must be surgically treated. Otherwise, skull fractures must heal on their own.

A concussion consists of a brief loss of consciousness from which there is total recovery. The person may have amnesia (a loss of memory) during the trauma or for a brief period following the trauma.

A contusion is characterized by edema or swelling and capillary hemorrhages in the area of damage. There is usually a loss of consciousness for a longer period. The amount of damage depends on the area and the severity of the injury. The contusion can occur at the site of the impact and/or at an area opposite the point of impact.

Patients with a head injury may have headaches afterward. They are often given analgesics, but stronger narcotic medications are usually avoided. This avoids the sedating effect of medications interfering with assessment of alertness and level of consciousness.

After a head injury, a **hematoma** (he″mah-to′mah) may occur, especially if contusion or fracture is present. A hematoma is a collection of blood between the meninges and the skull.

The bleeding is arterial or venous with the accumulated blood pressing on the brain disturbing vital areas of function and also causing increased intracranial pressure. The treatment is usually surgery to control the bleeding and remove the clot or blood. An epidural hematoma results from arterial bleeding. Symptoms of increased intracranial pressure occur rapidly. A subdural hematoma results from venous bleeding and symptoms develop gradually over several days.

A subarachnoid hemorrhage is bleeding into the meninges and ventricular system containing cerebrospinal fluid. This causes a sudden onset of severe headache, restlessness, agitation, and loss of consciousness. An intracerebral hemorrhage arises from bleeding deep within the brain causing increased intracranial pressure with rapidly occurring symptoms. Approximately one-half of patients with intracerebral hemorrhage die suddenly. Treatment includes supportive treatment to minimize the effect of blood in the brain causing edema and vasospasm of the other blood vessels, and to ensure adequate blood flow to the other areas of the brain.

Treatment varies from an emergency room visit to a lengthy hospitalization, often involving months of rehabilitation. The patient may have full recovery and be able to continue with regular activities or may have varying degrees of damage necessitating major changes in way of life. Some die as a result of their injury and complications. As in CVA, the best treatment is, of course, prevention of head injury. Examples of prevention include the use of restraints and helmets in moving vehicles, abstinence or responsible use with alcohol, and avoidance of high risk behaviors. These all help reduce the risk of head injury.

After minor head injury such as concussion or contusion, the patient may be discharged after examination and the family instructed about po-

Table 10–3. Symptoms of Serious Problems Following Head Injury

If any of the following develop, return to the hospital
1. Severe headache
2. Persistent vomiting
3. Convulsions
4. Paralysis or trouble walking
5. Clear or bloody fluid from ears or nose
6. Unequal pupils
7. Pupils that do not get smaller in a bright light
8. Increasing fever
9. Unusual drowsiness or confusion

tential signs and symptoms of complications. It is advisable that these instructions be written down and explained to the family. If the patient develops any symptoms, a physician needs to be seen for further evaluation. Problems that indicate further evaluation are listed in Table 10–3.

SPINAL CORD TRAUMA

The incidence of acute spinal cord injury in the United States each year has been conservatively estimated at 12,000 people. Another 4,000 die before ever reaching the hospital after the injury. Yearly, approximately 6,000 die from automobile accidents that cause high cervical fracture. One-third of these deaths result from not using seat belts. Spinal cord trauma has an unequal distribution between the sexes with males affected four times more frequently than females. The peak age for spinal cord trauma is 24 years for males and 25 to 29 years for females. In summary, spinal cord trauma greatly affects people and has a tremendous impact on their lives. The economic impacts of hospital care are approximately $81,000 per year for a quadriplegic and $67,000 per year for a paraplegic. The cost to provide care for these individuals is estimated at $2.4 billion annually.

The main causes of spinal cord trauma include vehicular accidents, with approximately a 50% mortality rate. Falls, sports injuries, and gunshot wounds are other causes. The use of alcohol or other substances also can play a role in the injury. Again, the most effective treatment is prevention.

Spinal cord injuries are similar to head injuries. Spinal cord injuries range from concussion, contusion, and physical tears or lacerations to transections where there has been complete or incomplete severing of the cord. Because the spinal cord is located in a small space and has a limited blood supply, great damage can arise from what appears to be a mild injury. If the spinal cord has been incompletely transected or damaged, there is a temporary suppression of reflexes below the level of the injury that may last from days to months. As the period of spinal shock begins to resolve, involuntary spastic movements may appear and deep tendon and perianal reflexes return. When the spinal cord has been completely transected, the initial response of spinal shock usually includes instability in blood pressure with cervical and upper thoracic injuries. Immediately after the injury in complete transection, there can be unpredictable preservation of the innervation below the level of the injury for specific types of sensation, perspiration, and bowel and bladder function. The long term effects of complete spinal cord transection include a flaccid and total paralysis of all skeletal muscles below the level of the injury. There is a loss of all spinal reflexes and sensation.

The rehabilitation potential following spinal cord injury depends on the level and extent of spinal cord damage. The cord is not capable of regeneration. Early intervention includes immobilization of the spine and intravenous administration of a high dose steroid to minimize spinal cord edema and swelling. Surgical decompression allows extra space for the swollen cord to minimize cellular damage. Surgical treatment may focus on stabilization of the spine to minimize further trauma.

Table 10–4 shows some functional activities for various spinal cord injuries. While this table may provide general information, it will not tell you about a specific individual. Patients can have a wide variety of incomplete injuries and are the best resource as to what they can and cannot do. Generally, patients with injuries between C1 and C4 require assisted ventilation for breathing. A C8 spinal cord injury is generally the dividing line between quadriplegia and paraplegia.

Patients with a spinal cord injury at T6 or above have the potential to develop problems with autonomic nervous system dysfunction, also known as autonomic hyperreflexia or dysreflexia. This results from an increased autonomic response usually to a noxious stimulus below the level of the injury. The noxious stimuli might include a distended bladder, bowel, or decubitus ulcer.

During dysreflexia, the patient may have a sudden severe headache as the blood pressure rises rapidly. The patient may appear flushed in the face and sweat above the level of the injury.

During dysreflexia, after a noxious stimulus, sensory receptors send afferent impulses to the cord and up to the level of the injury. The impulses are blocked because of the damage, and a reflex arteriolar spasm produced by way of a sympathetic ganglia occurs. This causes vasoconstriction in the blood vessels below the injury with an immediate increase in the blood pressure. The patient has a headache that develops as the blood pressure rises. In response, the vasomotor center in the brain sends parasympathetic impulses by way of the vagus in an attempt to lower the blood pressure. Vasodilatation results, causing the patient to become flushed and sweat profusely above the level of the injury.

The treatment for dysreflexia is prompt rec-

TABLE 10–4. General Guide of Spinal Cord Injury Level and Functional Abilities or Resulting Disability

C1-2-3	Mechanical ventilation, unable to turn head
C4	Able to shake head yes/no, still requires assistive ventilation as this level innervates the phrenic nerve
C5	Can use a rachet splint, allows for independent feeding, brushing teeth, and driving an electric wheel chair, otherwise dependent for other care needs, cannot do chair pushups
C6	Wears splints for finger motion, has wrist extension, can do transfers with special equipment, able to do chair pushups, can drive a car
C7	Should not need any adaptive devices for upper extremities, can transfer without any special equipment, able to put own wheelchair into a vehicle
C8	Has wrist flexion, able to move first three digits of hand, dividing line between quadriplegia and paraplegia
T1	Has excellent upper extremity function, has very poor balance for standing or sitting
L2	Wears long leg braces and uses crutches
L3	Wears short leg braces and uses crutches
L4-5	Probably able to walk without crutches

ognition of the problem and immediate treatment to lower the patient's blood pressure and identify and relieve the noxious stimulus. The patient needs to be closely observed and have blood pressure carefully monitored until the symptoms have subsided.

Often, patients with spinal cord injuries have dysfunction with bowel and bladder elimination. Individualized bowel and/or bladder management programs are instituted depending on the individual. Bladder management programs may include intermittent urinary catheterization every four, six, or eight hours to drain the bladder. The goal is to prevent over-distention of the bladder and retention of urine that can lead to urinary tract infection. For some patients, mechanical methods such as Credé's or manual pressure over the bladder area may be used to stimulate voiding. Indwelling urinary catheters are avoided if at all possible because of the frequency of recurrent infections. Bowel management programs may include digital stimulation, suppositories, or enemas on a continual basis in efforts to develop consistent elimination.

Other problems are related to recurring urinary complications such as bladder and kidney infections, which are discussed in more detail in Chapter 20. Those with cervical injuries may be more prone to developing pneumonia and other respiratory problems. All patients experience problems related to immobility and skin integrity. These issues are discussed in Chapter 3. While rehabilitation following spinal cord injury is lengthy and costly, it provides the best hope of maximizing recovery from the injury.

CENTRAL NERVOUS SYSTEM INFECTIONS

Meningitis (men-in-ji'tis) is an inflammation and/or infection of the meninges of the brain and spinal cord that is sudden in onset. It is caused by various organisms including bacteria, viruses, and fungi. Common causative organisms are the pneumococcus, streptococcus, staphylococcus, and meningococcus bacteria.

The patient has a severe headache, high fever, stiffness and pain in the neck, nausea, and vomiting. If untreated the patient gradually becomes comatose and seizures can occur. Diagnosis includes spinal tap to examine and culture the cerebrospinal fluid. The patient is started on several antibiotics, and these are fine-tuned after antibiotic sensitivities are determined for the offending organism. The patient receives supportive care to provide comfort and prevent complications.

Encephalitis (en"sef-ah-li′tis) is an inflammation and/or infection of the brain. It is caused by the same organisms that cause meningitis but may also be caused by other substances such as lead or arsenic. Viral encephalitis is the most common type. The symptoms develop several weeks after a primary infection and include headache, fever, vomiting, confusion, personality changes, and seizures. The patient may also have problems with speech, coordination, and motor control. The patient may become comatose and have deterioration in respirations. Encephalitis has a high mortality rate of 70% if patients are untreated. Patients who have coma, increased intracranial pressure, hemiparesis, and frequent seizures have the highest mortality rate.

Treatment of viral encephalitis includes giving intravenous acyclovir as early as possible. Supportive care focuses on managing and treating increased intracranial pressure, controlling seizures, and preventing other complications of immobility, and a prolonged hospitalization. In general, the prognosis is more guarded for encephalitis.

POLIOMYELITIS

Poliomyelitis is a viral disease that has declined since polio vaccines became available. The virus attacks the anterior horn of the spinal cord, causing a flaccid paralysis to the skeletal muscles. The onset is acute with fever, headache, vomiting, neck stiffness, and pain in the back and limbs. This may last two to four days and then subside completely and is called non-paralytic poliomyelitis. In a few cases, after the non-paralytic period, there is a 48-hour interval and then the paralytic stage begins with pain and extreme tenderness in various muscles. Following this, the muscles become rapidly weak or paralyzed. When respiratory and throat muscles become involved, swallowing, coughing, and breathing become impossible. Immediate intubation and mechanical ventilation are required. When the acute stage subsides, many muscles may recover completely but others may waste and atrophy. Considerable supportive care and physical therapy are needed to promote the best recovery from poliomyelitis.

HYDROCEPHALUS

Hydrocephalus (hi-dro-sef′ah-lus) occurs when there is an imbalance between cerebrospinal fluid (CSF) production and reabsorption with resulting accumulation of CSF. If the CSF cannot circulate or be reabsorbed, it accumulates within the ventricles, enlarging them and squeezing the soft brain tissue. If this occurs in an infant, the fontanels begin to bulge, the space between the cranial sutures widens, and the head enlarges to accommodate the increased volume of CSF. In an older child or adult, where soft spots are closed and cranial sutures have fused, signs include headache, nausea, and vomiting, changes in vision, and decrease in level of consciousness as intracranial pressure increases. If untreated, brain herniation and death result.

The causes of hydrocephalus fall into two groups: congenital and acquired. Congenital causes include developmental defects or anomalies that may obstruct or compromise the circulation of spinal fluid. Acquired causes of hydrocephalus include neoplasms or tumors that may directly or indirectly cause a blockage in the system. Infections such as meningitis are common causes of hydrocephalus. During meningitis, the increased cells and protein in the CSF can plug or block the arachnoid villi where the CSF is reabsorbed. Another acquired cause of hydrocephalus is blood in the ventricular system because of intraventricular hemorrhage or subarachnoid hemorrhage. The blood also plugs the arachnoid villi, the site of CSF reabsorption, thus causing an accumulation of CSF and subsequent hydrocephalus.

Hydrocephalus is diagnosed using CT or MRI scan. Ventricles appear enlarged and obstruction may be seen. The usual treatment for hydrocephalus is a surgical procedure in which a flexible tube called a shunt is placed. A shunt diverts spinal fluid from the ventricle to another area of the body to bypass an obstruction in the system or to augment the rate of spinal fluid drainage. The most common shunt is the ventriculoperitoneal shunt. This diverts spinal fluid from the lateral ventricle into the peritoneal cavity. A valve within the shunt system regulates the pressure at which the cerebrospinal fluid is allowed to flow into the peritoneum and prevents a backward flow of CSF. Other types of shunts include ventriculoatrial and lumboperitoneal shunts.

After the person has recovered from shunt surgery, there are no particular restrictions in daily activities. The patient usually resumes regular medical care with periodic neurosurgical follow up. The implanted shunt systems used to control hydrocephalus are made to perform reliably over a long period. For some patients, surgical revisions in the shunt may be necessary. Two common complications include shunt malfunction, which requires a second surgery or revision to correct the problem, and shunt infection, which also requires removal of the infected shunt, antibiotic treatment, and a shunt replacement.

MUSCULAR DYSTROPHY

Muscular dystrophy is not a single disease but a group of muscle-destroying disorders that vary in hereditary pattern, age of onset, the muscles attacked, and the rate of progression. As a general rule, it is often true that the earlier clinical symptoms appear, the more rapid is the progression of the disease. Few children who develop muscular dystrophy live a normal lifespan. Symptoms are characterized by weakness in the muscles and muscle wasting, with an otherwise normal nervous system. No treatment has been found to correct the underlying pathology or to arrest the progression of the disease. As muscles deteriorate, the patient becomes weaker and more helpless, unable to perform simple daily activities. Death usually results from recurrent infections and eventual respiratory failure. Physical therapy is often prescribed along with an individualized program of exercises after diagnosis to keep healthy muscles functioning and delay contractures.

PARKINSON'S DISEASE

Parkinson's disease is a slow, progressive disease that affects a small area of cells in the middle part of the brain called the basal ganglia. These cells gradually degenerate and die. Their loss produces a reduction in a vital neurotransmitter called dopamine, causing symptoms that include tremor, stiffness in the muscles (rigidity), loss of balance (postural dysfunction), and slowness of movement (bradykinesia). Patients with Parkinson's may have a mask-like facial expression, a slow shuffling gait, a stooped posture, a tendency to keep the arms fixed at the sides when walking, and difficulty with fine hand movements. The condition may affect one or both sides of the body.

The cause of Parkinson's disease remains a mystery. It is possible to develop a secondary form of Parkinson's that can be caused by drugs that interfere with the dopamine in the brain. These drugs may include some tranquilizers (haloperidol, thioridazine, or chlorpromazine) and high blood pressure drugs that contain reserpine. There are no medical or surgical treatments to cure or prevent the disease. Methods of treatment involve medications, rehabilitative measures like physical, occupational, and speech therapy, and consistent home exercise and activity programs.

The most desirable treatment for Parkinson's would be to increase the amount of dopamine in special areas of the brain. However, this is not possible. A cellular barrier between the blood and brain prevents dopamine from reaching brain cells unless it is manufactured in the brain itself. The medications used to treat Parkinson's contain the precursors, L-dopa, which enter the brain and are converted to dopamine. The medications must be taken daily as prescribed and require individualization in dose. Other medications used include anticholinergic drugs and drugs that improve the patient's ability to increase the production of dopamine. The anticholinergic drugs decrease the presence of acetylcholine, another neurotransmitter, whose effects are the opposite of dopamine. While several types of surgical procedures are helpful for a few patients, most treatment focuses on appropriate use of medication, physical therapy, and an active lifestyle.

MYASTHENIA GRAVIS

Myasthenia gravis (mi″as-the′ne-ah grav′-is) is an uncommon disease characterized by an abnormal fatigability of those muscles under voluntary control. This fatigability becomes worse by repeated use of the muscles and is repaired by rest and certain medications. The onset is gradual and the course varies greatly from one patient to another. Research has focused on myasthenia being a process of an autoimmune attack on the acetylcholine receptor site leading to skeletal muscles in the body.

In most patients the disease begins gradually with symptoms of double vision and drooping of one or both eyelids. It may progress to involve muscles of speech, chewing and swallowing, limb muscles, and respiratory muscles. In most patients, the symptoms are least evident on rising in the morning and grow worse with effort and as the day proceeds. Myasthenia is grouped into two main types: ocular and generalized. In ocular myasthenia, there is involvement of eye muscles only and symptoms tend to be mild. In generalized myasthenia, the severity can range from mild with good response to drug therapy and lack of respiratory muscle involvement to severe with rapid onset and progression of cranial nerve and skeletal muscle weakness with early respiratory muscle involvement. This last group may have frequent emergency crises, poorer response to drug therapy, poor prognosis, and high mortality rate. For all patients with myasthenia, ups and downs or remissions and exacerbations in the symptoms are common. Certain factors such as emotional crises, febrile illness, and pregnancy aggravate the symptoms.

The diagnosis is based on the clinical history and electromyographic studies that show characteristic muscle fiber degeneration. Other tests used for diagnosis include injecting a short-acting, anti-cholinesterase medication called edrophonium chloride or Tensilon. The patient is exercised until myasthenic symptoms appear, and Tensilon is then injected. If the patient has myasthenia, clear improvement within seconds after injection of the drug results. The drug clears the body within minutes. A new diagnostic test involves examining blood for the presence of acetylcholine receptor antibodies.

The treatment focuses on medications to treat the symptoms and normalize, at least partially, the acetylcholine receptor sites at the muscle junction. These drugs, called anticholinesterases, work to prolong the activity and effect of acetylcholine by decreasing the enzyme that breaks it down. This increases the time that acetylcholine acts at a receptor site on the muscle. Drugs such as neostigmine, Tensilon, mestinon, and mytelase all work in this fashion.

Other types of treatment include immunosuppressive therapy with drugs such as prednisone, cyclosporin, and imuran, although these are usually reserved for patients who have experienced severe symptoms such as myasthenia crisis with respiratory involvement. Plasmapheresis is another technique that has been added since the discovery of the receptor antibodies. This treatment involves exchanging the patients plasma to reduce the circulating antibody levels, thus reducing many myasthenic symptoms. Plasmapheresis can apparently decrease the antibody level by as much as 50% after only a few treatments. It has not led to a permanent cure, however.

Another form of treatment includes thymectomy. The role of the thymus gland with respect to immunity is not well understood. The patient with myasthenia gravis has a higher incidence of thymus cancer and other types of cancer, and thymectomy appears to have beneficial results in significantly reducing the subsequent occurrence of cancer.

Patients with myasthenia gravis must become well educated about the disease and its treatment. The drugs taken to treat the symptoms must be carefully managed. The patient must learn to monitor symptoms so as to play an active role with the physician in regulating the medications.

MULTIPLE SCLEROSIS

Multiple sclerosis is a demyelinating disease where patches of demyelinization or plaques develop in parts of the spinal cord, cerebellum, brain stem, cerebral hemispheres, or optic pathways. The peripheral nerves are not affected by this demyelinating process. Over time, the plaques can flare up, take weeks or months to settle down, and after an interval of months or years, may flare up again in another site. Scar tissue or gliosis forms in those places where the myelin has been destroyed. After several attacks, the process of gliosis causes permanent sclerosis and damage with resulting loss of function. The patient with multiple sclerosis has a history of intermittent neurological dysfunction that remits and then recurs over time. This may cause progressive disturbances in vision, speech, mental status, and ability to move. In the early stages of the disease, the patient may have periods of remission and exacerbation with mild symptoms. In the later stages, the patient may become severely handicapped.

There is no single diagnostic test for multiple sclerosis. Patients often undergo many diagnostic tests including CT scan, MRI scan, lumbar puncture for cerebrospinal fluid analysis, and visual evoked potentials. The diagnosis is based on clinical symptoms, evidence of plaques on MRI scan, prolonged latency on visual evoked potentials, elevated gamma globulin, and the presence of oligoclonal bands in the cerebrospinal fluid.

Although much research is being done concerning the cause and treatment of multiple sclerosis, at present the only treatment is symptomatic and supportive. Physical and occupational therapy help the patient remain independent and active as long as possible. Patients are encouraged to get plenty of rest, avoid situations that are emotionally upsetting, and eat a nourishing diet.

GUILLAIN–BARRÉ SYNDROME

Guillain–Barré (gil–an bar′a) **syndrome** is characterized by an abrupt onset of an ascending polyneuropathy. There is inflammation and demyelination in the peripheral nerves. The cause of the disease is not well understood but may represent one of the autoimmune diseases where the patient's own body defenses cause nerve sheath damage.

The syndrome develops rapidly, often after a few weeks of a vague febrile illness, usually an upper respiratory infection. The patient has symptoms of polyneuritis consisting of numbness, pins and needles, and burning feelings in the fingers, hands, toes, and feet. They begin to have a motor weakness or paralysis that is usually symmetrical and begins in the lower extremities and ascends to involve the trunk, upper limbs, and cranial nerves. Respiratory involvement may be seen about 7 to 12 days after the onset of the disease and may necessitate mechanical ventilatory support.

While there is no specific diagnostic test for the disease, the diagnosis is based on history, clinical symptoms, and an elevated protein in the CSF with a normal lymphocyte count.

The treatment for Guillain–Barré is supportive and symptomatic since most deaths are related to respiratory failure and complications of immobility. After two or three weeks of great disability, 75% of patients slowly make a complete recovery. Steroids may be used, although some physicians question their effectiveness. Ongoing physical and occupational therapy are useful during the recovery process.

SUMMARY QUESTIONS

1. List the main components in a neurological history and examination.
2. Describe the procedures involved for at least three neurological diagnostic tests.
3. Name at least three principles to consider when communicating with a confused or apprehensive patient.
4. Describe what to do when you are with a patient who experiences a seizure consisting of a fall with stiffening and jerky movements.
5. List at least three symptoms of increased intracranial pressure and discuss why it requires emergency treatment.
6. Discuss at least three risk factors for CVA and explain how they might be controlled for stroke prevention in a patient.
7. List three strategies to help decrease the incidence of head and spinal cord injuries.
8. Describe three causes of hydrocephalus, and explain how a shunt works.
9. Name at least three symptoms that might be seen in a patient with Parkinson's disease.
10. Discuss at least three differences between multiple sclerosis and Guillain–Barré syndrome.

KEY TERMS

angiogram

cerebrovascular accident

computerized tomography

electroencephalogram

electromyogram

encephalitis

epilepsy

evoked responses or potentials

Guillain–Barré syndrome

hematoma

hydrocephalus

intracranial pressure, increased

lumbar puncture

magnetic resonance imaging

meningitis

multiple sclerosis

muscular dystrophy

myasthenia gravis

myelogram

Parkinson's disease

seizures

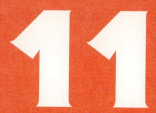

11

Sense Organs

OBJECTIVES

On completion of this chapter, you will be able to:

1. Describe the structures involved in the sensations of taste and smell.
2. Describe the structures of the outer, middle, and inner ear.
3. Explain how sound waves are converted to nerve impulses.
4. Discuss how equilibrium is maintained.
5. Describe the structure of the eye.
6. Explain the function of the canal of Schlemm.
7. Discuss how light rays are refracted.
8. Explain what is involved in the process of accommodation.
9. Discuss the general senses.

OVERVIEW

I. CHARACTERISTICS AND MECHANISMS
OF SENSATION
II. SPECIAL SENSES
   A. Taste
   B. Smell
   C. Hearing
   D. Equilibrium
   E. Vision
      1. Protection
      2. Layers of the Eyeball
      3. Focusing
      4. Visual Pathway
      5. Binocular Vision
III. GENERAL SENSES
   A. Cutaneous Senses
   B. Organic Sensations

Sensation is the result of processes taking place in the brain in response to nerve impulses from the sense receptors. The proper functioning of the sense organs is a major factor in keeping us aware of conditions in our environment as well as of the activities within our bodies. Accurate interpretation of the data from our sense organs assists us in making appropriate adjustments to environmental conditions as well as in attending to our bodily needs.

CHARACTERISTICS AND MECHANISMS OF SENSATION

Special senses are sight, hearing, equilibrium, taste, and smell. Cutaneous sensations, such as touch, heat, cold, and pain, and visceral sensations, such as hunger, nausea, and thirst, are considered general senses. For interpretation of a sensation, there must be a functioning receptor, a nerve pathway, and brain cortex. Most conventional forms of anesthesia are based on interrupting the functions of one of these structures. For example, some local anesthetics block the pathway, whereas others merely inhibit the nerve receptor. General anesthetics interfere with the ability of the cerebral cortex to interpret sensation.

The sense receptors, except those for pain, are specialized for a particular type of stimulus. The afferent pathways from sense receptors are over spinal or cranial nerves. As discussed in Chapter 9, the thalamus functions as a relay center for most afferent messages. Here, the sensory impulses are sorted and sent to the area of the brain cortex where the impulses can be interpreted. These cortical cells are prepared for the stimulation of these impulses by the reticular formation. Although we believe there are specialized centers in the brain cortex that are specific for each type of sensation, many areas of the cortex are involved in producing a meaningful sensory message.

Sensory adaptation results from prolonged stimulation of some receptors. Under these circumstances, there may be a temporary loss of irritability of the receptor. Removal of the stimulus for a short period of time will allow the receptor to resume response to the stimulus. Adaptation occurs more quickly in some receptors than in others. The olfactory receptors and those for touch and pressure are particularly subject to adaptation. We become adapted to odors, even unpleasant ones, rather quickly.

There is no sensory adaptation to the sensation of pain. You may hear the comment that someone has a high pain threshold, and the implication is that this person is not as sensitive to pain as most people. Actually, it is unlikely that there is any difference in the "pain threshold" of different people. How people demonstrate their response to pain and how it is reported to others differs, but the difference is the result of a learned pattern that has social and cultural aspects to it rather than a physiological difference.

As discussed in Chapter 9, receptors can be classified as extroceptors, enteroceptors, or proprioceptors, depending on whether they receive their stimulus from outside the body, from within the viscera, or in the joints and muscles. Receptors can also be classified according to the types of stimuli they respond to. Thermoreceptors respond to changes in temperature. Chemoreceptors respond to changes in the concentration of chemicals. Mechanoreceptors respond to mechanical changes such as changes in pressure or movement. Nociceptors (pain receptors) detect tissue damage. Photoreceptors respond to light and are found only in the eye.

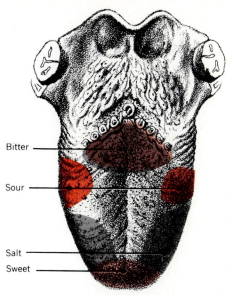

Bitter

Sour

Salt

Sweet

Figure 11-1. *Taste buds are located on the sides of the papillae of the tongue. The shaded areas indicate areas of the tongue that are the most sensitive to the different tastes as indicated.*

SPECIAL SENSES

TASTE

The receptors for the sensation of taste are the taste buds located on the sides of the papillae of the tongue. A few taste buds are located on the soft palate, epiglottis, and pharynx. Taste buds are classified according to the stimulus that causes the maximum response. There are four basic types of buds: those for bitter, sour, salt, and sweet. The taste buds serving the four sensations do not respond equally to the same degree of stimulus. Listing taste sensitivity from the greatest to the least, bitter is followed by sour, salt, and sweet.

Different areas of the tongue are more sensitive to some tastes than to others. The tip of the tongue is sensitive to sweet, the back to bitter, and the sides to sour, and both the tip and sides to salt (see Fig. 11-1). The anterior two-thirds of the tongue is innervated by a branch of the facial nerve and the posterior third by the glossopharyngeal. The vagus nerve receives impulses from the deeper recesses of the throat and pharynx.

Nerve impulses are conducted over these pathways to the taste center in the medulla. From the taste center, connections are made with the thalamus and cerebral cortex. In the cortex, impulses are interpreted as the sensation of taste. The taste sensation may stimulate the secretion of saliva and digestive juices.

To create the sensation of taste, a substance must be in solution in order to contact the receptors between the papillae of the tongue. One of the functions of saliva is to dissolve substances so that they can enter the taste pores and stimulate the receptors. The sensation of taste may be diminished if the flow of saliva is limited. Impairment of the sensation of taste can also be the result of poor oral hygiene if the papillae are covered over with a coating called **sordes** (sor′dez).

SMELL

The sensation of taste is closely related to that of smell. Odor often influences the selection of food and our enjoyment of certain dishes. For example, when you have a cold and nasal congestion, your food seems tasteless. The odor of food you like helps to initiate the flow of some digestive juices in much the same way as does taste.

The stimulus for the sensation of smell must be a gaseous substance that becomes dissolved in the fluid of the nasal chamber. The fluid stimulates the sensitive olfactory cells in the upper part of the nasal mucosa. The amount of stimulus reaching the olfactory area is greatly increased by sniffing. The pathway is the olfactory nerve and the cortical interpretation is in the temporal lobe (see Fig. 11-2).

Some fibers of the trigeminal nerve are also located in the olfactory mucous membrane. These respond to such irritating substances as ammonia or pepper and may cause sneezing, shortness of breath, or some other unpleasant sensation. It is because of this response that "smelling salts" may arouse someone who feels faint.

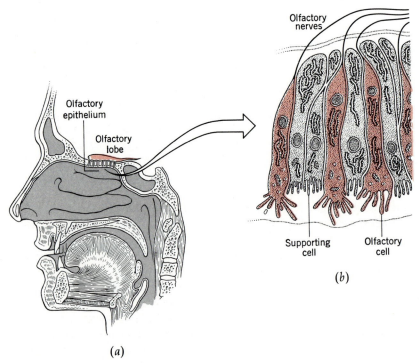

Figure 11-2. (a) Receptors for smell are located in the upper region of the nasal cavity. (b) These olfactory cells transmit the impulses over the olfactory nerve to the brain.

The olfactory receptors are easily fatigued and sensory adaptation for a specific odor can occur rapidly. The fatigue causes a loss of the ability to recognize a persistent odor, but a new odor may be detected at once.

Unlike taste, with only four stimuli recognized, there are a multitude of distinct odors. Individual odors in a mixed smell can be distinguished, and the memory for odors is very keen. People can often recall an odor that has been experienced only once before.

HEARING

There are many structures involved in the sensation of hearing. In people, the external ear, or auricle, is relatively unimportant, although it does help to funnel the sound waves into the more internal structures concerned with hearing. The external auditory or acoustic meatus is lined with skin and is directed inward, forward, and downward from the auricle to the **tympanic membrane**. There are ceruminous (se-ru'men-us) glands in this area that secrete ear wax or cerumen (se-ru'men). Although **cerumen** is a protective agent, excess amounts of it can partially obstruct the auditory canal and interfere with hearing. Excess cerumen can be removed by irrigating the canal with warm water.

The tympanic membrane vibrates in response to sound waves and transmits these vibrations into the middle ear. In the middle ear there are three small bones, the malleus, incus, and stapes (commonly called the hammer, anvil, and stirrup) that move in response to the vibrations of the tympanic membrane. These bones magnify the sound. Also in the middle ear is the opening of the **eustachian** (u-sta'ke-an) **tube**, which connects the middle ear with the nasopharynx. This tube helps equalize the pressure in the middle ear with that of the atmosphere (see Fig. 11-3). When these pressures are un-

equal, the tympanic membrane does not vibrate properly with the sound waves and there is impairment of hearing.

Because the mucous membrane of the throat is continuous with that of the middle ear, ear infections may be associated with upper respiratory infections. **Otitis** (o-ti'tis) **media**, or infection of the middle ear, may extend into the mastoid sinuses. Recall that the mastoid sinuses are air spaces that drain into the middle ear.

The inner ear, called the labyrinth, is concerned with the sensations of both hearing and equilibrium. The bony labyrinth is hollowed out of the petrous portion of the temporal bone. Parts of the bony labyrinth are the vestibule, semicircular canals, and cochlea (ko'kle-ah). The bony labyrinth is lined with a membranous labyrinth that is about the same shape. There is a small amount of fluid called perilymph (par'e-limf) between the bony and membranous labyrinths.

The movement of the malleus, incus, and stapes in response to the sound waves causes the oval window into the inner ear to move. The oval window presses against the fluid in the cochlear channel (endolymph) of the inner ear, causing ripplelike waves. These waves stimulate hair cells of the organs of Corti located on the basilar membrane within the membranous cochlea (see Fig. 11-4). The organs of Corti are the dendrites of the cochlear branch of the auditory nerve. The nerve impulses resulting from the stimulation of the organs of Corti travel to the temporal lobe of the brain where sound is interpreted.

Note that as the stapes pushes the oval window inward, there must be a corresponding outward bulge, because fluid cannot be compressed. The outward bulge is accomplished by the round window located just below the oval window.

Sound waves are vibrations of air. How loud a sound is and how high the pitch have to do

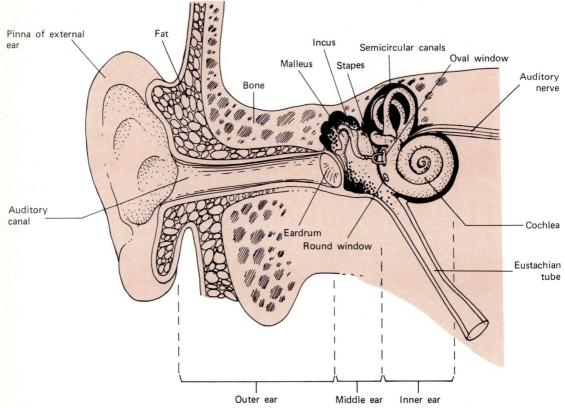

Figure 11-3. *Human ear showing the outer, middle, and inner ears and their various parts*

with the nature of the vibrations. The amplitude or loudness has to do with the force of the vibrations. This intensity of sound is usually expressed in decibels. Normal conversation is about 65 decibels (dB), a whisper is about 30, and the noise of heavy automobile traffic may reach 80 or 90 dB. People whose occupations require them to be exposed to intense sound waves should wear special ear shields to protect them from injury to the nerve cells in the inner ear.

The number of vibrations or frequency per second determines the pitch of the sound. The basilar membrane is thin and tight near the oval window. When dendrites in this region are stimulated, the tension of the basilar membrane here will result in a high frequency of vibrations and, therefore, a high pitch. At the other end, the membrane is thicker and loose; stimulation of the dendrites here will result in low-pitched sounds.

EQUILIBRIUM

The structures in the inner ear concerned with equilibrium are the semicircular canals that lie in three different planes, the utricle (u′tre-kl),

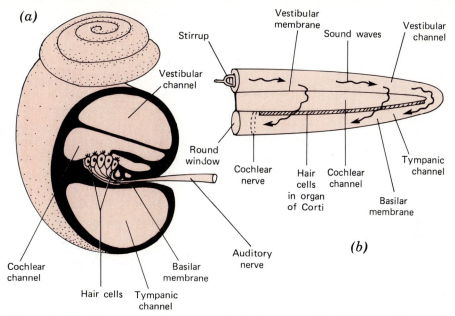

Figure 11-4. *(a) Cross section of the cochlea. Perilymph is in the vestibular and tympanic channels. Endolymph is in the cochlear channel. (b) Schematic representation shows these channels hypothetically unwound.*

and possibly the saccule (sak'yul). The utricle and saccule are membranous structures located in the vestibule of the inner ear.

In Chapter 9, we learned that the cerebellum is concerned with adjusting the position of the body so that equilibrium is maintained. The basal ganglia are involved in coordination and the reticular formation also contributes to coordination, at least for gross muscle activity.

Within the utricle are tiny hair cells that have small stones (calcium carbonate), or otoliths (o'to-liths), attached to their free surfaces. These hair cells bend backward when you begin to move forward. Their action gives you a sensation of falling off balance in a backward direction. As a result, you will bend forward to correct the sensation. A runner leans forward as he begins the race to correct the feeling of being off balance.

There are also hair cells in the membranous semicircular canals. These hair cells are stimulated by the movement of the endolymph in the canal. The result is a nerve impulse that travels over the vestibular branch of the auditory nerve and is interpreted as motion, assisting us in maintaining our balance. Any change in motion, acceleration, deceleration, or change in direction causes impulses to originate in the dendrites of the vestibular nerve.

Proprioceptors and visual receptors are also important in maintaining the sense of balance. These receptors send impulses directly to the cerebellum.

VISION

The receptors for vision are located in the retina of the eye, the pathway is over the optic or second cranial nerves, and the center for cortical localization is located in the occipital lobe of the brain.

Protection

The bony orbital cavity, formed by a union of the frontal, maxillary, zygomatic, lacrimal, sphenoid, and palatine bones, provides protection for the eyes. Also in the orbital cavity are the extrinsic muscles for movement of the eye, the lacrimal glands, and a large amount of adipose tissue (see Fig. 11-5). The adipose tissue functions as a protective cushion. Loss of the orbital fat causes the eyes to have a sunken appearance in people who have had a severe weight loss.

The lacrimal glands are a part of the lacrimal apparatus that also provides protection for the eyes. These glands are located at the upper outer angle of the eyes and secrete tears constantly to keep the cornea of the eye moist. The tears contain lysozyme (li′so-zim), a bactericidal enzyme. The cells of the cornea are living cells and must have a liquid cellular environment so they do not become cornified as the epidermis of the skin when exposed to air. The tears also wash away any particles of dust or other foreign material that may contact the eye. Normally, the tears drain into the lacrimal canals at the inner canthus (kan′thus) of the eye. From the lacrimal canal, the tears enter the lacrimal sac, then move to the nasolacrimal duct, and finally drain into the nasal cavity. With a respiratory infection, swelling of the nasal mucosa might partially obstruct this passageway and cause the eyes to water.

The eyelids or palpebrae (pal-pe′brah) form a protective movable shield in front of the eyeball. The lids are lined with a transparent mucous membrane called the **conjunctiva** (kon-junk-ti′vah). The meibomian (mi-bo′me-an) glands are sebaceous glands in the lids. These glands drain into small openings at the edge of the lid. A chalazion (kal-la′ze-on) is a small tumor that forms if the secretions accumulate in a meibomian gland. The eyelashes serve to protect the eyes from the entrance of foreign bodies. The sebaceous glands associated with the follicles of the eyelashes may become inflamed. This condition is called a hordeolum (hor-de′o-lum) or sty.

Layers of the Eyeball

The **sclera** (skla′rah), which is a dense fibrous membrane, is the outermost covering of the eyeball. The cornea is the transparent anterior part of this outer coat. The **cornea** (kor′ne-ah) contains no blood vessels and so must be nourished by the fluids that bathe its surface (see Fig. 11-6). The transparent cornea is the first medium to refract light rays as they enter the eyeball. Refraction means the bending of light rays as they pass through a medium of a different density, such as from air to the cornea.

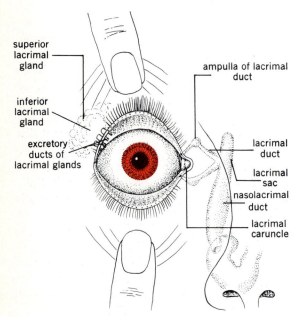

Figure 11-5. Lacrimal apparatus

superior lacrimal gland

inferior lacrimal gland

excretory ducts of lacrimal glands

ampulla of lacrimal duct

lacrimal duct

lacrimal sac

nasolacrimal duct

lacrimal caruncle

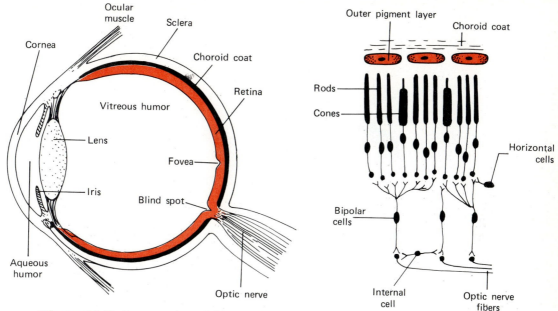

Figure 11-6. *Cross section of the eye (left), and detailed structure of the retina (right)*

Just posterior to the cornea is the anterior chamber, which is filled with **aqueous humor**, a clear fluid that is constantly being formed and leaves the eye to enter the bloodstream through the canal of Schlemm. The canal is located at the corneal-scleral junction (see Fig. 11-7). The aqueous humor is a watery fluid important to the nutrition of the cornea. The formation and reabsorption of the aqueous humor regulates the intraocular pressure.

Beneath the sclera is a vascular layer, the choroid (ko'rid). The anterior part of the choroid is the ciliary (sil'e-ar-e) body. Within the ciliary body is the ciliary muscle, which aids in the adjustment of the shape of the lens. The lens becomes more spherical (thereby increasing the refractive power) for viewing objects that are nearby. Attached to the ciliary body is the **iris**, a circular curtain that regulates the amount of light entering the lens.

The iris is made of two sheets of smooth muscle: a circular one called the sphincter muscle and a radial one called the dilator muscle. When the light is bright, the sphincter muscle contracts, constricting the pupil (the opening in the center of the iris). The pupil also constricts when a nearby object is viewed. In dim light or when a distant object is viewed the pupil becomes larger.

Just posterior to the iris and anterior to the ciliary body and ciliary ligaments is the posterior chamber. This chamber is also filled with aqueous humor, which drains into the canal of Schlemm. In Figure 11-7, notice the relationship of the iris to the canal of Schlemm. From this illustration, you can see that, when the pupil dilates, the iris will exert pressure on the canal of Schlemm and partially obstruct the flow of aqueous humor in the canal.

The innermost layer of the eyeball is the

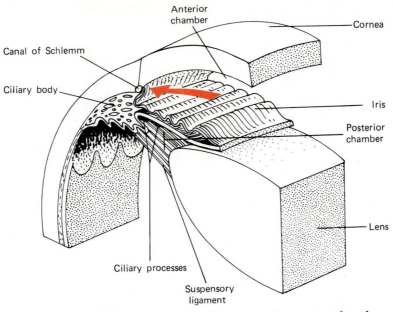

Figure 11-7. *Detailed view of the anterior and posterior chambers of the eye. The aqueous humor in these chambers drains into the canal of Schlemm. As shown with the arrow, dilatation of the pupil can put pressure on this canal and obstruct this drainage.*

retina (see Fig. 11-6). The retinal layer is held firmly to the choroid by a clear, jellylike substance called the **vitreous humor**. The rods and cones are photoreceptor cells in the retina. Rods are for dim-light vision and cones are for color and daylight vision. In the center of the posterior of the eyeball is the fovea centralis, which is a thinning of the retina and the area of most acute vision. Only cone cells are located in the foveal region, whereas rods are found concentrated in the periphery. A short distance to the nasal side of the fovea centralis is the **optic disc**. This structure is called the blind spot since there are neither rods nor cones in this area. The optic disc is also a relatively weak area since the scleral layer is absent. It is here that the optic nerve leaves the eyeball.

Focusing

All of the processes necessary for vision must be in perfect coordination. Refraction is the bending of the light rays. The speed of the light rays decreases with increasing density of the medium through which they pass. The refractive media are the cornea, aqueous humor, lens, and vitreous humor. The normal eye has refractive power that permits an object 20 feet away to form a clear image on the retina. To see an object at a closer range, the eye's refractive power must be increased. This process is accomplished by the contraction of the ciliary muscle pulling the choroid forward and lessening the tension on the suspensory ligaments of the lens (see Fig. 11-8). The lens then bulges or becomes more convex. Adjusting the refractory power of the lens is called accommodation.

Another process necessary for focusing is the regulation of the size of the pupil. This is a function of the muscles of the iris. For near vision, the pupil must constrict; for distant vision, the pupil must dilate. The pupil also constricts in response to bright light as illustrated in Figure 11-9.

Convergence is the process by which you see with both eyes but do not see double because the two images fall on corresponding parts of each retina. The nearer the object to be viewed, the more the eyes converge. Hold a pencil for one of your friends to view and slowly move the pencil toward the friend's eyes and then some distance away. You will be able to observe the process of convergence.

Visual Pathway

The nerve fibers from the rods and cones of the retina come together at the optic disc and leave the eyeball as the optic nerve. The two optic nerves meet at the optic chiasma (ki-az′mah) located just above and a little anterior to the pituitary gland. At the optic chiasma, the fibers from the nasal side of each eyeball cross to the opposite side while those that originate on the lateral sides remain uncrossed. The optic tracts carry the fibers from the optic chiasma to the occipital cortex.

The clinical significance of this crossing is that pressure on the optic chiasma might occur as a result of a pituitary tumor. This pressure will

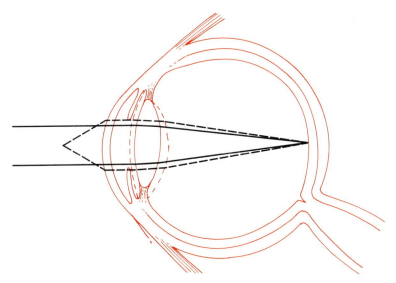

Figure 11-8. *The solid lines illustrate distance vision. The ciliary muscles relax causing tension on the suspensary ligaments and the lens becomes thin. The dotted lines represent rays of light and the shape of the lens for near vision.*

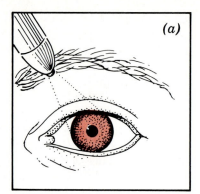 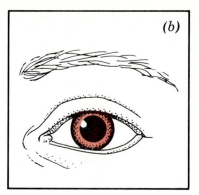

Figure 11-9. *Pupillary reflexes. (a) Pupil constricts when exposed to bright light for near vision. (b) Pupil dilates in dim light and for distance vision.*

interfere with peripheral vision but not with central vision since the fibers from the medial or nasal side receive the peripheral images. This type of visual defect is called tunnel vision.

Figure 12-2 shows the structures of the visual pathway and the fields of vision of each normal eye. The type of visual impairment resulting from various lesions is illustrated so that you will understand the function of each part of the pathway.

Binocular Vision

Binocular vision or vision with two eyes enables us to have a perception of depth and a larger visual field. A person who has one eye bandaged will have the impression that, although the visual field is limited, distance judgment within that field is accurate. The deficiency will be realized when the person attempts to put a key in a keyhole. Although believing the aim for the keyhole is correct, the person will be off by about an inch. People who have lost the sight of one eye will in time compensate for this deficiency.

GENERAL SENSES

CUTANEOUS SENSES

Touch, pressure, heat, cold, and pain are cutaneous senses. The receptors for these senses are widely distributed in the skin and many other tissues of the body. The number of receptors for each of the sensations varies greatly, and for this reason not all parts of the body are equally sensitive. For example, the tip of your tongue and your finger tips are quite sensitive, but the back of your neck is much less sensitive.

The receptors for touch and pressure are located in nerve endings around the hair follicles and in the papillary layer of the skin. The pathway for the nerve impulses is found in the cranial nerves going directly to the brain or in spinal nerves leading to the spinal cord and then to the brain. These impulses are interpreted in the general sensory area of the brain just posterior to the central fissure.

Receptors for the sensation of cold are near the surface of the skin; those for heat lie deep in the skin. The afferent pathways for these nerve impulses and their cortical localization are similar to those for touch and pressure.

Pain receptors in the skin, muscles, tendons, and joints are numerous and important because the sensation of pain warns you of danger so that you can protect yourself from extensive injury. The afferent pathways for this type of pain are similar to those for other cutaneous sensations. You may find it helpful to review the discussion in Chapter 9 concerning the tracts within the spinal cord for a more thorough understanding of how these sensations travel through the cord to the brain. Cortical localization of somatic (meaning that of the body rather than the viscera) pain is probably in the parietal lobes of the brain. However, since fear and anxiety are usually associated with pain, the prefrontal cortex and other areas of the cortex are probably involved. Visceral pain is discussed in Chapter 3.

ORGANIC SENSATIONS

Organic sensations such as hunger, thirst, nausea, and distention of the bowel and bladder are complex sensations. The stimuli for these sensations probably help determine the receptors and the pathway to the brain. For example, the sensation of nausea may result from having eaten spoiled food, but it may also result from the sight of something unpleasant. Thirst may be a sensation that results from a feeling of dryness in the pharynx and mouth. However, general dehydration resulting from vomiting, diarrhea, or hemorrhage may also cause thirst.

The pathways of these organic sensations involve the autonomic nerve fibers. The sensory areas in the brain have not been identified, but it is likely that more than one area of the cortex is responsible for the discrimination of each of the organic sensations.

SUMMARY QUESTIONS

1. Where is the nasolacrimal duct and what is its function?
2. Where are the semicircular canals and what is their function?
3. List the refractive media of the eye.
4. What structures are located in the membranous cochlea?
5. Where is the canal of Schlemm and what is its function?
6. What is the function of the organs of Corti?
7. Where are the receptors for the sensation of taste located?
8. What is the nerve pathway for the sensation of smell?
9. Into what structure do secretions from the mastoid sinuses drain?
10. List in sequence the structures through which a sound wave passes until the sound is interpreted by the cerebral cortex.
11. Where in the eye are the receptors for vision located?
12. What is the function of the iris?
13. What processes are involved in near vision?

14. Discuss cutaneous sensations.
15. Explain what is involved in the process of accommodation.
16. Where is the fovea centralis?
17. Explain the nerve pathways at the optic chiasma.

KEY TERMS

aqueous humor

cerumen

conjunctiva

cornea

eustachian tube

iris

optic disc

otitis media

retina

sclera

sordes

tympanic membrane

vitreous humor

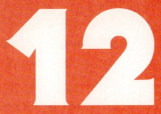

Disorders of the Sense Organs

OBJECTIVES

On completion of this chapter, you will be able to:

1. Discuss the difference between conductive and nerve deafness.
2. Differentiate between hyperopia and myopia.
3. Discuss the cause of presbyopia.
4. Discuss the treatment of cataracts.
5. List the signs and symptoms of a detached retina and explain how this condition is treated.
6. Explain how eye infections are managed.
7. Explain how to communicate with a person who experiences presbycusis.
8. Describe the parts used in the cochlear implant.
9. Discuss the diagnostic tests and treatment of glaucoma.

OVERVIEW

I. DIAGNOSTIC TESTS
   A. Hearing Tests
   B. Eye Examinations
II. IMPAIRED VISION AND DISEASES OF
    THE EYES
   A. Visual Field Defects
      1. Hyperopia
      2. Myopia
      3. Astigmatism
      4. Presbyopia
   B. Strabismus
   C. Cataracts
   D. Glaucoma
   E. Detached Retina
   F. Infections
      1. Conjunctivitis
      2. Hordeolum
      3. Chalazion
   G. Corneal Problems
III. DISEASES AND DISORDERS OF THE
     EARS
   A. Otitis Media
   B. Mastoiditis
   C. Impacted Cerumen
   D. Foreign Bodies in the Ear
   E. Impaired Hearing
      1. Conductive Hearing Loss
      2. Sensorineural Hearing Loss
      3. Presbycusis
   F. Cochlear Implants
      1. Labyrinthitis
   G. Vestibular Disease

This chapter was written by Jo Anne S. Maehling.

Because the function of our sense organs is an important aspect of our ability to adapt to our environment, some disease processes involving these structures can be serious handicaps if they are not properly diagnosed and treated. In this chapter, we shall consider some of the common diseases of the eyes and ears.

DIAGNOSTIC TESTS

HEARING TESTS

Simple tests such as whispering words to the patient in such a way that the examiner's lips cannot be seen and then having the patient repeat the whispered words can be helpful in screening large numbers of people for hearing defects. Tuning forks also help to determine whether a hearing defect is conductive (an obstruction of the sound wave in the outer or middle ear) or neural (a defect in the inner ear). The doctor or medical assistant sets the tuning fork into vibration and places it on the patient's forehead. The patient is asked to report in which ear the sound is heard. This test is called the Webber test. The Rinne test also uses the tuning fork but the tuning fork is placed on the mastoid process. The patient is asked when the sound is heard and when it no longer can be heard. When the patient reports that the sound has stopped, the tuning fork is quickly placed in front of the ear auricle. The patient is again asked to report when the sound is heard and when it stops. Under normal conditions, the sound should be heard twice as long when the tuning fork is placed over the ear auricle than when it is placed over the mastoid process.

More accurate hearing tests are achieved by using the audiometer, an instrument that produces pure tones of controlled loudness and pitch. The patient uses earphones and sits in a soundproof room and signals when the tone is heard and when it can no longer be heard.

EYE EXAMINATIONS

A physician's assistant, oculist, or optometrist can perform some eye examinations. Others are done by an ophthalmologist, a medical doctor specializing in the diagnosis and treatment of diseases of the eyes. Although not a medical doctor, an optometrist is highly skilled and qualified to diagnose and treat errors of refraction.

The Snellen chart consists of a series of letters or symbols of different sizes. People with unimpaired vision can read the largest letters at a distance of 200 feet. The smaller letters can be seen at 100, 50, and 20 feet. The patient usually sits 20 feet from the chart and is requested to read the letters in the smallest line that is visible. The patient's vision will be reported as 20/20 if he is able to read the letters with each eye that people with normal vision can read at 20 feet. If he can read at a distance of 20 feet letters no smaller than those a person with normal vision can see at 30 feet, his vision is described as 20/30. A person whose vision is reduced to 20/200 is usually considered legally blind.

To determine whether or not the refracting media of the eye bend light rays to focus normally on the retina, the ophthalmologist utilizes various lenses. This procedure can determine, for patients who have less than 20/20 vision, which lenses will offer the most effective correction of the refractive error. Frequently, before the refraction is done, the physician or assistant places eye drops in the patient's eyes to temporarily paralyze the muscle of accommodation. To administer eye drops, you hold the upper lid firmly against the frontal bone with your index finger and the lower lid firmly against the zygomatic with your thumb. Then place the drops in the lower conjunctival sac and instruct the patient to keep the eyes closed for a few minutes. Following the examination, the patient should wear dark glasses until the ability to accommodate to light and dark returns. You should never use these drops for patients who have glaucoma because they will dilate the pupils and thereby put pressure on the canal of Schlemm (see below under "Glaucoma").

The ophthalmologist can measure intraocular pressure with a tonometer (see Fig. 12-1). Before the test, some local anesthetic is placed into the eyes. This test is a valuable diagnostic aid in determining glaucoma, which is evidenced by increased intraocular pressure. This is a crude measurement of intraocular pressure. Advanced technology has provided instruments that quickly pass air across the cornea, measuring the resistance that is reflective of the intraocular pressure. Other than increased pressure, there may be no signs of the disease until it is quite advanced. Because glaucoma is one of the most common causes of blindness, all adults should have their intraocular pressure measured annually.

With an ophthalmoscope, the interior of the eye can be examined. This examination is usually done in a dark room. If the optic disc is cupped (bulges outward), there is increased intraocular pressure. If the disc is choked (appears squeezed), there is increased intracranial pressure. The doctor can also examine the condition of the blood vessels in the eye, a check that can be helpful in the early diagnosis of such diseases as arteriosclerosis.

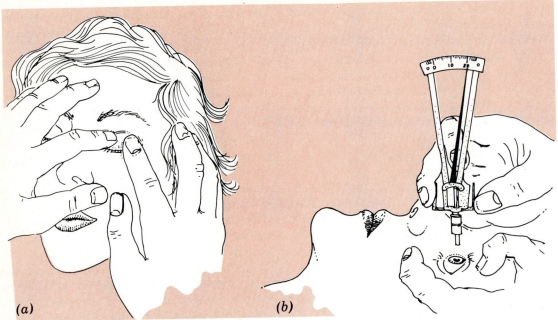

Figure 12-1. *Measuring intraocular pressure (a) by palpation and (b) with a Schiotz tonometer. The Schiotz tonometer is in common use; however, there are also electronic tonometers being used.*

IMPAIRED VISION AND DISEASES OF THE EYES

VISUAL FIELD DEFECTS

Figure 12-2 shows the pathway of nerve impulses that originate in the retina and are interpreted by the visual cortex in the occipital lobe of the brain. Damage to various parts of this pathway will result in different visual defects.

Hyperopia

Hyperopia (hi"per-o'pe-ah) (also called hypermetropia) is farsightedness. In this condition, the eyeball is too short and, thus, the light rays focus at a theoretical point behind the retina.

Lenses to correct this refractive error can be prescribed by an optometrist (see Fig. 12-3).

Myopia

Myopia (mi-o'pe-ah), or nearsightedness, usually results from an elongation of the eye. The light rays focus at a point in the vitreous humor in front of the retina. Proper lenses can also correct myopia.

Astigmatism

Astigmatism (ah-stig'mah-tizm) results from an irregularity in the shape of the cornea or, sometimes, of the lens. Vision is blurred, and the patient will need lenses to correct the refractive error.

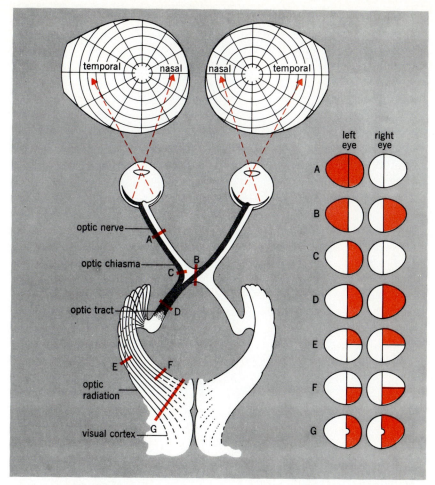

Figure 12-2. *Visual pathways with indications of the type of visual defect that will result from lesions in different parts of the system. The shaded areas at the right show the deficit of vision.*

Presbyopia

Presbyopia (pres-be-o'pe-ah), or elder vision, is caused by the gradual loss of elasticity of the lens and a weakening of the ciliary muscles as we grow older. The result is a decreased ability to accommodate for near vision. A person must hold reading matter farther away in order to see

clearly. Bifocal glasses in which the lower part of the glasses is used for near vision and the top for distant vision will correct this error. People who have never worn glasses frequently want "reading glasses" instead of bifocals, as they believe the bifocals will be a difficult adjustment for them. However, reading glasses will blur

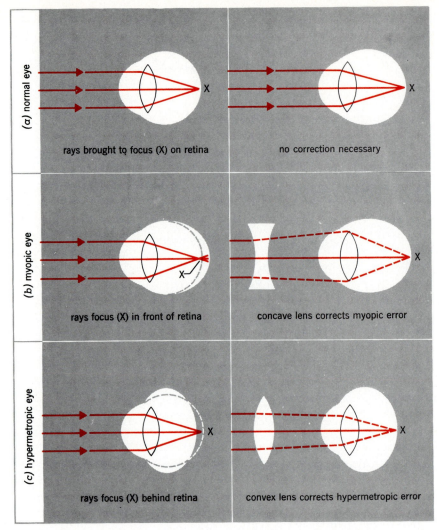

(a) normal eye

rays brought to focus (X) on retina

no correction necessary

(b) myopic eye

rays focus (X) in front of retina

concave lens corrects myopic error

(c) hypermetropic eye

rays focus (X) behind retina

convex lens corrects hypermetropic error

Figure 12-3. *(a) Normal vision, (b) nearsighted, and (c) farsighted eyes. The type of lens required to correct the vision is shown at the right.*

their distant vision, and they will find that they are constantly taking their reading glasses off and putting them back on. Thus, the short time of adjustment to bifocals is well worth the effort.

STRABISMUS

Strabismus (strah-biz′mus) is a deviation of one eye from the other in an outward, inward, upward, or downward manner. Strabismus is a common symptom of central nervous system, ocular, and other general systemic problems. It can be of the paralytic or nonparalytic types. Paralytic results from damage of the nerves controlling the extraocular muscles. Nonparalytic is a result of a defect in the position of the two eyes.

Intervention to treat strabismus includes surgical procedures that will advance, resect, or tuck muscles that support the eye. The goal is to align the eyes equally. This is primarily used for the nonparalytic type of strabismus. Treatment of paralytic strabismus is aimed at correcting the underlying cause of neural damage.

CATARACTS

Cataracts (kat'ah-rakts) are an opacity of the lens. This condition can be treated surgically by removing the lens. There are two types of procedures. The procedure of choice is to remove the lens and leave a portion of the capsule intact. An intraocular lens implant is then inserted into the capsule. This procedure is called an extracapsular cataract extraction followed by an intraocular lens implant. With the lens implant, vision is usually fine tuned with the use of glasses. Bifocal glasses also may be used for close work. The lens implant eliminates the use of thick, heavy glasses that had been previously necessary.

Intracapsular cataract extraction is complete removal of the lens with its capsule. Patients are required to wear thick lenses to correct their vision.

Today, cataract surgery is done in a day surgery unit with the patient going home the same day surgery is done. Postoperative patients need to be instructed to initially wear their eye shield to protect the eye. Also, they may need to be instructed on the correct way to administer their eye medication. They should be instructed to avoid straining the eye, for example, lifting heavy objects, or straining with bowel movements. Discomfort is usually mild after surgery, but pain can be a sign of a serious complication. If pain is associated with nausea and vomiting, this could indicate increased intraocular pressure and hemorrhage. The physician should be notified and treatment initiated immediately.

GLAUCOMA

Glaucoma (glaw-ko'mah) results from a disturbance of the normal balance between the production and the drainage of aqueous humor. The increased intraocular pressure, if it is not relieved, can result in blindness. Although it can occur at any age, glaucoma is most common in people over 40. Early diagnosis and treatment are most important in preventing loss of vision.

In acute glaucoma, the patient has attacks of severe pain in and around the eyes, sees halos, particularly around lights, and has blurred vision. These attacks usually occur suddenly. The patient should be given miotics (mi-ot'iks), which are drugs that constrict the pupil to relieve the pressure on the canal of Schlemm. Other drugs, such as diuretics, are given to slow the production of the aqueous humor. Patients need analgesics and complete rest. The surgical treatment is to relieve the pressure by removing a piece of the iris (iridectomy). This allows the aqueous humor to flow through the anterior chamber.

Chronic glaucoma occurs more frequently than the acute type. Patients often have no symptoms until their disease process is fairly well advanced; then the symptoms are similar to those of acute glaucoma. The treatment of chronic glaucoma is to maintain intraocular pressure at a level that prevents further damage to the structures of the eye. This is accomplished medically by the use of miotics. Another approach used prior to the use of surgery is to use a pneumatic eye softner (Honan balloon). The

Honan intraocular pressure reducer applied to the eye decreases intraocular pressure faster than medications and eliminates the side effects of systemic medications.

Surgery or laser therapy may be done if medical treatment is not effective. A trabeculectomy is the surgical procedure. This is the removal of a piece of the sclera containing the trabecular network along with an iridectomy. This is done to improve the flow of aqueous humor through the subconjunctival tissue. More frequently, a laser is used to perform the trabeculectomy. This procedure is less invasive and only takes 30 minutes to perform. Postoperative patients are required to use topical steroids.

All patients with glaucoma should avoid coffee, tea, and other caffeine products and must also limit their total fluid intake. It is important that they avoid lifting heavy objects which can cause increased intraocular pressure, and limit activities that cause eye strain and fatigue.

DETACHED RETINA

In a detached retina, the nerve layer of the retina becomes separated from the pigmented layer and deprives the nerve layer of blood supply. Thus, vision is lost in the affected area. The symptoms depend on the size of the affected area, but generally, the patient reports seeing flashes of light or a sensation of seeing spots or moving particles. The patient also may describe his vision as if a curtain or shade is being pulled over the eye. Pain is usually not present. The detachment may be treated surgically, or if it is a relatively small area it can be corrected by photocoagulation (fo"to-ko-ag"u-la'shun). Photocoagulation is a procedure in which a beam of light is directed toward the area of detachment causing the retina at that point to adhere to the choroid. Other surgical procedures include scleral buckling (suturing a small silicone sponge onto the sclera over the break or

hole) and banding with a silicone strap or band placed under the extraocular muscles around the globe. An invasive procedure is to remove the vitreous humor, replacing it with air or inert gas. This creates a bubble to provide countertraction to assist in reattaching the retina.

INFECTIONS

Conjunctivitis

Conjunctivitis (kon-junk-ti-vi′tis), or pink eye, is an inflammation of the conjunctiva due to allergy or microorganisms. If the etiology is allergy, the patient may be treated with antihistamines or perhaps can be desensitized to the particular allergen. If it is due to bacteria, it may be treated with appropriate antibiotics.

Hordeolum

A **hordeolum** (hor-de′o-lum) is a sty, or infection at the edge of the eyelid in a lash follicle. Hot wet compresses help to localize the infection. Within a few days, the lesion will drain and require no further treatment. Occasionally, it is necessary to incise and drain the lesion. If a person is subject to frequent recurrences of this type of infection, it may be helpful to wash the face three or four times a day with antibacterial soap. Because this preventative measure will very likely cause dry skin, the patient should be told that cold cream to combat the unpleasant dryness will also counteract the efforts to minimize the population of bacteria on the face.

Chalazion

Small sebaceous glands are located within the upper eyelids. An infection of these glands, called a **chalazion** (kah-la′ze-on), can be quite painful and require surgical treatment.

CORNEAL PROBLEMS

If corneal scarring occurs, causing opacities of the cornea and decreased visual acuity, it may be necessary to do a corneal transplant. Since the cornea does not contain blood vessels, these transplants are rarely rejected.

Keratitis (ker"ah-ti'tis) is an inflammation of the cornea. It can be caused by microorganisms or by chemical or mechanical injuries to the epithelium of the cornea. If there are repeated attacks of keratitis there may be scarring and opacities with decreased visual acuity. Parenteral antibiotics are usually given for the infection and topical corticosteroids are used to decrease the inflammatory response and scarring of the cornea. Eye pads are contraindicated, as organism growth is increased in dark environments.

DISEASES AND DISORDERS OF THE EARS

OTITIS MEDIA

Otitis (o-ti'tis) **media** is an inflammation in the middle ear. It is a common condition in young children and infants because their eustachian tubes are short and straight and almost any upper respiratory infection can spread to the middle ear if it is not recognized and treated early.

The condition is characterized by decreased hearing and a throbbing pain in the affected ear. A child may tug on the ear and an infant may roll the head from side to side. The fever may run as high as 40 to 41.1 degrees Centigrade. Antipyretics can be used to reduce the fever. Pain is managed with aspirin, codeine, and acetaminophen.

Pus in the middle ear causes the eardrum to bulge. If the infection is not readily relieved with antibiotic treatment, a **myringotomy** (mir-in-got'o-me), which is an incision into the eardrum, may be performed to drain the ear. Petrolatum may be placed around the outer ear to prevent the skin from becoming **excoriated** (eks-ko're-a"ted) or irritated.

If a child who has had a myringotomy becomes drowsy or unusually irritable, complains of severe headache, or has a rise in temperature, the doctor should be notified since these symptoms may indicate that the eardrum needs to be reopened because the mastoid cells, brain, or meninges are becoming infected. A myringotomy incision usually heals completely and does not affect hearing.

MASTOIDITIS

If the middle ear infection is not treated early or if the infection is particularly virulent, mastoiditis can occur. An abscess forms in the mastoid cells and there is pain, fever, and profuse discharge from the affected ear. The treatment consists of antibiotics, bed rest, medication for pain, and increased fluid intake. Surgery is rarely necessary unless symptoms persist or become worse.

IMPACTED CERUMEN

A certain amount of wax, or cerumen, in the ear canal is normal. Without wax, there is itching and scaling of the skin in the ear canal. If the wax becomes dry and impacted, however, it can cause discomfort and temporary deafness. These problems can also be caused by getting water in the ear which will cause the cerumen to swell.

The doctor may recommend instilling a few drops of warm oil or hydrogen peroxide into the ear daily for three or four days in order to soften the wax prior to removing it by irrigation.

FOREIGN BODIES IN THE EAR

Children or mentally disturbed adults occasionally put small objects into their ears. These should be removed by a physician because there is danger of traumatizing the canal or eardrum while probing for them. Insects may also get into the ear. A few drops of mineral oil or alcohol placed in the ear will either kill or anesthetize the insect, which can then be removed with a forceps or washed out.

IMPAIRED HEARING

Conductive Hearing Loss

Conductive hearing loss is the inability of sounds to pass through the external and middle ear. A ruptured eardrum, otitis media, or **otosclerosis** (o"to-skle-ro′sis) can cause conductive hearing loss. Otosclerosis is a condition in which the ossicles of the middle ear do not move freely and, therefore, cannot transmit the sound waves into the oval window. Large amounts of wax in the ear canal can also impair hearing. This wax should be removed by a doctor or his or her assistant. Attempts on the part of the patient to clean the wax out will most likely result in pushing the wax further into the ear and possibly damaging the tympanic membrane. Regardless of the cause of conductive hearing loss, it usually can be corrected by repairing the defect or by using a hearing aid. Hearing aids do not improve the ability to hear but do make sounds louder.

Sensorineural Hearing Loss

Sensorineural hearing loss involves pathology that leads to loss of function of the cochlear or the acoustic branch of the eighth cranial nerve. This type of "nerve deafness" can result from a variety of conditions. These include infections (e.g., measles), ototoxic drugs, trauma, tumors of the acoustic nerve, continued exposure to loud noises (e.g., machinery in factories), and the aging process. Treatment for sensorineural hearing loss is difficult if nerve tissue is permanently damaged. New techniques, such as cochlear implants, offer patients new hope in restoring their hearing.

PRESBYCUSIS

Presbycusis is the gradual decline of hearing frequently seen in the aged. It is classified as a type of sensorineural hearing loss that affects people usually in their fifth decade. Most people past their sixth decade have some degree of presbycusis. Structural degenerative changes occurring in both ears lead to the hearing loss. Often the individual cannot hear mid- to high-pitched sounds as the condition progresses. The person will hear some words and messages but not others.

Unfortunately, this condition cannot be treated. Hearing aids or cochlear implants have been helpful in improving the ability to communicate. However, social isolation is often a problem for people with presbycusis. This is not a psychological disorder and it is cruel to imply that these people hear only what they want to hear and when they want to hear. Efforts should be made to try to communicate with these individuals by speaking clearly and slowly. Shouting is not necessary and often raises the pitch of the voice. Rephrasing and lowering the pitch of the voice is the best technique.

COCHLEAR IMPLANTS

Cochlear implants have been used to help people with profound deafness and complete loss of hearing. There are several types of implants used. Each has four basic features that include: a microphone that picks up the sound transmitted; a microelectronic processer that converts the sound to an electrical impulse; a system that transmits the signal to the implanted components; and an enlongated slender electrode that is placed into the cochlea (see Fig. 12-4). The electrode delivers the electrical signal

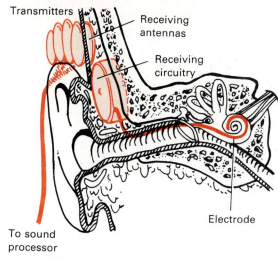

Transmitters

Receiving antennas

Receiving circuitry

Electrode

To sound processor

Figure 12-4. Cochlear implant

to the auditory nerve for sound interpretation. The implants are surgically placed with few postoperative complications. Patients should be informed that the implant will not completely restore their hearing, but will help them hear sounds that they would not have otherwise heard. Implants can have a single channel or multiple channels. The multichannel implants permit a variety of pitches to be heard. These implants enable some people to hear words, whereas the single channel implants may restore a broad sense of pitch, like a telephone ringing. Regardless of the type of cochlear implant, this procedure has been helpful to those with complete hearing loss.

Labyrinthitis

Infection or inflammation of the inner ear may involve the cochlea or vestibular portion of the labyrinth or both. Patients are likely to have **vertigo** (ver′ti-go″) which is severe dizziness, tin-

nitus (tin′i-tus) or ringing in the ears, and some hearing loss. They are also likely to have nystagmus (nis-tag′mus), an abnormal jerking movement of the eye. The nystagmus associated with labyrinthitis has a horizontal beat, whereas nystagmus indicative of brainstem disease is vertical.

If the problem is caused by an infection, the patient will usually recover in about a week and there will be no hearing loss. If the process lasts for more than a week, it may progress until the cochlea is destroyed and possibly vestibular function as well.

VESTIBULAR DISEASE

There are a variety of diseases of the inner ear that are characterized by vertigo, tinnitus, and deafness. The vertigo is often so severe that there is nausea and vomiting, blurred vision, a tendency to fall in a certain direction, and nystagmus. Electronystagmography (e-lek″tro-nis-tag′mo-gra″fe) is a diagnostic test that is useful in identifying vestibular diseases. Electrodes are placed on each side of the face to measure movements of the eyes while they are closed.

Menieres (men′e-arz) disease is the most common of the vestibular diseases. The cause is unknown. There are many types of treatment prescribed to help limit the severity of the attacks. The patients are usually told to limit their fluid and salt intake because this type of vertigo seems to be associated with an accumulation of fluid. Diuretic drugs may also be used. The nausea and dizziness may be relieved with motion-sickness drugs.

When vestibular disease is severe but limited to one ear, surgical removal of the membranous labyrinth can be done, resulting both in the removal of the vertigo and in the loss of hearing in that ear.

SUMMARY QUESTIONS

1. Differentiate between hyperopia and myopia.
2. What causes presbyopia?
3. What treatment is used for patients with cataracts?
4. What is the diagnostic test used to detect glaucoma?
5. What causes astigmatism?
6. How is a hordeolum treated?
7. What are the symptoms of a detached retina?
8. Explain how hearing tests are done.
9. What is the difference between conductive hearing loss and sensorineural hearing loss?
10. How can you best communicate with a patient who has presbycusis?
11. What are the four parts of the cochlear implant?

KEY TERMS

astigmatism
chalazion
conjunctivitis
excoriated
glaucoma
hordeolum

myopia
myringotomy
otitis media
otosclerosus
presbyopia
vertigo

13

The Cardiovascular System

OBJECTIVES

On completion of this chapter, you will be able to:

1. Explain the gross structure of the heart.
2. Discuss the functions of the four heart valves.
3. Tell what cardiac events produce the heart sounds.
4. Describe the internal conduction system of the heart.
5. Explain in detail the phases of the cardiac cycle.
6. Discuss the factors that influence cardiac output.
7. Explain what causes variations in the blood pressure in the different parts of the circulatory system.
8. Trace a drop of blood from the heart to the capillaries of all of the major organs and back to the right side of the heart.
9. Discuss the functions of the different types of blood cells.
10. Describe the functions of the lymphatic system.

OVERVIEW

I. THE HEART
   A. Heart Valves
   B. Blood Supply to the Heart
   C. Nerve Supply
   D. Intrinsic Conduction System
II. PHYSIOLOGY OF CIRCULATION
   A. Cardiac Cycle
   B. Electrical Changes
   C. Circulation
   D. Stroke Volume and Cardiac Output
   E. Cardiac Reflexes
      1. Pressure Receptors
      2. Chemoreceptors
   F. Blood Flow
   G. Resistance to Flow
   H. Velocity
   I. Blood Pressure
III. ARTERIAL CIRCULATION
IV. CAPILLARIES
V. VENOUS RETURN
VI. FETAL CIRCULATION
VII. THE COMPOSITION OF BLOOD
VIII. IMMUNITY
   A. Humoral Immunity
   B. Cellular Immunity
IX. BLOOD GROUPS
   A. Blood Typing
X. THE LYMPHATIC SYSTEM

Highly specialized cells are not capable of carrying on an independent existence. They cannot search for food or distribute the goods they manufacture, such as enzymes and hormones, needed by other cells of the body, nor can they move away from their waste products. For this reason, we need the circulatory system, which functions as the body's transport mechanism. There are two divisions of this system: the lymphatic, which helps to return tissue fluid to blood, and the blood. The blood division is a closed circuit. Thus, pathology in any part, be it a blockage in the flow or a leak, will lead to easily predictable symptoms.

THE HEART

We shall first consider some of the major structures of the blood circulatory system. The heart is the pump for the blood. It is located in the thoracic cavity, medial to the lungs, in the **mediastinum** (me″de-as-ti′num). The sternum is anterior to the heart, and four thoracic vertebrae (T2 through T6) are posterior. The base of the heart is directed upward and to the right and its apex is directed downward and to the left of the midline.

The heart is surrounded by a sac called the **pericardium** (per-i-kar′de-um). This sac has two layers, the parietal, which is fibrous, and the visceral, which is serous membrane. Between the layers is a small amount of fluid that serves as a lubricant. The visceral pericardium, also known as the **epicardium**, is closely attached to the cardiac muscle or **myocardium**. The lining of the heart is called the **endocardium**, which is endothelial tissue continuous with the lining of the blood vessels.

The upper chambers of the heart, or the atria (a′tre-ah), have thin walls and a smooth, shiny inner surface. The septum between the right and left atria has a scar on it that is called the fossa ovale (fos′ah o-va′le). This fossa was the foramen ovale in fetal life and functioned to allow some blood to flow directly from the right atrium to the left, bypassing the nonfunctioning lungs of the unborn child. The right atrium receives venous blood from the superior and inferior vena cava and also from the coronary sinus. The coronary sinus receives its blood from the coronary veins, which are returning blood from the capillaries of the myocardium. Some coronary veins empty directly into the right atrium. The right atrium sends its blood to the right ventricle. The left atrium receives blood from four pulmonary veins and also from the bronchial vein. From the left atrium the blood goes to the left ventricle.

The lower chambers of the heart are the ventricles, which have much thicker walls than do the atria. Their inner surfaces are irregular because they contain several papillary (pap'i-lar-e) muscles as well as stringlike structures, or chordae tendineae (kor'de ten-din'i), that are attached to the papillary muscles and to the valve flaps that are located between the upper and lower chambers. The chordae tendineae prevent the valves from turning inside out when the ventricles contract and force the blood upward. The right ventricle sends its blood to the pulmonary artery and then to the capillaries of the lungs to be oxygenated and to eliminate carbon dioxide. The left ventricle, with walls normally about three times as thick as the walls of the right ventricle, forms the apex of the heart. Pulsations of the apex can be heard between the fifth and sixth ribs, about 5 cm below the left nipple in the male. The function of the left ventricle is to pump blood into the aorta and to all parts of the body (see Fig. 13-1).

HEART VALVES

The valves of the heart, which are made of tough fibrous tissue, all function to prevent the backflow of blood. Between the right atrium and ventricle is the tricuspid (tri-kus'pid) valve. It has three triangular flaps, which are attached to the chordae tendineae. Between the left atrium and ventricle is the bicuspid (bi-kus'pid) or mitral (mi'tral) valve. When the ventricles contract, blood is forced upward and closes these valves. Semilunar valves prevent the blood from flowing

back into the ventricles once it has been pumped out either into the pulmonary artery or into the aorta. Both the aortic and pulmonary semilunar valves are composed of three halfmoon-shaped pockets that catch the blood and balloon out to close the orifices. It is the closure of the heart valves that makes the heart sounds. When the atrioventricular (a"tre-o-ven-trik'u-lar) valves close, the first sound (lupp) is heard; when the semilunars close, the second sound (dupp) is heard. Abnormal heart sounds or murmurs, therefore, may be indicative of some valvular pathology. Clinically, you will frequently see the heart sounds abbreviated as S_1 for the sound of the closure of the AV valves and S_2 for the sound of the semilunar valves. Likewise, murmurs are abbreviated M_1 and M_2.

BLOOD SUPPLY TO THE HEART

The blood supply to the myocardium travels via the coronary arteries. Right and left coronary arteries are the first branches off the ascending aorta. They go to a rich capillary network throughout the myocardium, from there to coronary veins, and then to the coronary sinus and right atrium. Some coronary veins drain directly into the right atrium. The endocardium receives its nourishment from the blood passing through the chambers. Blood can flow through the coronary circuit only during the relaxation phase of the cardiac cycle since these vessels are greatly constricted while the heart is contracting. Occlusion, or blockage of the coronary blood supply, can result in a heart attack if collateral circulation is not adequate.

NERVE SUPPLY

The nerve supply of the heart is responsible for altering the rate and force of the cardiac contraction to meet the needs of the body. Efferent nerves going to the heart originate in the cardiac center in the medulla of the brain. The vagus,

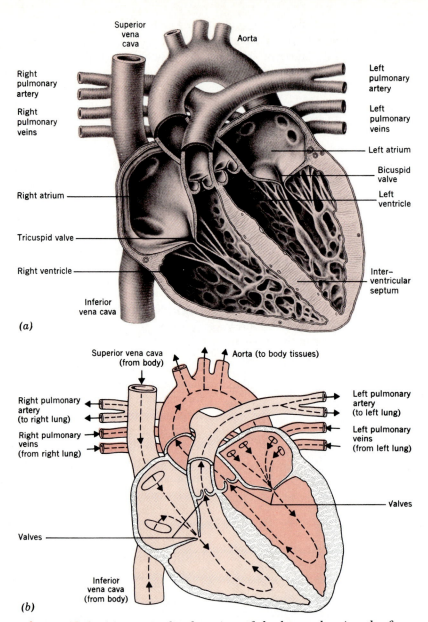

Figure 13-1. (a) *Longitudinal section of the heart showing the four chambers and the major arteries and veins.* (b) *Blood flow through the heart. The blood on the right side of the heart contains more carbon dioxide than oxygen and the blood on the left contains more oxygen than carbon dioxide.*

a parasympathetic nerve, will slow the heart rate; branches from the sympathetic nerves will increase the rate depending on the needs of the body. See Chapter 9 for a more detailed discussion of the nervous system. Epinephrine and norepinephrine, hormones from the adrenal glands, will also increase the rate of cardiac contractions.

When the walls of the right atrium are stretched because of an increased amount of blood being returned to the heart, afferent, or sensory, nerves are stimulated. These fibers send impulses to the medullary center in the brain causing it to increase the rate and strength of contraction.

Other afferent nerve fibers can be stimulated by a lack of oxygen. If coronary blood flow is inadequate, the cells of the myocardium are not receiving sufficient oxygen. This condition can cause chest pain or angina (an-ji'nah) pectoris.

INTRINSIC CONDUCTION SYSTEM

The heart has specialized tissue that enables it to contract rhythmically and continuously without any motor (efferent) nerve impulses. Structures involved in this specialized conducting system are the sinoatrial (or SA) node, the atrioventricular (or AV) node, and the bundle of His (see Fig. 13-2). The SA node is the pacemaker that initiates the beat. The myocardial cells of the SA node leak sodium faster than do the other myocardial cells and so depolarize first. The SA node is located approximately at

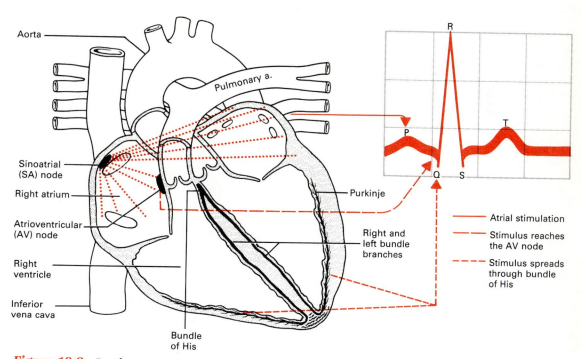

Figure 13-2. *Conduction system of the heart showing the source of electrical impulses produced on an ECG*

the place where the superior and inferior venae cavae (ve′ne ca′ve) enter the right atrium, and it sends electrical impulses via the atrial myocardium to the AV node, located just below the coronary sinus in the septum. The AV node sends the impulses to the bundle that branches throughout the walls of the ventricles.

Damaged myocardial cells may leak sodium faster than the SA node. Under these circumstances, there will be abnormal pacemakers, and the patient will have an **arrhythmia** (ah-rith′me-ah), or an irregular heart beat. This is also called **dysrhythmia** and is discussed in Chapter 14.

PHYSIOLOGY OF CIRCULATION

The work of the heart is to pump blood into the arterial circulation. The right side of the heart receives blood from the venae cavae and coronary circulation. This poorly oxygenated blood is sent from the right side of the heart into the pulmonary circulation. The left side of the heart receives the oxygenated blood from the pulmonary circuit and unoxygenated blood from the bronchial vein and pumps the blood into the aorta.

CARDIAC CYCLE

One cardiac cycle is one contraction of the heart and the relaxation period that follows. The contraction of the heart is called **systole** (sis′to-le) and the relaxation is called **diastole** (di-as′to-le). During the ventricular systole, blood from both ventricles is forced out of the heart through the two semilunar valves into the pulmonary artery and aorta. At the same time, the force of the blood against the atrioventricular valves causes them to close. It is the closure of these

atrioventricular valves during systole that causes the first heart sound.

During ventricular diastole, the atrioventricular valves open and the ventricles fill with blood from the atria, which is in systole. While the ventricles relax, blood in the pulmonary artery and aorta begins to flow back toward the ventricles. The force of this blood against the semilunar valves causes them to close. The second heart sound, indicating the closure of the semilunar valves, is heard during ventricular diastole.

ELECTRICAL CHANGES

Electrical changes take place during the cardiac cycle. These changes can be visualized and recorded with an electrocardiograph, or ECG. Both the size of the wave and the length of time consumed by each event in the cardiac cycle are important (see Fig. 13-3). The waves are designated the P wave, QRS complex, and the T wave. The letters were arbitrarily assigned and do not stand for any words.

The P wave occurs when the impulse has been received by the SA node and represents the depolarization of the atria. An enlarged P wave indicates an enlarged atrium, as can occur if the AV valve is stenosed (ste-nost′) (will not open wide enough). The QRS complex occurs when the impulse is passing through the ventricles. An enlarged Q is seen with a myocardial infarct (in′farkt) or heart attack. An enlarged R indicates enlarged ventricles. The T wave represents repolarization of the ventricles while they are in diastole. The PR interval should be 0.12 to 0.2 seconds. If it is too long, there is a conduction delay at the AV node, as may occur with rheumatic heart disease or hardening of the arteries. The ST segment is elevated in an acute myocardial infarct. It is depressed if there is insufficient

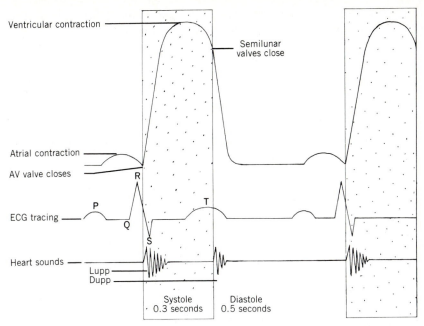

Ventricular contraction

Semilunar valves close

Atrial contraction

AV valve closes

R

ECG tracing

P

T

Q

S

Heart sounds

Lupp
Dupp

Systole
0.3 seconds

Diastole
0.5 seconds

Figure 13-3. *Relationship between the closure of the heart valves, heart sounds, systole, diastole, and an ECG tracing*

oxygen getting to the heart. This will also cause a flattened T wave. There will be an elevated T wave if the patient's blood potassium is too high.

The entire cardiac cycle takes 0.8 second if the heart is beating at 75 beats per minute. The systole, or contraction, of the ventricles takes 0.3 second and the diastole takes 0.5 second. Because the heart, like other muscles, abides by the All or None Law, the only way the rate of contraction can be increased is to shorten the diastole. The significance of this increase in rate with the shortening of the diastole is that greater work is being required of the heart and less rest time is being provided.

Figure 13-3 will help you understand the relationship between the contraction of the ventricles, the heart sounds, and the electrical changes taking place during the cardiac cycle.

CIRCULATION

Circulation depends primarily on the action of the heart, the condition of the blood vessels, and the viscosity of the blood. It can, however, be influenced by temperature, body size, activity, and by some drugs. The average rate is 65 to 70 beats per minute for men and 70 to 80 beats per minute for women. Age also is an important factor. An infant's heart beats at about 120 times per minute, and a fetus has a heart rate of about 150 beats per minute. Fever will increase the heart rate because the metabolism has increased. Drugs that stimulate the sympathetic nervous system will increase the heart rate, whereas parasympathetic agents and sedatives will decrease the rate. Thyroxin from the thyroid gland and epinephrine from the adrenal glands will increase the rate of the heart. An elevated blood potassium will depress the rate and an elevated blood calcium will increase the rate.

STROKE VOLUME AND CARDIAC OUTPUT

Stroke volume is the amount of blood pumped by each beat of the heart. Cardiac output is the stroke volume multiplied by the number of heart beats per minute. At a rate of 75 beats per minute, 70 ml of blood are ejected by each ventricle per beat. This calculation amounts to 5 liters per minute, which is the total volume of blood in a 150-pound person. During exercise, the cardiac output can easily be doubled. A weak heart must pump faster to make up for a low stroke volume. A well-trained athlete has a relatively slow pulse because he will have a good stroke volume. Young elastic vessels can tolerate a great increase in stroke volume. As you get older, your vessels lose their elasticity and an increased stroke volume can cause a weakened vessel to rupture.

There are several factors that influence cardiac output. The rate and force of heart contraction is controlled by the cardiac center in the brain. This center is one of the mechanisms that regulates the cardiac output so that the needs of the body for blood are met.

Under normal conditions, the amount of blood being returned to the right side of the heart will determine the output of the left ventricle. When the cardiac muscle fibers are stretched as they are when a large amount of blood has entered the heart, the force of the contraction that follows will be increased. This direct relationship between the volume of blood and the force of the contraction is Starling's Law of the Heart.

During exercise, there is an increased venous return to the heart and, therefore, an increased cardiac output. There is also an increase in the carbon dioxide produced by the active skeletal muscles. Carbon dioxide dilates the blood vessels, thereby reducing the resistance to the blood flow and further increasing venous return to the heart. The cardiac reserve is the percentage that the cardiac output can be increased above normal. Ordinarily, with exercise, the cardiac output can be increased 300%; however, the cardiac reserve of a well trained athlete will be as much as 500%.

Figure 13-4 illustrates the interrelationship of some of the factors responsible for an increase in cardiac output.

CARDIAC REFLEXES

There are some important reflexes that influence circulation. These respond either to pressure or to the amount of carbon dioxide and oxygen in the blood.

Pressure Receptors

The pressure receptors are also called baroreceptors. These are located in the bifurcation of each carotid artery near the carotid pressure point described in Figure 3-3 and also in the arch of the aorta. These receptors are called the carotid and aortic sinuses and they respond to pressure. An elevation in the blood pressure will stimulate these receptors and cause a reflex slowing of the heart and a decrease in the force of contraction. The carotid sinus functions primarily to monitor the blood pressure in the vessels of the brain. The aortic sinus monitors general systemic blood pressure.

Chemoreceptors

The chemoreceptors are also located in the carotid and aorta. Although the primary effect of these receptors is on the rate and depth of breathing, they also influence the heart. When the blood oxygen level is low, these receptors

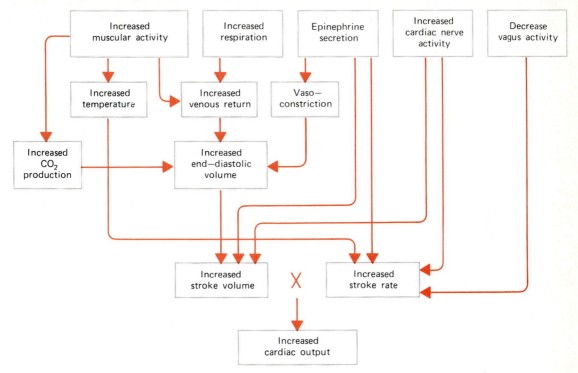

Figure 13-4. *Some factors responsible for an increase in cardiac output*

respond by causing vasoconstriction, elevating the blood pressure and increasing the pulse rate. Similarly, an increased level of carbon dioxide in the blood will increase the rate and force of cardiac contraction. However, excessive amounts of carbon dioxide will depress the cardiac muscle.

BLOOD FLOW

Blood flow is the quantity of blood moving through a vessel or vessels at a given period of time. Normally, at rest, the vessels of the skeletal muscles contain only about 15% of our blood; however, during exercise, the muscles can command as much as 75% of the blood. This dramatic change would seem to suggest that during

exercise the demands of the skeletal muscles must require blood to be "stolen" from some area. Fortunately, this is not the case. There is a very sizable quantity of blood in the venous reservoirs of the intestines where, although it is in circulation, it is not serving any purpose other than being held in reserve. The spleen and skin also function as blood reservoirs.

Brain, kidneys, and liver represent only a small fraction of the total body mass. However, under basal conditions, these organs command over 60% of the blood flow. When you compare this figure with the 15% going to the resting skeletal muscles, which represent 35 to 40% of the body mass, you realize that the body is very efficient in the manner in which it distributes its blood according to metabolic need rather than mass. It is interesting to note that the brain receives about 15% of the total volume of blood whether the person is sleeping or involved in some complex thought processes.

The blood always flows from higher pressure to lower pressure. This pressure is highest in the aorta and falls greatly by the time it reaches the capillaries. From the capillary bed, the pressure continues to drop as the blood flows into the veins. The drop on the venous side is not so great as that on the arterial side.

The rate of the flow is determined by the pressure gradient. There is a tremendous drop, approximately 100 mm Hg (millimeters of mercury), in the pressure between the aorta and the capillaries and, therefore, the blood flows very rapidly. The flow rate here is about 40 to 50 cm/sec. From the arterial end of the capillary to the venous end, the drop is only about 10 mm Hg so the blood will be moving very slowly, allowing enough time for the gases and nutrients to move between the capillaries and the tissue cells. Capillary blood moves at about 0.7 mm/sec. It will pick up a little speed on the venous side, between the capillaries and right atrium, where the pressure gradient is about 20 mm Hg.

RESISTANCE TO FLOW

Friction causes resistance to blood flow. The resistance to the blood flow is directly proportional to the length of the vessel. Since blood is retarded only by the surface of the vessel, the diameter of the vessel must be considered in estimating the amount of resistance to the blood flow. When blood vessels are constricted, resistance to flow increases. The thicker or more viscous the blood, the greater the resistance to the flow. Following hemorrhage, when there has been an increased return of tissue fluid to the vascular compartment, the blood will decrease in viscosity and the flow rate will increase as is evident from the rapid pulse.

The viscosity will increase when there is a great deal of edema such as there is during the first 48 to 72 hours following a massive burn.

VELOCITY

The velocity of the flow of blood is the distance that it travels in a given period of time. Measurement of this velocity is called circulation time. One of two substances, either decholin (de-ko'lin), which has a bitter taste, or ether, is injected into an arm vein. The time that it takes the substance to get to the capillaries of the tongue and be tasted or to the lungs from which the exhaled air will have the odor of ether is measured. The normal value for arm-to-tongue circulation time is about 10 to 16 seconds and for the arm-to-lung circulation time about 4 to 8 seconds. A prolonged circulation time suggests some increased resistance to the flow of blood.

BLOOD PRESSURE

Arterial blood pressure is determined by cardiac output and resistance to the flow of blood. It falls progressively from the time the blood leaves the left ventricle until it returns to the right atrium. In the aorta, the pressure is normally about 120 mm Hg. By the time it gets back to the right atrium, it is near 0 mm Hg. Systolic pressure measures the force of the ventricular contraction. It is this pressure that forces blood into the arterial circulation and to some extent through the circuit.

In a healthy young person, the chief factor moving blood through the arterial circulation is the alternate stretching and recoil of the elastic vessel walls. The flow of blood through aging vessels that have lost some of their elasticity is increasingly dependent on the force of systole. Therefore, high blood pressure is fairly common in people of advanced years.

On the capillary level, blood pressure pushes fluid rich in nutrients from the capillary into the tissue spaces (see Fig. 13-5). Peripheral cellular nutrition, therefore, is dependent on blood pressure.

Recall that the rate of blood flow between any two points in the circuit depends on the difference between the pressures at these points. Since the difference is much greater on the arterial side of the circuit, the blood is flowing much more rapidly there than it is in either the capillaries or the veins.

When you take a person's blood pressure, you wrap a blood pressure cuff around the upper arm and place a stethoscope over the brachial artery, which is on the medial aspect of the antecubital (an"te-ku'be-tal) fossa. You then pump the cuff up either until the gauge reads higher than you expect the patient's pressure to be or until you can no longer feel a radial pulse. You

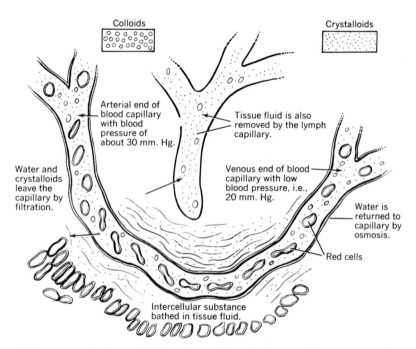

Figure 13-5. Tissue fluid is formed by a process of filtration at the arterial end of the blood capillary where the blood pressure exceeds the colloidal osmotic pressure. The fluid is absorbed by the blood capillaries and lymphatics. It will be returned to the venous end of the capillary when the colloidal osmotic pressure exceeds the blood pressure. The fluid is absorbed into the lymphatic capillary when the interstitial fluid pressure is greater than the pressure within the lymphatic capillary. Normally, only very little colloid escapes from the blood capillary. The escaped colloid is returned to the blood circulation by the lymphatics. (From Burke, S.R., Composition and Function of Body Fluids, 3rd ed. St. Louis: The C.V. Mosby Co., 1980)

should deflate the cuff slowly and listen for the first sound. This sound will be the systolic pressure, ordinarily about 120 mm Hg. You then continue deflating the cuff slowly until there is a change in the tone of the sound or until the sound disappears. Usually, the change in the tone and the disappearance of sounds are at the same reading, which is the diastolic pressure. In the healthy young adult, this is usually about 80 mm Hg. You would record this as 120/80. If the change in the tone and the disappearance of the sounds do not occur together, then you record all three numbers; for example, 120/80/60.

Occasionally, when a person is in shock, you may not be able to hear any sounds. When this happens, palpate the pulse and pump up the cuff until you can no longer feel the pulse. Slowly deflate the cuff until you again feel the pulse. This reading on the gauge will be the systolic pressure. You cannot get a diastolic pressure using this technique. Record this pressure reading and make a note that it was obtained by palpation.

Diastolic pressure is a measure of the peripheral resistance to blood flow and represents the force that must be overcome by the left ventricle before any blood can enter the aorta. For this reason, it is usually considered of greater clinical significance than the systolic pressure unless the patient is in shock. Mean pressure (approximately the arithmetic average of the systolic and diastolic pressures) is more important than either the systolic or diastolic alone since it represents the average rate at which the blood is circulated.

Venous pressure is also measured. Pressure in an arm vein is normally about 10 to 0 mm Hg. However, venous pressure is measured with a water manometer, not a mercury manometer. The water values are about 100 to 60 mm. The pressure is measured by inserting a needle into an arm vein. A manometer is attached to the needle by means of a three-way stopcock. The arm of the stopcock is arranged so that the venous blood will flow into the manometer. The height of the column of blood indicates the venous pressure.

If frequent venous pressure readings are required, central venous pressure (CVP) measurements are used. A polyethylene catheter is passed through a vein and into the entrance of the right atrium. This catheter is attached by means of a three-way stopcock to a manometer and a continuous intravenous infusion. When a reading is made, the infusion is stopped, and the fluid is allowed to enter the manometer. The fluid rises in the manometer and slowly falls. The level to which it falls and starts fluctuating is the CVP reading.

Pressure in the pulmonary circuit can also be measured. This is done by inserting a Swan-Ganz catheter into a peripheral vein through the right side of the heart and into the pulmonary artery. A balloon at the tip of this catheter is inflated to obtain pressure readings, which are reflected by means of a transducer to a monitor. Normal pulmonary artery pressure (PAP) is 8 to 18 mm Hg. Pressure changes here reflect changes in left ventricular activity. It is important that the pressure in the pulmonary circuit be much lower than it is in the periphery since fluid should not be filtered out into the alveoli. The function of the pulmonary circuit is for the exchange of gases, not nutrition to the lungs.

You can learn something about venous pressure by allowing your hand to hang down at your side until the superficial veins of the hand become distended; then raise the hand slowly until the veins are no longer distended. Normally, there will be no distention when the hand is raised to the level of the heart. When the venous pressure is elevated, the distention will not disappear until the hand is substantially above the level of the heart.

ARTERIAL CIRCULATION

Arteries carry blood from the heart to the capillaries. They are more muscular and elastic than veins and do not collapse when cut. The arteries are generally deeper in the body and have smaller diameters than their corresponding veins. Capillaries are the microscopic connections between the arterioles and venules (very small arteries and veins). It is here that the work of the blood is done. Veins differ from arteries in that they are thin-walled and collapse when cut. Most veins have valves to prevent the backflow of blood.

The pulmonary circulation arises from the pulmonary artery and branches down to capillaries that surround the alveoli in which the blood gases (oxygen and carbon dioxide) are exchanged. Once the blood is oxygenated and most of the carbon dioxide has been removed, the blood is returned to the left side of the heart via the pulmonary veins.

The systemic circulation begins in the aorta. From the arch of the aorta there are three branches: the left common carotid, the left subclavian, and the innominate, or brachiocephalic, which gives rise to the right common carotid and right subclavian (see Figs. 13-6 and 13-7). A short cord, the ligamentum arteriosum (lig"ah-men'tum ar-te-re-o'sum) extends from the undersurface of the aortic arch to the pulmonary artery. In fetal life, this structure was the ductus arteriosus, which permitted blood to flow from the pulmonary artery into the aorta and, thus, bypass the pulmonary circuit.

Circulation to the head and neck begins with the common carotid arteries, which subdivide at about the angle of the mandible into the external carotid supplying the superficial structures of the head and the internal carotid supplying the deeper structures. The internal carotid

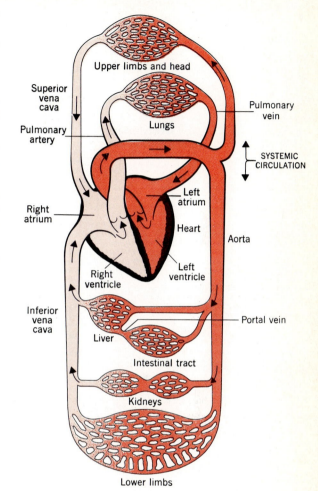

Figure 13-6. *The circulatory system*

feeds into the circle of Willis at the base of the brain. This circle is an important **anastamosis** (ah-nas"to-mo'sis), or joining, of vessels that provides for collateral circulation to this vital area in the event of blocking of the blood supply to the brain.

The vertebral arteries that branch off the subclavians also feed into the circle of Willis (see

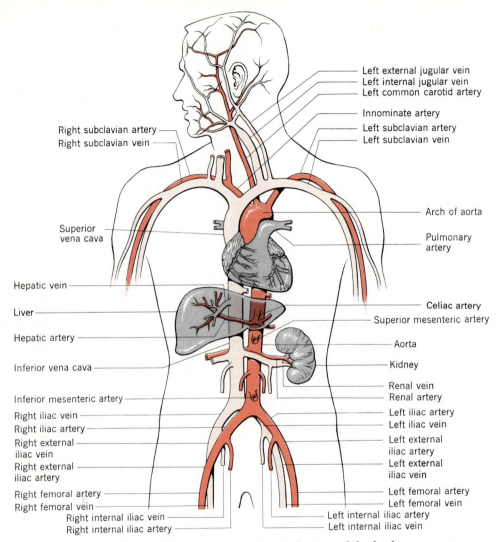

Figure 13-7. *Major arteries and veins of the body*

Figs. 13-8 and 13-9). You can feel pulsations in these subclavian arteries just above the clavicles. The subclavian changes its name as it proceeds toward the upper extremities. It first becomes the axillary and then the brachial, which divides to form the radial and ulnar arteries. You can feel pulsations in the radial artery on the lateral, distal, anterior aspect of your forearm. This is the radial pulse. The radial and ulnar arteries anastomose to form the volar arch in the hand.

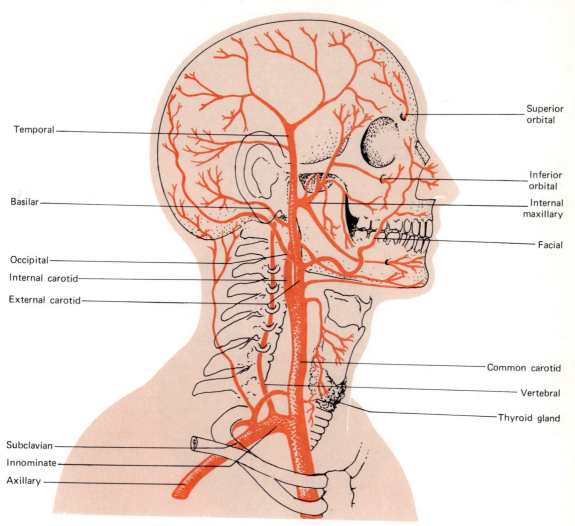

Figure 13-8. *Arterial circulation to the head*

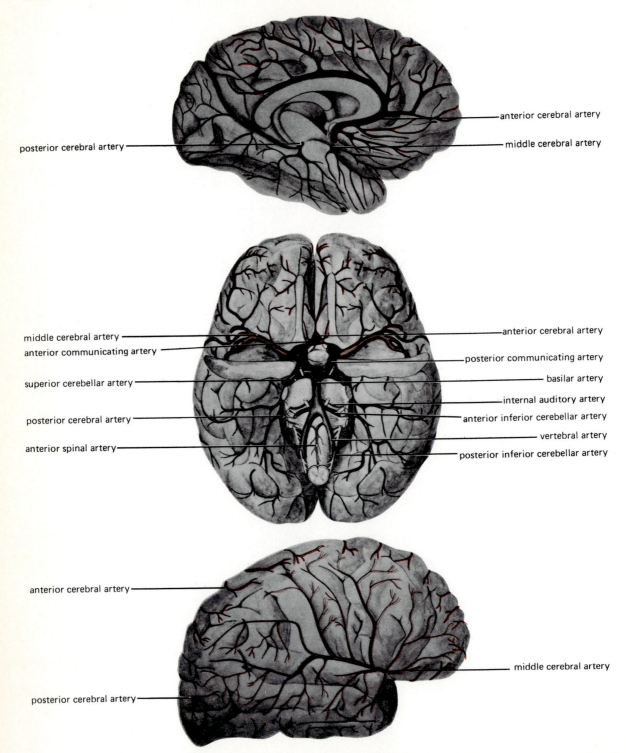

Figure 13-9. Blood vessels of the brain

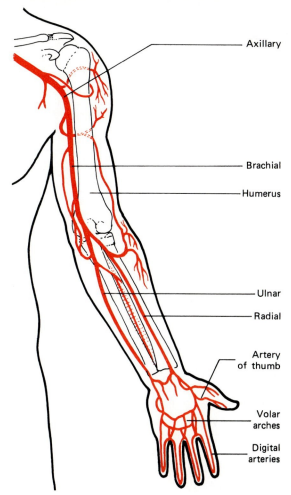

Figure 13-10. *Major arteries of the upper extremity*

rietal branches are the intercostals, which supply the intercostal muscles, and the superior phrenics, which supply the upper surface of the diaphragm.

The first visceral branch off the abdominal aorta is the celiac, lying just below the diaphragm. This artery feeds into a complex anastomosis that has several branches to supply the stomach, spleen, pancreas, liver, gall bladder, and the first part of the small intestine. Other visceral branches of the abdominal aorta are as follows: the superior mesenteric, which supplies the small intestines and the first half of the large bowel; the suprarenals; the renals; the inferior mesenteric, which supplies the last half of the large bowel; and the spermatics or ovarians. The parietal branches of the abdominal aorta include four lumbars and a middle sacral (see Fig. 13-11).

At about the level of the fourth lumbar vertebra, the aorta divides to form the common iliac arteries. These arteries in turn, divide to become the internal iliac, which supplies the pelvic viscera, the external genitalia, and the buttocks; and the external iliac, which goes down the lower extremity and becomes the femoral. From the femoral artery, the blood flows into the popliteal artery, which divides to become the anterior and posterior tibial arteries. The anterior tibial extends down to the foot where it becomes the dorsalis pedis artery. The deep plantar artery, one of the branches of the dorsalis pedis, descends into the sole of the foot where it unites with a branch of the posterior tibial artery and forms the plantar arch. Metatarsal and digital arteries branch from this arch (see Fig. 13-12).

It is important to note that the blood vessels themselves, like any organ, must have a blood supply. These blood vessels are call vasa vasorum (meaning vessels of the vessels).

This arch gives off small digital arteries to the fingers (see Fig. 13-10).

Two major visceral arteries come off the thoracic aorta: the bronchial, which is the nutrient artery to the lungs, and the esophageal. The pa-

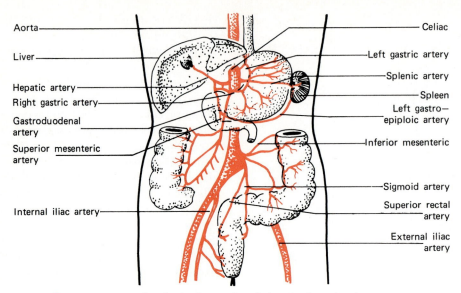

Figure 13-11. Blood supply to the abdominal and pelvic viscera

CAPILLARIES

The arteries branch to smaller and smaller arterioles and finally to microscopic capillaries. It is in the capillaries that the work of the circulatory system is accomplished. Into the tissue spaces, the blood pressure filters water and crystalline substances such as glucose, amino acids, and electrolytes needed by the cells for their metabolism. Oxygen, which is in greater concentrations in the capillaries than it is in the intercellular spaces, diffuses from the blood to the cells. Carbon dioxide, which is in greater concentrations in the tissue spaces than it is in the blood, diffuses into the bloodstream to be returned to the pulmonary circuit where it can be eliminated in the expired air. Excess water in

the tissues can be returned to the blood capillary by osmosis or to the lymph capillary (see Fig. 13-5). Any products such as hormones and enzymes manufactured by the cells can enter the capillaries and be carried to other cells where they are needed. Proteins and foreign particles that cannot easily enter the blood capillary from the interstitial spaces will be removed by the lymph capillaries.

VENOUS RETURN

As we consider the venous circulation, we shall begin in the periphery, where the veins are the smallest, and trace the blood as it moves into

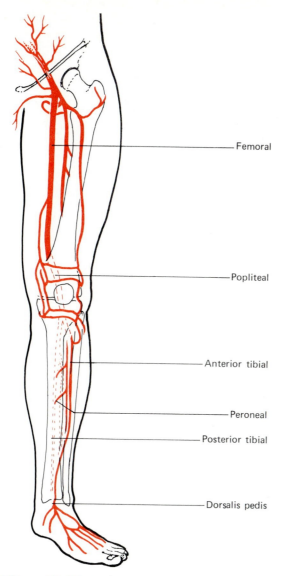

Figure 13-12. *Major arteries of the lower extremity*

— Femoral

— Popliteal

— Anterior tibial

— Peroneal

— Posterior tibial

— Dorsalis pedis

the larger and larger veins until finally it is returned to the right atrium.

The external and internal jugular veins are the chief veins returning blood from the head. They receive their blood from the cranial venous sinuses and return it to the subclavians and then into the right or left innominates. The innominates empty into the superior vena cava, which enters the right atrium (see Fig. 13-13).

Both deep and superficial veins are found in the upper extremity. The deep veins have the same names as their corresponding arteries. However, the superficial ones have different names. They begin in the dorsal network of the hand. The cephalic goes up the lateral side of the forearm and empties into the axillary. The basilic, which is on the ulnar side of the forearm, also empties into the axillary. The prominent superficial vein at the elbow is the median cubital (see Fig. 13-14).

Veins of the thorax include the innominates, which receive from the jugulars, subclavians, and others. Blood flows into the superior vena cava from these vessels and is returned to the right atrium. Small azygos veins, which also empty into the superior vena cava, bring venous blood from the lower parts of the body (see Fig. 13-15).

The veins of the lower extremities have the most valves. The deep veins have the same names as their corresponding arteries. The superficial veins, called the great and small saphenous veins, are those that are most likely to become varicosed (see Fig. 13-16). The great saphenous empties into the femoral vein and the small saphenous into the popliteal vein in back of the knee.

Veins of the abdomen and pelvis include the external iliac, which is a continuation of the femoral, and the internal iliac, which drains the pelvis and flows into the common iliac. The inferior vena cava receives blood from four lum-

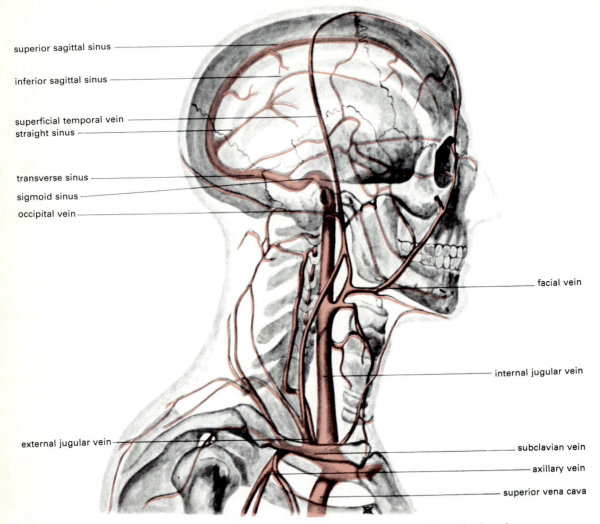

superior sagittal sinus

inferior sagittal sinus

superficial temporal vein
straight sinus

transverse sinus

sigmoid sinus

occipital vein

facial vein

internal jugular vein

external jugular vein

subclavian vein

axillary vein

superior vena cava

Figure 13-13. *Cranial venous sinuses and venous return from the head*

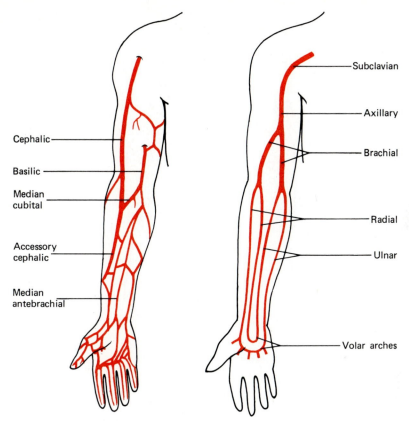

Figure 13-14. Venous return of the upper extremity showing super-ficial veins (left) and deep veins (right)

bars; the spermatics or ovarians; the renal, which drains the kidney; the suprarenals from the adrenal glands; and the hepatic, which drains the liver.

The portal system is very important. It receives blood from the organs of digestion and the spleen and takes it to the liver so that the liver can perform many important functions on the substances contained in this blood (see Fig. 13-17). The superior mesenteric, inferior mes-

enteric, spleenic, gastric, and esophageal venous blood flows into the portal vein, and after entering the liver, branches to smaller and smaller vessels until the blood finally comes into contact with the liver cells in the sinusoids. Here blood glucose can be converted to glycogen and stored for future use. Blood proteins are made in the liver from amino acids in this blood. In Chapter 17, we will discuss further the vital functions occurring here. Also flowing into the sinusoids

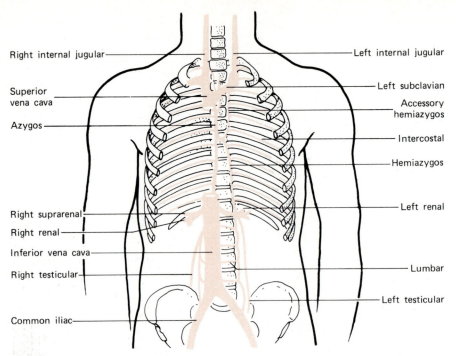

Figure 13-15. *The azygos system of veins. The superior and inferior vena cava and some of their tributaries are also shown.*

is the blood from the hepatic artery, which is nutrient to the cells of the liver. From the sinusoids the blood flows into the central veins and then into the hepatic vein. The hepatic vein empties into the inferior vena cava.

You should note that the portal vein differs from other veins in that it does not have valves to prevent the backflow of blood. Thus, in certain liver diseases in which some of the sinusoids become blocked, there may be large accumulations of blood in the mesenteric veins and a great increase in venous pressure here. Figure 13-18 illustrates how valves within most veins help maintain the proper direction of blood flow.

FETAL CIRCULATION

The gastrointestinal system, kidneys, and lungs do not perform the same functions in the fetus as they do after the baby is born. The fetus receives its nourishment and oxygen from its mother and also depends on her for the elimination of its waste products and carbon dioxide. The placenta, or afterbirth, is where this exchange takes place. There is, however, no direct connection between the circulatory systems of the mother and the fetus.

Two umbilical arteries and an umbilical vein

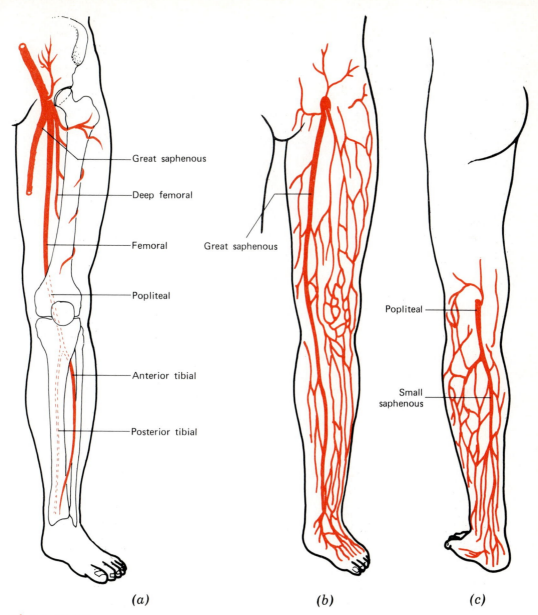

Great saphenous

Deep femoral

Femoral

Popliteal

Anterior tibial

Posterior tibial

Great saphenous

Popliteal

Small
saphenous

(a)

(b)

(c)

Figure 13-16. *(a) Deep veins of the lower extremity. (b) Anterior view of the superficial veins of the leg. (c) Posterior view of the superficial veins of the leg.*

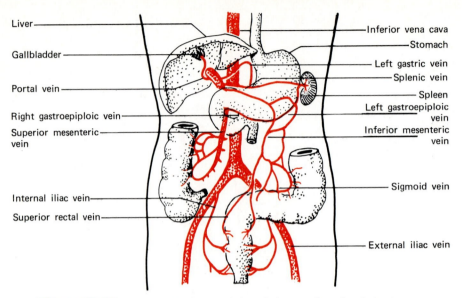

Figure 13-17. *Venous drainage of the abdominal and pelvic viscera*

connect the fetus with the placenta. These blood vessels are in the umbilical cord (see Fig. 13-19). Blood enters the placenta by way of the umbilical arteries, which branch off the internal iliac arteries of the fetus. After circulating through

the capillaries of the placenta, where it picks up nutrients and oxygen and eliminates waste, the blood returns to the fetus by way of the umbilical vein and goes directly to the liver where it divides into two branches. One branch joins the portal vein and enters the liver. The other branch, called the ductus venosus, goes on to the inferior vena cava. The ductus venosus and the umbilical vein are obliterated a few days after the baby is born.

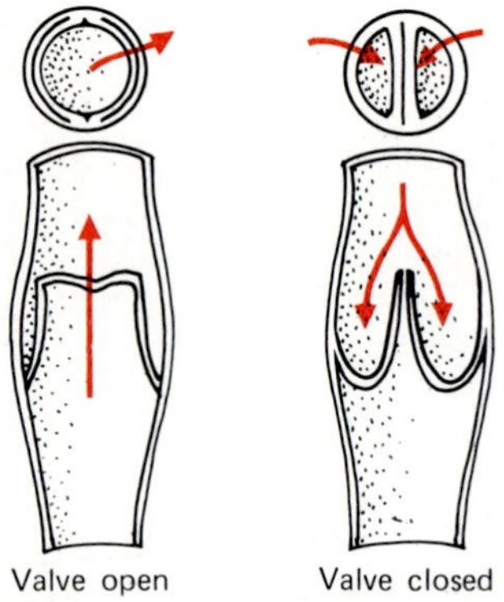

As blood from the lower part of the fetus returns to the inferior vena cava it is mixed with the blood rich in oxygen and nutrients returning from the placenta. This blood then enters the right atrium. A valve in the inferior vena cava guides a steady stream of blood from the right atrium through the foramen ovale and into the left atrium, thus bypassing the pulmonary circuit. Blood from the upper portion of the body enters the right atrium by way of the superior vena cava. Some of this blood may also enter the foramen ovale. However, any blood that de-

Valve open   Valve closed

Figure 13-18. *Veins contain valves that open in the direction of blood flow and prevent backflow of blood when closed.*

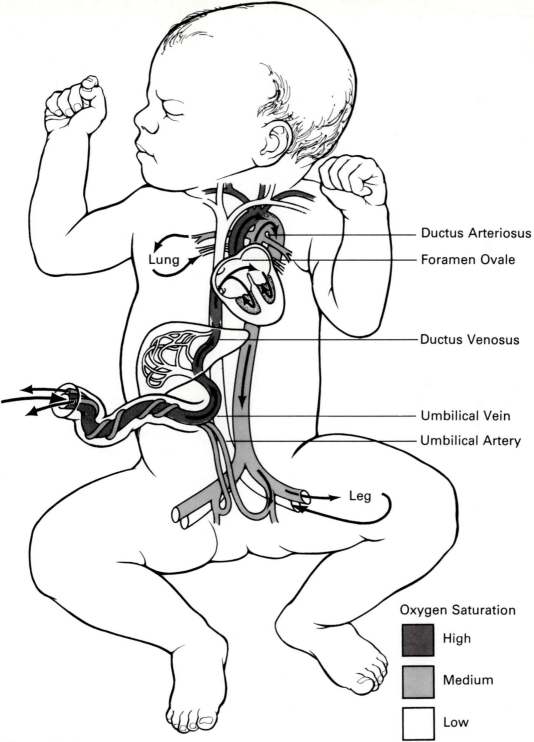

Labels on figure:
Lung
Ductus Arteriosus
Foramen Ovale
Ductus Venosus
Umbilical Vein
Umbilical Artery
Leg

Oxygen Saturation
High
Medium
Low

Figure 13-19. *Placental circulation (From Butnareseu, G., and Tillutson, D., Maternity Nursing Theory to Practice. New York: John Wiley & Sons, 1983)*

scends into the right ventricle is pumped into the pulmonary artery, but since the lungs of the fetus are collapsed, from the pulmonary artery it will go through the ductus arteriosus, which opens into the arch of the aorta. Normally, the foramen ovale and the ductus arteriosus close soon after the baby is born.

The blood in the aorta and other arteries of the fetus is a mixture of oxygenated and poorly oxygenated blood. The umbilical vein is the only fetal vessel that carries fully oxygenated blood.

THE COMPOSITION OF BLOOD

The liquid portion of the circulating blood is called **plasma**. The formed elements of the blood are the platelets and blood cells. Although red blood cells are very small, they are biconcave disks that are thin near the center and thicker around the rims, providing a large surface area through which gases can diffuse. These cells are manufactured in the red bone marrow and have a life span of about 120 days. Proper production and maturation of these cells depend on adequate supplies of vitamin B_{12}, also known as an "extrinsic factor," since it is ingested in the food we eat. The absorption of this vitamin is dependent on the "intrinsic factor," a substance produced by the lining of the stomach. Production of red blood cells is also dependent on renal erythropoietin (er-ith"ro-po-e'tin). This hormone from the kidney and liver is produced in response to oxygen lack and stimulates the bone marrow to produce red blood cells. Red blood cells contain **hemoglobin**, which contains iron for oxygen transport. Each cell is about one-third hemoglobin by volume. When hemoglobin combines with oxygen the resulting oxyhemoglobin is bright red. When the oxygen is released deoxyhemoglobin is formed and the cell is a darker red. Blood that is rich in deoxyhemoglobin may appear blue when seen through the vessel walls. A person with a prolonged deficiency of oxygen will have **cyanosis** (si-ah-no'sis), a condition in which the skin and mucous membranes appear bluish because of a high concentration of deoxyhemoglobin.

Normal hemoglobin is about 15 g/100 ml. It is normally a little higher in men than in women. The number of red blood cells is about 4.5 to 5 million cells/cu mm. The **hematocrit** (he-mah'to-krit) is the fraction of the total volume of blood that consists of cells, normally about 40% to 45%. Patients who are hemorrhaging have low hematocrits. Patients who are losing the fluid portion of their blood (for example, in burns with a great deal of edema) have high hematocrits, and their blood has a much greater tendency to clot. Old, worn-out red blood cells are destroyed in the **reticuloendothelial system** (the liver, spleen, and bone marrow). The iron from these cells is saved and reused.

The leukocytes, or white blood cells, are formed in both the red bone marrow and lymphatic tissue. The normal white blood cell count, called the absolute count, is about 5,000 to 10,000 cells/cu mm.

The percentage of each type of white cell is known as a differential count. The neutrophils make up about 65% of the total white blood count (WBC). These increase in acute infections. Monocytes make up about 5% of the absolute count. Their numbers increase in chronic infections. Lymphocytes, which account for about 27.5% of the total, are important in helping to develop immunity. The circulating lymphocytes do little to help fight infections. However, they are powerful phagocytes while they are in the lymph nodes. Eosinophils and basophils together comprise about 2.5% of the total white cell count (see Fig. 13-20). Eosinophils detoxify foreign proteins, break down antigen-antibody complexes after immune reactions have oc-

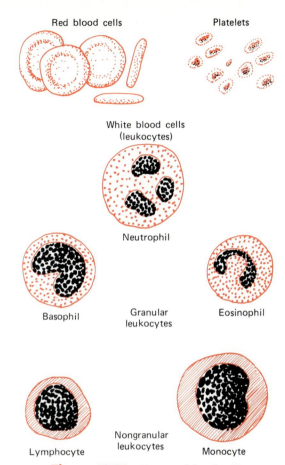

Red blood cells

Platelets

White blood cells
(leukocytes)

Neutrophil

Basophil

Granular
leukocytes

Eosinophil

Lymphocyte

Nongranular
leukocytes

Monocyte

Figure 13-20. Human blood cells

curred, and turn off inflammatory reactions. Basophils, though not phagocytic, do play a role in the body's defense mechanisms. They release histamine into injured tissue and, thereby, initiate the inflammatory process.

The thrombocytes (throm'bo-sits), or platelets, which are smaller than the red blood cells, play an important role in blood clotting. Because they are sticky and will adhere to a damaged vessel wall, they help to plug the leak and also allow other cells to stick to them and to form a clot.

Clotting time is normally about seven to ten minutes. If this time is prolonged, the patient will have a bleeding tendency. If the clotting time is less than normal, he will have a tendency toward intravascular clots.

An intravascular clot is called a **thrombus**; if the clot moves, it is called an **embolus**. Intravascular clotting is promoted by injury to the vessel wall, prolonged bed rest, foreign material in the blood, or trauma to the components of the blood itself. It is hindered by early ambulation, stable platelets, and the presence of heparin or other anticoagulants. Vitamin K deficiency is not a common clinical problem except in newborns, who are normally vitamin K deficient. Normally, the bacteria in the large bowel form vitamin K. But because the bowel of the newborn is sterile, the infant has no vitamin K unless the mother has had an injection of vitamin K shortly before delivery or the infant has received an injection.

Prothrombin (pro-throm'bin) time, the time it takes plasma to clot, is normally about 12 to 13 seconds. If it is much longer, the person will have a bleeding tendency. People who are on anticoagulants because they have thrombosis or have had a heart attack must have frequent prothrombin time checkups done to be sure that their prothrombin time does not become too prolonged. These people should have the name and the dose of anticoagulant with their identification card, since in case of an accident, the emergency room staff will need to take this into account in the treatment of the wounds.

Extravascular clotting is hastened by contact with a rough surface such as gauze and is hindered by oxalates (ok'sah-latz) and citrates (sit'ratz), which remove the calcium from the blood.

For a more complete picture of the composition of blood and types of clinical studies done on blood, see Tables 13-1 and 13-2.

Table 13-1. Hematology Findings in Health and Disease

Normal Range	Conditions in Which Variations from Normal May Occur
Volume 7–9% of body weight (4000–6000 ml)	Decreased: hemorrhage, surgical shock, burns
Erythrocytes 4.5–5 million/mm³	Increased: polycythemia, anoxia, chronic pulmonary disease, high altitudes, renal disease with increased secretion of erythropoietin, Cushing's Syndrome Decreased: anemia, hemorrhage, leukemia
Reticulocytes 0.8–1% of rbc (red blood cells)	Increased: hemolytic jaundice, anemia with increased bone marrow activity
Leukocytes 5,000–10,000 mm³	Increased: infections and tissue destruction, leukemia, metabolic disorders Decreased: irradiation, bone marrow aplasia
Neutrophils (PMN) 60–70% of wbc (white blood cells)	Increased: acute infections, gout, uremia, neoplastic diseases of the bone marrow, diabetic ketosis, massive necrosis, poisoning by mercury, lead, or digitalis Decreased: agranulocytosis, acute leukemia, measles, malaria, overwhelming bacterial infections
Lymphocytes 25–33% of wbc	Increased: whooping cough, chronic infections, infectious mononucleosis, chronic lymphatic leukemia, thyrotoxicosis Decreased: Hodgkin's Disease, in response to adrenal cortical steroids, whole-body irradiation
Monocytes 2–6% of wbc	Increased: chronic bacterial diseases, tetrachlorethane poisoning, monocytic leukemia
Eosinophils 1–3% of wbc	Increased: hypersensitivity (hay fever, asthma, chronic skin diseases), helminthic infestations, leukemia Decreased: steroid therapy
Basophils 0.05–0.5% of PMN	Increased: acute severe infections, leukemia
Metamyelocytes 5% of PMN	Increased: acute severe infections, leukemia
Platelets 250,000–350,000	Increased: after trauma or surgery, after massive hemorrhage, polycythemia Decreased: thrombocytopenic purpura, lupus erythematosus, following massive blood transfusions
Hemoglobin 14–16 gm/100 ml	Increased: conditions in which there is an increase in erythrocytes Decreased: anemia, hemorrhage, leukemia
Hematocrit 42–47%	Increased: dehydration, plasma loss, burns, conditions in which there is an increase in erythrocytes Decreased: hemorrhage, anemia

Sedimentation rate
  Men 0–12 mm/hr
  Women 0–20 mm/hr
	Increased: infection, coronary thrombosis, leukemia, anemia, hemorrhage, malignancy, hyperthyroidism, kidney disease
	Decreased: severe liver disease, malaria, erythemia, sickle-cell anemia

Bleeding time 1–3 min	Increased: thrombocytopenia, acute leukemia, Hodgkin's Disease, hemorrhagic disease of the newborn, hemophilia, thrombocytopenia
Coagulation time 6–12 min	Increased: hemophilia, anticoagulant therapy

Clot retraction time
  Begins in 1 hr
  Completes in 24 hr
	Increased: thrombocytopenia, acute leukemia, pernicious anemia, multiple myeloma, malignant granuloma, hemorrhagic disease of the newborn

Prothrombin time 10–15 sec	Increased: treatment with anticoagulants, hemorrhagic disease of the newborn, liver disease, hemophilia

From Shirley R. Burke, *The Composition and Function of Body Fluids*, 2nd ed., St. Louis: The C. V. Mosby Co., 1976.

Table 13-2. Blood Chemistry Findings in Health and Disease*

Normal Range	Conditions in Which Variations From Normal May Occur
Albumin 3.5–5.5 g/dl	Increased: dehydration
	Decreased: renal disease, liver disease, malnutrition
Aldolase 3–8 units/ml	Increased: muscular atrophy, cancer, acute or chronic disease
Ammonia 20–160 μg/dl (diffusion)	Increased: liver disease
Amylase 60–160 Somogyi units/dl	Increased: pancreatitis, postgastrectomy, cholecystitis, salivary gland disease
	Decreased: hepatitis, thyrotoxicosis, severe burns, toxemia of pregnancy
Bicarbonate 21–28 mM/L	Increased: metabolic alkalosis
	Decreased: metabolic acidosis
Bilirubin	Increased: biliary obstruction, impaired liver function, hemolytic disease
Total 0.3–1.5 mg/dl	
Direct 0.1–0.3 mg/dl	
Blood gases	
pH arterial 7.35–7.45	Increased: alkalosis
pH venous 7.3–7.41	Decreased: acidosis
Po_2 arterial 95–100 mm Hg	Increased: administration of high concentrations of oxygen
	Decreased: hypovolemia, decreased cardiac output, chronic pulmonary diseases
Pco_2 arterial 36–44 mm Hg	Increased: respiratory acidosis, metabolic alkalosis
Pco_2 venous 40–45 mm Hg	Decreased: respiratory alkalosis, metabolic acidosis, hypothermia
Blood urea nitrogen (BUN) 8–18 mg/dl (adult)	Increased: fever, excess body protein catabolism, renal failure, congestive heart failure with decreased renal blood supply, obstructive uropathy
	Decreased: growing infant
Calcium	Increased: hyperparathyroidism, vitamin D excess, multiple myeloma, thyrotoxicosis, sarcoidosis, bone cancer, fractures
Ionized 2.1–2.6 mEq/L	
Total 4.5–5.3 mEq/L	Decreased: hypoparathyroidism, acute pancreatitis, vitamin D deficiency, steatorrhea, nephrosis, rickets, Paget's disease, malabsorption, pregnancy, respiratory alkalosis
Infants 11–13 mg/dl	
CO_2 combining power	Increased: emphysema, metabolic alkalosis
45–70 vol%	Decreased: respiratory alkalosis, metabolic acidosis
21–28 mEq/L	
CO_2 (measured as HCO_3	Increased: respiratory acidosis, metabolic alkalosis
25–35 mEq/L	Decreased: respiratory alkalosis, metabolic acidosis
Carboxyhemoglobin	Increased: industrial pollution, smoking
Suburban nonsmokers less than 1.5% saturation of hemoglobin	
Smokers 1.5%–5.0%	
Heavy smokers 5.0%–9.0%	

*Values depend to a certain extent on the technique used for the determination; therefore occasional discrepancies may occur when comparing different normal value charts.

Table 13-2. Blood Chemistry Findings in Health and Disease—Cont'd

Normal Range	Conditions in Which Variations From Normal May Occur
Chloride 95–105 mEq/L	Increased: dehydration, hyperchloremic acidosis, brain injury, steroid therapy, respiratory alkalosis, hyperparathyroidism Decreased: gastrointestinal loss, potassium depletion associated with alkalosis, diabetic ketosis, Addison's disease, respiratory acidosis, mercurial diuretic therapy
Cholesterol 150–250 mg/dl (varies with age and diet)	Increased: obstructive jaundice, renal disease, pancreatic disease, hypothyroidism, untreated diabetes mellitus, chronic pancreatitis, familial hypercholesterolemia Decreased: severe liver disease, starvation, terminal uremia, hyperthyroidism, cortisone therapy, anemia
Creatine phosphokinase Males 55–170 units/L Females 30–135 units/L	Increased: myocardial infarction, crush injury, hypothyroidism, tissue transplant rejection, cerebral vascular accident
Creatinine 0.6–1.2 mg/dl	Increased: acromegaly, renal failure
Fibrinogen 200–400 mg/dl	Increased: inflammatory processes Decreased: liver disease, hemorrhagic disease
Gastrin 40–150 pg/ml	Increased: peptic ulcers, gastric carcinoma, pernicious anemia
Globulin 2.5–3.0 g/dl	Increased: chronic infectious diseases, chronic hepatitis, sarcoidosis
Glucose 70–120 mg/dl (fasting)	Increased: diabetes mellitus, severe thyrotoxicosis, burns, shock, stress, after norepinephrine injection, pheochromocytoma (during attack), Cushing's syndrome, pancreatic insufficiency, diuretics Decreased: insulin overdosage, hyperplasia of islet cells, hypothalamic lesions, postgastrectomy dumping syndrome, liver disease, Addison's disease
Glutamic-oxaloacetic transaminase (SGOT) less than 40 units/ml	Increased: myocardial infarction, acute rheumatic carditis, cardiac surgery, cirrhosis, hepatitis, pulmonary infarction, acute pancreatitis, trauma, shock, skeletal muscle disease
Glutamic-pyruvic transaminase (SGPT) less than 30 units/ml	Increased: acute hepatitis, cirrhosis of liver, myocardial infarction, infectious mononucleosis
Glutathione reductase 10–70 units/ml	Increased: cancer, hepatitis
Hydroxybutyric dehydrogenase 140–350 units/ml	Increased: myocardial infarction, myocarditis, liver disease
Iodine (PBI) 4.0–8.0 µg/dl	Increased: hyperthyroidism, exogenous iodine intake, elevated serum protein Decreased: hypothyroidism, low serum protein
Iron, total 50–150 µg/dl	Decreased: hypochromic anemia, hemoglobinopathies
Isocitric dehydrogenase (ICD) 60–290 units/ml	Increased: hepatitis, pancreatic malignancy, preeclamptic toxemia, carcinomatosis of liver
Lactic acid Venous 5–20 mg/dl Arterial 3–7 mg/dl	Increased: lactic acidosis

Table 13-2. Blood Chemistry Findings in Health and Disease—Cont'd

Normal Range	Conditions in Which Variations From Normal May Occur
Lactic dehydrogenase (LDH) 200–425 units/ml LDH$_1$ 17%–27% LDH$_2$ 27%–37% LDH$_3$ 18%–25% LDH$_4$ 3%–8% LDH$_5$ 0%–5%	Increased: myocardial infarction (LDH in heart muscle is stable so that when specimen is incubated, level remains elevated), hepatitis, skeletal muscle damage (LDH in liver and muscle is heat labile so that elevated levels return to normal after incubation), renal tissue destruction, pulmonary emboli, pneumonia, pernicious anemia, cerebral vascular accident
Lipids (values increase with age) Total 400–800 mg/dl Cholesterol 150–250 mg/dl (age 35 yr)	Increased: familial hypercholesterolemia, obstructive jaundice, renal disease, pancreatic disease, hypothyroidism, pancreatitis, untreated diabetes mellitus Decreased: severe liver disease, starvation, uremia, hyperthyroidism, cortisone therapy, anemia
Triglycerides 10–150 mg/dl (age 35 yr)	Increased: atherosclerosis, hyperlipemia, diabetes mellitus, lipid metabolism abnormality Decreased: deficient bile production, liver damage, poor intestinal absorption, lipid metabolism abnormality
Phospholipids 150–380 mg/dl (age 35 yr)	Increased: hyperlipidemia, atherosclerosis, lipid metabolism abnormality, diabetes mellitus Decreased: severe liver disease, malabsorption
Low-density lipoproteins (LDL) 45%–50% of total lipids	Increased: hyperlipidemia, coronary artery disease
Magnesium 1.5–2.4 mEq/L	Increased: administration of magnesium compounds in presence of renal failure Decreased: severe malabsorption
Nonprotein nitrogen (NPN) 20–35 mg/dl	Increased: renal insufficiency
Osmolality 280–295 mOsm/L	Increased: water loss, diabetes, azotemia, sepsis, lactic acidosis, liver failure, drug intoxication Decreased: water excess, sodium loss
Oxygen pressure Po$_2$ arterial 95–100 mm Hg	Increased: administration of high concentrations of oxygen Decreased: hypovolemia, decreased cardiac output, chronic pulmonary disease
pH Arterial 7.35–7.45 Venous 7.3–7.41	Increased: alkalosis Decreased: acidosis
Phosphatase Acid 0.13–0.63 units/L (Bessey-Lowry)	Increased: prostatic malignancy
Alkaline Adults 0.8–2.3 units/L (Bessey-Lowry) Children 3.4–9.0 units/L (Bessey-Lowry)	Increased: bone diseases and malignancies, liver disease, hyperparathyroidism, obstructive jaundice

Table 13-2. Blood Chemistry Findings in Health and Disease—Cont'd

Normal Range	*Conditions in Which Variations From Normal May Occur*
Phospholipids 150–380 mg/dl	Increased: hyperlipidemia, coronary artery disease, atherosclerosis, lipid metabolism abnormality
Phosphorus Adult 1.8–2.6 mEq/L	Increased: vitamin D excess, healing fractures, renal failure, hypoparathyroidism, diabetic ketosis, hyperthyroidism
Children 2.3–4.1 mEq/L	Decreased: hyperparathyroidism, rickets, osteomalacia
Potassium 3.0–4.5 mEq/L	Increased: shock, crush syndrome, anuria, Addison's disease, renal failure, diabetic ketosis
	Decreased: severe diarrhea, bowel fistula, diuretic therapy, Cushing's syndrome
Protein Total 6.0–7.8 g/dl	Increased: dehydration
	Decreased: renal disease, malnutrition, liver disease, severe burns
Albumin 3.5–5.5 g/dl	Increased: dehydration
	Decreased: renal disease, liver disease, malnutrition
Globulin 2.5–3.0 g/dl	Increased: chronic infectious diseases, sarcoidosis, Hodgkin's disease
Sodium 133–143 mEq/L	Increased: steroid therapy, hypothalamic lesions, head injury, hyperosmolar states
	Decreased: gastrointestinal loss, sweating, renal tubular damage, water intoxication, Addison's disease, diuretics, metabolic acidosis, inappropriate ADH syndrome, bronchogenic carcinoma, pulmonary infections

Thyroid hormone tests
    (expressed as thyroxin)
    T_4 (Murphy-Pattee)
    6.0–11.8 μg/dl
	Increased: hyperthyroidism
	Decreased: hypothyroidism

T_3 (resin uptake) 25%–35% uptake	Increased: hyperthyroidism, thyrotoxicosis Decreased: hypothyroidism
Triglycerides (age 35 yr) 10–150 mg/dl	Increased: atherosclerosis, hyperlipemia, diabetes mellitus, lipid metabolism abnormality
	Decreased: deficient bile production, liver damage, poor intestinal absorption, lipid metabolism abnormality
Urea nitrogen (BUN) 8–18 mg/dl	Increased: renal failure, obstructive uropathy, congestive heart failure with decreased renal blood supply fever, excess body protein catabolism
	Decreased: growing infant
Uric acid 1.5–4.5 mg/dl	Increased: gout, gross tissue destruction, renal failure, hypoparathyroidism
	Decreased: administration of uricosuric drugs (cortisone, salicylates)

IMMUNITY

Immunity is an important defense against pathogens, cancer, and many foreign substances. There are two types of immunity. One type involves a chemical reaction and is called humoral immunity. The other relates to activities of certain cells and is called cell-mediated immunity or cellular immunity. Lymphoid tissue is responsible for both types of protection.

HUMORAL IMMUNITY

A kind of lymphocyte called B cells initiates the humoral immune response. This type of immunity is the main defense against bacterial and viral infections. When activated by **antigens** (an'ti-jenz), B cells become plasma cells that secrete antibodies or immune bodies to neutralize or remove the antigen as a threat. Antigens are foreign agents that, if introduced into the body, stimulate the production of antibodies. In the humoral immune system, the antigens are usually bacteria or viruses. The antibodies produced are proteins specific to the particular organism. This is the basis of immunization.

Immunity is the result of the development within the body of antibodies capable of destroying or inactivating the causative agent of the disease should it enter the body at a later time. For example, immunization against measles is produced by injecting a preparation of the live but weakened organisms. For typhoid immunization, a preparation of killed organisms is used. Table 13-3 gives an immunization schedule.

CELLULAR IMMUNITY

The cellular immune response is particularly effective against fungi, parasites, some cancer cells, and foreign tissue. This immunity is mediated by a type of lymphocyte called **T cells**. These cells require a hormone, **thymosin**, produced by the thymus gland, to make them capable of responding to antigens.

Some of these thymosin-dependent cells become killer cells that recognize the antigen as foreign, attack, and destroy the object that does not belong. An example of this type of immune response is the rejection of a tissue or organ transplant.

Other T cells become primed cells capable of responding to a second exposure to a given antigen. With primed cells, the first exposure sen-

Table 13-3. Recommended Immunization Schedule

	2 Months	4 Months	6 Months	15 Months	2 Years	4–6 Years	14–16 Years
DTP	*	*	*	*		*	Td ADULT
Polio	*	*		*		*	
Measles				*		*	
Rubella				*			
Mumps				*			
Hib					*		

DTP = Combined diphtheria, tetanus, and pertussis
Td = Combined tetanus and diphtheria given every 10 years throughout life.
Hib = Hemophilus Influenzae b

sitizes the cell, and the subsequent exposure produces the immune reaction. Tuberculin testing is an example of this type of immune response.

In cell-mediated immunity, the response can occur without the production of demonstrable antibodies. If antibodies are formed, they remain fixed to the sensitized lymphocytes that produced them.

BLOOD GROUPS

The blood groups are examples of genetically determined antigens. There are two main groups: the ABO system of antigens and the Rh system of antigens. Rh antigens are present in blood that is Rh positive. In the ABO system, the antigens, called A and B, may be present in the red blood cells. Neither is present in the red blood cells of people with type O blood. A is present in type A blood, B is present in type B blood, and both A and B antigens are present in type AB blood.

Which antigens are present is determined by the person's genes. The combination of genes a person has for a particular trait is called the genotype. Each individual has two genes that determine the ABO blood type from among the three kinds that may be present, genes A, B, and O. Genes A and B cause the synthesis of antigens A and B. Gene O lacks the information needed to make any antigen. The possible genotypes therefore are: AA, AO, BB, BO, AB, and OO. Genotypes AA and AO produce type A blood, BB and BO produce type B blood, genotype AB produces AB, and genotype OO produces type O. The observable characteristic produced by a genotype is called the phenotype. Therefore, the type of blood you have is your phenotype for that trait.

If a child's mother is type A and the child is type AB, then the father must have either type B or AB blood. Tests involving only ABO blood types may prove a man **not** to be the child's father, but they cannot prove he is the father. Antigens from infant and maternal tissues other than blood provide more precise information about the antigens the father must have.

BLOOD TYPING

Blood typing is done to help assure that a person who needs a blood transfusion will receive compatible blood. The administration of incompatible blood can lead to a very serious reaction or even a fatal transfusion reaction. Typing helps but does not assure that a patient will not have a transfusion reaction. The ABO typing system is most commonly used. Type O is called the universal donor. In theory, a person with type O blood can give blood to anyone but can only receive from type O donors. Type O blood will not agglutinate (ah-gloo"tin-ate), or clump, with either anti-A or anti-B sera. Type AB is the universal recipient. People with type AB can receive blood from anyone but give only to type AB recipients. This blood agglutinates with both anti-B and anti-A sera. Type A blood agglutinates with anti-A serum. People with type A blood can receive from donors of either type A or type O and can give to recipients of either type A or AB. Type B blood agglutinates with anti-B serum. People with type B blood can give to people with either type B or AB blood and can receive from either type B or type O donors.

More than 85% of humans are Rh-positive. The remaining few, who are Rh-negative, are susceptible to trouble if they receive an Rh-positive blood transfusion. This factor is probably overrated as a troublemaker in pregnancy. An Rh-negative mother must be carrying an Rh-positive baby and a placental leak must take place in order for the mother to form antibodies against the Rh factor. No problems occur with the first baby. In subsequent pregnancies, if the baby is Rh-positive, these antibodies can cross the placenta and destroy the baby's red blood cells. This condition is called erythroblastosis fetalis (e-rith"ro-blas-to'sis fe-tal'is). The baby must have a complete exchange transfusion. Rhogam, a drug that can be given to an Rh-negative mother after the birth of an Rh-positive baby, will destroy the mother's antibodies and prevent damage to the blood cells of her next baby. Rhogam should also be given to an Rh-negative woman after a miscarriage since there is a possibility that the aborted fetus had Rh-positive blood.

Blood transfusion reactions can be extremely dangerous. Because the signs and symptoms of a reaction usually occur within the first ten minutes of the transfusion, all transfusions should be started at a very slow flow rate until it is reasonably certain that a reaction is not going to occur. With the transfusion going slowly, if a reaction does occur, the patient will have received a relatively small amount of the incompatible blood thereby decreasing the severity of the reaction. Symptoms of a transfusion reaction include chills and fever. There may be a rash and itching, shortness of breath, nausea, and pain, usually in the kidney region, chest, or legs. **Hematuria** (he"mah-tu're-ah) (blood in the urine) and shock are present if the reaction is severe. Because such a reaction is an emergency situation, the transfusion should be stopped immediately. However, the needle should not be removed except by the blood bank personnel as the transfusion equipment should be examined by them in order to help determine the cause of the reaction. Urine specimens should be collected and examined for hemoglobin.

THE LYMPHATIC SYSTEM

The general functions of the lymphatic system are to return tissue fluid to the bloodstream and to filter the tissue fluid. In contrast to the blood system, these vessels begin in the tissues and end in a vein in the chest. There is no pump as such. The movement of lymph is slow; it depends on the contractions of muscles and pulsations in nearby arteries. The many valves in the lymphatic vessels prevent the backflow of the fluid.

Lymph capillaries open into the tissue spaces and lead to larger lymph vessels. The lymph capillaries originating in the villi of the small intestine are called lacteals (lak'te-alz). The milky lymph found in the lacteals after digestion contains 1% to 2% fat and is called chyle (kil). The large vessels penetrate lymph nodes as they proceed toward the subclavian vein where the tissue fluid is returned to the bloodstream. Lymph nodes function as filters to trap bacteria or foreign substances so that they will not be poured into the bloodstream. If there is a severe infection, the lymph nodes proximal to the site can become enlarged because they are filled with the bacteria that are being destroyed by the lymphocytes there.

The lymphatic collecting vessels that receive lymph from the capillaries eventually empty into one of two terminal ducts. The thoracic duct is terminal for the upper left part of the body and all of the lower parts of the body. It begins in a dilatation known as the cisterna chyli (sis-ter'nah ki'li), which is located at about the level of the second lumbar vertebra. It ascends with the aorta and receives lymph from intercostal lymphatic trunks and subclavian trunks. It ends in the left subclavian vein. The right lymphatic duct drains the rest of the body and empties into the right subclavian vein (see Fig. 13-21).

The thymus, spleen, and tonsils are also a part of the lymphatic system. The thymus is relatively large during infancy and early childhood. After puberty, it atrophies and by adulthood it is very small.

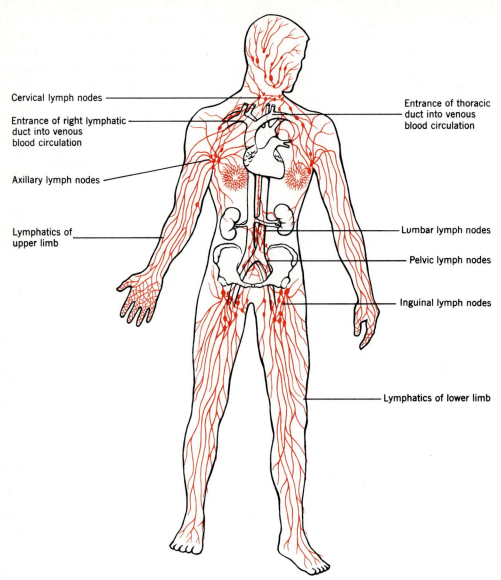

Cervical lymph nodes

Entrance of right lymphatic duct into venous blood circulation

Axillary lymph nodes

Lymphatics of upper limb

Entrance of thoracic duct into venous blood circulation

Lumbar lymph nodes

Pelvic lymph nodes

Inguinal lymph nodes

Lymphatics of lower limb

Figure 13-21. Lymphatic circulation. Tissue fluid collected by lymphatic vessels is carried either to the right lymphatic or thoracic ducts. These lymphatic ducts return the fluid to the subclavian veins.

SUMMARY QUESTIONS

1. Trace a drop of blood from the time it enters the right atrium until it enters the aorta.
2. What is the function of the valves of the heart?
3. What are the names of the valves located between the atria and ventricles?
4. How does the heart receive its blood supply?
5. What causes the heart sounds lupp and dupp?
6. Describe the intrinsic conduction mechanism of the heart.
7. What causes the closure of the semilunar valves?
8. Why must blood pressure in the pulmonary circuit be so much lower than the blood pressure in the peripheral arteries?
9. What are the functions of the lymphatic system?
10. Trace a drop of blood from the time it leaves the aorta until it gets to the capillaries of the small intestine and then returns to the right atrium.
11. Describe the functions of the different types of blood cells.
12. Discuss the events in the cardiac cycle and the electrical changes that take place during the cycle.
13. Describe the changes in blood pressure as the blood flows through the peripheral circuit and relate these to the rate of blood flow.
14. Discuss the factors influencing cardiac output.
15. What is the function of the azygos system of veins?
16. What is the function of lymph nodes?
17. Discuss two ways that tissue fluid is returned to the blood stream.

KEY TERMS

anastamosis
antigens
arrhythmia
cyanosis
diastole
dysrhythmia
embolus
endocardium
epicardium
hematocrit
hematuria

hemoglobin
mediastinum
myocardium
pericardium
plasma
reticuloendothelial system
systole
T cells
thrombus
thymosin

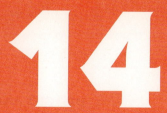

14

Diseases of the Cardiovascular System

OBJECTIVES

On completion of this chapter, you will be able to:

1. List the symptoms that suggest cardiac and/or cardiovascular disease.
2. Explain various diagnostic procedures that are designed to assess the structure and function of the cardiovascular system.
3. Describe the effects of hypertension on the heart and vascular system.
4. List risk factors for atherosclerosis that can be modified or controlled.
5. Explain the basis of chest pain associated with ischemic heart disease.
6. Discuss the pathophysiology of heart valve stenosis and insufficiency.
7. Outline the principles for treating congestive heart failure.

OVERVIEW

I. DIAGNOSTIC PROCEDURES
   A. History and Physical Examination
   B. Electrocardiogram
   C. Phonocardiogram
   D. Echocardiogram
   E. Doppler Ultrasound Studies
   F. Arteriography
   G. Cardiac Catheterization
   H. Radionuclide Studies
II. CARDIOVASCULAR DISEASE
   A. Atherosclerosis
   B. Hypertension
III. HEART DISEASE
   A. Ischemic Heart Disease
   B. Cardiac Disrhythmias
   C. Infective Endocarditis
   D. Valvular Heart Disease
   E. Congenital Heart Disease
   F. Congestive Heart Failure
IV. VASCULAR DISEASES
   A. Peripheral Arterial Disease
   B. Arterial Aneurysms
   C. Varicose Veins
V. DISEASES OF THE BLOOD CELLS
   A. Anemia
   B. Polycythemia Vera
   C. Hemorrhagic Disorders

In general, diseases of the circulatory system will result in impaired body function because supplies such as oxygen and nutrients necessary for cellular work are not delivered in adequate amounts. First we shall consider diagnostic techniques that assist in the process of determining the type and degree of circulatory problem and then we will discuss some of the common disorders of the circulatory system.

This chapter was written by Patricia Bohachick.

DIAGNOSTIC PROCEDURES

HISTORY AND PHYSICAL EXAMINATION

It is important to obtain the patient's account of present and past health, paying particular attention to reports of symptoms that suggest cardiovascular disease such as chest pain, shortness of breath, awareness of heart beat (palpitation), fatigue, dizziness or loss of consciousness, edema, and pain in the legs when walking. Inquiries about personal habits and about family health may help identify risk factors. In addition to a thorough physical examination, there are several procedures that may give rather specific information concerning the adequacy of the structures and functioning of the cardiovascular system.

ELECTROCARDIOGRAM

The electrocardiogram (ECG) is a graphic recording of the electrical currents produced by the heart. Electrodes that pick up these currents are positioned on the body surface and a graphic recording of the phases of the cardiac cycle will be produced. This procedure is useful in identifying abnormalities of heart rate and rhythm as well as enlargement of the heart, ischemia, and damage to the heart. However, the ECG may be normal in the presence of heart disease.

Since in some cases ECG abnormalities may occur only under certain circumstances, it may be helpful to do an ambulatory electrocardiogram. Ambulatory electrocardiography is useful in evaluating the cardiac response to daily activities. The person being tested carries a small recorder that registers a continuous ECG. As the person goes through a normal daily routine, a diary is kept documenting the time, activity, and any symptoms that occurred during the recording.

Exercise stress electrocardiography is used to uncover myocardial ischemia triggered during exertion. Blood pressure and heart rate are monitored and the ECG continuously recorded while the patient walks on a treadmill or pedals a stationary bicycle. The patient is observed for signs of effort intolerance and instructed to report any discomfort. The stress is increased until it reaches the maximum level for that patient or an abnormal response is demonstrated.

PHONOCARDIOGRAM

The phonocardiogram is a graphic recording of heart sounds. A microphone, positioned in different locations on the chest, picks up the sounds that are transmitted to a graph marker and the ECG is simultaneously recorded. Pulse waves of arteries in the neck may also be simultaneously recorded.

ECHOCARDIOGRAM

An echocardiogram (ek"o-kar'de-o-gram) uses ultrasound to measure the size and movements of various structures of the heart. Sound waves directed at the heart are reflected back to a transducer (a device that changes one form of energy to another) as they bounce off cardiac structures and are converted to electric signals. The data appear as lines and spaces on an oscilloscope and can also be recorded on a permanent record.

DOPPLER ULTRASOUND STUDIES

Ultrasound can be used to measure blood flow through vessels. The ultrasound beam is reflected off the blood cells moving through the vessels, and pulsations in arteries can be amplified enough to be heard. This procedure is useful in detecting pulses that are too faint to be felt.

ARTERIOGRAPHY

Arteriography (ar'te-re-og'rah-fe) is a radiographic examination of arteries (see Fig. 14-1). A radiopaque, thin, hollow tube (catheter) is inserted into the artery, a radiopaque dye is injected, and X-rays or a rapid series of X-rays are taken of the blood flow. Venography is a similar technique used to view the venous system. These studies are used to detect vascular abnormalities and evaluate blood flow.

CARDIAC CATHETERIZATION

Cardiac catheterization is done by passing a radiopaque catheter into chambers of the heart. To study the right side of the heart, a vein is used and the catheter is threaded via the vena cava into the right side of the heart and up the pulmonary artery. For a left heart catheterization, the catheter is threaded through an artery into the left ventricle. Through the catheter blood samples are taken, pressures are measured, and cardiac output is measured. Radiopaque dye may be introduced into heart chambers, and moving X-ray pictures of blood flow in the chambers can be taken, called cineangiography.

Coronary arteriography is usually done with a left heart catheterization. With the catheter positioned at the orifices of the coronary arteries, radiopaque dye is injected and cineangiograms are taken of the dye moving through the vessels. These films show the exact location and extent of any obstructive lesions in these vessels.

RADIONUCLIDE STUDIES

In nuclear studies of the heart, radionuclides such as thallium or technitium are injected intravenously. As these substances disintegrate, they emit small amounts of energy in the form of gamma rays that can be detected outside of

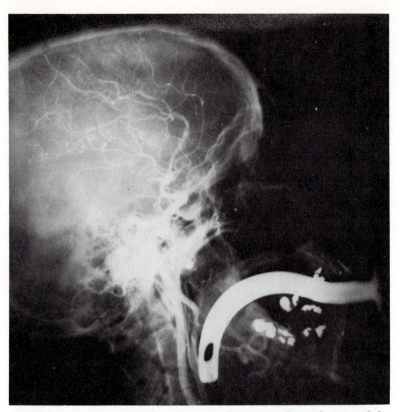

Figure 14-1. *A carotid arteriogram showing a lateral view of the cerebral arterial circulation. The procedure was done while the patient was under general anesthesia so there is an airway in the patient's mouth. The small opaque spots near the airway are dental fillings. (Courtesy of Mercy Hospital, Pittsburgh, PA)*

the body by a gamma scintillation camera. Readings from the camera are fed into a computer and translated into an image or scan (scintogram). Information can be obtained about blood flow to the myocardium, the motion of the heart wall, ventricular function, and the presence of abnormalities such as myocardial infarction.

CARDIOVASCULAR DISEASE

Cardiovascular disease afflicts nearly 67 million Americans and is the largest single cause of death in the United States, accounting for 46% of all deaths. Figure 14-2 presents estimated

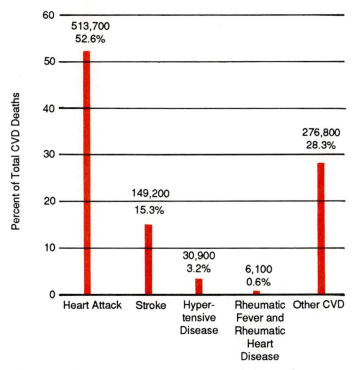

Estimated Deaths Due to Major Cardiovascular Diseases

United States: 1987 Estimate

Figure 14-2. From 1990 Heart and Stroke Facts *(Courtesy of the American Heart Association. Reproduced with permission.)*

deaths due to cardiovascular disease by the major types of disorder.

ATHEROSCLEROSIS

The major underlying cause for the high incidence of cardiovascular disease is **atherosclerosis** (ath′er-o-skle-ro′sis), a form of **arteriosclerosis** (ar-te-re-o-skle-ro′sis). Arteriosclerosis is a general term referring to a variety of entities that cause thickening and loss of elasticity in arterial walls. With atherosclerosis, the inner layer of the artery wall is made thick and irregular by deposits of a fatty substance that progressively narrows the lumen of the artery. Complications of atherosclerosis depend on which organ the diseased artery supplies (see Fig. 14-3).

While the exact cause of atherosclerosis is unknown, we do know several factors that con-

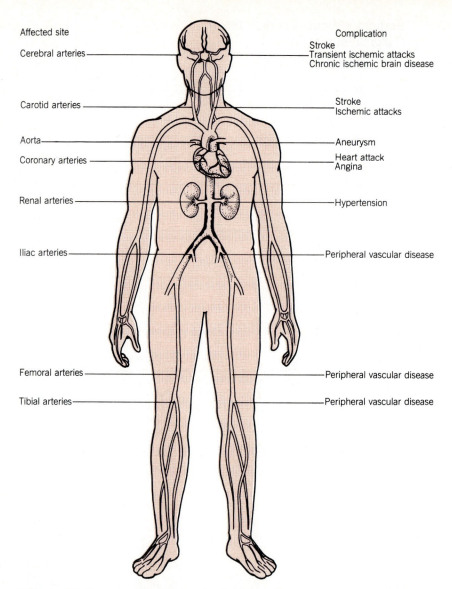

Figure 14-3. Major blood vessels that may be affected by atherosclerosis and some resulting complications (Courtesy of National Heart, Lung and Blood Institute of the National Institutes of Health)

tribute to an increased risk such as an elevation of blood lipids, high blood pressure, and cigarette smoking. Obesity, physical inactivity, and a tense, anxious approach to life are also contributing factors to the disease. Both the prevention and treatment of atherosclerosis must include limiting or eliminating as many of these contributing factors as possible.

HYPERTENSION

Hypertension is a condition in which the blood circulates at a pressure higher than normal. Although there is no clear-cut dividing line between what are normal and abnormal blood pressures, readings above 140 mm Hg for systolic pressure and 90 mm Hg for diastolic pressure are considered abnormal for adults. Hypertension is a major health problem in our society because of its prevalence and its being a leading cause of disability and premature death.

It is estimated that one in four adult Americans have high blood pressure. In 90% of these cases, no specific cause can be found and so a diagnosis of essential hypertension is made. In the remaining 10%, high blood pressure is a symptom of a disease such as adrenal tumors or kidney disease. This type of high blood pressure is referred to as secondary hypertension. The term malignant hypertension is used to describe a severe, rapidly accelerating, and life-threatening rise in blood pressure that results in vascular and organ damage. This problem can develop in persons with essential or secondary hypertension.

High blood pressure adds to the workload of the heart, causing hypertrophy of the left ventricular wall and eventually heart failure. High blood pressure ultimately causes structural changes in the walls of arteries and arterioles, accelerates the development of atherosclerosis, and reduces life expectancy as a result of cere-

bral vascular accidents, renal failure, peripheral vascular disease, and heart attacks.

Substantial evidence indicates that reduction of blood pressure to normal or near normal levels dramatically reduces complications and thus improves prognosis. In most cases, hypertension cannot be cured, but blood pressure can be kept under control with medication. Drugs used in the treatment of hypertension include **diuretics**, which increase the excretion of sodium by the kidneys; sympatholytic drugs that decrease the activity of the sympathetic nervous system; and **vasodilators** that relax arteriolar smooth muscle. Weight reduction and a decrease in the amount of salt (sodium) ingested may help to lower the blood pressure. Screening programs to detect hypertension and education of patients with hypertension on the importance of adhering to life-long therapy is vital since hypertension rarely causes symptoms until a complication occurs.

HEART DISEASE

ISCHEMIC HEART DISEASE

The leading cause of death in the United States is ischemic heart disease. Atherosclerosis of the coronary arteries is the most common cause of this disease.

To maintain proper functioning, the heart must have a continuous supply of oxygen. When the heart pumps against an elevated blood pressure or pumps more forcefully or faster, more oxygen is required by the myocardium. This requirement should be met by an increased flow of oxygen-rich blood through the coronary arteries. With atherosclerosis and a narrowing of the lumen of the coronary arteries, this requirement may not be met. When the oxygen supply becomes inadequate, varying degrees of ischemia appear and **angina pectoris** (an-ji′nah pek′to-ris), **myocardial infarction**, or sudden death may occur.

Angina pectoris is transient chest pain or discomfort owing to temporary and reversible ischemia of the myocardium. Most commonly the discomfort is described as heaviness, tightness, or aching in the center of the chest, usually substernal. See Figure 14-4 for other possible locations of anginal pain. Any circumstance that increases myocardial oxygen demand or reduces the oxygen supply is capable of inducing angina. As would be anticipated, angina is most commonly noted with strenous physical effort or emotional upsets. When the activity stops, oxygen demand falls and the pain subsides within a few minutes. As the disease progresses, angina may change from its usual pattern to a more unstable one with an increase in the frequency or severity of episodes or inconsistent relief of pain despite therapy.

Management of angina is directed toward minimizing the imbalance between myocardial oxygen supply and demand. This process includes avoiding factors that precipitate attacks, and taking drugs such as nitroglycerine (a vasodilator) or drugs that reduce the oxygen requirements of the heart. Because unstable angina is frequently a forewarning of myocardial

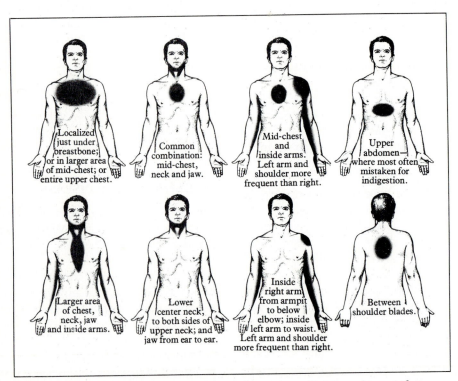

Figure 14-4. *Locations of anginal pain (Courtesy of Metropolitan Life Insurance Company)*

infarction, patients are instructed to seek medical attention in the event of a change in their anginal pattern. In some cases, angioplasty or coronary artery bypass surgery may be indicated to increase blood supply to the heart muscle.

Percutaneous transluminal coronary angioplasty (PTCA) is a nonsurgical procedure used to dilate a stenotic segment of a coronary artery. A catheter with a deflated balloon on its tip is passed through the femoral or subclavian artery into the aorta and then into the targeted segment of the coronary artery. Once in position, the balloon is inflated to compress the atherosclerotic plaque against the vessel wall and widen the narrowed segment (see Figure 14-5). Complications of this procedure, such as arterial dissection or arterial occlusion from atheromatous material, may necessitate emergency coronary artery bypass surgery. Therefore, the person undergoing PTCA must also be a suitable candidate for open heart surgery.

In coronary artery bypass graft surgery, a section of a vein is removed and one end is sewn onto the aorta and the other to the diseased coronary artery distal to the site of narrowing. Blood may then flow from the aorta through the vein graft to the nonobstructed portion of the coronary artery (see Fig. 14-6).

When the ischemia is profound and sustained, necrosis of myocardial tissue (myocardial infarction or heart attack) ensues. Often, myocardial infarction results from occlusion of a coronary artery by thrombus formation at the site of an atherosclerotic plaque. Coronary artery occlusion produces myocardial ischemia, injury, and eventually necrosis.

Chest pain is the principal symptom of a myocardial infarction. The pain is not necessarily associated with exertion and is not relieved with rest. The person who experiences warning signs of a heart attack requires immediate medical attention (see Fig. 14-7).

Goals in managing the patient with myocardial infarction include (1) limiting heart muscle

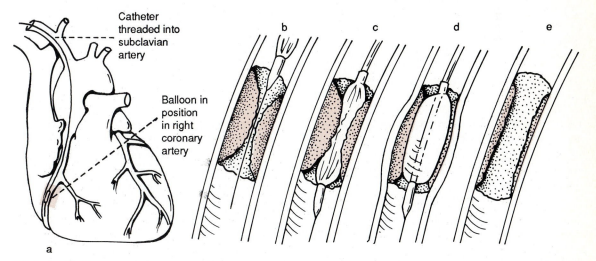

Figure 14-5. *Percutaneous transluminal coronary angioplasty (PTCA). (a) Balloon-tipped catheter positioned in blocked artery. (b) Balloon is centered in blockage, and (c) inflated. Pressure of balloon, (d) flattens blockage, and (e) reopens artery. (From: Luckmann, J. & Sorensen, K.C., Medical-Surgical Nursing—A Psychophysiologic Approach, 3rd ed., Philadelphia: W.B. Saunders Company, 1987)*

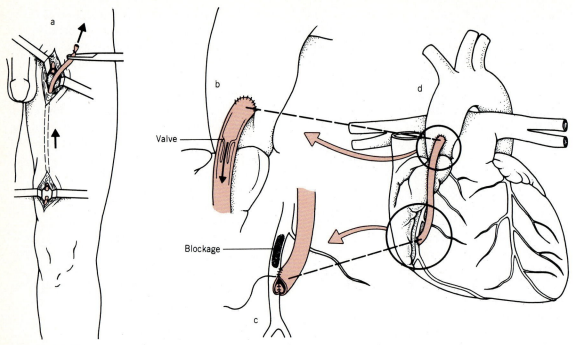

Figure 14-6. *Saphenous vein revascularization procedure. (a) Saphenous vein is removed from the patient's leg. The vein is reversed so that valves will not interfere with blood flow. (b) The distal end of the vein is sutured to the ascending aorta. (c) At a point distal to the blockage, the vein is sutured to the coronary artery by end-to-end anastomosis. (d) The completed bypass reestablishes the flow distal to the blockage. (From Brunner, L.S., and Suddarth, D.S.,* Textbook of Medical-Surgical Nursing, *4th ed. Philadelphia: J.B. Lippincott, 1980)*

damage by decreasing the workload of the heart and increasing the blood supply to the myocardium, and (2) preventing complications or detecting them early so appropriate treatment may be given.

Oxygen therapy will be needed. An intravenous line should be established to provide a route for emergency medications, and a cardiac monitor attached for constant surveillance. Relief of pain is essential and may require intravenous administration of a narcotic. Cardiac workload is reduced by physical and mental rest and by medications. Also, thrombolytic (clot-dissolving) therapy is used early in the course of infarction to dissolve the thrombus in the coronary artery and restore some blood flow.

Sudden death in patients with ischemic heart disease is almost always due to disturbances in the electrical activity of the heart. In these instances the heart either stops abruptly (cardiac arrest) or ventricular fibrillation (fi-bri-la′shun) (rapid, irregular contractions of the ventricle) occurs. Death is inevitable unless cardiopulmonary resuscitation (kar′de-o-pul′mo-ne-re re-sus′i-ta′shun) is immediately administered (see Fig. 14-8).

EARLY WARNINGS OF A HEART ATTACK

PAIN, in one form or another, almost always accompanies a heart attack. Ranges from a mild ache to one of unbearable severity. When severe, pain is often felt as constricting, like vise on chest. Pain also often includes the burning and bloated sensations that usually accompany indigestion. Pain may be continuous and then might subside—but don't ignore if it does. Could be in any one or combination of locations shown below.

Checklist of Other Heart Attack Early Warnings.

None of the symptoms below is conclusive proof of a heart attack. But the more of them present, the more likely it is that the patient *is* undergoing a heart attack.

DIFFICULTY BREATHING
PALPITATIONS
NAUSEA
VOMITING

COLD SWEAT
PALENESS
WEAKNESS
ANXIETY

How to Help a Possible Heart Attack Victim.

You can best help—possibly save a life—if you know in advance: 1) The nearest hospital equipped to handle heart attack emergencies. 2) How to do Cardiopulmonary Resuscitation (CPR).* 3) How quickly to call a doctor, the hospital and/or an ambulance. 4) The fastest route to the hospital. Knowing these things, you should:

1 Help victim to least painful position—usually sitting, with legs up and bent at knees. Loosen clothing around neck and midriff. Be calm, reassuring.

2 Call ambulance to get victim to hospital via your local Rescue Squad, police or whatever other method available. Speed is vital. Once the ambulance is on the way, notify family physician, if known.

3 If ambulance will arrive in a few minutes, wait, comforting victim. Otherwise, help victim to car, trying to keep victim's exertion to minimum. If possible, take another CPR-trained person with you. Victim should sit up.

4 Drive cautiously to hospital. Keep close watch on victim (or have passenger do so). If victim loses consciousness, stop car, pull victim to hard surface outside, perform CPR. Call for help. Keep up CPR until resuscitator or ambulance arrives.

5 If patient retains consciousness to hospital, make sure he is carried, not walked, to emergency room.

* Taught by local chapters of the American Heart Association and the American Red Cross.

✢ Metropolitan
Where the future is now

T. 15135—Printed in U.S.A.

Figure 14-7. Early warnings of a heart attack (Courtesy of Metropolitan Life Insurance Company)

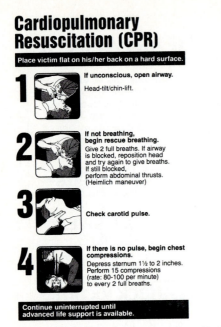

Figure 14-8. Cardiopulmonary resuscitation (Courtesy of the American Heart Association)

CARDIAC DYSRHYTHMIAS

A dysrhythmia (dis-rith'me-ah) is an abnormality in the rate, rhythm, or conduction of the heart beat. Such irregularities of heart beat may be simply a normal physiological response or they may be a sign of some disease.

Dysrhythmias may be classified on the basis of the site of origin of the arrhythmia (SA node, atria, AV node, ventricle) and on the basis of the mechanism responsible for the disorder (**tachy**-**lia** (tak-e-kar'de-ah), which is an abnormally rapid heart rate (160 to 190 beats per minute); **bradycardia** (brad-e-kar'de-ah), a pulse rate of less than 60 beats per minute; premature beats; flutter; fibrillation; or conduction defects). For example, an atrial premature beat is an abnormal impulse that originates in the

atria and causes a heart beat earlier than the next expected beat; a ventricular premature beat describes a similar event but the early beat originates in the ventricles.

Sinus tachycardia is a rhythm originating normally in the SA node but the rate is rapid, greater than 100 beats per minute. Sinus bradycardia is a pulse rate of less than 60 beats per minute that originates in the SA node.

Atrial fibrillation is rapid, irregular contractions of the atria at a rate of 400 to 600 beats per minute. At this rate, there is no coordinated contraction and the atria appear to quiver. Fortunately, most of the atrial impulses are unable to pass through the AV node so the ventricles beat at a rate much slower than the atria, usually between 100 and 160 beats per minute, and with an irregular rhythm. With some beats, there may not be time for adequate filling of the ventricles, and the ventricles will not be able to expel a sufficient amount of blood to produce a palpable radial pulse. In this situation, there will be a pulse deficit; the radial pulse rate will be slower than the contractions of the heart. Atrial fibrillation is a frequent complication of mitral valve disease and may also occur with ischemic heart disease.

With ventricular fibrillation, individual muscle fibers of the ventricles contract in a disorganized, quivering fashion that is ineffective in expelling blood from the heart. The patient loses consciousness, no heart beat can be heard, and there are no pulses. Respirations are initially gasping, then absent. Ventricular fibrillation is a lethal dysrhythmia that requires immediate treatment with electric shock to "defibrillate" the ventricles. If this treatment is not immediately available, cardiopulmonary resuscitation must be quickly instituted.

Atrioventricular (A-V) block is a disturbance in the conduction of impulses across the AV node. The defect in conduction may be incomplete, in which case there is a simple delay in conduction of impulses or some impulses may fail to be transmitted. In complete blocks, none of the atrial impulses are transmitted to the ventricles. In this situation, the heart beat may be initiated by an impulse originating in the ventricular conducting system. As a result, the atria and ventricles beat independently of each other and the pulse rate is slow, about 30 to 40 beats per minute. This condition requires treatment with an artificial cardiac pacemaker.

Treatment for dysrhythmias include therapy for the underlying cause of the dysrhythmia, antidysrhythmic drugs, and electrical interventions such as cardioversion (kar'de-o-ver'zhun), pacemakers, and implantable electrical devices.

Cardioversion is a method for restoring heart rhythm by delivering a brief electrical shock to the heart via electrode paddles applied to the surface of the chest. The electrical current causes all cells of the heart to depolarize simultaneously and, thereby, interrupts all abnormal impulse formation. The sinus node can then take over and restore normal heart rhythm.

An artificial cardiac pacemaker is a device designed to deliver an electrical stimulus to the heart muscle to initiate a heart beat. The system has two components: a pulse generator (the power source and electronic circuitry for sensing intrinsic electrical activity and sending out the appropriate electrical stimulus) and a lead-electrode system (catheter with sensing and stimulating electrodes). The lead electrode system relays information about intrinsic electrical activity back to the pulse generator and delivers electrical stimuli.

The method most commonly used for pacemaker implantation is to pass the catheter electrode through a vein in the neck and into the right ventricle, positioning the electrode against the endocardium. For temporary pacing, the catheter electrode is attached to an external pulse generator. For permanent pacing, the pulse generator is implanted under the skin, usually in the chest area below the clavicle, and connected to the catheter electrodes (see Fig. 14-9).

The automatic implantable cardioverter-defibrillator (AICD) represents a recent development in the treatment of patients at risk of sudden death from lethal cardiac dysrhythmias. The AICD system is designed to detect ventricular tachycardia or ventricular fibrillation and automatically deliver a countershock to terminate the dysrhythmia. The device consists of a pulse generator and two lead systems with electrodes for sensing electrical activity and delivering current. The electrodes are surgically placed in and on the heart. The pulse generator is implanted subcutaneously in the left upper quadrant of the abdomen.

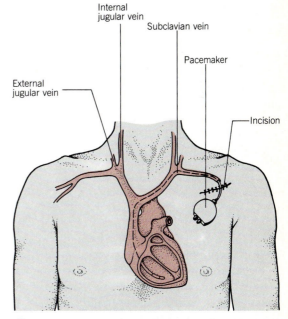

Figure 14-9. A permanent pacemaker. Note site of insertion and location of power source. (From Beyers, M., and Dudas, S., The Clinical Practice of Medical-Surgical Nursing. Boston: Little, Brown, 1977)

INFECTIVE ENDOCARDITIS

Infective endocarditis is an infection of the lining of the heart, generally on a heart valve. The disorder occurs most often in people with underlying valve disease or congenital heart defects but can also occur in people without evident heart disease. The infecting organisms attack the endocardium and form vegetations composed of fibrin, platelets, and bacteria. Bacteria from the vegetations are constantly being swept into the bloodstream and are responsible for fever and toxemia manifestations. Vegetations on the valves can lead to valvular deformity. Since the vegetations are fragile, bits can break off and enter the circulation as emboli and obstruct arteries.

In the early stages of infective endocarditis, the patient has fever, chills, sweating, weakness, malaise, and other nonspecific signs. Most patients also have a cardiac murmur of some type.

Endocarditis is managed by administration of appropriate antibiotics. The prognosis of the patient who has undergone successful treatment generally depends on the residual valvular damage. People with structural abnormalities of the heart or great vessels should receive preventive antibiotic therapy before dental work such as cleaning the teeth or any procedure that could result in bacteria entering the bloodstream.

VALVULAR HEART DISEASE

The most common cause of valvular heart disease is rheumatic fever. Rheumatic fever is an inflammatory reaction to infection by Group A betahemolytic streptococcus. The body reacts to the infection by producing antibodies to combat the invading organism. In some people for unknown reasons, these antibodies not only react with the streptococcus but also with certain tissues of the body, such as the heart valves, and cause an inflammatory reaction. Damage to the heart due to rheumatic fever is termed rheumatic heart disease. Inflammation and scarring leave hardened, stiff valves that either will not open wide enough (stenosis) or will not close completely (insufficiency), or both.

Mitral stenosis impedes blood flow from the left atrium to the left ventricle. More pressure must be exerted by the left atrium to force blood through the narrowed valve. The increase in the left atrial pressure is reflected backward to the blood vessels of the lungs. The work of breathing increases as vessels in the lungs become distended with blood and the patient will be short of breath. The patient may also get pulmonary edema should the pressure in the pulmonary capillaries exceed the osmotic pressure of these capillaries. A restriction of blood flow to the left ventricle limits the ability of the heart to increase blood flow to the tissues on demand. As a result, activity tolerance decreases and fatigue is common. With long-standing mitral stenosis, there will be sclerotic changes in the pulmonary arterioles, and resistance to blood flow through the pulmonary circuit increases. The right side of the heart must work harder to pump blood through the lungs and eventually fails.

With mitral insufficiency, some of the blood that should be pumped out of the heart leaks back into the left atrium when the left ventricle contracts. When the ventricle relaxes, the blood that leaked into the atrium plus normally flowing blood enters the left ventricle. This increased volume of blood in the left ventricle causes dilation of this chamber and hypertrophy of its wall. The left atrium also enlarges. If the leak is large, pressure in the left atrium and pulmonary vessels increases (just as with mitral stenosis) and there will be dyspnea. Effort tolerance is greatly limited and there is pronounced fatigue. Eventually, because of long-standing overwork, the muscle of the left ventricle fails.

Aortic stenosis impedes blood flow from the left ventricle into the aorta. The left ventricle must generate a high pressure to expel blood; the ventricular muscle hypertrophies in response to the pressure overload. With severe stenosis, the amount of blood pumped out of the heart will decrease and since the pressure overload and hypertrophy increase oxygen requirements of the myocardium, ischemia of the heart muscle may occur. Symptoms of aortic stenosis may include angina pectoris, fainting, and sudden death owing most probably to dysrhythmias. Deterioration is often rapid after the appearance of symptoms, and life expectancy is limited.

With aortic insufficiency, some of the blood that is pumped into the aorta when the left ventricle contracts leaks back into the left ventricle during diastole. The left ventricle must then try to pump forward an extra amount of blood as well as the normal quantity. Because of this increased volume of blood, the chamber dilates and the muscle hypertrophies. The left ventricle is usually able to deliver adequate amounts of blood to the body for a relatively long period. Patients with aortic insufficiency often live many years without significant disturbance. However, with severe prolonged aortic insufficiency, the volume load becomes excessive and the left ventricle fails.

Damaged valves may be surgically repaired or replaced. When valvular damage is moderate, or when symptoms are mild, surgical intervention may not be indicated and the patient can be treated medically. Management of valvular disease includes precautions against streptococcal infections, a balanced diet, and preventive antibiotics under special circumstances. One goal of therapy is the prevention and relief of heart failure. In some cases, a low-salt diet, diuretics, and medications such as digitalis to strengthen the heart muscle are prescribed. Complications, such as atrial fibrillation, require special treatment.

CONGENITAL HEART DISEASE

Congenital heart defects are abnormalities of the heart that are present at birth. Congenital defects such as narrowing of the heart valve or coarctation of the aorta obstruct the flow of blood. Coarctation of the aorta, characterized by a localized constriction of the aorta, most commonly occurs in the aortic arch distal to the insertion of the ductus arteriosus. The narrowing of the aortic lumen produces an increased blood pressure proximal to the obstruction (upper extremities) and a relatively decreased blood pressure in the lower extremities.

Some congenital heart defects, such as a septal defect or a patent ductus arteriosus, reroute blood from the left side of the heart to the right side. For example, in a patent ductus arteriosus, some of the oxygenated blood leaving the aorta enters the ductus and returns to the pulmonary circuit. As a result, although the peripheral circulation does not receive as much blood as it should, what blood it does receive is well oxygenated. The pulmonary circuit, on the other hand, receives more blood than it should. When the ductus is large, the left ventricle must pump an excess amount of blood and may eventually fail.

An atrial septal defect is an abnormal opening between the atria. In this defect, some of the blood that has returned from the lungs to the left atrium is shunted into the right atrium instead of flowing into the left ventricle. Thus, blood is recirculated through the right heart and pulmonary circuit, increasing the workload on the right ventricle.

In a ventricular septal defect, an abnormal opening exists in the interventricular septum. As with atrial septal defects, the flow of blood through the opening is from left to right because of the higher pressure in the left ventricle. The functional consequences of ventricular defects depend on the size of the opening and presence of other cardiac anomalies. Approximately one-quarter to one-half of medium or small defects close spontaneously.

Congenital heart defects that reroute blood from the right side of the heart to the left prevent this blood from getting oxygenated. If the defect is severe, **cyanosis** (si-ah-no'sis) will result because the peripheral tissues will not receive adequate amounts of oxygen. An infant with this condition is commonly called a "blue baby" because of the blue tinge of the skin.

Tetralogy of Fallot is a congenital heart defect that causes cyanosis by restricting pulmonary blood flow. It consists of four abnormalities: (1) right ventricular outflow obstruction that impedes blood flow from the right ventricle to the lungs; (2) ventricular septal defect; (3) dextroposition of the aorta so that it lies over the septal defect; and (4) hypertrophy of the right ventricle.

Some congenital heart defects require surgical correction. Others may be treated medically. Although the cause of most congenital heart defects is unknown, there is an association between German measles (rubella) in the mother during the early months of pregnancy and congenital heart defects. For this reason, immunization against this disease is important.

CONGESTIVE HEART FAILURE

Congestive heart failure is a state in which the pumping ability of the heart is diminished and excess fluid is retained in the tissues. Normally, the heart is able to pump as much blood as is delivered to it and to pump sufficient blood to meet the needs of the body under varying degrees of activity. In heart failure, the heart does not pump blood adequately.

Causes of heart failure include long-standing overwork of the heart muscle, impairment of blood flow through the chambers of the heart, disease of the myocardium, or actual loss of myocardium (as with a heart attack). The body compensates for heart failure in several ways. Unfortunately, each of the compensatory mechanisms has limitations or disadvantages as well

as advantages and can be responsible for some of the symptoms the patient experiences.

One of the earliest compensations is increased sympathetic nervous system activity that results in an increase in heart rate and a greater force of contraction of the heart muscle. There will also be arterial vasoconstriction and constriction of the veins, which enhances venous return, thereby augmenting cardiac output. Through arteriolar constriction, there may be a redistribution of peripheral blood flow from the skin and kidneys to vital organs. Sympathetic stimulation may result in an excessively rapid heart rate, sweating, cool skin, and decreased urinary output.

A second compensation in heart failure is retention of fluid by the kidneys. With a fall in cardiac output, there is decreased blood flow to the kidneys and less sodium and water are excreted. Blood volume increases; more blood is returned to the heart and, in turn, cardiac output is increased. However, if the heart is unable to satisfactorily pump this extra blood, venous pressure increases and edema occurs. Figure 14-10 shows the capillary dynamics associated with the edema of heart failure. You should compare this illustration with the normal capillary dynamics in Figure 13-5.

Another compensation is enlargement of the heart. Initially, the chambers of the heart dilate. Later, the muscle fibers of the heart hypertrophy. Stretching of the heart muscle and greater muscle mass leads to a stronger contraction of the heart. However, with excessive stretching, the contractions become weaker. Additionally, the larger heart requires more oxygen for its work. The coronary circulation may not be able to supply sufficient blood to the enlarged heart and myocardial ischemia will result.

When these mechanisms compensate for the failing heart and effectively maintain an adequate blood flow to the body, the patient is said to be in compensated heart failure. Decompen-

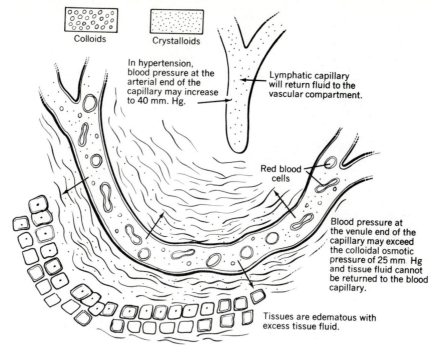

Colloids   Crystalloids

In hypertension, blood pressure at the arterial end of the capillary may increase to 40 mm. Hg.

Lymphatic capillary will return fluid to the vascular compartment.

Red blood cells

Blood pressure at the venule end of the capillary may exceed the colloidal osmotic pressure of 25 mm. Hg and tissue fluid cannot be returned to the blood capillary.

Tissues are edematous with excess tissue fluid.

Figure 14-10. Capillary dynamics in congestive heart failure that will result in edema (From Burke, S.R., Composition and Function of Body Fluids, 3rd ed. St. Louis: The C.V. Mosby Co., 1980)

sated heart failure occurs when the limits of compensation are reached. In this state, the patient experiences fatigue, rapid heart rate, and diminished urine output because of insufficient systemic blood flow. Additional symptoms related to excessive fluid retention develop.

Inadequate pumping of the left ventricle leads to an excess volume of blood and an increased blood pressure in the pulmonary circuit. The normally elastic lungs become stiffened, the work of breathing increases, and the patient has dyspnea. Dyspnea may occur when the patient lies down, which is called orthopnea (or"thop-ne'ah), or the patient may awaken at night with an attack of shortness of breath (paroxysmal nocturnal dyspnea). If the elevation of capillary pressure is severe, fluid from the capillary may filter out into the alveoli (pulmonary edema) producing a life-threatening condition.

Impaired pumping of the right ventricle results in increased pressure in the systemic venous system. The elevated venous pressure often results in peripheral edema, which is described as dependent edema and pitting (see Fig. 14-11). Elevated pressure in the veins of the liver will cause that organ to be distended with blood and enlarged, called hepatomegaly (hep"ah-to-meg'ah-le). Less commonly, fluid may accumulate in the pleural, pericardial, or peritoneal cavities.

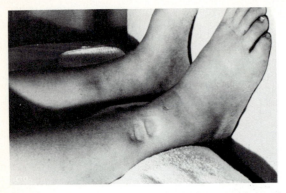

Figure 14-11. *Edema is called pitting when, if the edematous area is pressed, an indentation remains for a few seconds after the pressure is removed. Dependent edema refers to an excess amount of tissue fluid in the lower parts of the body. (From Roe, A. and Sherwood, M.,* Learning Experience Guides for Nursing Students, *Volume 2, 3rd ed. New York: John Wiley & Sons, Inc., 1978)*

Principles of treatment of congestive heart failure include: (1) correcting the underlying cause when possible; (2) controlling any factors that may precipitate decompensation such as anemia, disrhythmia, or infection; (3) reducing the workload of the heart by physical rest, and in some cases, by medications; (4) enhancing myocardial contractility with drug therapy; (5) controlling edema formation with diuretics and sodium restriction.

Heart transplantation is a therapeutic option for selected patients with end-stage heart disease, a poor six-month prognosis for survival, and no possibility of improvement with medical or other surgical therapy. Additionally, candidates must be free of conditions that might limit survival after transplantation. Most candidates for heart transplantation have end-stage heart failure from ischemic heart disease or cardiomyopathy (heart muscle disease). The operative technique for heart transplantation is illustrated

in Figure 14-12. Recipients must be on life-long immunosuppressive therapy. Major problems after transplant surgery include rejection of the transplanted organ, infection, and complications of immunosuppressive therapy.

Heart-lung transplantation has been performed as therapy for advanced pulmonary vascular disease. This surgery involves removing the recipient's diseased lungs and heart as a unit and replacing them with the heart and lungs of a brain-dead donor. Major limitations of heart-lung transplantation include the unavailability of suitable donor organs and relatively high mortality as compared to heart-alone transplantation.

VASCULAR DISEASES

PERIPHERAL ARTERIAL DISEASE

There are a variety of types of peripheral arterial disease and each one has some distinctive features. They all have in common a decreased blood flow.

Decreased blood flow to the lower extremities causes pain on walking, particularly when walking upstairs or up a hill. This condition is called claudication (klaw-de-ka'shun). With poor blood supply in the legs, patients often develop leg ulcers that are difficult to treat because wounds are dependent on a good blood supply for healing (see Fig. 14-13).

For the most part, these diseases are treated palliatively (symptomatically). To achieve vasodilatation, surgeons may do a sympathectomy (the removal of some of the sympathetic nerve chain). The results of this procedure are often disappointing, particularly if the disease is advanced. When there is a localized area of arterial blockage with decreased patency of vessels distal to the obstruction, a bypass graft may be at-

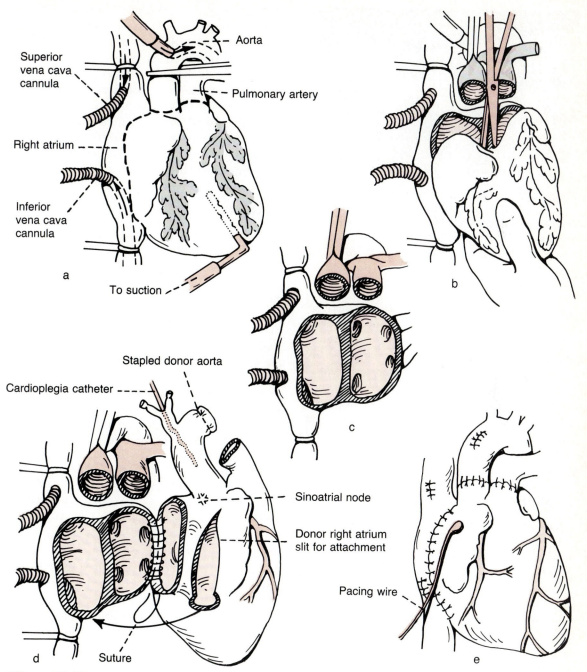

Figure 14-12. *Heart transplantation. (a) Person placed on cardiopulmonary bypass. (b) Recipient's heart removed. (c) Exposed heart ready for transplantation. (d) Initial attachment of left atrium of donor heart. (e) Transplanted heart, off bypass, with pacing wire in place. Adapted and redrawn from Simmons, R.L., et al.,* Manual of Vascular Access, Organ Donation, and Transplantation. *New York: Springer-Verlag, 1984. (From Luckmann, J., and Sorenson, K.C.,* Medical-Surgical Nursing: A Physiologic Approach, *3rd ed. Philadelphia: W.B. Saunders Company, 1987)*

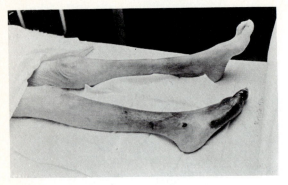

Figure 14-13. Poor arterial circulation to the legs can result in ulcerations and necrosis. (From Roe, A., and Sherwood, M., Learning Experience Guides for Nursing Students, *Volume 2, 3rd ed. New York: John Wiley & Sons, Inc., 1978)*

tached above and below the blocked segment of the artery. Blood may then flow around the area of obstruction. Recently, efforts to press plaques against the vessel wall and thus enlarge the lumen of the vessel by means of an arterial catheter and balloon (angioplasty) have been successful. Since one commonly occurring type of peripheral arterial disease is caused by atherosclerosis, efforts to limit or prevent the disease include modification of risk factors for atherosclerosis.

ARTERIAL ANEURYSMS

An **aneurysm** is a localized dilatation of an artery caused by weakness in the wall by trauma, disease, or congenital defects. Most aneurysms are caused by atherosclerosis and occur in the thoracic or abdominal aorta. Aneurysms may be fusiform (encompassing the entire aortic circumference) or saccular (localized outpouching). A dissecting aneurysm results from a tear in the intimal wall that allows blood under pressure to enter and strip the intima from the adventitia for variable distances.

Clinical manifestations of an aneurysm result from compression on adjacent structures, impaired blood flow, and dissection or rupture of the aneurysm. The major symptom of a dissecting aneurysm is the sudden onset of excruciating pain in the anterior and posterior chest (thoracic aortic aneurysm) or in the abdomen and lower back (abdominal aortic aneurysm). Apprehension, profuse sweating, and faintness commonly accompany the pain. Dissecting aneurysms require emergency treatment.

VARICOSE VEINS

Varicose veins are abnormally dilated veins with incompetent valves. They occur most frequently in the lower extremities. There seems to be a hereditary tendency to varicose veins, but occupations that involve prolonged standing in one place cause strain on the valves and, therefore, may predispose one to the development of varicose veins. Since the superficial veins of the legs are not supported by strong muscles, these are the most vulnerable. Even before there are symptoms of discomfort, these veins may appear darkened, tortuous, and more prominent when the patient stands or assumes positions that cause congestion, such as sitting with the knees crossed.

Varicose veins promote stasis of blood, a predisposing factor in blood clotting. At the site of clot formation, the vein may become inflamed (thrombophlebitis), break off (thromboembolism), and travel through the great veins, the right side of the heart, the pulmonary artery, and occlude a branch of the artery (pulmonary embolism).

People who have varicose veins, or those who are predisposed either by heredity or by occupation, should not wear constricting garters. When practical, they should elevate their feet for a few minutes every two or three hours during the day. If obliged to stand for long periods of time in one place, they should exercise the leg muscles by moving up and down on their toes. The activity of these muscles will help prevent venous pooling in the leg veins. Support hose, properly applied, can be a great help in preventing venous pooling and varicosities and in relieving discomfort of varicose veins.

DISEASES OF THE BLOOD CELLS

ANEMIA

Anemia is a condition where there is a reduction in the amount of hemoglobin or of red blood cells, or both. Anemia can be caused by loss, destruction, or faulty production of red blood cells and hemoglobin. Symptoms of anemia are similar regardless of the cause and are mainly the result of the inability of the blood to transport sufficient oxygen to the tissues. Patients may feel faint, tire easily, and have pallor. They are particularly sensitive to chilling and usually complain of being cold when others find the temperature comfortable. They have a rapid pulse. Exertional dyspnea occurs when the anemia is severe.

The treatment is directed toward correcting the cause of the anemia. If it is due to blood loss, the bleeding must be controlled and blood transfusions may be necessary. For pernicious anemia, caused by faulty production of red blood cells, the treatment is dietary, with supplements of vitamin B$_{12}$. Iron deficiency anemia may also respond to dietary treatment that should include extra citrus fruits because vitamin C is necessary for the proper utilization of dietary iron. It may also be necessary to give iron supplements.

POLYCYTHEMIA VERA

In polycythemia (pol"e-si-the'me-ah) vera, there is an excessive production of red blood cells, white cells, and platelets. The red blood count may rise to eight or twelve million per cubic millimeter; the patient has a reddish-purple complexion, weakness, dyspnea, and headache. There is an increased tendency for clot formation and death may occur owing to thrombosis. The treatment of this disease includes therapy to suppress bone marrow function and phlebotomy (fle-bot'o-me), the removal of blood from a vein.

HEMORRHAGIC DISORDERS

Diseases characterized by bleeding tendencies are usually related to a hereditary deficiency of some clotting factor, such as in hemophilia, or some abnormality in the blood platelets called purpura (pur'pu-rah). Treatment of hemorrhagic disorders is directed toward removing or controlling the cause of the disease and controlling bleeding.

SUMMARY QUESTIONS

1. List seven symptoms that suggest cardiac and/or cardiovascular disease.
2. Discuss the value of ambulatory and exercise stress electrocardiography.
3. What information can be gathered from cardiac catheterization?
4. List five risk factors for atherosclerosis.
5. Describe the effects of hypertension on the heart and vascular system.

6. Explain the basis for chest pain that occurs with ischemic heart disease.

7. List signs and symptoms that would lead you to suspect a myocardial infarction.

8. Discuss the pathophysiology of aortic stenosis and aortic insufficiency.

9. Describe the treatment of valvular heart disease.

10. Describe the compensatory mechanisms for heart failure including the value, disadvantages, and possible symptoms associated with each mechanism.

11. Outline the principles for treatment of congestive heart failure.

KEY TERMS

aneurysm
angina pectoris
arteriosclerosis
atherosclerosis
atrioventricular (A-V) block
bradycardia

cyanosis
diuretics
myocardial infarction
tachycardia
vasodilators

15

The Respiratory System

OBJECTIVES

On completion of this chapter, you will be able to:

1. Describe seven structures of the respiratory tract.
2. Explain the structure and functions of the paranasal sinuses.
3. Describe the muscle actions in inspiration and expiration.
4. Discuss the mechanism of internal and external respirations.
5. Discuss the pressures involved in external respirations.
6. Discuss the factors involved in the association and dissociation of oxygen and hemoglobin.
7. Explain how both oxygen and carbon dioxide are transported in the bloodstream.
8. Discuss the major factors that stimulate respirations.
9. Discuss Boyle's and Dalton's laws concerning gases.
10. Describe the compensatory mechanisms for respiratory pH imbalances.
11. Explain the causes of respiratory acidosis and alkalosis.

OVERVIEW

I. STRUCTURES OF THE RESPIRATORY
   SYSTEM
   A. Nasal Cavities and Related Structures
   B. Pharynx and Tonsils
   C. Larynx and Voice Production
   D. Trachea
   E. Bronchi and Bronchioles
   F. Alveoli
   G. Lungs and Pleura
II. PHYSIOLOGY OF RESPIRATIONS
   A. Pressures Involved
   B. External and Internal Respirations
   C. Factors Facilitating the Combining of
      Oxygen with Hemoglobin
   D. Gas Transport
   E. Regulation of Breathing
III. AIR VOLUMES
IV. GAS LAWS
V. RESPIRATORY REGULATION OF ACID-
   BASE BALANCE

Oxygen is essential for most of the chemical reactions taking place in our body. Carbon dioxide is a major waste product resulting from metabolism. It is the role of the respiratory system to help the circulatory system in the exchange of these gases. Because the respiratory system and circulatory system are so closely related, patients whose disease is actually respiratory in nature may have complaints that suggest circulatory problems, whereas those who have pathology of the circulatory system may complain mostly of respiratory symptoms, such as shortness of breath. We shall examine the structure of the respiratory system and consider the functions of these vital structures (see Fig. 15-1).

STRUCTURES OF THE RESPIRATORY SYSTEM

The mucous membrane lining most of the respiratory tract is highly vascular and moist. The inhaled air is warmed by the blood flowing through the vessels of this membrane. As the air passes over the moist membrane, it is moistened and dust may be collected in the mucus. The nasal cavity and pharynx are lined with ciliated columnar epithelium. The cilia in this part of the tract beat downward toward the pharynx so that mucus, along with debris trapped in it, is moved into the pharynx where it is swallowed or ejected. A similar epithelium lines the bronchial tubes, but here the cilia beat upward toward the pharynx so that mucus and debris are moved away from the lungs. In the smallest bronchioles and alveolar ducts, the cells are cuboidal and lack cilia.

NASAL CAVITIES AND RELATED STRUCTURES

Air enters the tract through the nose. The internal surface of the nose is greatly increased by the three nasal conchae that project from the lateral wall of each nasal cavity. The nasal septum separating the nasal cavities is mostly cartilage covered by mucous membrane. The posterior part of the septum is bone, the vomer, and the perpendicular plate of the ethmoid. The olfactory (ol-fak'to-re) region of the nasal mucosa is located on the superior part of the nasal cavity and the superior conchae (see Fig. 15-2). The sense of smell is discussed in Chapter 11.

The paranasal sinuses are air spaces in some of the skull bones that open into the nose. These sinuses are lined with mucous membrane that is contiguous with that of the respiratory tract.

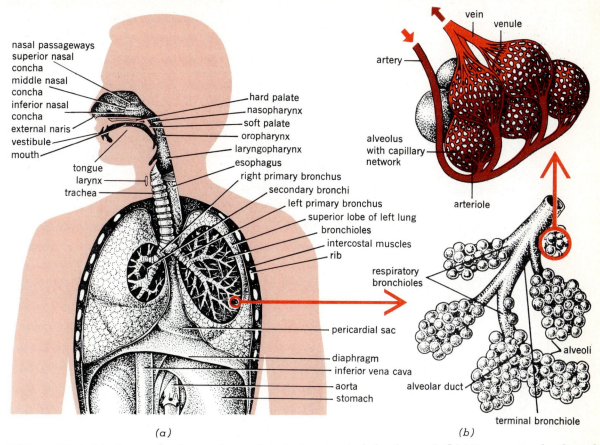

Figure 15-1. *(a) The conduction pathway for air (anatomical dead space). (b) Microscopic alveoli and pulmonary capillaries where oxygen and carbon dioxide are exchanged between the lungs and bloodstream.*

The sinuses give resonance to the voice and lightness to the head. If the sinuses are infected and filled with mucus, some of the resonance is lost. The paranasal sinuses take the names of the bones in which they are located: frontal, ethmoid, maxillary, and sphenoid (see Fig. 7-21).

The nasolacrimal ducts, which open into the nasal cavity, are also lined with mucous membrane. These ducts convey tears into the nose. Tears are constantly being produced by the lacrimal glands to cleanse the surface of the eye. These tears also serve as an added source of moisture to humidify the air. Tears, as well as the secretions of the mucous membrane, contain lysozyme, an enzyme that helps to destroy bacteria that we inhale.

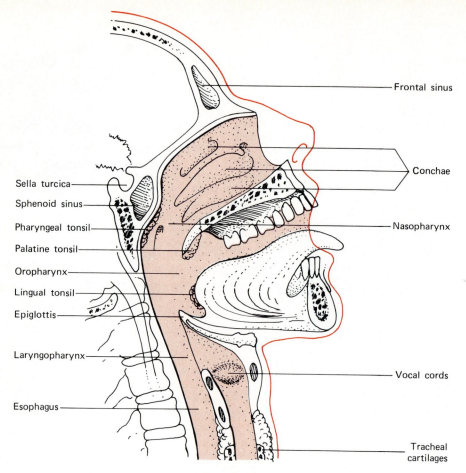

Sella turcica

Sphenoid sinus

Pharyngeal tonsil

Palatine tonsil

Oropharynx

Lingual tonsil

Epiglottis

Laryngopharynx

Esophagus

Frontal sinus

Conchae

Nasopharynx

Vocal cords

Tracheal cartilages

Figure 15-2. *Structures of the upper respiratory tract ·*

PHARNYX AND TONSILS

From the nose, the air passes into the naso-pharynx, a tubular passageway posterior to the nasal cavities and the mouth. The walls of the **pharynx** (far'inks) are skeletal muscle, and the lining is mucous membrane. The pharynx is subdivided into three parts: nasal, oral, and laryngeal.

The **eustachian** (u-sta'ke-an) **tube** from the middle ear opens into the nasopharynx. This tube helps to equalize the pressure in the ear with that of the atmosphere. Upper respiratory infections—particularly those in children—can spread through the tube to the ear and cause an ear infection.

The pharyngeal (fah-rin'je-al) tonsil is lym-phatic tissue located in the posterior part of the nasopharynx. This lymphatic tissue, as well as others elsewhere, plays an important role in protecting the body from bacterial invasion. If enlargement of the pharyngeal tonsil obstructs the upper air passage to such an extent that the person is obliged to breathe through the mouth, the air will not be properly moistened, warmed, and filtered before it reaches the lungs.

The oropharynx, which is inferior to the nasopharynx, serves as a passageway not only for air but also for food. Lymphatic tissue in the oropharynx includes the palatine (pal′ah-tin) and lingual (lin′gwal) tonsils. From the oropharynx, the air passes into the laryngopharynx. The laryngopharynx opens posteriorly into the esophagus and anteriorly into the *larynx* (lar′inks).

LARYNX AND VOICE PRODUCTION

The larynx, or voice box, is made of nine cartilages joined together by ligaments and lined with mucous membrane. The larynx is controlled by skeletal muscle. The thyroid cartilage is the largest of the laryngeal cartilages. It forms the laryngeal prominence, or "Adam's apple." Just inferior to the thyroid cartilage is the cricoid (kri′koid) cartilage. The epiglottis (ep-e-glat′is) is a leaf-shaped cartilage that closes the opening to the remainder of the respiratory tract during the act of swallowing.

At the upper end of the larynx are the vocal folds, cordlike structures that can vibrate as expired air passes over them. In this way, sound is produced. The loudness of the sound depends on the force of the vibration, and the pitch depends on the frequency of the vibrations. Because children and women usually have shorter vocal cords than men, their voices tend to be higher pitched. The glottis, the space between the vocal folds, is the narrowest part of the laryngeal cavity. Any obstruction, such as a foreign body (for example, a piece of food), can cause suffocation if it is not promptly removed.

TRACHEA

The **trachea** (tra′ke-ah) is a cylindrical tube extending from the larynx to the bronchi. It is about 12 cm (4.5 inches) long extending from the level of the sixth cervical vertebra to the fifth thoracic vertebra. The anterior and lateral aspects of the tube are composed of fibrous membrane and C-shaped cartilages. The cartilage rings keep the trachea open for the passage of air to and from the lungs. Smooth muscle layers and connective tissue fill in the posterior interval of the tube. During the act of swallowing, the esophagus (e-sof′ah-gus) which is posterior to the trachea, can bulge into this smooth muscle. The trachea is lined with a ciliated mucous membrane, which contains goblet cells for the production of mucus. The mucus produced by these goblet cells will trap dust and other small particles entering with the air.

From the trachea, the air enters the primary **bronchi** (brong′ki). The primary bronchi are lined with ciliated mucous membranes and are held open by hyaline cartilaginous rings. There are two primary bronchi, one entering each lung. The right bronchus is shorter, wider, and more vertical than the left. For this reason, any foreign body that has been aspirated is more likely to enter the right bronchus than the left.

BRONCHI AND BRONCHIOLES

The bronchi are similar to the trachea in structure. Each primary bronchus makes 23 branchings. The first 16 form the bronchi, bronchioles, and terminal bronchioles. The last seven form the respiratory bronchioles, alveolar ducts, and alveolar sacs, which all form the portion of the system where the exchange of gases takes place. This complex branching arrangement greatly increases the surface area exposed to air flowing into and out of the lungs. The air flow is fairly rapid in the bronchi but owing to the great increase in cross-sectional area, flow is much slower in the smaller branches.

As the bronchi branch into smaller and smaller bronchioles, the cartilaginous rings begin to disappear, and the walls are mostly smooth muscle. The wall of the terminal bronchioles are entirely smooth muscle passageways. The respiratory bronchioles and alveoli are surrounded by pulmonary capillaries. This is where the exchange of gases between the respiratory system and the bloodstream takes place. Beginning in the respiratory bronchioles, the ciliated columnar epithelium and mucus secreting cells are replaced with cuboidal epithelium and with simple squamous epithelium in the alveoli. The respiratory structures leading to the respiratory bronchioles comprise what is known as the anatomical dead space because air contained in these structures following inspiration does not reach the alveoli and will be exhaled. During a normal quiet inspiration, about 500 ml of air is inhaled. About 150 ml of this air remains in the anatomical dead space until expiration.

ALVEOLI

Each microscopic alveolus is surrounded with a rich capillary network arising from the pulmonary artery. The blood pressure in the pulmonary capillaries is very low so that, normally, no fluid filters into the alveoli. The chief reason for the blood pressure in these pulmonary capillaries being so much lower than it is in most other capillaries is the enormous size of the capillary bed and the small amount of blood contained within the capillaries at any one time. The capillary bed covers an area of about 60 square meters in a normal-sized adult. This is about half the size of a tennis court. The total quantity of blood in these capillaries at any one time is about 60 to 70 ml. With such a small amount of blood spread over such an enormous area, it is easy to understand why the diffusion of gases

across the pulmonary membrane is so rapid. The pulmonary membrane, sometimes called the respiratory membrane, is the area between the alveoli and the pulmonary capillaries. Normally this membrane is 0.004 mm thick.

The blood in the arteriole end of the pulmonary capillary is high in carbon dioxide and low in oxygen. Most of the carbon dioxide in this blood diffuses into the alveoli, and oxygen from the alveoli diffuses into the blood capillary. Diffusion is the process of particles moving from an area of greater concentration to an area of lesser concentration (recall the discussion of diffusion in Chapter 1). Therefore, the exchange of gases here depends on the differences in the concentration of the gases on each side of the pulmonary membrane, the enormous surface area of the pulmonary membrane, and the permeability of this very thin membrane (see Fig. 15-3).

The inner surface of the alveoli produces surfactant (sur′fakt-ant), which has a detergentlike action and lowers the alveolar surface tension. As a result, when the alveoli become smaller during expiration, the surface tension does not increase. Because of this process, the alveoli are less likely to collapse when deflated, and the tendency of one alveolus to empty into an adjacent alveolus is minimized. A few newborn babies do not secrete adequate quantities of surfactant, which makes lung expansion difficult. This condition is known as hyaline membrane disease.

From the previous discussion, you will recall that blood pressure in the arterial end of peripheral capillaries is higher than the colloidal osmotic pressure. Therefore, fluid is filtered out of the capillary to nourish peripheral capillaries. In the pulmonary capillaries, osmotic pressure is normally higher than the blood pressure on both the arterial and venous ends of the capillary. There is no filtration of fluid into the alveoli as long as the pulmonary blood pressure is nor-

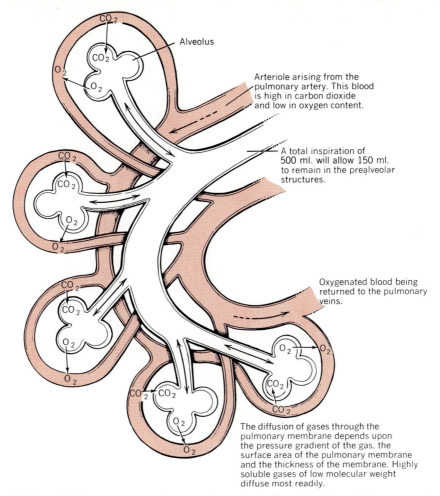

Alveolus

Arteriole arising from the pulmonary artery. This blood is high in carbon dioxide and low in oxygen content.

A total inspiration of 500 ml. will allow 150 ml. to remain in the prealveolar structures.

Oxygenated blood being returned to the pulmonary veins.

The diffusion of gases through the pulmonary membrane depends upon the pressure gradient of the gas, the surface area of the pulmonary membrane and the thickness of the membrane. Highly soluble gases of low molecular weight diffuse most readily.

Figure 15-3. *Normal exchange of oxygen and carbon dioxide between alveoli and the pulmonary capillaries (From Burke, S.R.,* Composition and Function of Body Fluids, *3rd ed. St. Louis: The C.V. Mosby Co., 1980)*

mal. In the pulmonary artery, the pressure is about 25/10 mm Hg and as the blood enters the left atrium, the systolic pressure has dropped to about 8 mm Hg. With pulmonary hypertension, fluid may be pushed into the alveoli, causing pulmonary edema, which was discussed in Chapter 14.

Oxygenated blood containing nutrients for the supporting tissues of the lungs is carried by the bronchial arteries. After the bronchial arterial blood has passed through its capillaries and collected carbon dioxide from the lung tissues, it empties into the left atrium (not the right). The significance of this action is that the cardiac output of the left ventricle is normally slightly greater than that of the right and also the carbon dioxide content of the blood leaving the left side of the heart is somewhat higher than that in the pulmonary veins.

LUNGS AND PLEURA

The two lungs are located in the thoracic cavity, one on either side of the heart (see Fig. 15-1). The apex of the lung is about 4 cm above the first rib, and the base of the lung rests on the diaphragm. The right lung has three lobes, and the left has two. The pleura is a serous membrane covering the lungs. The visceral layer of this membrane closely covers the lungs, and the parietal layer lies on the inner surface of the chest wall, the diaphragm, and the lateral aspect of the **mediastinum** (me"de-as-ti′num) or the space between the two lungs containing the heart, blood vessels, trachea, esophagus, thymus, lymphatic tissue, and vessels. A small amount of serous fluid in the space between the visceral and parietal pleura prevents friction.

PHYSIOLOGY OF RESPIRATIONS

Air flows from an area of higher pressure or concentration to an area of lower pressure or concentration. Involved in the mechanics of respiration are the atmospheric pressure, intrapulmonic pressure, and intrapleural or intrathoracic pressure.

PRESSURES INVOLVED

The atmospheric pressure is that of the air around us. At sea level, this pressure is 760 mm Hg. The intrapulmonic pressure is the pressure of the air within the bronchi and bronchioles. This pressure varies above and below 760 mm Hg, depending on the size of the thorax. The

intrapleural, or intrathoracic, pressure is the pressure in the pleural space. It is normally less than atmospheric, about 751 to 754 mm Hg. This pressure, however, may exceed atmospheric pressure when a person coughs or strains at stool.

During inspiration, the size of the thorax increases chiefly because of the contraction and descent of the diaphragm. The external intercostal muscles also contract to increase the size of the thorax by raising the ribs. The sternum pushes forward to increase the anterior-posterior diameter of the thoracic cavity. As the volume of the thorax increases, the intrapulmonic and intrapleural pressures decrease. Thus, air enters the lungs until the intrapulmonic pressure is equal to atmospheric pressure (see Fig. 15-4). In essence, air is being pulled in because the pressures within the respiratory tract are less than the atmospheric pressure.

Air pressure inside the viscoelastic alveoli as they expand produces pressure on the bony thorax and causes it to expand. This expansibility is called compliance. Specifically, compliance is the volume increase per unit of intraalveolar pressure. The compliance of the normal lungs and thorax combined is 0.13 liter per centimeter of water pressure. That is, every time the alveolar pressure is increased by 1 cm water, the lungs expand 130 ml. During inspiration, the intraalveolar pressure becomes slightly negative with respect to atmospheric pressure, normally less than -3 mm Hg. During expiration, on the other hand, the intraalveolar pressure rises to almost $+3$ mm Hg. Very little pressure is required to move air into and out of the lungs.

In general, the normal expansion and contraction of the chest are opposed by airway resistance and nonelastic tissue resistance. Abnormal conditions that decrease compliance are destruction of lung tissue, fibrotic alveoli, blocked alveoli, pulmonary edema, chest deformity, and muscular weakness.

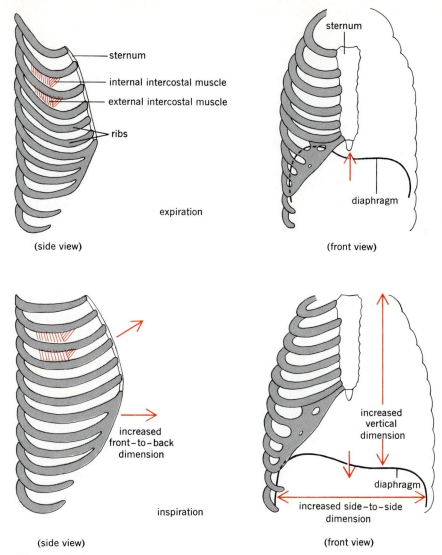

Figure 15-4. *Changes in the dimensions of the thorax during respirations*

EXTERNAL AND INTERNAL RESPIRATIONS

The drop in intrapleural pressure during normal inspiration favors venous return of blood to the right side of the heart. This respiratory effect on the circulation is sometimes called the thoracic pump factor. In addition to favoring venous return to the heart, it helps expand the pulmonary blood flow and increase left heart filling and cardiac output.

Expiration is mainly a passive action. The relaxation of the diaphragm and external intercostal muscles decreases the size of the thorax. As these muscles return to their resting state, the elastic lungs recoil. This recoil increases the intrapulmonic pressure slightly above the atmospheric pressure, and the air is forced out of the lungs.

External respiration involves the exchange of gases between the circulating blood in the alveolar capillaries and the air in the alveoli. Internal respiration involves the exchange of gases between the circulating blood in the peripheral capillaries and the tissue cells as they use oxygen and produce waste carbon dioxide.

FACTORS FACILITATING THE COMBINING OF OXYGEN WITH HEMOGLOBIN

In a mixture of gases, the combination of the pressures exerted by all of the gases is called the total pressure. The pressure exerted by a single gas is called the partial pressure. The partial pressure of oxygen in the lungs is greater than that in the bloodstream. Therefore, oxygen goes from the lungs to the blood. The partial pressure of oxygen in the blood is higher than that in the peripheral tissues, so oxygen diffuses from the blood into the tissues.

A small amount of oxygen is dissolved in the plasma and transported in this manner. However, most of the oxygen in the blood combines with hemoglobin to form **oxyhemoglobin** (ok"se-he-mo-glo′bin) in the pulmonary capillaries. Hemoglobin's ability to transport oxygen resides in its iron atoms. When metallic iron and oxygen are combined, as in iron ore, it takes a blast furnace to separate them. But the iron of hemoglobin can react with oxygen at body temperatures and with considerable speed. Let us explore how this is done. This combination of

oxygen with hemoglobin in the pulmonary capillaries and the dissociation of the oxygen from the hemoglobin in the peripheral capillaries are chemical reactions. The ease and speed of these reactions is influenced by both the pH and temperature of the blood. One of the main factors determining blood pH is the amount of carbon dioxide present. Carbon dioxide and water combine to form carbonic acid, thereby favoring acidity. Blood temperature is influenced by the heat generated by skeletal muscle activity.

A pH toward the alkaline side favors the combining of oxygen with hemoglobin, whereas a pH toward the acid side favors the dissociation of oxygen from hemoglobin. In the pulmonary circuit, because carbon dioxide and water are being expelled, the blood is slightly more alkaline; here, oxygen readily combines with hemoglobin. In the active peripheral tissues, carbon dioxide is being produced. Therefore, because carbon dioxide combines with water to produce carbonic acid, blood in these capillaries is slightly more acid. This acidity favors the release of oxygen from hemoglobin.

Increased metabolism produces slightly higher temperatures in the active peripheral tissues than in the pulmonary circuit, favoring the dissociation of oxygen from hemoglobin in the periphery and the association of oxygen with hemoglobin in the pulmonary circuit.

GAS TRANSPORT

Oxygen is transported mainly as potassium oxyhemoglobin in the red blood cells. However, a small amount is dissolved in the plasma. Carbon dioxide is mainly carried in the plasma in the form of bicarbonate. Some of the carbon dioxide in the plasma is carried as carbonic acid. In the red blood cells, carbon dioxide is carried in the form of **carbaminohemoglobin** (kar-bam"in-o-hem-o-glo′bin) and as bicarbonate.

REGULATION OF BREATHING

The respiratory center in the medulla of the brain controls the rate and depth of respiration according to the needs of the body. This medullary center is the rhythmicity center that allows two seconds for inspiration and three for expiration. Normal respiratory rates are about 14 to 20 respirations per minute. Obviously, vigorous exercise can greatly increase the rate of respirations, since active skeletal muscles require more oxygen than do resting muscles.

When the medullary respiratory center is stimulated, it sends efferent (motor) nerve impulses via the phrenic (fren'ik) nerves to the diaphragm to increase the rate of contractions. Various stimuli affect this respiratory center, but the most powerful and important is an increased level of carbon dioxide in the blood. Excess oxygen or decreased amounts of carbon dioxide will depress this respiratory center and respirations will become slower.

Pressoreceptors in the alveoli are stimulated by the expansion of the lung during inspiration. They send afferent (sensory) messages to the brain to inhibit respirations, preventing over-distention of the lungs. As the lung deflates, the pressoreceptors cease sending their impulses and the diaphragm contracts. This is called the Hering-Breuer reflex.

The pneumotaxic (nu"mo-tax'ik) center is located in the pons. When stimulated, the pneumotaxic center increases the rate of respirations but simultaneously decreases the depth of respirations. The apneustic (ap'nu"stik) center is also in the pons. This center prolongs inspiration by allowing the medullary inspiratory neurons to continue to send signals.

As discussed in Chapter 13, in the aorta and carotid arteries, chemoreceptors respond to oxygen lack and to increased levels of carbon dioxide. As the oxygen level in the blood falls, these chemoreceptors are stimulated, and nerve impulses are sent to the respiratory center to increase the rate and depth of respirations. Although these chemoreceptors are not of major importance in the regulation of respirations in the normal healthy person, they may be very important in patients with serious respiratory diseases (see Chapter 16).

Other factors, such as fever and pain, can also modify the rate and depth of respiration. Fever increases the body metabolism, which in turn increases respiration. Pain may also cause an increase in the rate of respiration. However, if the pain is due to thoracic surgery or high abdominal surgery, the patient is likely to have slow, shallow respirations because the respiratory movements will be painful. As a result of shallow respirations following this type of surgery, the patient may develop pneumonia. To help prevent this, the patient should be encouraged to cough and breathe deeply while the incision is supported.

AIR VOLUMES

Lung air volumes are graphically illustrated in Figure 15-5. **Tidal air** is the air that is moved during quiet inspiration and expiration. Normally, the volume of this air is about 500 ml. Of the 500 ml, about 150 ml stays in the anatomical dead space, the bronchi, bronchioles, and other prealveolar structures until the following expiration, when it is exhaled.

The inspiratory reserve is the amount of air that can be forcibly inspired after a normal inspiration. This volume is about 2,000 to 3,000 ml. The expiratory reserve is the amount of air that can be forcibly expired after a normal expiration. The normal expiratory reserve volume, somewhat less than the inspiratory reserve, is about 1,200 ml.

Residual air, which is about 1,000 to 1,200 ml,

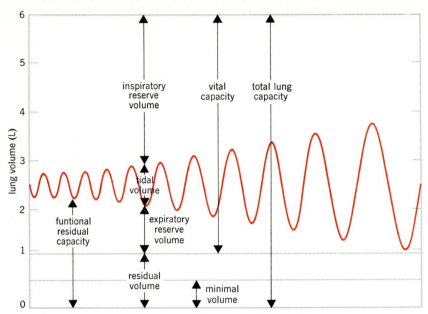

Figure 15-5. Subdivision of lung volume

is the air that remains in the lung as long as the thorax is airtight. It cannot be removed from the lungs even by forceful expiration. The purpose of this air is to aerate the blood between breaths. Were it not for the residual air, the amounts of oxygen and carbon dioxide in the blood would rise and fall markedly with each respiration, intermittently allowing oxygen-poor blood to traverse vital capillaries.

Vital capacity is the quantity of air moved on deepest inspiration and expiration. On the average, vital capacity is about 3,000 to 5,000 ml, although in a healthy young adult it may be much greater. Other than the anatomical build of a person, vital capacity is affected by (1) the position of the person during measurement of vital capacity, (2) the strength of the respiratory muscles, and (3) the distensibility of the lungs

and chest cage, which is called pulmonary compliance. Disease processes that affect any or all of these three factors will result in a decreased vital capacity.

Inspiratory capacity is the maximum amount of air an individual can inspire after a normal expiration. This is equal to the sum of the tidal volume and the inspiratory reserve volume or about 2,500 to 3,500 ml.

All pulmonary volumes and capacities are about 20 to 25% less in women than in men, and they are obviously greater in the large, athletic person than in the small, unathletic one.

Once the alveoli have been inflated with air, a certain amount of air remains in the alveoli even if the lung has collapsed because of trauma. This is minimal air. Minimal air represents about 40% of the residual volume.

GAS LAWS

Boyle's law concerning gases states that at a constant temperature the volume of a gas is inversely proportional to the pressure of the gas. Dalton's law states that each gas exerts its pressure independently of other gases. All of the chemical and physiological activities of gases are determined by the pressure under which the gas is maintained. These pressures, which can be measured, yield valuable diagnostic information.

Table 15-1. Gas Pressures as Measured in mm Hg

	Atmosphere	Arterial	Venous
pO_2	160	100	37
pCO_2	0.3	40	46

As mentioned above, in a mixture of gases such as the oxygen and carbon dioxide in the bloodstream, the combination of the pressures is called the total pressure. Clinically, we are concerned with the pressure of each gas, which is called the partial pressure. The partial pressure of oxygen, or the pO_2, in arterial blood is about 100 mm Hg. It is obviously influenced by the oxygen content of the inspired air and by blood volume. The partial pressure of carbon dioxide, or the pCO_2, of arterial blood is 40 mm Hg. The pCO_2 decreases with hyperventilation as more and more carbon dioxide is blown off. The pressure is increased with shallow respirations and diseases of the respiratory system that decrease the ventilatory space. The activity of carbon dioxide is of particular clinical concern because of its ability to combine with water and form carbonic acid. The formation of too much carbonic acid owing to decreased lung volume in a patient with diseased lungs will disturb the normal pH of the blood, and the patient may develop acidosis.

RESPIRATORY REGULATION OF ACID-BASE BALANCE

As mentioned briefly in Chapter 1, the stability of the blood pH is very important to health. The respiratory system automatically helps to maintain this pH very close to the normal of 7.4, regardless of factors such as diet and exercise that would tend to alter the pH.

Carbon dioxide is one of the major products resulting from cellular metabolism. As we have seen, carbon dioxide and water combine to form carbonic acid. This is a reversible reaction that is catalized by carbonic anhydrase. The carbonic acid can ionize to form hydrogen and bicarbonate. Clearly, retention of excess amounts of carbon dioxide will increase the partial pressure of the gas and cause the formation of carbonic acid, increasing the relative acidity of the blood. Under normal healthy conditions, this does not happen because carbon dioxide itself is the most important stimulus for respirations. Hold your breath for a few moments and soon the stimulus of carbon dioxide will be so great that you must breathe. You will breathe rapidly until the excess accumulation of carbon dioxide is eliminated, and then your respiratory rate will return to normal. The respiratory system has adjusted its lowered pH back to the normal 7.4.

You can also explore how the respiratory system will react if the pH moves a little to the alkaline side of normal. Breathe rapidly for a few moments eliminating more carbon dioxide than would be eliminated with ordinary respirations. After a brief period of voluntary hyperventilation, your respirations will automatically become slower and more shallow, retaining enough carbon dioxide to adjust the blood pH.

Let us examine some of the clinical indicators of acid-base balance and see how these may be altered in acidosis and alkalosis. Normally, most of the carbon dioxide is transported as bicarbonate; however, a smaller amount is transported as carbonic acid. Actually, we normally have a 20:1 ratio of bicarbonate to carbonic acid (24 mEq/liter as bicarbonate and 1.2 mEq/liter as carbonic acid). Under these circumstances with a pCO_2 of 40 mm Hg, there will be a blood pH of 7.4. If we retain too much carbon dioxide, the pCO_2 will increase. Therefore, more carbonic acid will be formed and the blood pH will be reduced. To compensate for this imbalance, we will attempt to eliminate more of the carbon dioxide and lower our pCO_2. However, the efficiency of this compensatory mechanism will be limited by whatever it was that caused the retention of the carbon dioxide in the first place.

The kidneys also help to regulate acid-base balance. However, this regulatory mechanism is slow. It may take three to five days for the kidneys to compensate for an imbalance. Respiratory regulation of acid-base balance is rapid. Respirations can alter blood pH from 7.2 to 7.8 in about one minute.

The most likely cause of respiratory acidosis is pulmonary disease, such as emphysema or bronchitis, that has caused an increase in the anatomical dead space. Diseased lungs with a decreased functioning pulmonary membrane are unable to eliminate adequate amounts of carbon dioxide so the blood carbon dioxide content increases.

Respiratory alkalosis is not very common, but it can occur in inexperienced people who attempt mountain climbing. The rarefied atmosphere of the high altitude and the strenuous exercise can induce alkalosis as can hyperventilation. Also, if not properly performed, the breathing exercises for natural childbirth can cause alkalosis. Anxiety can also cause hyperventilation severe enough to result in alkalosis. In this instance, too much carbon dioxide is eliminated, thereby lowering the pCO_2. The normal 20:1 ratio of bicarbonate to carbonic acid will become more like 40:1 and the pH will rise. To compensate, one will, of course, try to stop the hyperventilating; however, it is unlikely that this will be very successful. Having the patient breathe into and out of a paper bag will help.

SUMMARY QUESTIONS

1. Discuss internal and external respirations.
2. List in sequence all of the structures through which inhaled air passes from the time it enters the nose until it reaches the alveoli.
3. What are the functions of the nose?
4. List the paranasal sinuses.
5. What are the functions of the paranasal sinuses?
6. Discuss the pressures involved in the process of external respiration.
7. What muscle action is involved in normal inspiration?
8. What muscle action is involved in normal expiration?
9. Discuss the factors that facilitate the combining of oxygen with hemoglobin.
10. Where is the rhythmicity respiratory center located and how is this center stimulated?

11. How is carbon dioxide transported in the bloodstream?
12. Discuss Boyle's and Dalton's laws concerning gases.
13. What is the cause of respiratory acidosis?
14. Explain the compensatory mechanisms involved in respiratory alkalosis.
15. Where is the pneumotaxic center and explain what happens when it is stimulated.
16. Where is the apneustic center and what does it do?

KEY TERMS

bronchi
carbaminohemoglobin
eustachian tube
mediastinum
oxyhemoglobin

pharynx
tidal air
trachea
vital capacity

16

Diseases of the Respiratory System

OBJECTIVES

On completion of this chapter, you will be able to:

1. List eight procedures used to evaluate respiratory diseases.
2. Explain the preparations necessary before a bronchoscopy.
3. Give five reasons for pulmonary function testing.
4. Differentiate between restrictive and obstructive lung diseases and give examples of each.
5. List the eight upper respiratory tract diseases and their treatments.
6. Describe the treatment for cancer of the larynx.
7. Describe the pathogenesis, diagnosis, and treatment of tuberculosis.
8. Differentiate between pulmonary embolism and pulmonary infarction.
9. List five chronic obstructive lung diseases and their treatments.
10. Explain the role of chest physical therapy, vibration, and postural drainage in pulmonary hygiene.
11. Give three examples of environmentally related lung disorders.
12. List risk factors associated with the development of lung cancer.
13. Describe the pathophysiology of IRDS.
14. Describe the pathophysiology of ARDS.
15. Differentiate between a spontaneous and a traumatic pneumothorax.

OVERVIEW

I. DIAGNOSTIC PROCEDURES
  A. Roentgenography
    1. Lung Scans
    2. Pulmonary Angiography
    3. Computerized Tomography
  B. Sputum Specimens
  C. Bronchoscopy
  D. Tuberculin Tests
  E. Pulmonary Function Tests
II. DISEASES OF THE UPPER RESPIRATORY
   TRACT
  A. Sinusitis
  B. Epistaxis
  C. Tonsillitis
  D. The Common Cold
  E. Influenza
  F. Cancer of the Larynx
  G. Croup
  H. Epiglottitis
III. DISEASES OF THE LUNGS AND PLEURA
  A. Pneumonia
  B. Pleurisy
  C. Tuberculosis
  D. Pulmonary Embolism and Pulmonary
     Infarction
  E. Chronic Obstructive Pulmonary Disease
    1. Chronic Bronchitis
    2. Emphysema
    3. Bronchiectasis
    4. Bronchial Asthma
    5. Cystic Fibrosis
    6. Treatment of Chronic Obstructive
       Pulmonary Diseases
  F. Environmental Lung Disorders
  G. Cancer of the Lung
IV. LIFE-THREATENING LUNG DISORDERS
  A. Infant Respiratory Distress Syndrome
     (IRDS)
  B. Adult Respiratory Distress Syndrome
     (ARDS)
  C. Chest Trauma
  D. Pneumothorax

This chapter was written by Wayne C. Anderson.

Diagnosis of respiratory system diseases begins when the patient notices a deviation from his normal state of health and seeks medical help. Symptoms the patient may describe include chest pain, cough, shortness of breath, hemoptysis, and wheezing. Based on this information plus a thorough physical examination, the physician may proceed to more sophisticated procedures in order to make a firm diagnosis and provide optimal therapy.

DIAGNOSTIC PROCEDURES

ROENTGENOGRAPHY

Roentgenography (rent-gen-og′rah-fe), or X-rays of the chest, helps in the diagnosis of many types of chest diseases. Usually both posteroanterior (PA) and lateral views are taken, since the view of some lesions in a single X-ray may be obstructed by surrounding structures (see Figs. 16-1 and 16-2). In addition, special views of the lungs may be obtained by placing the patient in various positions for better visualization of certain areas.

Tomography, or body section X-rays, facilitates the study of suspicious areas by focusing at different depths in the thoracic cavity. With a series of pictures, the tomogram can define the shape, size, and borders of lesions.

Lung Scans

For a lung scan, the patient either inhales or is given intravenously a gamma-ray-emitting ma-

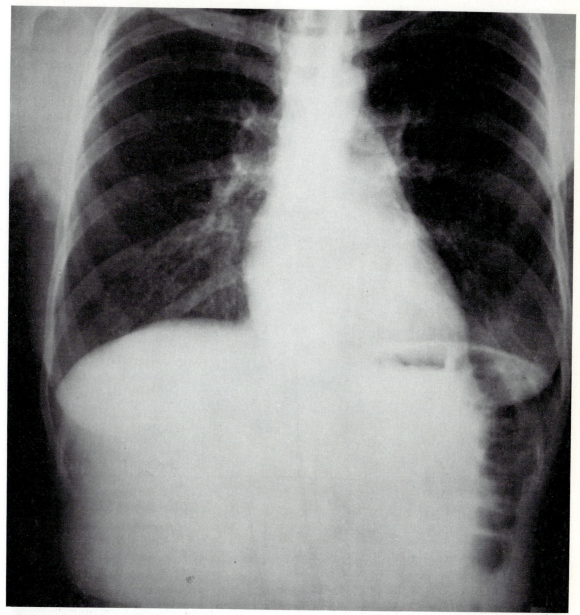

Figure 16-1. *Normal PA chest X-ray (Courtesy of University of Pittsburgh Medical Center, Pittsburgh, PA)*

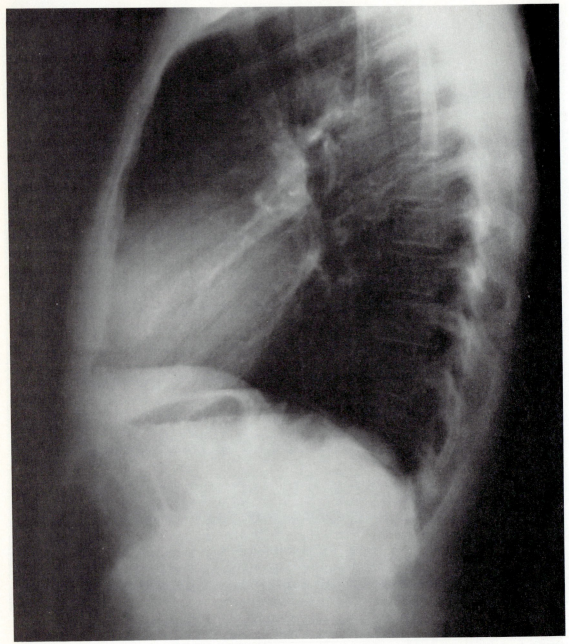

Figure 16-2. *Normal lateral chest X-ray (Courtesy of University of Pittsburgh Medical Center, Pittsburgh, PA)*

terial. Then a scanning device records patterns of the pulmonary radioactivity. The visual pattern produced provides information concerning ventilation and is helpful in the diagnosis of lung and pulmonary vascular disorders.

Pulmonary Angiography

If a pulmonary embolus (or if pulmonary emboli) is suspected, a catheter can be passed through the right side of the heart and into the pulmonary artery. A radiopaque dye is injected into the artery and a rapid series of X-rays is taken. The embolus will create a filling defect in the blood vessel since the clot keeps the blood from flowing past the point of obstruction.

Computerized Tomography

A relatively recent innovation used in the assessment of chest disease is computerized tomographic scanning (CT scan). In this technique, radiologic and computer technologies combine to produce pictures showing thin, transverse cross sections of the body, allowing for better localization and identification of certain chest disorders (see Fig. 16-3).

SPUTUM SPECIMENS

Sputum specimens help in the diagnosis of infections of the respiratory system. Abnormal cells from tumors are also sometimes present in the sputum and sputum cytological examinations may be done.

With infections, the causative organism can be cultured and tested for its sensitivity to a variety of antibiotics. If a sputum sample is not generated spontaneously by the patient, the instillation of hypertonic saline (3% sodium chloride) via a nebulizer into the bronchial tree is irritating and may induce a productive cough.

Efforts should be made to ensure that the sputum sample is from the lungs and not the upper respiratory tract. Color, odor, consistency, and volume of sputum should all be noted.

BRONCHOSCOPY

Bronchoscopy (brong-kos′ko-pe) can be used to visualize directly the upper airway and bronchi and to obtain a specimen of tissue for microscopic examination if a tumor is suspected. The procedure can also be used to remove foreign bodies, such as a toy or a piece of food, that have been aspirated.

The bronchoscope, a rigid, hollow instrument used for this examination, is passed into the trachea and on to the bronchi. To avoid the danger of aspirating vomitus, the patient should have nothing to eat or drink for 8 to 12 hours before the bronchoscopy. The patient will be sedated for the procedure and given a local anesthetic. Because the patient's gag reflex will be absent for a few hours following the examination, the period of fasting must be continued until the gag reflex has returned.

A fiberoptic (fi′ber-optic) bronchoscope is a flexible instrument that allows better visualization of the lower airway than the rigid bronchoscope (see Fig. 16-4). Forceps may extend from the tip of the instrument and secure tissue samples for examination, thus possibly eliminating the need for an open lung biopsy. With the suction mechanism activated, mucus plugs can be removed from the airway and sputum samples obtained. A brush may be inserted through the bronchoscope to scrape or brush the mucosa. These samples are then examined with various cytologic and microbiologic stains. Because the bronchoscope actually draws air out of the lung during some of the procedures, supplemental oxygen should be given and vital signs monitored.

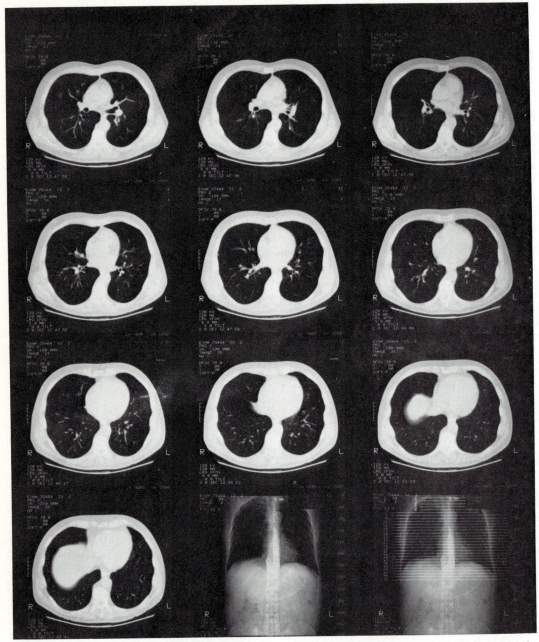

Figure 16-3. *Normal CT scan of the chest. (Courtesy of University of Pittsburgh Medical Center, Pittsburgh, PA)*

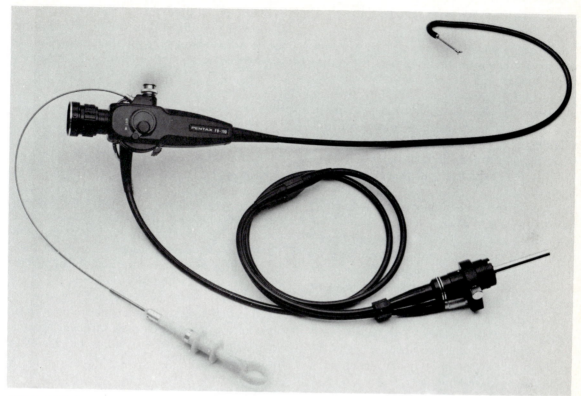

Figure 16-4. *A flexible fiberoptic bronchoscope. Samples of tissue from the periphery of the lung may be obtained by use of the biopsy forceps. (Courtesy of Pentax Precision Instrument Corporation, Orangeburg, NY)*

TUBERCULIN TESTS

Several different types of tuberculin skin tests are used. All are based on the fact that about six to eight weeks after the body has been invaded by the tubercle bacillus, the body develops an allergy to the organism. About 48 to 72 hours after an intradermal injection of tuberculin, if the test is positive, a person will develop an area of induration (swelling and redness) at the site of the injection.

A positive reaction does not necessarily mean that the person has tuberculosis. False positives can occur if the person is allergic to the protein derivative used in testing. The induration can also mean that although the bacillus has invaded the body, a primary healed lesion has developed. If the person has recently converted from a negative to a positive tuberculin reaction, a chest X-ray should be taken. Frequently, isoniazid is prescribed to help prevent the development of clinical tuberculosis.

PULMONARY FUNCTION TESTS

Pulmonary function tests are performed to assess lung function related either to the movement of air in and out of the lungs (ventilation) or to the diffusion of gases across the alveolar-capillary membrane. Localized diseases, such as tuberculosis or lung abscesses, may have little effect on pulmonary function, whereas generalized diseases like emphysema or chronic bronchitis produce significant changes in pulmonary performance.

Although the primary reason for pulmonary function tests is to determine the cause of dyspnea, it may also be used for preoperative evaluation to pinpoint patients at high risk for postoperative respiratory complications, or for screening to detect pulmonary disease at an early stage. The effectiveness of drug therapy may be evaluated by serial testing before and after administration of the drug. These procedures may also be used to evaluate workers' disability in the case of an occupation-related disease, such as black lung disease.

Spirometry measures the various lung volumes discussed in Chapter 15 as well as flow rates of air. Lung diseases can be classified into two categories by the results of spirometry: restrictive disorders and obstructive disorders. In restrictive diseases, total lung capacity is reduced, while obstructive disease is characterized by reduced expiratory flow rates. Neuromuscular disorders, such as Myasthenia gravis and Guillain-Barré syndrome, that cause weakness or paralysis of the respiratory muscles are classified as restrictive diseases.

In an obstructive disease such as emphysema or bronchiectasis, there is an impedance to air flow owing to retained secretions or destruction of lung tissue. One person may simultaneously have an obstructive disorder such as asthma and a restrictive disorder such as pneumonia. Spirometric studies can be used to assess the degree of both types of dysfunction. The physician can also use the results of these studies in directing the treatment and rehabilitation program toward maximizing the remaining lung function.

DISEASES OF THE UPPER RESPIRATORY TRACT

SINUSITIS

Sinusitis is an infection of the paranasal sinuses. Because the mucous membrane that lines these sinuses is continuous with that of the nose and throat, sinusitis is a fairly common complication of any upper respiratory infection. It can be particularly painful if the mucosa lining the ducts leading from these sinuses into the nose is so swollen that there is little or no drainage from the sinuses. Nose drops such as phenylephrine may help decrease the swelling and facilitate drainage.

EPISTAXIS

Epistaxis (ep-e-stak′sis) is a nosebleed that may be caused by trauma or ulceration of the lining of the nose. Breathing excessively dry air, small tumors, or polyps can also cause epistaxis. Epistaxis also may be a symptom of hypertension.

Epistaxis usually can be controlled if the patient remains quiet with the head elevated. Because cold causes vasoconstriction, cold compresses may be helpful. In some cases, the nasal cavity may have to be packed with gauze to apply pressure on the bleeding vessels. In extreme cases, to stop the bleeding vessels may have to be cauterized (extreme heat is applied).

TONSILLITIS

Tonsillitis commonly affects children between the ages of five and ten. Symptoms of tonsillitis include a sore throat causing painful swallowing, fever, chills, malaise, and swelling of the lymph glands. Acute tonsillitis is treated with rest, analgesics, increased fluid intake, and appropriate antibiotics.

Although tonsillitis is usually self-limiting, serious complications such as otitis media, scarlet fever, bacteremia, and rheumatic fever may occur. Chronic tonsillitis may require a tonsillectomy.

THE COMMON COLD

The common cold is an acute viral infection that causes inflammation of the upper respiratory tract. Symptoms include pharyngitis, headache, nasal congestion, malaise, and lethargy. One characteristic of the cold virus is it usually fails to produce an immunity and some people suffer one cold after another. Treatment of the common cold is symptomatic; analgesics for the pain, increased fluid intake, nasal decongestants such as phenylephrine, and bed rest. At the current time, there is no known cure or way to prevent this disorder.

INFLUENZA

Influenza is a highly contagious viral infection of the respiratory tract characterized by fever, chills, cough, headache, and malaise. Transmission of this disorder occurs through inhalation of respiratory droplets from an infected person or by use of contaminated articles, such as a drinking glass or silverware. Influenza has caused many deaths in the elderly and in patients with chronic pulmonary and cardiac disease. Treatment includes bed rest, increased fluid intake, and aspirin to treat the fever and muscle ache.

CANCER OF THE LARYNX

Anatomically, the larynx marks the division between the upper and lower airways. It performs a protective function by closing off the glottis during swallowing, thereby preventing food or fluid from entering the lower airway. The larynx also participates in both the cough and speech mechanisms.

Major predisposing factors for laryngeal cancer include cigarette smoking and alcoholism. Early symptoms include persistent hoarseness and difficulty in swallowing. The treatment of this disease includes radiation therapy, surgery, or both. If the tumor is large, it may be necessary to do a laryngectomy (lar-in-jek'to-me). If the tumor is discovered while it is still relatively small, sometimes it can be removed by cordectomy or partial laryngectomy.

If a laryngectomy is necessary, the patient will have a permanent **tracheostomy** (tra-ke-os'to-me) and will not be able to speak normally. Many cities have Lost Chord Clubs, groups of people who have had this surgery and who help one another cope with the disability. In addition to providing emotional support, club members are often able to teach new members esophageal speech. The patient learns to swallow and to regurgitate air and gradually is able to reproduce speech. With practice, the speech becomes less jerky and is understandable.

CROUP

Croup is an upper respiratory tract disease that most frequently affects children between three months and four years of age. Croup is usually viral in origin and frequently follows an upper respiratory tract infection.

Clinical symptoms that suggest croup include respiratory distress, inspiratory stridor, and a characteristic "barking" cough. These symptoms are caused by inflammatory edema and spasm of the upper airway. Diphtheria and epiglottitis should be ruled out as a diagnosis as well as foreign body obstruction.

Treatment includes adequate hydration, aerosol therapy with vasoconstrictors such as ra-cemic epinephrine to reduce mucosal swelling, cool mist inhalation, and acetaminophen. An-tibiotics are not indicated unless bacterial infec-tion is a complication.

EPIGLOTTITIS

Epiglottitis is an acute bacterial inflammation of the epiglottis that can induce life-threatening airway obstruction. Epiglottitis is frequently seen in children between the ages of two and twelve. It is more common in males.

Diagnosis of epiglottitis is made by two meth-ods: (1) direct observation of a swollen, cherry-red epiglottis or (2) a lateral neck X-ray that shows an enlarged epiglottis. Direct visualiza-tion is a risky procedure because total obstruc-tion may be precipitated.

Symptoms include fever, sore throat, difficulty in swallowing, drooling, and stridor. Patients frequently assume a characteristic sitting up po-sition with neck hyperextended, mouth open, and tongue protruding. This position tends to reduce airway obstruction.

The first step in the management of epiglot-titis is the placement of an artificial airway. Be-cause of the danger of sudden total obstruction, observation alone is unsafe. Usually, nasotra-cheal intubation is necessary for only a few days until the inflammation and edema are relieved. Also, antibiotics and oxygen therapy are given.

DISEASES OF THE LUNGS AND PLEURA

PNEUMONIA

Pneumonia is an acute inflammatory process of the lungs and has many possible causes. Community-acquired pneumonias are most fre-quently pneumococcal in origin, although other bacteria, viruses, and protozoa may be impli-cated. Many of these organisms frequently can be cultured from the noses and throats of healthy people. With decreased resistance, how-ever, these individuals are likely to develop pneumonia. For this reason, pneumonia is a common complication of other diseases. At high risk are transplant patients, patients who have aspirated, patients undergoing chemotherapy, and people with acquired immune deficiency syndrome (AIDS). An opportunistic pneumonia commonly associated with AIDS is Pneumocys-tis carinini.

Pneumonia may be either **lobar**, involving an entire lobe of a lung, or **bronchopneumonia**, with the disease scattered throughout the lung. In both types, there is copious sputum, chest pain, dyspnea, and fever.

Treatment of pneumonia depends on the cau-sative organism. Supportive measures include bed rest, analgesics, oxygen to treat hypoxia, and adequate fluid intake.

PLEURISY

Pleurisy, which usually is secondary to some other respiratory disease, is an inflammation of the pleurae. It takes two forms: pleurisy with effusion, in which large amounts of a fluid col-lect in the pleural space and may have to be removed by a **thoracentesis** (tho"rah-sen-te'sis) (see Fig. 16-5), and dry pleurisy, in which little fluid is produced. Sharp pain occurs as the vis-ceral and parietal pleurae rub together during respirations. Treatment of pleurisy is based on the underlying cause, but symptomatic relief may be obtained with bed rest, antiinflamma-tory agents, and analgesics.

TUBERCULOSIS

Tuberculosis is a chronic disease caused by the bacillus Mycobacterium tuberculosis or other mycobacteria. The organism is usually trans-

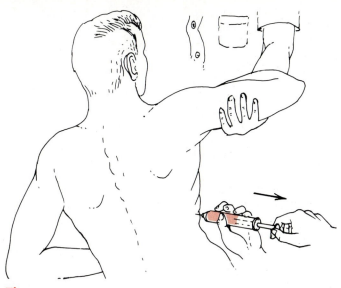

Figure 16-5. *Fluid being removed from the pleural cavity by means of a thoracentesis. If there is a large amount of fluid to be removed, tubing will be attached to the three-way stopcock between the needle and syringe. This allows the fluid to drain into a container.*

mitted by droplet infection. When a person with active tuberculosis sneezes or coughs, the organisms spread through the air and may be inhaled by someone else.

Pulmonary tuberculosis develops directly following implantation of the tubercle bacillus in the lung. This stage is known as the primary phase of the disease. If the patient's resistance is high, the lesion may heal by fibrosis and calcification. The remnants of the healed primary focus are usually visible on X-ray. They may contain viable bacilli that are walled off and cannot spread to other lung tissue unless there is a marked decrease in resistance at some subsequent time. The patient will have a positive tuberculin test and some degree of immunity to subsequent exposure to the organism.

At times, the primary complex does not heal but goes on to a progressive form of the disease. The focus of the infection may enlarge and undergo caseation (ka-se-a'shun), a form of necrosis with a cheeselike appearance. This area may slough away and leave a cavity in the lung. In miliary tuberculosis, there is a general spread of the bacillus into body organs and tissue with the production of countless minute tubercle lesions.

The disease is insidious and often produces no symptoms at all until the disease is fairly advanced, at which time there is a low-grade fever in the evening, night sweats, increased fatigue, and a cough that produces purulent sputum that may be blood streaked. **Hemoptysis** (he-mop'tis-is), the coughing up of blood, may also occur, and later there is marked wasting, weakness, and dyspnea. There may be chest pain if the infection has spread to the pleura.

Treatment of tuberculosis is centered around multiple-drug chemotherapy. Combinations of two or more of the following drugs are administered for different durations of therapy: isoniazid (INH), rifampin, ethambutol, streptomycin, and pyrazinamide. Many of these drugs have toxic side effects that may require a change in treatment regimen. Complications include hepatitis, optic neuritis, upset stomach, and thrombocytopenia (abnormal decrease in number of blood platelets).

PULMONARY EMBOLISM AND PULMONARY INFARCTION

Pulmonary embolism is a frequent complication of hospitalized patients. A conservative estimate of 50,000 deaths from pulmonary embolism occur each year.

Pulmonary embolism is defined as an obstruction of the pulmonary circulatory system caused by a dislodged thrombus (blood clot at its origin), air, fat, tumor cells, or other foreign material. Pulmonary infarction is the necrosis of lung tissue due to an interruption of blood supply, usually as the result of an embolism.

The most likely source of the embolism is the large leg veins. If you trace the pathway of any venous blood except that coming from the organs of digestion, you will find it flows to vessels of increasing diameter that are not likely to stop the movement of the clot until it reaches the pulmonary circuit where the blood proceeds to flow to smaller and smaller branches (see Fig. 16-6).

Postsurgical patients, and particularly those who have had pelvic or abdominal surgery, are most vulnerable to thrombus formation because of decreased activity. Early ambulation helps to prevent this complication.

If a clot does form in a vein and begins to move, it goes rapidly to the pulmonary circuit, which acts as a filter to prevent the clot from reaching the systemic circulatory system where more serious consequences may occur. The size of the occluded artery and the number of emboli will determine the severity of the problem and the prognosis.

Diagnosis begins with a high degree of suspicion and observation of clinical symptoms such as tachycardia, dyspnea, pleuritic chest pain, and productive cough. Pulmonary angiography is the definitive test for diagnosis of pulmonary embolism.

Treatment of pulmonary embolism may be medical or surgical. Medical treatment includes anticoagulation with heparin to prevent new thrombus formation. Thrombolytic agents such as streptokinase and urokinase are controversial and carry significant risk in addition to high costs. Surgical treatment includes embolectomy, ligation of the inferior vena cava, and insertion of an inverted umbrella-shaped filter into the inferior vena cava that prevents any clots from reaching the pulmonary vessels.

CHRONIC OBSTRUCTIVE PULMONARY DISEASE

Respiratory diseases in which there is a decrease in expiratory flow rates are classified as obstructive lung diseases. In turn, obstructive lung diseases are subcategorized into reversible disorders and irreversible disorders. Examples of irreversible disorders include **emphysema** (em″fi-se′mah), chronic bronchitis, and cystic fibrosis. A reversible obstructive lung disorder is asthma.

Patients with obstructive lung disease normally have characteristics of more than one of these diseases. Because of this, clinicians may say that the patient has chronic obstructive pulmonary disease (COPD) instead of emphysema

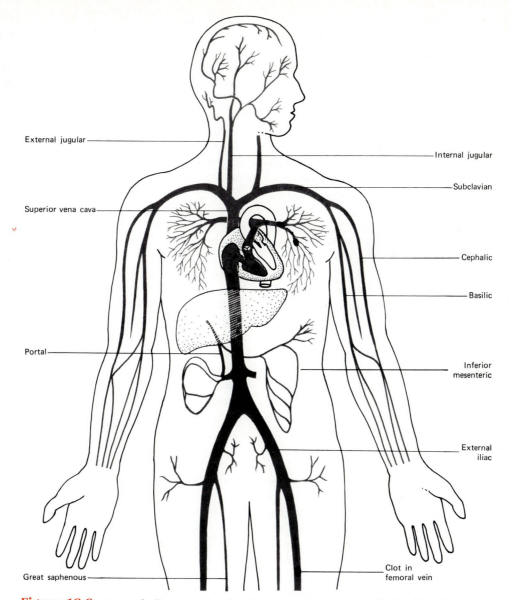

External jugular

Internal jugular

Subclavian

Superior vena cava

Cephalic

Basilic

Portal

Inferior mesenteric

External iliac

Great saphenous

Clot in femoral vein

Figure 16-6. *An embolism originating in any vein moves with the blood flow to larger and larger veins. The route will not obstruct the movement of the clot until the diameter of the vessel is smaller than the clot. This will occur in branches of the pulmonary artery and result in a pulmonary infarction unless the thrombus develops in veins draining the organs of digestion. In this instance, the movement of the clot will be obstructed in small branches of the portal vein.*

or chronic bronchitis. Synonyms include COLD (chronic obstructive lung disease) and CAO (chronic airway obstruction). For the purposes of this chapter, each disease will be discussed as if it were a pure disorder.

Chronic Bronchitis

Chronic bronchitis is defined in clinical terms. In chronic bronchitis, there is an increase in coughing and mucus production for at least three months per year for two consecutive years. The increased secretions are caused by an increase in both number and size of mucus-secreting glands in the airways. These airway changes are usually associated with heavy cigarette smoking.

A productive cough along with an acute lower respiratory tract infection is the most common cause for the patient to seek medical attention. The patient with chronic bronchitis frequently has a history of respiratory tract infections and often has a poor work record. Prolonged expiratory times and wheezing are frequent findings on physical examination. Patients who have pure chronic bronchitis tend to be overweight compared with patients who have pure emphysema.

A frequent complication of chronic bronchitis is **cor pulmonale** or right-sided heart enlargement. The cause of this heart enlargement is the respiratory acidosis and hypoxemia that are often seen with chronic bronchitis. An increased pCO_2 and a decreased pO_2 act upon the pulmonary circulatory system by causing vasoconstriction. This vasoconstriction increases resistance to blood flow through the lungs, and the right side of the heart enlarges in an attempt to maintain a normal output. If the right side of the heart is unable to maintain a normal flow to the lungs, fluid may accumulate in the lower extremities causing them to swell. This is another common reason for the patient to seek medical help.

Emphysema

Emphysema is defined in anatomic terms compared to the clinical definition of chronic bronchitis. Emphysema is a disease in which the airways distal to the terminal nonrespiratory bronchioles are enlarged in association with destruction of the alveolar walls. There is a relationship between cigarette smoking and emphysema. However, genetic factors also may be involved since not everyone who develops emphysema is a smoker.

On physical examination, there are differences between the patient with emphysema and one with chronic bronchitis. The patient with emphysema is older, is not usually as heavy, and has an increased anterior-posterior (A-P) diameter of the chest. Breath sounds heard with a stethoscope are diminished as well as cardiac sounds because with the increased A-P diameter there is more air between the chest wall and the heart. Normally, the patient does not produce much sputum unless chronic bronchitis is also present. In addition, since arterial blood gases are close to normal, the patient with emphysema is not as likely to develop cor pulmonale as is the patient with chronic bronchitis.

As the disease progresses, expiration becomes more prolonged. The patient often assumes a characteristic breathing position to minimize the work of breathing. The patient sits up, leaning forward for support with arms rigid, exhaling slowly through closely approximated lips. This "pursed-lip" breathing prevents the airways from collapsing and allows for more complete emptying of the lungs. With advanced disease, a deterioration in the arterial blood gases occurs. Carbon dioxide retention and hypoxemia indicate severe disease.

Bronchiectasis

In bronchiectasis, there is an irreversible dilation of the bronchial tree. There are two types of bronchiectasis: saccular and cylindrical. In saccular bronchiectasis, there are "sacs" in the bronchial walls. In cylindrical bronchiectasis, the bronchi fail to taper in diameter as they branch towards the periphery. Both forms develop as the result of repeated pulmonary infections that may be traced back to childhood.

Many patients have proven bronchiectasis as seen by CT scan but have no symptoms and may require no treatment. Other patients may produce a large amount of sputum that interferes with carbon dioxide and oxygen exchange. Postural drainage helps to remove the secretions by gravity (see Fig. 16-7). The exact position of the patient during this treatment depends on the segments of the lung that need to be drained. The general principle involves positioning the patient so the area to be drained is higher than the bronchi and other passageways through which the sputum must pass to be expectorated.

Bronchial Asthma

Asthma is defined in both clinical and physiological terms. Asthma is a disease characterized by an increased tracheal and bronchial responsiveness to various stimuli, resulting in wheezing, mucosal edema, and hypersecretion of mu-

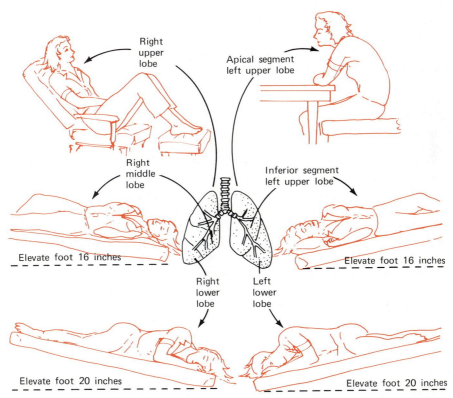

Figure 16-7. Elimination of secretions in the respiratory passageway is facilitated by positioning. The drawing shows the positions that favor the drainage of various parts of the lungs.

cus. It may reverse itself spontaneously or as a result of therapy.

There are two types of asthma: extrinsic or allergic asthma and intrinsic or nonallergic asthma. Extrinsic asthma usually begins in childhood and has specific allergenic stimuli, such as ragweed pollen or dust. Patients with intrinsic asthma are usually older, lack a family history of asthma, and do not have demonstrable allergenic stimuli. Provoking factors that may cause intrinsic asthma include infection, emotions, and exercise.

Clinical findings during an asthmatic attack include diaphoresis, wheezing, shortness of breath, and a cough that is initially unproductive of sputum but later produces large amounts of mucus. Other clinical symptoms include tachycardia, tachypnea, and use of the accessory muscles of ventilation. The absence of wheezing on chest auscultation is not necessarily good. If the chest is silent, it may mean the patient is deteriorating and no ventilation is taking place.

Most patients with chronic asthma respond to therapy rapidly. A patient who does not respond to conventional therapy within a few hours is said to be in **status asthmaticus**. Such a patient should be immediately admitted to the hospital and closely monitored for signs of respiratory failure because a high mortality rate is associated with this disorder. Endotracheal intubation and mechanical ventilation may become necessary to treat the severe hypoxemia and respiratory acidosis that may develop in this situation.

Pathologic findings include hypertrophy of bronchial smooth muscle and mucus glands. The volume of secretions may be so great that it may totally obstruct the airways. Interestingly, nasal polyps are also a frequent finding.

Treatment of asthma is symptomatic and preventative. Bronchodilators such as epinephrine and **aminophylline** not only relieve the bronchospasm but also reduce the mucosal edema. Drugs such as albuterol administered via a nebulizer and deposited directly into the lungs give rapid relief. These drugs may cause unpleasant side effects such as nausea, tachycardia, anxiety, and tremors.

Drug therapy may also include steroids, cromolyn sodium, and oxygen. Steroids reduce inflammation and cause bronchodilation but have numerous serious side effects. Cromolyn sodium prevents bronchospasm but is not a bronchodilator and should not be administered during an acute attack. Oxygen therapy may be indicated if hypoxemia is present. If oxygen is given, it is best to use an oxygen cannula rather than a face mask. A face mask may intensify the patient's anxiety by creating a suffocating feeling.

If the asthma is associated with allergy, it may be possible to desensitize the patient to the allergen. If this is not possible, measures must be taken to avoid exposure to dust, pollens, and animal danders.

Cystic Fibrosis

Cystic fibrosis is the most common cause of severe chronic respiratory disease in children and young adults. Approximately one in two thousand are born with this genetic disorder that affects other organs as well as the lungs. Pulmonary complications of cystic fibrosis include an increase in the quantity and viscosity of secretions, massive hemoptysis, cor pulmonale, and pneumothorax. Other problems associated with this usually fatal disease include pancreatic dysfunction, gastrointestinal blockage, malnutrition, abnormal sweat gland function, and sterility in males.

Diagnosis of cystic fibrosis is made by finding a highly increased chloride concentration in a sample of the patient's sweat. Parents may first become suspicious of this disease if they notice a salty taste when they kiss their children.

Treatment of cystic fibrosis is symptomatic and preventative. Chest physical therapy and vibration are useful when there is increased sputum production or viscosity. With the patient lying prone on his side, the practitioner cups his hands and claps rhythmically over the chest wall, dislodging secretions adhering to the airways. Following this action, the therapist places both hands on the chest and creates vibrations that further mobilize tenacious secretions. If the patient's cough reflex is absent or impaired, the dislodged mucus must be removed by suctioning so the airway will not be obstructed by the mucus.

Bronchodilators and antibiotics are indicated to treat the frequent respiratory tract infections and bronchospasms. Oxygen is also indicated if hypoxemia is present.

Treatment of Chronic Obstructive Pulmonary Diseases

Compare Figures 15-3 and 16-8. Figure 15-3 illustrates the normal exchange of gases between the alveoli and the bloodstream. Figure 16-8 shows some of the pathologic changes that occur in COPD. Although the pathologic changes that occur in COPD are for the most part irreversible, much can be done to slow the progressive deterioration of the respiratory system and to relieve the symptoms of these crippling diseases.

Treatment of obstructive lung disorders is symptomatic and includes techniques such as chest physical therapy and postural drainage to assist in the removal of secretions. Oxygen therapy is frequently necessary to treat hypoxemia, but care should be taken to limit the concentration and duration to the absolute minimum required. Oxygen should be treated like other drugs that have significant side effects.

Bronchodilators are administered to treat bronchospasm, relieve mucosal edema, and in-crease the strength of contraction of the diaphragm. Adequate hydration helps keep secretions thin so they can be more easily expectorated.

Only if more conservative therapy fails and arterial blood gases deteriorate should endotracheal intubation and mechanical ventilation be considered. There is no evidence that mechanical ventilation increases life expectancy in obstructive lung diseases.

ENVIRONMENTAL LUNG DISORDERS

Environmental lung diseases result from the inhalation of a variety of pathogenic gases or forms of particulate matter. Normally the lung's defense mechanisms either prevent these agents from entering the respiratory tract or rapidly remove them. However, some of these defense mechanisms act slowly. Thus, the inhaled agents may have time to exert their toxic effects.

Pneumoconiosis (nu″mo-ko-ne-o′sis) is a group of pulmonary problems resulting from the inhalation of dust particles. Asymptomatic retention of particulate matter is characteristic of all lungs. However, some particles, such as dust from silica (quartz) or asbestos, when inhaled over a long period of time can cause the lungs to become stiff and fibrotic.

Silicosis (sil-e-ko′sis) is a disease caused by the inhalation of silica dust over a prolonged period. Workers who operate sandblasting equipment and miners are at risk of developing this disorder.

Symptoms of silicosis include dyspnea and cough. Chest pain and hemoptysis also may be present if the patient has a secondary pulmonary infection. There is no effective treatment for silicosis. Therefore, efforts should be made to prevent its development by limiting exposure.

Asbestosis (as-bes-to′sis) results from the inhalation of asbestos fiber dust. Complications of asbestosis inhalation include lung cancer, pul-

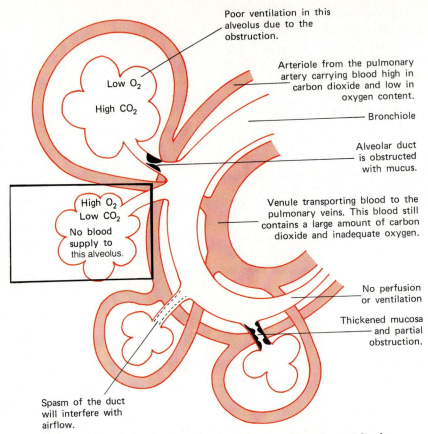

Figure 16-8. *Some pathologic changes that interfere with the exchange of gases between the alveoli and pulmonary capillaries in chronic obstructive pulmonary disease (From Burke, S. R., Composition and Function Of Body Fluids, 3rd ed. St. Louis: The C.V. Mosby Co., 1980)*

monary fibrosis, and mesothelioma. This form of usually fatal cancer develops almost exclusively in patients with a history of exposure to asbestos.

Many other inhaled dusts and noxious gases have been associated with the development of respiratory symptoms. Some of these agents include anthracite coal (coal worker's pneumoconiosis), inhalation of spores that grow in moldy hay or silage, and gases such as nitrogen dioxide and sulfur dioxide.

CANCER OF THE LUNG

Tumors in the lung usually produce no symptoms until the growth is fairly advanced. At this

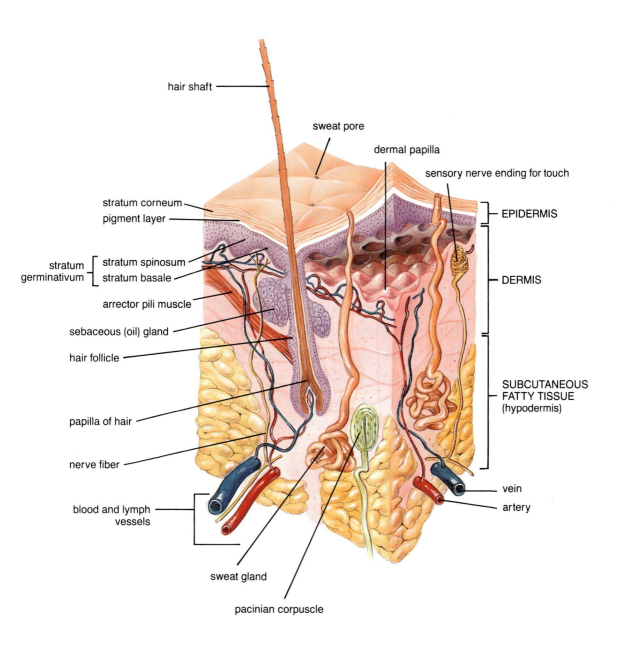

hair shaft

sweat pore

dermal papilla

sensory nerve ending for touch

stratum corneum

pigment layer

EPIDERMIS

stratum germinativum

stratum spinosum

stratum basale

DERMIS

arrector pili muscle

sebaceous (oil) gland

hair follicle

SUBCUTANEOUS FATTY TISSUE (hypodermis)

papilla of hair

nerve fiber

vein

artery

blood and lymph vessels

sweat gland

pacinian corpuscle

Plate 1 Cross Section of Skin

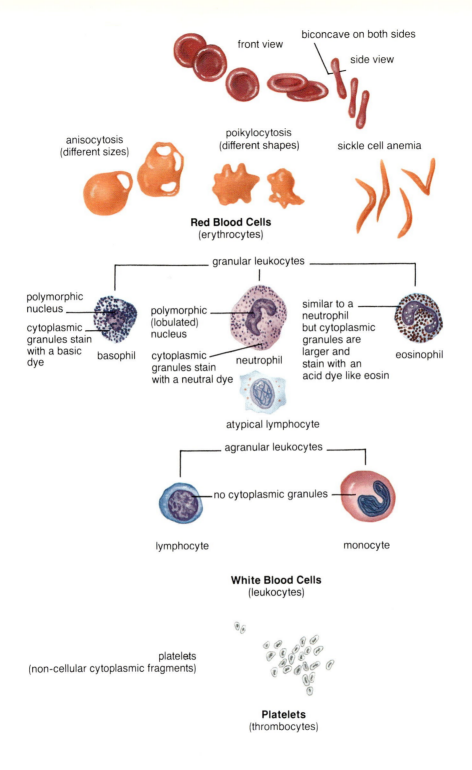

front view

biconcave on both sides

side view

anisocytosis
(different sizes)

poikylocytosis
(different shapes)

sickle cell anemia

Red Blood Cells
(erythrocytes)

granular leukocytes

polymorphic
nucleus

cytoplasmic
granules stain
with a basic
dye

basophil

polymorphic
(lobulated)
nucleus

cytoplasmic
granules stain
with a neutral dye

neutrophil

similar to a
neutrophil
but cytoplasmic
granules are
larger and
stain with an
acid dye like eosin

eosinophil

atypical lymphocyte

agranular leukocytes

no cytoplasmic granules

lymphocyte

monocyte

White Blood Cells
(leukocytes)

platelets
(non-cellular cytoplasmic fragments)

Platelets
(thrombocytes)

Plate 2 Blood Cells and Platelets

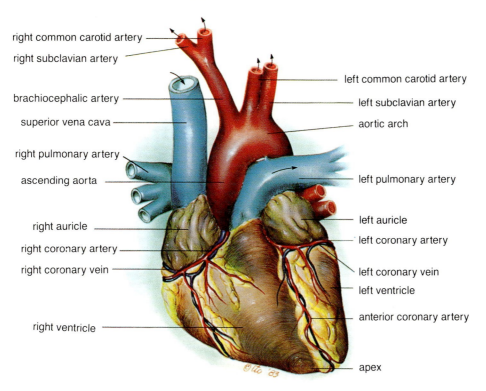

right common carotid artery
right subclavian artery
brachiocephalic artery
superior vena cava
right pulmonary artery
ascending aorta
right auricle
right coronary artery
right coronary vein
right ventricle

left common carotid artery
left subclavian artery
aortic arch
left pulmonary artery
left auricle
left coronary artery
left coronary vein
left ventricle
anterior coronary artery
apex

Otto '83

Plate 3 Front View of Heart

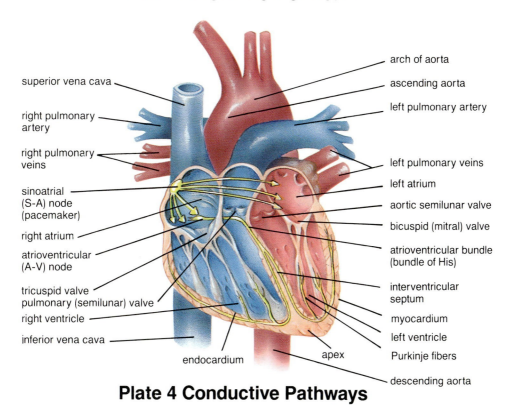

superior vena cava
right pulmonary artery
right pulmonary veins
sinoatrial (S-A) node (pacemaker)
right atrium
atrioventricular (A-V) node
tricuspid valve
pulmonary (semilunar) valve
right ventricle
inferior vena cava
endocardium

arch of aorta
ascending aorta
left pulmonary artery
left pulmonary veins
left atrium
aortic semilunar valve
bicuspid (mitral) valve
atrioventricular bundle (bundle of His)
interventricular septum
myocardium
left ventricle
Purkinje fibers
descending aorta
apex

Plate 4 Conductive Pathways

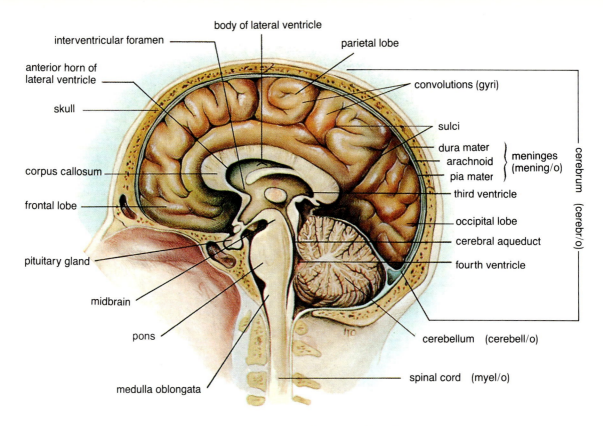

interventricular foramen

body of lateral ventricle

parietal lobe

anterior horn of
lateral ventricle

skull

corpus callosum

frontal lobe

pituitary gland

midbrain

pons

medulla oblongata

convolutions (gyri)

sulci

dura mater
arachnoid — } meninges (mening/o)
pia mater

third ventricle

occipital lobe

cerebral aqueduct

fourth ventricle

cerebrum (cerebr/o)

cerebellum (cerebell/o)

spinal cord (myel/o)

Plate 5A Section of Brain

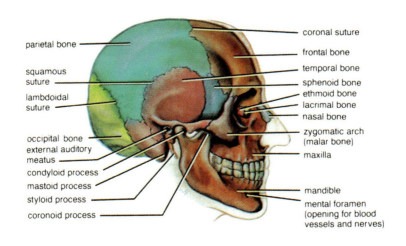

parietal bone

squamous
suture

lambdoidal
suture

occipital bone
external auditory
meatus
condyloid process
mastoid process
styloid process
coronoid process

coronal suture

frontal bone

temporal bone

sphenoid bone
ethmoid bone
lacrimal bone
nasal bone

zygomatic arch
(malar bone)

maxilla

mandible

mental foramen
(opening for blood
vessels and nerves)

Plate 5B Lateral View of Cranium

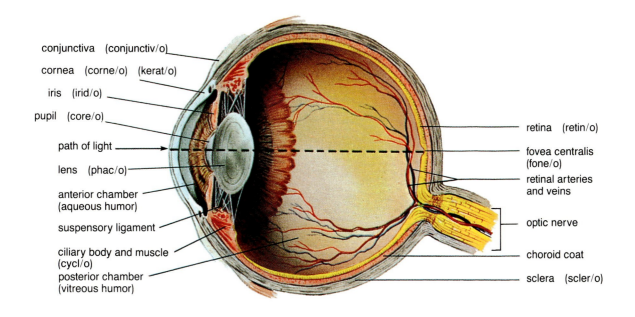

conjunctiva (conjunctiv/o)

cornea (corne/o) (kerat/o)

iris (irid/o)

pupil (core/o)

path of light

lens (phac/o)

anterior chamber
(aqueous humor)

suspensory ligament

ciliary body and muscle
(cycl/o)

posterior chamber
(vitreous humor)

retina (retin/o)

fovea centralis
(fone/o)

retinal arteries
and veins

optic nerve

choroid coat

sclera (scler/o)

Plate 6A Eye Structure

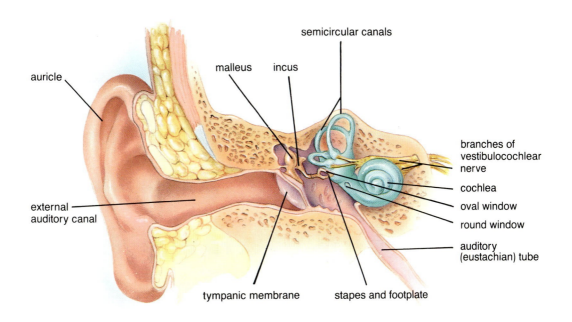

semicircular canals

auricle

malleus   incus

branches of
vestibulocochlear
nerve

cochlea

oval window

round window

external
auditory canal

auditory
(eustachian) tube

tympanic membrane   stapes and footplate

Plate 6B Ear Structure

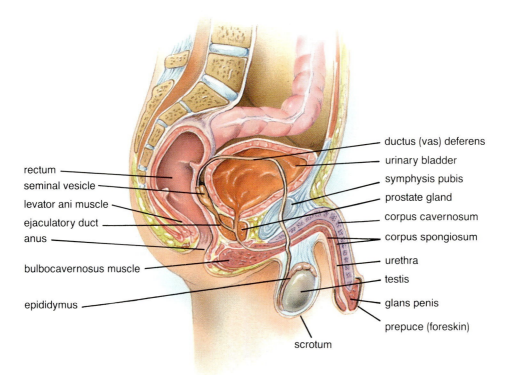

rectum

seminal vesicle

levator ani muscle

ejaculatory duct

anus

bulbocavernosus muscle

epididymus

ductus (vas) deferens

urinary bladder

symphysis pubis

prostate gland

corpus cavernosum

corpus spongiosum

urethra

testis

glans penis

prepuce (foreskin)

scrotum

Plate 7A Male Reproductive

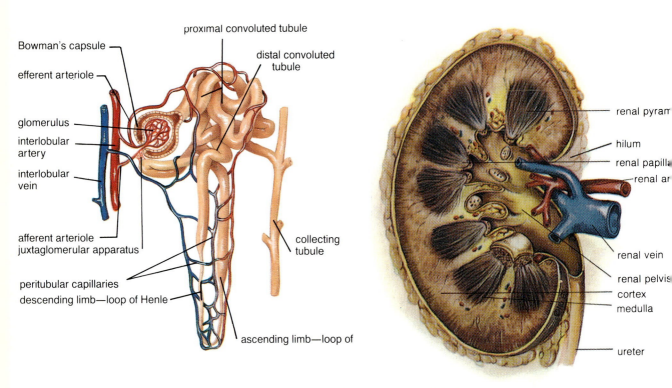

proximal convoluted tubule

Bowman's capsule

efferent arteriole

distal convoluted tubule

glomerulus

interlobular artery

interlobular vein

afferent arteriole
juxtaglomerular apparatus

peritubular capillaries

descending limb—loop of Henle

collecting tubule

ascending limb—loop of

renal pyram

hilum

renal papilla

renal ar

renal vein

renal pelvis

cortex

medulla

ureter

Plate 7B Nephron and Cross Section of Kidney

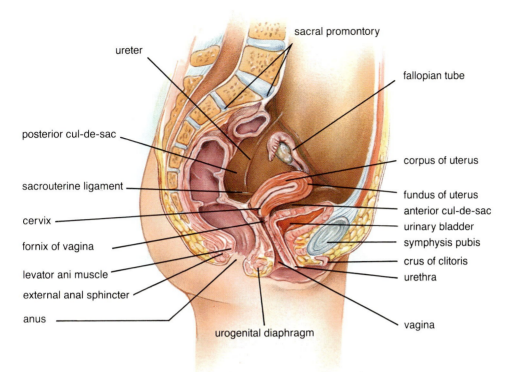

Plate 8A Female Reproductive

ureter
sacral promontory
fallopian tube
posterior cul-de-sac
corpus of uterus
sacrouterine ligament
fundus of uterus
anterior cul-de-sac
cervix
urinary bladder
fornix of vagina
symphysis pubis
levator ani muscle
crus of clitoris
external anal sphincter
urethra
anus
urogenital diaphragm
vagina

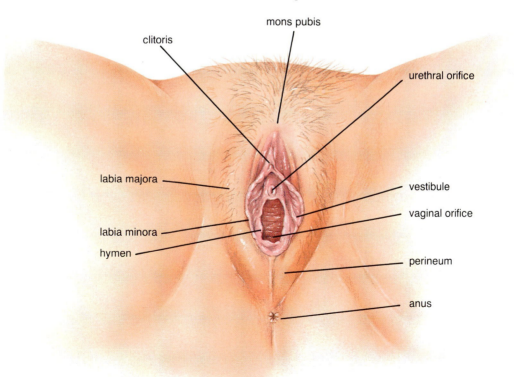

Plate 8B Female External Genitalia

clitoris
mons pubis
urethral orifice
labia majora
vestibule
vaginal orifice
labia minora
hymen
perineum
anus

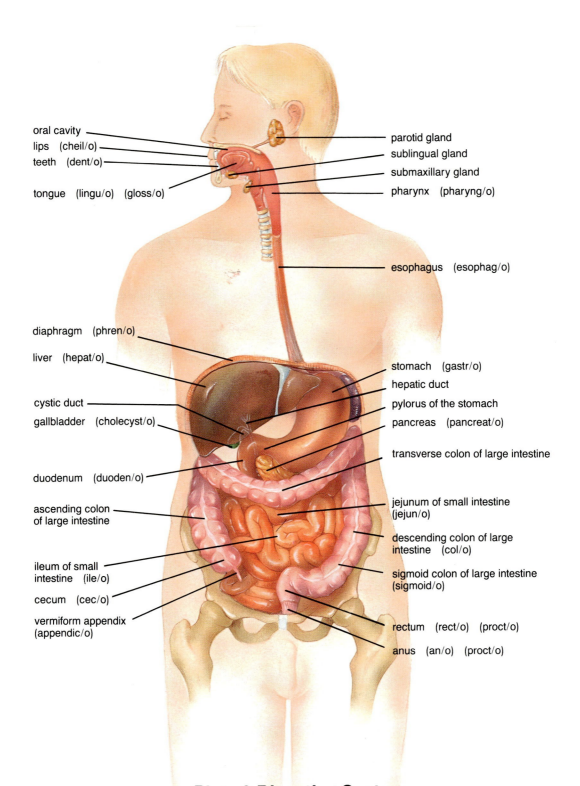

oral cavity

lips   (cheil/o)

teeth   (dent/o)

tongue   (lingu/o)   (gloss/o)

parotid gland

sublingual gland

submaxillary gland

pharynx   (pharyng/o)

esophagus   (esophag/o)

diaphragm   (phren/o)

liver   (hepat/o)

cystic duct

gallbladder   (cholecyst/o)

duodenum   (duoden/o)

ascending colon
of large intestine

ileum of small
intestine   (ile/o)

cecum   (cec/o)

vermiform appendix
(appendic/o)

stomach   (gastr/o)

hepatic duct

pylorus of the stomach

pancreas   (pancreat/o)

transverse colon of large intestine

jejunum of small intestine
(jejun/o)

descending colon of large
intestine   (col/o)

sigmoid colon of large intestine
(sigmoid/o)

rectum   (rect/o)   (proct/o)

anus   (an/o)   (proct/o)

Plate 9 Digestive System

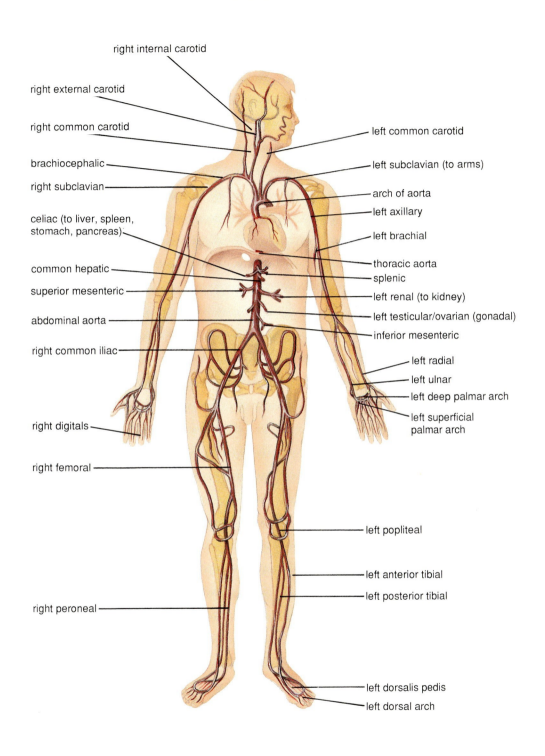

right internal carotid

right external carotid

right common carotid

brachiocephalic

right subclavian

celiac (to liver, spleen, stomach, pancreas)

common hepatic

superior mesenteric

abdominal aorta

right common iliac

right digitals

right femoral

right peroneal

left common carotid

left subclavian (to arms)

arch of aorta

left axillary

left brachial

thoracic aorta

splenic

left renal (to kidney)

left testicular/ovarian (gonadal)

inferior mesenteric

left radial

left ulnar

left deep palmar arch

left superficial palmar arch

left popliteal

left anterior tibial

left posterior tibial

left dorsalis pedis

left dorsal arch

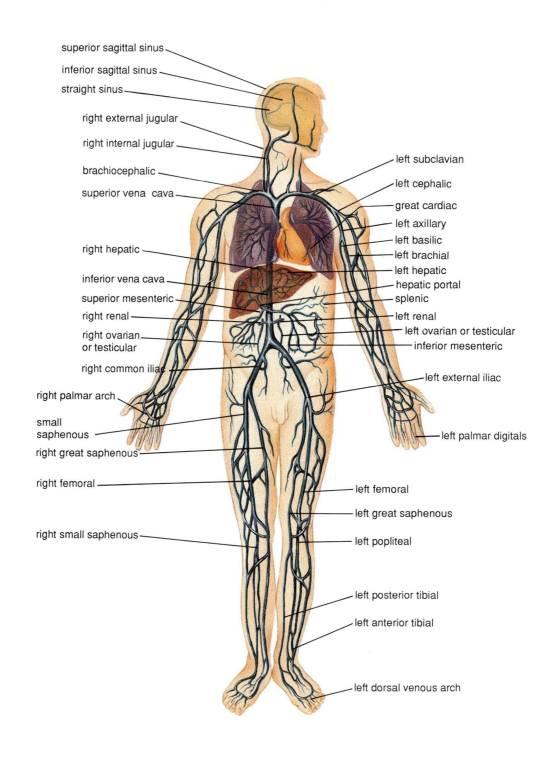

superior sagittal sinus

inferior sagittal sinus

straight sinus

right external jugular

right internal jugular

brachiocephalic

superior vena cava

right hepatic

inferior vena cava

superior mesenteric

right renal

right ovarian or testicular

right common iliac

right palmar arch

small saphenous

right great saphenous

right femoral

right small saphenous

left subclavian

left cephalic

great cardiac

left axillary

left basilic

left brachial

left hepatic

hepatic portal

splenic

left renal

left ovarian or testicular

inferior mesenteric

left external iliac

left palmar digitals

left femoral

left great saphenous

left popliteal

left posterior tibial

left anterior tibial

left dorsal venous arch

Plate 10B Venous Distribution

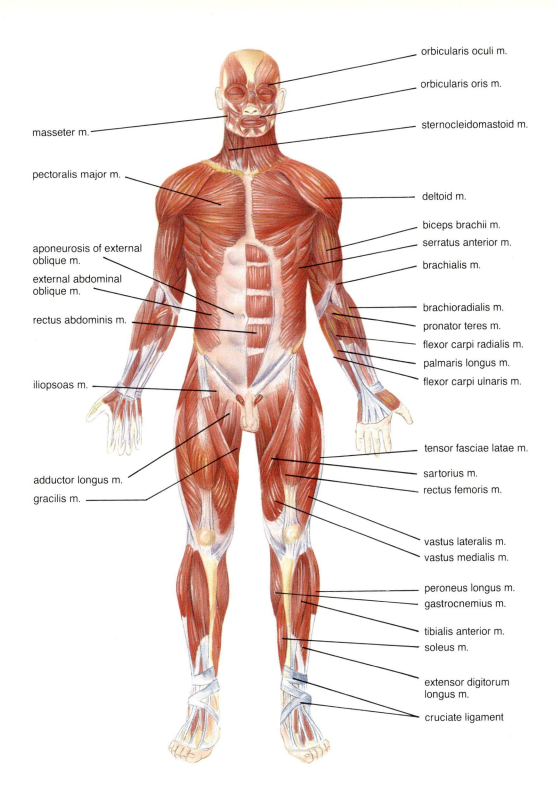

orbicularis oculi m.

orbicularis oris m.

sternocleidomastoid m.

masseter m.

pectoralis major m.

deltoid m.

biceps brachii m.

serratus anterior m.

brachialis m.

aponeurosis of external oblique m.

external abdominal oblique m.

rectus abdominis m.

brachioradialis m.

pronator teres m.

flexor carpi radialis m.

palmaris longus m.

flexor carpi ulnaris m.

iliopsoas m.

tensor fasciae latae m.

sartorius m.

rectus femoris m.

adductor longus m.

gracilis m.

vastus lateralis m.

vastus medialis m.

peroneus longus m.

gastrocnemius m.

tibialis anterior m.

soleus m.

extensor digitorum longus m.

cruciate ligament

Plate 11A Muscular System, Anterior

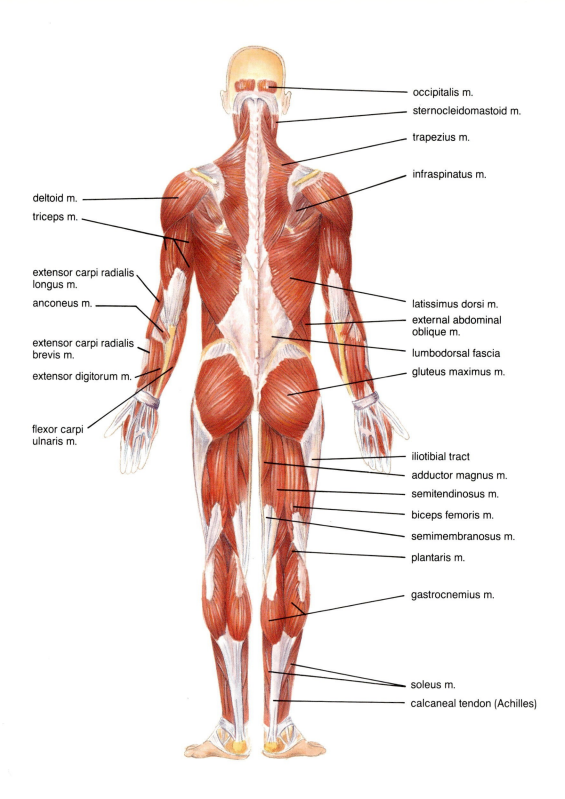

occipitalis m.

sternocleidomastoid m.

trapezius m.

infraspinatus m.

deltoid m.

triceps m.

extensor carpi radialis
longus m.

anconeus m.

extensor carpi radialis
brevis m.

extensor digitorum m.

flexor carpi
ulnaris m.

latissimus dorsi m.

external abdominal
oblique m.

lumbodorsal fascia

gluteus maximus m.

iliotibial tract

adductor magnus m.

semitendinosus m.

biceps femoris m.

semimembranosus m.

plantaris m.

gastrocnemius m.

soleus m.

calcaneal tendon (Achilles)

Plate 11B Muscular System, Posterior

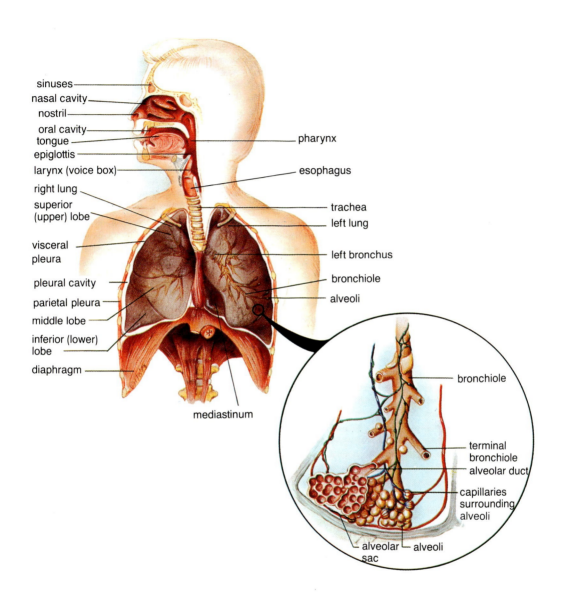

sinuses

nasal cavity

nostril

oral cavity

tongue

epiglottis

larynx (voice box)

right lung

superior
(upper) lobe

visceral
pleura

pleural cavity

parietal pleura

middle lobe

inferior (lower)
lobe

diaphragm

pharynx

esophagus

trachea

left lung

left bronchus

bronchiole

alveoli

mediastinum

bronchiole

terminal
bronchiole

alveolar duct

capillaries
surrounding
alveoli

alveolar
sac

alveoli

Plate 12 Respiratory System

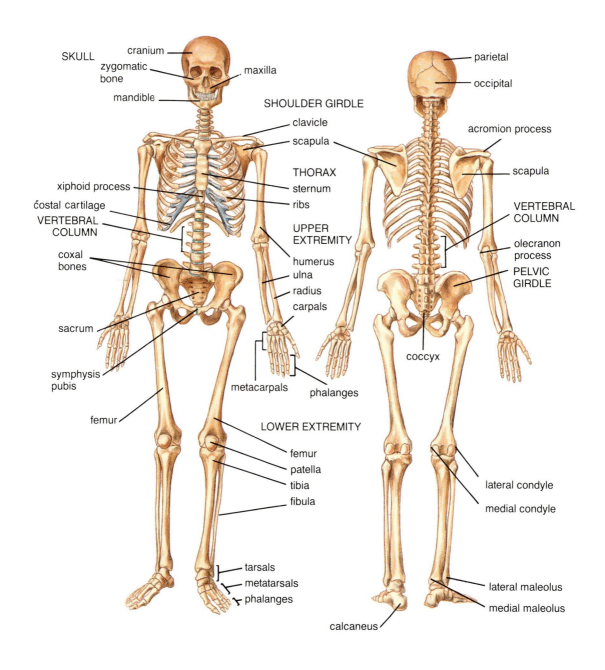

SKULL

cranium
zygomatic bone
maxilla
mandible

parietal
occipital

SHOULDER GIRDLE
clavicle
scapula

acromion process
scapula

THORAX
sternum
ribs

xiphoid process
costal cartilage
VERTEBRAL COLUMN

VERTEBRAL COLUMN
olecranon process

UPPER EXTREMITY
humerus
ulna
radius
carpals

coxal bones

sacrum

PELVIC GIRDLE

coccyx

symphysis pubis

metacarpals
phalanges

femur

LOWER EXTREMITY
femur
patella
tibia
fibula

lateral condyle
medial condyle

tarsals
metatarsals
phalanges

lateral maleolus
medial maleolus

calcaneus

Plate 13 Skeletal System

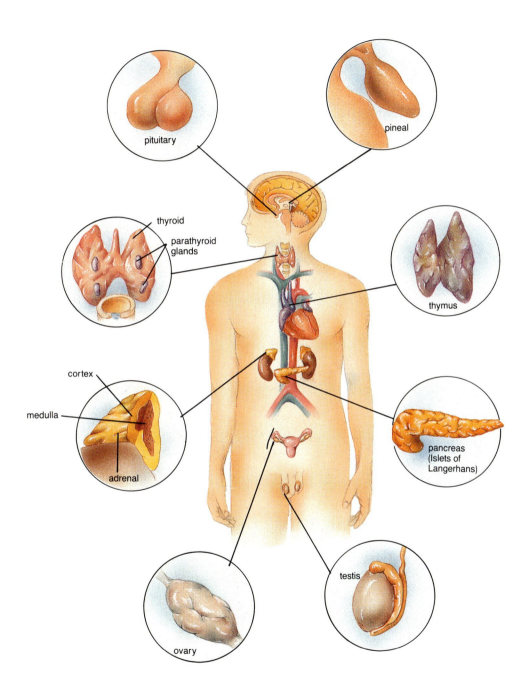

Plate 14 Endocrine System

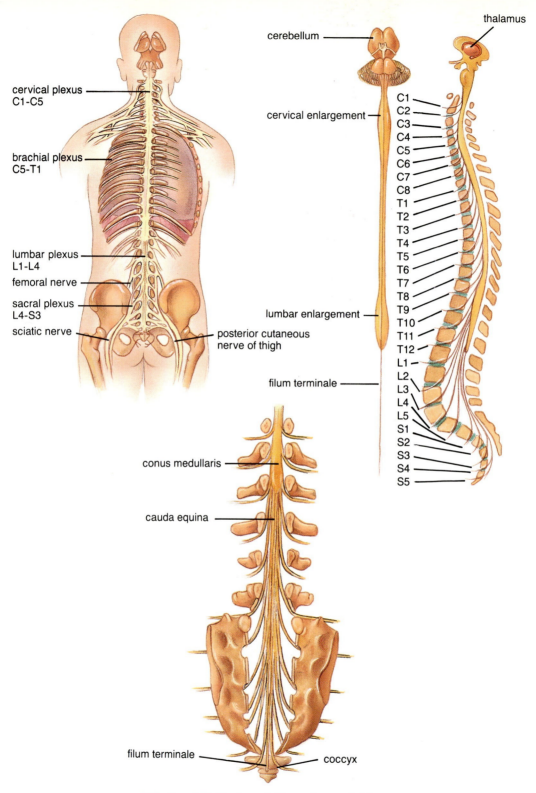

cerebellum

thalamus

cervical plexus
C1-C5

cervical enlargement

brachial plexus
C5-T1

C1
C2
C3
C4
C5
C6
C7
C8
T1
T2
T3
T4
T5
T6
T7
T8
T9
T10
T11
T12
L1
L2
L3
L4
L5
S1
S2
S3
S4
S5

lumbar plexus
L1-L4

femoral nerve

lumbar enlargement

sacral plexus
L4-S3

sciatic nerve

posterior cutaneous
nerve of thigh

filum terminale

conus medullaris

cauda equina

filum terminale

coccyx

Plate 15 Spinal Cord and Nerves

point, the patient may have a cough producing mucopurulent or blood-streaked sputum. The patient will have fatigue, anorexia, and weight loss. Dyspnea, chest pain, and hemoptysis are late symptoms of lung cancer.

Risk factors for development of lung cancer are many and varied. Asbestos, vinyl chloride, paints, and synthetic rubber have been implicated in the development of lung cancer. Cigarette smoking has been shown to be the most common risk factor. Heavy smokers have a risk 20 times as great as nonsmokers.

There are many different types of lung cancer, and they are categorized according to cell type. Each type has its own optimum treatment regimen that may include any combination of chemotherapy, radiation therapy, and surgical intervention. Prognosis for most forms of lung cancer remains grim.

INFANT RESPIRATORY DISTRESS SYNDROME (IRDS)

Also known as hyaline membrane disease, IRDS is the leading cause of death in the neonate. At high risk are premature infants, infants delivered by cesarean section, and the baby born to a mother with diabetes. IRDS is seldom seen in the infant born at term.

The cause of IRDS is immaturity of the lungs and a corresponding deficiency of surfactant (ser-fak'tant). Surfactant is a phospholipid produced by cells in the alveoli that prevents the alveoli from collapsing on expiration. If surfactant is deficient, the alveoli collapse and require tremendous effort by the neonate for reinflation. Diffuse atelectasis, pulmonary edema, and hya-

line membrane formation cause severe hypoxemia, carbon dioxide retention, and acidosis. Other complications of this disorder include pneumothorax, oxygen toxicity, and intracranial hemorrhage.

Clinically, the baby has tachypnea (rapid respirations), cyanosis, intercostal retractions, and commonly demonstrates expiratory "grunting." This "grunting" is an attempt by the neonate to keep the alveoli from collapsing on expiration.

Treatment of IRDS includes oxygen therapy to treat the hypoxemia and, frequently, the use of continuous positive airway pressure (CPAP). CPAP is the application of a positive pressure to the alveoli in an attempt to prevent their collapse on expiration. Endotracheal intubation and mechanical ventilation may also become necessary if respiratory failure develops. The administration of artificial surfactant offers considerable hope for treatment of this syndrome.

ADULT RESPIRATORY DISTRESS SYNDROME (ARDS)

The adult respiratory distress syndrome (ARDS) is a form of acute respiratory failure with numerous causes. These numerous etiologies are indicated in the different synonyms for ARDS including "shock lung," "posttraumatic pulmonary insufficiency," "noncardiogenic pulmonary edema," and "Da Nang Lung." The name "Da Nang Lung" was originated during the Vietnam conflict when wounded soldiers developed severe pulmonary complications.

There is a common pattern of clinical and pathophysiologic abnormalities in each of these forms of respiratory failure. This common pattern in each disorder led to the current usage of the term ARDS.

Clinical manifestations of ARDS begin with a period of relatively normal pulmonary function. Within 24 hours, the patient develops progressive dyspnea, tachypnea, and "grunting" respirations. As the syndrome progresses, cyanosis and intercostal retractions develop.

The primary pathophysiologic disorder is a leaky alveolar-capillary membrane. Fluid from the pulmonary blood vessels enters the alveoli and interferes with oxygenation. Surfactant is inactivated, causing the alveoli to collapse, contributing to the oxygenation difficulties. In spite of the administration of increasing concentrations of oxygen, the arterial pO_2 remains low. In the early stages of the syndrome, the arterial pCO_2 is low, but as it progresses, carbon dioxide retention occurs. At autopsy, the lungs are very "wet," heavy, and often are described as being "liverlike" in appearance.

Treatment involves ensuring adequate delivery of oxygen to the tissues and avoidance of complications. Since high concentrations of oxygen are not effective, positive end expiratory pressure (PEEP) or CPAP is usually indicated. Endotracheal intubation and mechanical ventilation may be necessary. Complications of ARDS are numerous and include pneumothorax, oxygen toxicity, sepsis, and multiple organ failure.

Despite therapy, approximately 50% of patients with ARDS will not survive. Of those who do survive, very few have long-term complications.

CHEST TRAUMA

Blunt chest trauma, such as occurs in an automobile accident, normally causes minimal pulmonary complications other than pain and tenderness in the affected area. Occasionally, the lungs themselves are "bruised" by the accident, and respiratory failure with carbon dioxide and hypoxemia may result.

Broken ribs are a frequent complication of blunt chest trauma. Single broken ribs are not usually a problem, but multiple adjacent broken ribs may create a condition known as a "flail chest." Steering wheel injuries and cardiopul-

monary resuscitation (CPR) are frequent causes of flail chest. With a flail chest, the flail segment of the chest wall moves paradoxically to the rest of the chest wall. During inspiration, the flail segment moves inward. During expiration, it bulges outward. The associated pain, ineffective cough, accumulation of secretions, and underlying lung damage lead to hypoxemia and carbon dioxide retention. Treatment of flail chest includes analgesics, oxygen for the treatment of hypoxemia, and deep breathing exercises to prevent "pooling" of secretions. CPAP or mechanical ventilation with PEEP may become necessary if respiratory failure should occur.

PNEUMOTHORAX

A pneumothorax is an abnormal accumulation of air in the pleural space separating the visceral and parietal pleura. There are two major categories of pneumothorax, spontaneous and traumatic. A spontaneous pneumothorax that occurs in healthy individuals is termed an idiopathic spontaneous pneumothorax. This occurs most commonly in tall, thin, young males with long, narrow chests. Most of these patients have blebs (blisters) on the lungs that rupture, causing the pneumothorax. Spontaneous pneumothorax is also frequently associated with COPD.

A traumatic pneumothorax is the result of chest injury, such as a stab wound or broken ribs. With a stab wound, there is free communication between the pleural space and the atmosphere. Since the intrapleural pressure is normally subatmospheric, air rushes into the pleural space. In an open pneumothorax, the air moves back and forth between the pleural space and the atmosphere.

A tension pneumothorax is a life-threatening situation in which air can enter the pleural space but cannot escape. As air accumulates, pressure in the pleural space increases, causing the lungs to collapse and the mediastinum to shift toward the unaffected side of the chest. This mediastinal shift can impede the return of blood to the right side of the heart and cause a decrease in blood pressure and cardiac output. Tension pneumothorax requires immediate insertion of a chest tube to remove the air if circulatory collapse is to be avoided.

SUMMARY QUESTIONS

1. Differentiate between a standard chest roentgenogram and computerized tomography.
2. For what purpose might sputum specimens be required?
3. How is a patient prepared for a bronchoscopy?
4. Why is pulmonary function testing done?
5. What are the symptoms of chronic tonsillitis?
6. Describe the treatment of epiglottitis.
7. Describe the treatment of tuberculosis.
8. Differentiate between chronic bronchitis and emphysema.
9. How is chronic obstructive lung disease treated?
10. Contrast the two primary types of asthma.
11. What newborns are at high risk for IRDS and how is it treated?
12. Trace a blood clot originating in the saphenous vein until it obstructs blood flow. Do the same for a clot starting in the brachial vein, the jugular vein, and the superior mesenteric vein.
13. Describe a tension pneumothorax and its treatment.
14. Describe the pathophysiology of ARDS.
15. Describe the treatment for cancer of the larynx.
16. Discuss the environmental lung disorders.

KEY TERMS

aminophylline
bronchopneumonia
bronchoscopy
cor pulmonale
emphysema
epistaxis
hemoptysis

lobar
pneumoconiosis
silicosis
spirometry
status asthmaticus
thoracentesis
tracheostomy

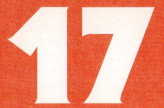

The Gastrointestinal System

OBJECTIVES

On completion of this chapter, you will be able to:

1. Define nitrogen balance.
2. Explain the roles of vitamins and minerals in the diet.
3. Describe the processes involved in mechanical digestion.
4. Explain the chemical digestion of each of the macronutrients.
5. Beginning with the mouth, list in sequence the structures of the alimentary canal.
6. Describe the structure of each of the organs of the alimentary canal.
7. Discuss the roles of the local hormones produced by the alimentary canal.
8. Explain the function of gastric hydrochloric acid.
9. Explain how the liver regulates the blood sugar level.
10. Describe at least five other functions of the liver.
11. Explain the function of pancreatic sodium bicarbonate.
12. Discuss the endocrine functions of the pancreas.
13. Explain the major factors involved in the process of absorption of foodstuffs.

OVERVIEW

I. FOODSTUFFS
   A. Carbohydrates
   B. Lipids
   C. Proteins
   D. Vitamins
   E. Minerals
II. DIGESTIVE PROCESSES
III. ALIMENTARY CANAL AND ACCESSORY
    ORGANS
   A. Mouth
   B. Pharynx and Esophagus
   C. Stomach
   D. Small Intestine and Accessory Organs
   E. Large Intestine
IV. METABOLISM
   A. Carbohydrate Metabolism
   B. Fat Metabolism
   C. Protein Metabolism

The general function of the digestive system is to break down and absorb foods and eliminate some of the waste products produced in the process of metabolism. Foods are any substances taken into the body for the purpose of yielding energy, building tissues, or regulating body processes. These substances must be rendered into simple diffusible forms that can be absorbed into the bloodstream or lymphatics and ultimately used by the body cells. About two-thirds of all the foods we consume is water, which is vital for all cellular activity.

FOODSTUFFS

Macronutrients are foods that can build body tissues and produce energy. These are carbohydrates, lipids, and proteins.

CARBOHYDRATES

Carbohydrates are the most abundant and economical foods. They are not only economical from the point of view of the price we pay for them but also from the point of view of the ease with which the body can utilize them and the energy they produce. Carbohydrates produce four calories per gram.

Carbohydrates are organic compounds containing carbon, hydrogen, and oxygen. They are widely distributed in such easily grown plants as grains, vegetables, and fruits. Compared with other types of food, carbohydrate foods can be kept in dry storage for relatively long periods of time without spoilage. Classified according to how chemically complex they are, there are three groups of carbohydrates.

Monosaccharides (mon-o-sak′ah-rides) are the simplest form of carbohydrate. These simple sugars are glucose (gloo′kos), fructose (fruk′tos), and galactose (gah-lak′tos); all are soluble in water. Glucose is the form in which sugar circulates in the bloodstream and it is oxidized to give energy. Fructose and galactose must be converted to glucose in order to be utilized by the body cells.

Disaccharides (di-sak′ah-rides) are also water soluble. These double sugars include sucrose (soo′kros), or cane sugar, lactose (lak′tos), or milk sugar, and maltose (mal′tose).

Polysaccharides (pol-e-sak′ah-rides) are complex molecules, such as plant starches, glycogen, and cellulose, that are not soluble in water. Cellulose is resistant to the digestive enzymes in man. It remains in the digestive tract and contributes important bulk to the diet. This bulk stimulates peristalsis and helps to move the food through the digestive tract.

LIPIDS

Lipids (lip′ids) are fats and fat-related substances not soluble in water. They are a concentrated form of fuel yielding nine calories per gram. However, they are not as easily utilized by the body as carbohydrates. They also are organic compounds containing carbon, hydrogen, and oxygen; however, they contain much more hydrogen than do carbohydrates. Whether a fat is saturated or unsaturated is determined by the amount of hydrogen the compound contains. The fewer hydrogens, the less saturated the fat is and the more liquid it is. Saturated fats are animal fats, and the unsaturated fats are of plant origin and usually are free-flowing oils that do not solidify even at low temperatures.

Emulsified fats are fats that are broken into fine particles and kept separated so they have a large surface area. In order for the body to chemically digest fats, they must first be emulsified by bile. Egg yolk is a naturally emulsified fat, and homogenized milk is mechanically emulsified.

The absorbable forms of fat are fatty acids and glycerols. In addition to producing energy, fat provides general padding and insulates the body against rapid temperature changes. Other important functions are those associated with fat-related compounds. Several important hormones are steroids that are lipids. Brain and nerve tissue are rich in phospholipids.

PROTEINS

The basic unit of protein is an **amino** (a″me′no) **acid**. Proteins yield four calories per gram. Like carbohydrates and fats, proteins contain carbon, hydrogen, and oxygen, but they also contain nitrogen and often other elements such as sulfur and phosphorus. Entirely free protein, such as albumin in egg white, is rare. Usually protein foods are found in combination with fats or carbohydrates. Animal protein is usually associated with fat, and plant protein is usually associated with carbohydrates. Important roles of proteins are to build and repair tissues; however, they

are frequently classified according to their other functions in the body:

1. Structural proteins—collagens
2. Contractile proteins—muscle
3. Blood proteins—albumin, fibrinogen, and hemoglobin
4. Antibodies—gammaglobulin
5. Enzymes
6. Hormones
7. Nutrient proteins—food sources of essential amino acids

If the diet is deficient in certain amino acids, the body may be able to synthesize that amino acid from others that are available in the diet. These amino acids are labeled as nonessential. If the body cannot synthesize the particular amino acid it is classified as essential. There are eight essential amino acids and twelve nonessential amino acids.

Enzymes are organic catalysts that control the rates of chemical reactions in the body. The action of most enzymes is fairly specific; they can usually only work on one substrate and cause one type of chemical activity. In addition to acting as catalysts for chemical reactions, enzymes also provide a surface on which the reaction takes place. An active site is the site where the enzyme forms a loose association with its substrate. The enzyme and substrate form a complex, the substrate undergoes a chemical change, and the product or products of the reaction are formed (see Fig. 17-1). If some other molecule has a structure similar to the substrate, it can occupy the active site, competing with the substrate and, thereby, preventing the reaction from taking place. This process is called competitive inhibition. This phenomenon is often used in pharmacology. Some antibiotics function by competitively inhibiting one of the bacterial enzymes, and certain chemotherapeu-

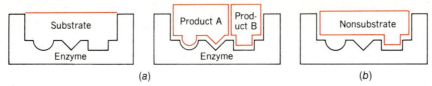

Figure 17-1. *(a) An enzyme can make two new products from its substrate; for example, the enzyme lipase can cause some lipids to become fatty acid and glycerol. (b) Competitive inhibition. Some other molecule looks enough like the true substrate to occupy the active site and prevent the enzyme from accomplishing the reaction.*

tic agents used to treat cancer inhibit enzymes in rapidly dividing cells.

Unlike carbohydrates and fats, proteins are not stored in significant amounts in our bodies. Nitrogen balance refers to the balance between intake and output of nitrogen. Although there are nonprotein sources of nitrogen, we commonly consider the nitrogen balance as an indicator of the protein homeostasis. Healthy adults are in nitrogen equilibrium. Growing children have a positive nitrogen balance; their intake of nitrogen exceeds their output. Someone with a wasting illness will have a negative nitrogen balance; their output exceeds their intake of nitrogen.

VITAMINS

Vitamins and minerals do not have caloric values, but they are important in regulating body metabolism. They both can function as coenzymes or enzyme activators.

Vitamins are organic compounds synthesized by plants and animals. Some vitamins are fat soluble and some are water soluble. Vitamins A, D, E, and K are fat soluble, whereas B and C are water soluble.

Proper fat metabolism is essential in the utilization of the fat-soluble vitamins. Vitamin A is found in milk, butter, egg yolk, liver, and most yellow fruits and vegetables. It prevents night blindness and helps restore epithelium, thereby increasing our resistance to infection. Vitamin D is the antirachitic (an"te-rah-kit'ik) vitamin, promoting the absorption of calcium from the gastrointestinal tract and thus preventing rickets. The best sources of vitamin D are fish liver oil, egg yolk, butter, and fortified milk. Although sunlight causes the synthesis of some vitamin D by the skin, overexposure to sunlight is not without its hazards. Prolonged overexposure to sunlight not only causes early aging but also predisposes one to skin cancer. Vitamin K, found in green leafy vegetables, is also synthesized by intestinal bacteria. It is needed for normal blood clotting and proper functioning of the cellular mitochondria. Circumstances that might lead to a deficiency of vitamin K are the absence of bile, the suppression of bacterial flora with antibiotics, and ulcerative colitis with poor absorption of the vitamin. The newborn is vitamin K deficient because there are no bacteria in the infant's intestines. Vitamin E is an antioxidant that helps prevent oxygen damage to fat-containing membranes, such as the myelin covering some nerves. It also favors the union of oxygen and hemoglobin and therefore may be helpful in the treatment of some types of anemia. Sources of vitamin E are wheat, corn, and leafy vegetables.

Vitamins B and C are water soluble. Vitamin C, or ascorbic acid, is important in protein and iron metabolism. It helps in the formation and maintenance of supporting tissues (bone, cartilage, and the intercellular substances of capillaries). A deficiency of vitamin C will cause scurvy, which is characterized by bleeding tendencies and poor wound healing. Sources of vitamin C are chiefly citrus fruits and tomatoes. If you do not eat breakfast (since tomato and citrus juices are usually breakfast drinks), you are probably vitamin C deficient. The degree of the deficiency may not be sufficient to cause scurvy, but it may be sufficient to reduce your ability to utilize dietary iron. Many iron deficiency anemias may not be related to insufficient iron intake, but instead to the inability to utilize the iron.

There are about a dozen members of the vitamin B complex, all of which are fairly stable when cooked. They are found in grain cereals, pork, milk, eggs, fruit, and vegetables. Deficiencies are characterized by weight loss, weakness, sores on the lips, and (in the case of a deficiency of vitamin B_1) neuritis (nu-ri′tis) or inflammation of nerve tissue.

MINERALS

Minerals are important nutrients that function as builders, activators, regulators, transmitters, and controllers. The minerals found in the body can be grouped according to whether they are present in large amounts (major minerals) or in small amounts (trace minerals). The quantity of the particular mineral, however, does not necessarily reflect its importance. For example, iron is a trace mineral but, as we know, it is essential for the transport of oxygen in the bloodstream. The functions of some of the trace minerals, however, are not as yet understood.

Major minerals include calcium, magnesium, sodium, potassium, phosphorus, sulfur, and chlorine. The trace minerals that have known functions are iron, copper, iodine, manganese, cobalt, zinc, and molybdenum. Vital functions of the minerals include:

1. Maintaining acid-base balance, which is essential to the activity of the cellular enzymes
2. Acting as catalysts for many biological reactions
3. Acting as components of essential body compounds, such as hormones, enzymes, and other compounds synthesized in the body
4. Maintaining and regulating water balance
5. Regulating excitability of nerve and muscle tissue
6. Acting in growth and repair.

DIGESTIVE PROCESSES

The digestive processes are both mechanical and chemical. In mechanical digestion, the food is chopped and ground into smaller and smaller particles, liquified, and moved along at the proper speed to allow time for whatever chemical processes take place in each area of the digestive tract. In chemical digestion, enzymes assist in breaking the foodstuffs down into their simplest diffusible forms. With enzyme action, carbohydrates are rendered into glucose, galactose, and fructose, proteins are broken down to amino acids, and lipids to fatty acids and glycerol. These simple substances can then be absorbed. Absorption depends on the size of the surface area, the length of time the foodstuffs are exposed to the surface area, and the rich capillary network of the mucosa of the small intestines.

The alimentary (al-e-men′ta-re) canal, which is about 30 feet long, and accessory organs such as the teeth, salivary glands, pancreas, and liver function to accomplish both the chemical and mechanical digestive processes (see Fig. 17-2).

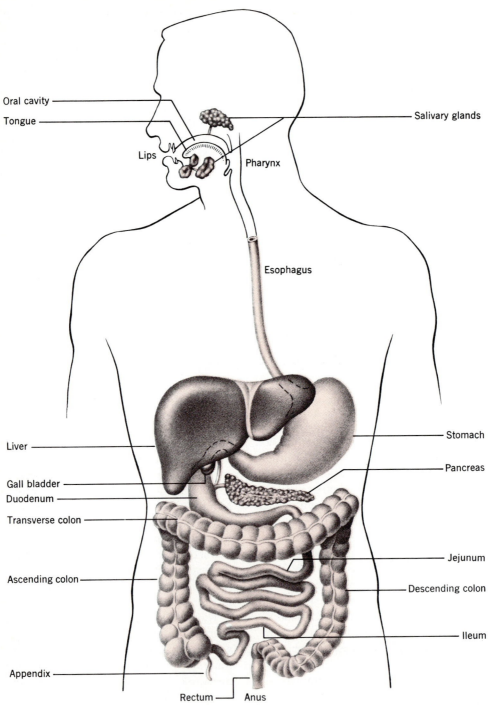

Figure 17-2. *Organs of the digestive system. The small intestine, consisting of the duodenum, jejunum, and ileum, is actually much longer than pictured here.*

The canal has four layers: a mucous membrane lining; a submucous coat that is very vascular; a smooth muscle layer that has both circular and longitudinal muscle layers; and, in the case of the stomach, an additional oblique layer of smooth muscle fibers. The outer coat of the alimentary tract above the diaphragm is fibrous tissue; below the diaphragm, is serous membrane, the **peritoneum** (per"i-to-ne'um).

You should be familiar with some special parts of the peritoneum. The greater omentum (o-men'tum) is attached to the greater curvature of the stomach and hangs like an apron over the intestines. Varying amounts of fats are deposited in the greater omentum. It provides protection and insulation to the structures that it covers. The lesser omentum extends from the lesser curvature of the stomach to the liver. The mesentery is a fan-shaped membrane that attaches the loops of small intestine together and to the posterior abdominal wall. There is also a peritoneal cavity, which actually is only a potential cavity, because normally the two layers of the peritoneum (the visceral and the parietal) are separated by only a small amount of lubricating serous fluid. The functions of the peritoneum are to prevent friction between the organs, to hold the organs in place, and, in the case of the greater omentum, to store fat and help insulate the organs.

ALIMENTARY CANAL AND ACCESSORY ORGANS

MOUTH

Digestive processes of the mouth are mostly concerned with grinding the food into smaller pieces and lubricating it so it will have a smooth passage into the esophagus and stomach. The salivary (sal'i-va-re) glands of the mouth pour salivary juices into the mouth for lubrication of the food. These juices contain salivary amylase, which is capable of breaking down polysaccharides to disaccharides. However, we usually do not keep the food in our mouths long enough for this to happen.

The **parotid** (pah-rot'id) **gland** is located anterior and inferior to the ear. Its duct opens into the upper jaw where the dentist puts the cotton roll to absorb the saliva from this gland. There are also submandibular salivary glands located near the inner surface of the mandible, and sublingual salivary glands, located beneath the tongue. All of these glands secrete saliva.

The tongue contains taste buds (see Fig. 11-1). These taste buds are located on the sides of the small papillae of the tongue. For this reason, a patient whose tongue is coated with sordes (thick mucus) will be unable to taste his food and is quite likely to have **anorexia** (an"o-rek'se-ah) or loss of appetite. There are also some taste buds under the tongue, and in children some are on the inner surfaces of the cheeks. The tongue assists in chewing and swallowing as well as in speech.

We are born with buds for two sets of teeth. The milk or deciduous set has 20 teeth. These start to erupt by the age of about 6 months and all 20 are usually in by the age of 2 years. The permanent set has 32 teeth, which begin to appear at about 5 to 7 years and are usually complete with the wisdom teeth at about 25 years of age (see Fig. 17-3).

Bacteria multiply rapidly in the moist, warm, dark environment of the mouth, particularly if particles of food are lodged between the teeth. Although brushing the teeth after eating is very important, a toothbrush scarcely reaches between the teeth. For this reason, you should use dental floss to prevent decay of the teeth and, most important, to prevent gum infections. For details of these potential problems refer to the discussion in Chapter 18. The importance of

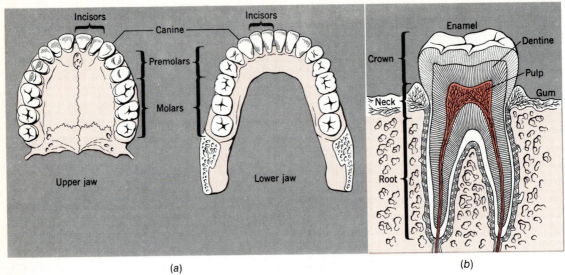

Figure 17-3. *(a) Adult teeth and (b) the main parts of a tooth*

good dental care for children can hardly be over-emphasized, not only because it can help to form lifelong habits of good dental hygiene but also because premature loss of the deciduous teeth can lead to deformity and poor occlusion of the permanent teeth.

PHARYNX AND ESOPHAGUS

After leaving the mouth, the food goes to the pharynx, the esophagus, and then to the stomach. For all practical purposes, no chemical changes take place in the pharynx or esophagus.

Mechanical changes move food at the proper rate. Swallowing is accomplished by contraction of striated muscles in the pharynx. The contraction of the smooth muscles in the walls of the esophagus moves the food toward the stomach. This type of smooth muscle contraction is called **peristalsis** (par-a-stal′sis), which means to contract around. It takes about four to eight sec-

onds for the food to go from the mouth to the stomach.

STOMACH

The stomach, which is a hollow muscular structure, is found in the upper left quadrant of the abdomen. It contains gastric fluid and mucus at all times. The cardiac sphincter is located between the stomach and the esophagus; the central portion or major part of the stomach is called the body. The fundus of the stomach is the rounded, upper portion above the esophageal opening. At the distal portion is the pyloric (pi-lor′ik) valve, which remains closed until the stomach has completed its work on the food.

The mucous membrane lining of the stomach has many folds or **rugae** (ru′gi) in it to allow for expansion of the stomach. This membrane secretes a great deal of alkaline mucus and some gastric juices to aid in digestion. The stomach produces a local hormone, gastrin, which stimulates the secretion of gastric juices, mainly hydrochloric acid. The hydrochloric acid, which provides a low pH unfavorable to the growth of bacteria, also functions to activate pepsinogen (pep-sin'o-jen) to become pepsin. Pepsin begins the chemical breakdown of proteins. The gastric juice also contains gastric lipase. The gastric lipase can begin the chemical digestion of emulsified fats. However, as a rule, we do not eat many emulsified fats. (Emulsified fats are finely dispersed in water as opposed to those occurring as large globules.) All enzymes are pH specific, and the activity of lipase is limited by the acidity of the stomach. There are also small amounts of gastric amylase; however, the amylase is inhibited by the acid pH of the stomach. In infants, the stomach produces rennin (ren'in), which coagulates the protein of milk. The purpose of this is to slow the emptying time of the stomach since most of the food of infants is already in liquid form. As you recall from Chapter 13, the stomach also produces the intrinsic factor that is essential for the proper maturation of red blood cells.

The stomach absorbs very little food because (with the exception of water, inorganic salts, a few drugs, and alcohol) the food is not yet in its diffusible form. In addition, the mucus coating the lining of the stomach is so thick that little food comes into contact with the stomach wall. The mucus is important in preventing the hydrochloric acid from coming into contact with and eroding the stomach wall. Some types of peptic ulcers may be associated with an excess amount of hydrochloric acid or to a lack of protective mucus in the stomach (see Fig. 17-4).

Normally, an average meal will stay in the stomach about three to four hours. During this time it is churned and mixed with the gastric juices and becomes quite liquid. The acid liquid is called chyme (kim). The churning is accomplished by the contractions of the smooth muscles of the stomach walls. The innermost layer of the smooth muscle has oblique fibers, the middle layer is made of circular fibers, and the outer muscle layer has longitudinal fibers. The circular and longitudinal fibers are mostly for peristalsis and the obliques do most of the churning (see Fig. 17-5).

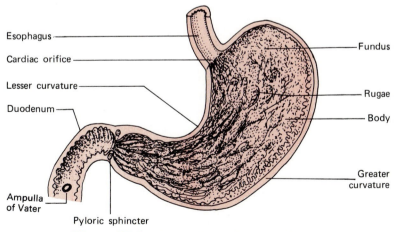

Figure 17-4. The inside of the stomach

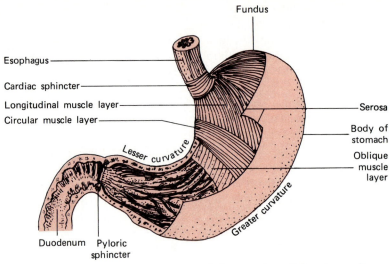

Figure 17-5. *Muscle layers and the interior of the stomach*

SMALL INTESTINE AND ACCESSORY ORGANS

After the pyloric valve opens, the food leaves the stomach and enters the small intestine, a narrow tube about 20 feet long. It has three divisions. The first is the **duodenum** (du-od′a-num), which is about 25 cm long or 9 to 10 inches. Its name, however, means twelve. The duodenum is about 12 fingerbreadths long. This is a common method used to measure things clinically. The **jejunum** (je-ju′num) is about 2.5 m (8 feet). Finally the distal portion of the small intestine is the ileum (il′e-um) which is about 3.5 m (12 feet). The inner mucosal surface of the small intestine is about 600 times the size of the serosal surface. This mucous membrane has washboard like circular folds, which greatly increase the surface area. On these folds are small protuberances, called villi (vil′e), which give the lining a velvety appearance (see Fig. 17-6).

The villi contain a blood capillary loop for the absorption of monosaccharides and amino acids, and a lymph capillary, or lacteal, for the absorption of fatty acids and glycerol. These folds and villi give the small intestine a tremendous surface area, which is important in the absorption of foodstuffs.

Accessory organs of the small intestine include the liver, the gall bladder, and the pancreas. Local hormones, secretin and chole-cystokinin-pancreozymin (ko″le-sis″to-kin′in-pan′kre″o″zi″min), or CCK-PZ, produced by the duodenal mucosa regulate the digestive functions of these organs and coordinate their activities with those of the digestive tract itself. Originally cholecystokinin and pancreozymin were discovered independently of each other and considered to be two separate hormones but now we believe they are two parts of the same hormone. The duodenal mucosa also produces enterogastrone which inhibits the secretions and motility of the stomach.

The liver is the largest and busiest gland in the body. It is often referred to as the chemical

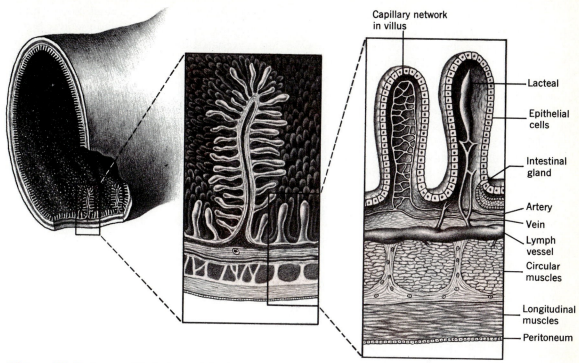

Figure 17-6. *A magnified view of the lining of the small intestine, showing the villi with blood and lymphatic capillaries for the absorption of the products of digestion*

capital of the body. It is covered with a tough fibrous covering, Glisson's capsule, which provides protection. The metabolic functions of the liver are so numerous and intricate that no attempt will be made to go into complete detail concerning liver functions. There are, however, a few that are particularly important for you to know. The liver helps to regulate the blood sugar level by converting fructose and galactose to glucose. Although fructose and galactose are simple sugars, the body can only utilize glucose. If the blood sugar level is adequate, the monosaccharides will be changed to glycogen, which the liver can store and release as glucose when the blood sugar level decreases. Another aspect of the liver's role in regulating the blood sugar level

is that it inactivates unneeded insulin. The liver also regulates the amino acid concentrations in the blood. It deaminizes (de-am′in-i-zes) amino acids that are not needed for protein synthesis and makes glucose out of these proteins. This process is called **gluconeogenesis** (gloo-ko-ne′o-jen″e-sis). The liver forms bile, which it sends to the gall bladder for concentration and storage. It helps in the destruction of old red blood cells, saves the iron for reuse, and eliminates the remainder of the old red cells in the bile. The liver uses fatty acids to synthesize triglycerides, lipoproteins, phospholipids, and cholesterol. The liver uses cholesterol to produce bile salts. There are at least two kinds of cholesterol; high density lipoprotein (HDL) and low density lipoprotein (LDL). The HDL helps prevent plaques from forming in the blood vessels. The LDL favors the formation of these plaques. The liver also forms blood proteins such as albumin, globulin, fibrinogen (fi-brin′o-jen), and prothrombin (pro-throm′bin). A final and important function of the liver is to detoxify harmful substances, such as alcohol and some sleeping pills, that may be ingested in excessive quantities. Harmful substances that the liver cannot detoxify, such as DDT, it will store, preventing their free circulation throughout the body.

Recall that the liver has a dual blood supply. The hepatic artery is nutrient to the liver bringing oxygenated blood to the liver cells, and the portal vein brings blood rich in the products of digestion so that the liver can perform its functions on these foodstuffs. Both the portal vein and the hepatic artery lead to the liver sinusoids, where their blood comes into contact with the liver cells. From the sinusoids, the blood goes into the central veins, then to the hepatic vein, and finally into the inferior vena cava (see Fig. 17-7).

In Figure 17-8 you can see how the hepatic

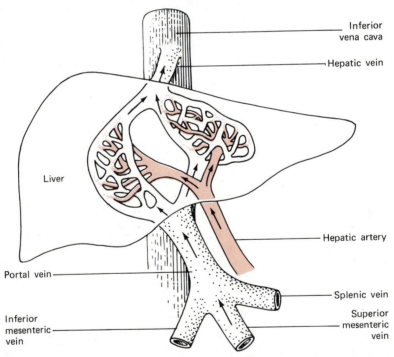

Figure 17-7. *Blood circulation through the liver. In order for the liver to perform its functions, venous blood from the organs of digestion that is rich in amino acids, monosaccharides, and other products of digestion is carried to the microscopic sinusoids by branches of the portal vein. Oxygenated blood is brought to these sinusoids by branches of the hepatic artery. Blood leaves the liver through the hepatic vein.*

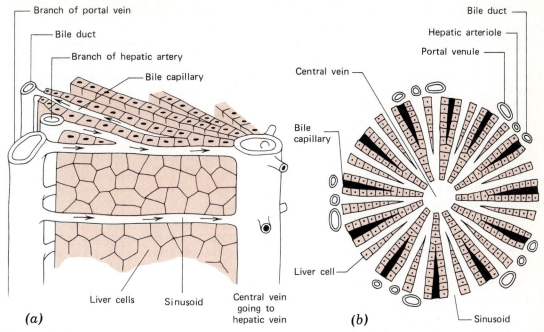

Figure 17-8. *(a) Arrangement of blood sinusoids and bile capillaries between rows of liver cells, and (b) cross section of a liver lobule*

arterial blood and that from the portal vein mixes in the liver sinusoids, and also the relationship of the bile capillaries to the liver cells and the blood sinusoids. The bile ducts unite to form the hepatic bile duct, which carries the bile to the cystic duct and then to the gall bladder.

The gall bladder is a small pear-shaped sac that can hold about 50 ml of bile, which it stores and concentrates. When fatty food enters the duodenum, CCK-PZ is released from the duodenal mucosa and sent to the gall bladder to cause it to evacuate the bile. The common bile duct receives the bile from the cystic duct and empties the bile into the duodenum through the ampulla of Vater shown in Figure 17-4. Bile has a detergent action that will emulsify dietary fats so they can be **hydrolyzed** (hi′drol-ized) by lipases. The results of the hydrolysis are fatty

acids and glycerol, which will be absorbed into the lacteals of the intestinal villi.

The pancreas is located behind the stomach at about the level of the first and second lumbar vertebrae. The head of the pancreas is found in the curve of the duodenum and the tail of the pancreas extends left laterally to the spleen. The pancreas is both an endocrine (en′do-krin) gland and an exocrine gland. The exocrine portion produces sodium bicarbonate to alkalinize the acid chyme. The sodium bicarbonate is produced in response to the local hormone secretin produced by the mucosa of the duodenum. The exocrine portion also produces digestive enzymes: trypsin (trip′sin), to complete the chemical digestion of proteins, and amylase to convert polysaccharides to disaccharides—maltose, sucrose, and lactose. The pancreas also produces lipase for fat digestion. All of these exocrine products enter the duodenum through a duct that opens at the ampulla of Vater. Once in the duodenum, the trypsin is activated to complete the chemical digestion of protein.

The endocrine portion produces insulin to lower the blood sugar level by causing increased utilization of carbohydrates by the peripheral tissue cells, stimulates the storage of glycogen from glucose and the formation of fat from glucose, and decreases gluconeogenesis. Insulin is degraded in the liver and to a somewhat lesser degree in the kidneys. Insulin is antagonized by epinephrine, by the **glucocorticoids** (gloo"ko-kor'te-koids), by the diabetogenic (di-ah-bet"o-jen'ik) factor from the anterior pituitary, and by **glucagon** (gloo'ka-gon). Glucagon is another hormone produced by the pancreas. It causes the liver to convert glycogen to glucose, thereby raising the blood sugar level.

The mechanical actions in the small intestine are segmental mixing contractions as well as propulsive movements of peristalsis. The segmentation consists of squeezing and mixing of the food with the digestive juices. Peristalsis causes a slow onward movement of the intestinal contents. The chemical actions are numerous. The bile emulsifies the fats, and the presence of bile in the large intestine enables bacteria there to produce vitamin K. In the absence of bile, a patient's stools will be clay-colored and he may have bleeding tendencies because of the deficiency of vitamin K.

The sodium bicarbonate from the pancreas produces an alkaline medium, so that the otherwise acid chyme will not cause erosion of the mucosa of the small intestines. This mucosa is not protected by as much mucus as is found in the stomach.

Pancreatic trypsin breaks proteins down to amino acids. Pancreatic amylase reduces polysaccharides to disaccharides, and pancreatic li-

pase reduces emulsified fats to fatty acids and glycerol.

The secretions of the intestinal glands are called succus entericus (suk'us en"ter'i-cus). The enzymes contained in the succus entericus are active in an alkaline pH. Erepsin (e-rep'sin) converts partially digested proteins to amino acids. **Maltase** (mal'tase), **sucrase** (su'krase), and **lactase** act on the disaccharides, forming the monosaccharides glucose, fructose, and galactose. Table 17-1 summarizes the chemicals involved in the digestion of foodstuffs.

The greatest amount (about 80%) of the absorption of food takes place in the small intestine because it is here that the foodstuffs are in their diffusible form, the surface area is so great, and peristalsis is slow enough to allow time for chemical digestion and absorption.

LARGE INTESTINE

The large intestine, which is about 1.5 meters (five feet) long, begins at the ileocecal (il"e-o-se'kal) valve and extends to the anus. The cecum is the first part of the large intestine. The appendix, which is about 8 cm (3 inches) long, is a narrow tube closed at one end and attached to the cecum. It has a relatively poor blood supply, which makes it particularly vulnerable to infection.

The colon is one continuous tube subdivided into four parts: ascending colon, transverse colon, descending colon, and sigmoid colon. Most of its action is that of peristalsis and the absorption of water and electrolytes. Severe diarrhea can result not only in serious dehydration but also in electrolyte imbalance because the rapid peristalsis does not allow enough time for the absorption of fluids and electrolytes, and so the patient will be dehydrated and also acidotic since the pancreatic sodium bicarbonate has not been reabsorbed.

Table 17-1. Chemicals of the Digestive System

Structure	Secretion	Acts On	Products Formed or Effect
Mouth	amylase	carbohydrates	disaccharides
	saliva	food	lubricates and liquefies
Stomach	hydrochloric acid	pepsinogen	pepsin
		gastric fluid	favorable pH for pepsin
	pepsin	proteins	partially digested proteins
	lipase	emulsified fats	fatty acids and glycerol
	gastrin	stomach glands	gastric juice
	mucus	mucosa	lubricates and protects from hydrochloric acid
Liver	bile	fat globules	emulsified fats
Pancreas	sodium bicarbonate	intestinal fluid	favorable pH for alkaline specific enzymes
	amylase	carbohydrates	disaccharides
	lipase	emulsified fats	fatty acids and glycerol
	trypsin	proteins	amino acids
Small intestine	enterogastrone	stomach	inhibits secretions and motility
	secretin	pancreas	sodium bicarbonate
	pancreozymin	pancreas	secretion of enzymes
	cholecystokinin	gall bladder	expulsion of bile
	mucus	mucosa	lubricates
	enterokinase	trypsinogen	trypsin
	erepsin	partly digested proteins	amino acids
	maltase	maltose	glucose
	sucrase	sucrose	glucose and fructose
	lactase	lactose	glucose and galactose

Failure to evacuate the bowel promptly may result in constipation because too much water is absorbed, and the feces become dehydrated and hard. Cathartic salts are relatively nonabsorbable and tend to pull tissue fluid into the bowel softening the feces and increasing the bulk in the bowel. Since mineral oil is a lubricant it is also a laxative. Some other types of laxatives work because they act as nonabsorbable bulk and stimulate peristalsis. Others stimulate peristalsis by chemical irritation.

Bacteria in the large intestine act on the undigested residues. They cause the fermentation of carbohydrates and putrefaction of proteins. These bacteria also synthesize vitamin K and some vitamin B, provided bile is present in the intestine. If a sufficient number of these helpful bacteria are destroyed by antibiotics taken for the purpose of treating some systemic infection, a vitamin deficiency can develop and the patient may also have diarrhea.

The sigmoid colon leads to the rectum, which

is about 20 cm (five inches) long and empties into the anal canal. The rectal sphincter protects the external orifice.

METABOLISM

Metabolism is the changes in foodstuffs from the time they are absorbed until they are excreted as wastes. These changes are accomplished by enzyme systems within the cells. The action of each enzyme is specific and depends on the action of the enzyme preceding it in the system. For this reason, if one enzyme in a chain of enzymes is missing or malfunctioning, the metabolic processes involved will be faulty. People with such conditions have inborn errors of metabolism.

Many enzymatic reactions depend on the presence of certain vitamins or minerals. Hormones produced by the endocrine glands influence the actions of some enzyme systems. It is also important to remember that enzyme action depends on a relatively narrow range of pH and temperature.

There are two phases of metabolism, **anabolism** (ah-nab'o-lizm) and **catabolism** (kah-tab'o-lizm). During anabolism substances are built up; for example, adipose tissue is formed from foodstuffs. During catabolism, substances are broken down by oxidation and energy is released.

CARBOHYDRATE METABOLISM

Although a small amount of carbohydrate is utilized in building tissues, the main purpose of carbohydrate metabolism is to provide energy. Glucose is the major product of carbohydrate digestion, and following its absorption there are several possible metabolic pathways available (see Fig. 17-9).

1. Glucose can enter the tissues and be oxidized to form carbon dioxide, water, and energy.

2. Glucose can be converted to glycogen and stored in the liver and muscle. This process is called **glycogenesis** (gli"ko-jen'e-sis).

3. When adequate carbohydrates have been stored as glycogen, any additional glucose is changed to fat and stored as adipose tissue.

4. **Glycogenolysis** (gli"ko-jen-ol'is-is) is the breakdown of glycogen to reform glucose. This occurs when the blood sugar falls, as it usually does between meals.

5. The liver can produce glucose from noncarbohydrate sources in response to a low blood sugar. This process is called gluconeogenesis. The **lactic** (lak'tik) and **pyruvic** (pi'roo-vik) **acids** produced by muscle contraction are converted to glucose. The liver can remove an amino group from certain amino acids and convert the remaining carboxyl portion to glucose. This process is called **deamination** (de-am"in-a'shun). Glycerol can also be converted to glucose by the liver. Gluconeogenesis is initiated largely by hormones from the adrenal gland in response to a low blood sugar, **hypoglycemia** (hi"po-gli-se'me-ah).

6. If there is a large intake of carbohydrate in a short period of time, some of the glucose may be eliminated by the kidneys. This also happens in uncontrolled diabetes mellitus.

The utilization of glucose by the cells and the ultimate production of energy from the oxidation of this fuel requires insulin. As discussed in Chapter 4, energy results from the breakdown of ATP in the cellular mitochondria. We can follow a glucose molecule through the processes involved in this production of energy by the cell.

First, the glucose combines with phosphate forming a large, activated, six-carbon sugar, which must be reduced in size in order to enter the mitochondrion. The breakdown of this large

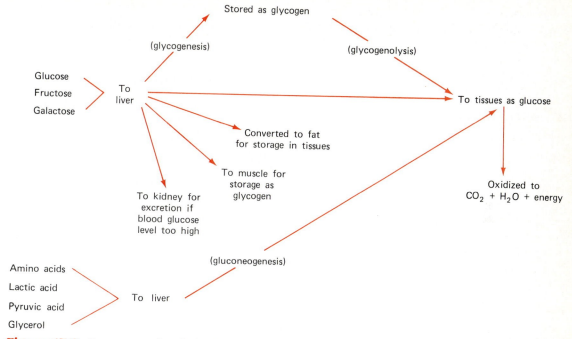

Figure 17-9. *Summary of carbohydrate metabolism. When blood sugar level decreases, the liver converts glycogen to glucose and releases it into the bloodstream. Blood sugar is also increased by gluconeogenesis. When the blood sugar level rises above normal, glucose is stored as glycogen or fat; in extreme cases, it is eliminated by the kidneys.*

molecule into two three-carbon pyruvic acid molecules is accomplished by enzymes. This process is anaerobic (requiring no oxygen) and is called **glycolysis** (gli-kol'is-is). Two molecules of ATP are formed during glycolysis.

The two pyruvic acid molecules are then converted to an acetic acid, which enters the mitochondrion. There, citric acid is formed and, through a series of steps called the citric acid cycle, large amounts of ATP are formed. At various steps in this cycle, which is also called the Krebs cycle, hydrogens with their energy are released and transferred to hydrogen acceptors. This part of the sequence is called the electron transport system.

The reactions taking place within the mitochondrion produce 36 molecules of ATP. This phase of energy production requires six molecules of oxygen. This is important because life processes require energy and there must be a continuous supply of oxygen to produce this energy. Note that only two molecules of ATP were produced during the anaerobic glycolysis, and an additional 36 are produced with the citric acid cycle.

Summarizing the changes of catabolism in equation form we see:

Glycolysis:
$$\text{glucose} \rightarrow 2 \text{ pyruvic acid} + 2 \text{ ATP} + \Delta$$

Citric acid cycle:
$$2 \text{ pyruvic acid} + 6O_2 \rightarrow$$
$$6 \text{ CO}_2 + 6 \text{ H}_2\text{O} + 36 \text{ ATP} + \Delta$$

About 40% of the energy resulting from catabolism of one molecule of glucose is represented in the total 38 molecules of ATP. The remaining 60% liberated as heat is distributed to all parts of the body by way of the bloodstream.

FAT METABOLISM

The catabolism of one gram of fat, a more concentrated form of fuel, yields nine kilocalories of heat as opposed to four kilocalories from the oxidation of one gram of carbohydrate. Fat catabolism is called ketogenesis (ke-to-jen'e-sis) because ketone bodies are formed. The absorbed fat is converted to an acetic acid (which is classified as a ketone body) in the liver. It then enters the citric acid cycle and is oxidized, producing carbon dioxide, water, and energy.

Fat anabolism is the storage of fat as adipose tissue. Fat stored in the fat deposits represents the body's largest reserve energy source. As long as carbohydrate catabolism supplies the energy needs, stored fats are not used to supply energy. If carbohydrates are not available in sufficient quantities to meet the energy requirements, adipose stores are used to supply energy needs.

Ketosis is an excess accumulation of ketones in the bloodstream as a result of the metabolism of large amounts of fats in the absence of carbohydrates. This can occur in uncontrolled diabetes mellitus because adequate amounts of insulin are not available for the utilization of carbohydrates (see Chapter 24). Ketosis can also result from a very low-calorie diet lacking in carbohydrates, and thus fad diets intended for weight reduction are very dangerous when they eliminate carbohydrates. With ketosis there is a disturbance in the body's ability to maintain the proper blood pH, and metabolic acidosis may occur.

PROTEIN METABOLISM

Proteins are primarily tissue-building foods; carbohydrates and fats are energy-supplying foods. For this reason, in considering protein metabolism our chief concern is anabolism rather than catabolism.

Protein anabolism or protein synthesis results in many essential substances such as enzymes, antibodies, body secretions, and blood constituents. Body growth and wound repair are dependent on protein anabolism.

One aspect of protein catabolism is deamination of amino acids, which takes place in the liver. This process is a type of gluconeogenesis. The oxidation of one gram of protein, as for carbohydrate, yields four kilocalories of heat.

Normally protein anabolism and catabolism go on continually but at different rates. The healthy adult body is usually in a state of protein or nitrogen balance. This means that the nitrogen intake (in the form of protein foods) equals the nitrogen excreted in urine, feces, and sweat.

A positive nitrogen balance exists when the intake of protein is greater than the nitrogen excretion, indicating protein anabolism is going on faster than protein catabolism. This occurs in growing children, during pregnancy, and during convalescence.

When protein catabolism exceeds anabolism, as in starvation and debilitating diseases, there is a negative nitrogen balance. Tissue wasting is indicative of a negative nitrogen balance.

SUMMARY QUESTIONS

1. Explain the roles of vitamins and minerals in the diet.
2. What are the purposes of mechanical digestion?

3. What is the purpose of chemical digestion?

4. What enzymes work on carbohydrates?

5. What enzymes work on fats?

6. What enzymes work on proteins?

7. Name the simplest forms of proteins, carbohydrates, and fats.

8. Beginning with the mouth, list in sequence and describe the structures of the alimentary canal.

9. What is the function of the greater omentum, and where is it located?

10. What type of membrane lines the alimentary canal?

11. What is the function of the hydrochloric acid in the stomach?

12. What chemical digestive processes take place in the stomach?

13. Why is there so little absorption of foodstuffs in the stomach?

14. Discuss at least five functions of the liver.

15. What are the secretions from the exocrine portion of the pancreas and what does each of these secretions accomplish?

16. What are the secretions from the endocrine portion of the pancreas and what are the functions of these hormones?

17. Absorption of the products of digestion depends on what factors?

18. What is nitrogen balance?

19. Discuss the roles of the local hormones produced by the alimentary canal.

KEY TERMS

amino acid
anabolism
anorexia
catabolism
deamination
disaccharides
duodenum
glucagon
glucocorticoids
gluconeogenesis
glycogenesis
glycogenolysis
glycolysis
hydrolyzed

hypoglycemia
jejunum
lactase
lactic acid
lipids
maltase
monosaccharides
parotid gland
peristalsis
peritoneum
pyruvic acid
rugae
sucrase

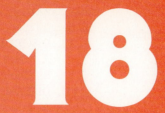

18

Diseases of the Gastrointestinal System

OBJECTIVES

On completion of this chapter, you will be able to:

1. Discuss the various tests used for diagnosing diseases of the gastrointestinal system.
2. List the signs and symptoms of peptic ulcers.
3. Describe the treatment of peptic ulcers.
4. Discuss the symptoms and treatment of gallbladder disease.
5. Explain the causes of the different types of hepatitis.
6. List the signs and symptoms of cirrhosis of the liver.
7. Discuss the causes and management of poisoning.

OVERVIEW

I. DIAGNOSTIC PROCEDURES
   A. Fecal Occult Blood
   B. Radiographic Studies
      1. Barium Swallow
      2. Upper Gastrointestinal and Small Bowel Series
      3. Barium Enema
      4. Oral Cholecystogram
   C. Endoscopy
   D. Ultrasonography
   E. Computerized Tomography
   F. Nuclear Medicine
II. FUNCTIONAL DISORDERS OF THE GASTROINTESTINAL SYSTEM
   A. Abdominal Pain
   B. Constipation
   C. Diarrhea
   D. Nausea and Vomiting
III. DISORDERS OF THE ORAL CAVITY
   A. Stomatitis
   B. Dental Caries
   C. Tumors of the Mouth
IV. DISORDERS OF THE STOMACH AND DUODENUM
   A. Gastritis
   B. Peptic Ulcer Disease
V. DISEASES OF THE LOWER GASTROINTESTINAL TRACT
   A. Diverticular Disease
   B. Peritonitis
      1. Ulcerative Colitis
      2. Crohn's Disease (Regional Enteritis)
   C. Inflammatory Bowel Disease
   D. Appendicitis
   E. Cancer of the Colon and Rectum
   F. Intestinal Obstruction
   G. Hemorrhoids

VI. DISORDERS OF THE GALLBLADDER
   A. Cholelithiasis
   B. Cholecystitis
VII. DISEASES OF THE PANCREAS
   A. Pancreatitis
VIII. DISEASES OF THE LIVER
   A. Hepatitis
   B. Cirrhosis
IX. POISON
   A. Food Poisoning
   B. Ingested Poisons
   C. General Principles for the Treatment of Poisoning

Most diseases of the gastrointestinal tract involve alterations in the the digestion and absorption of nutrients. Many of these diseases produce similar signs and symptoms. Extensive testing, therefore, is often necessary in order to make a diagnosis.

First we shall consider some of the diagnostic tests and then discuss the common disease processes of the gastrointestinal system.

This chapter was written by Linda M. Goodfellow.

DIAGNOSTIC PROCEDURES

FECAL OCCULT BLOOD

Blood in the feces is often invisible. Minute quantities of fecal **occult** (ok-kult') **blood** can be detected by tests for hemoglobin, such as the guaiac test. Examinations of stool specimens for occult blood is useful in the detection of gastrointestinal (GI) bleeding and aids in the diagnosis of colorectal cancer.

Three stool specimens are collected and tested. The specimens should be labeled with the patient's name and whatever other information is required by the particular laboratory. For two or three days before the tests and during the time of collection, the patient should refrain from eating red meat, poultry, fish, turnips, and horseradish. Some medications may also alter the results of the test and therefore should be withheld.

RADIOGRAPHIC STUDIES

Radiography is the passage of radiation beams through the patient to create X-ray films. Different densities appear as various shades on the films. The denser the structure, the lighter the picture. Consequently, air appears as black, fat is dark gray, soft tissue is light gray, and bone appears as white. In some procedures, a contrast medium may be used to accentuate the density.

Cineradiography films the motion of a contrast medium by a rapid sequence X-ray.

Barium Swallow

For this examination, the patient is required to swallow barium sulfate during a fluoroscopic examination. The esophagus is observed as the patient swallows the barium. The patient will be required to assume different positions to observe the reflux of barium and esophageal peristalsis.

This procedure is indicated in patients with complaints of regurgitation or **dysphagia** (dis-fa′zhe-ah) or difficulty in swallowing. A barium swallow should be done after radiographic studies of the lower parts of the tract are done since this ingested barium will move lower in the tract and impede X-ray visualization of the other structures. A barium swallow is not performed if a GI performation is suspected, since a leak of the barium would produce an acute inflammatory reaction.

Upper Gastrointestinal and Small Bowel Series

Upper gastrointestinal and small bowel series are X-ray examinations of the esophagus, stomach, and small intestine after the patient swallows barium sulfate. The barium serves as a contrast medium, outlining mucosal contours and peristalsis. Indications for these studies include dysphagia, regurgitation, burning or gnawing epigastric pain, diarrhea, weight loss, and GI bleeding.

The patient should have a low-residue diet for two or three days prior to the test. The patient should not eat, drink, or smoke after midnight the night prior to the test. After the barium has been ingested, the patient's body is rotated so that the barium fills the tract. X-rays are taken at various intervals until the barium reaches the cecum. The procedure may take up to six hours to complete. Esophageal abnormalities, motility disorders, gastric reflux, stomach ulcers or tumors, and disorders of the small intestine, such as regional enteritis, malabsorption syndrome, and tumors, may be revealed by these studies.

Barium Enema

A barium enema is an X-ray visualization of the large intestine after rectal instillation of barium sulfate alone or with air. Barium sulfate instilled alone is the single-contrast technique providing a profile view of the large intestine (see Fig. 18-1). Barium sulfate instilled with air is the double-contrast technique that provides profile and frontal views.

The bowel must be cleansed of all fecal material before the barium enema is given. Patients must comply with the prescribed dietary restrictions and bowel preparation. Protocol for bowel preparations may vary, but generally the patient should have a low-residue diet for two or three days prior to the test. A clear liquid supper is given the evening before the test. The patient is encouraged to drink plenty of water and clear liquids the day before the test. A laxative is given the afternoon of the day before the test. Cleansing enemas are given the morning of the barium enema. The patient may have a clear liquid breakfast that morning.

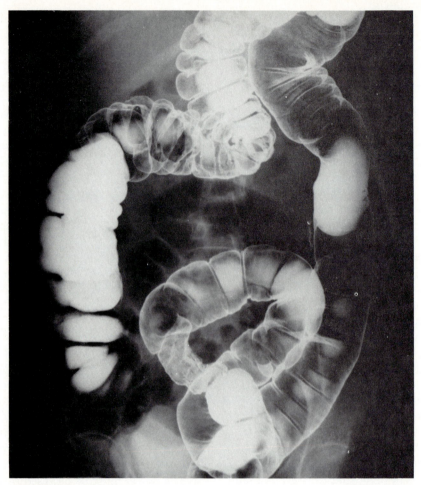

Figure 18-1. *X-ray of the lower gastrointestinal tract (Courtesy of Mercy Hospital, Radiology Department, Pittsburgh, PA)*

A rectal tube is inserted for instillation of the barium. A retaining balloon on the rectal tube may be inflated if the patient is unable to retain the barium. As the barium is instilled, the patient assumes different positions to assure complete filling of the bowel. After the X-rays are taken, the rectal tube is removed and the patient is asked to expel as much barium as possible in the toilet or a bedpan. Following any barium study, it is important to empty the bowel of any residual barium and to make sure the patient has daily bowel movements for the next few days since retained barium may be constipating.

Barium enema studies are useful in evaluating the colon for malignancies, polyps, diverticulitis, and inflammatory bowel disease.

Oral Cholecystogram

An oral cholecystogram is an X-ray visualization of the gallbladder after the patient injests a contrast medium. The patient eats a fatty meal at noon and a fat-free dinner the day prior to the test. Two or three hours after the evening meal, the patient ingests six tablets of the contrast material. These tablets are taken at five minute intervals with a total of eight ounces of water. After the tablets are taken, the patient is not allowed food or fluid until completion of the test the next morning. After the X-ray, occasionally a fatty meal is given and a second X-ray taken to determine the adequacy of the emptying of the gallbladder.

This test is indicated for patients complaining of right-sided epigastric pain, fatty food intolerance, and jaundice. Cholelithiasis, cholecystitis, and tumors of the gallbladder can be detected by this examination. Cholecystography is contraindicated in patients who are allergic to iodine dye or who are in early pregnancy.

ENDOSCOPY

Endoscopic examinations provide direct visualization of the lining of the gastrointestinal tract. These procedures frequently cause discomfort. The endoscope contains a cable-like cluster of glass fibers that transmits light into the area being examined and then returns an image to the scope's optical head. Endoscopic examination is used to detect inflammatory, ulcerative, and infective diseases as well as malignant and benign neoplasms.

Proctoscopy, sigmoidoscopy, and colonoscopy are the most frequently performed endoscopic examinations of the GI tract. Proctoscopy is the direct visualization of the lining of the rectum and anus. The proctoscope is a rigid scope approximately 7 cm long and is inserted through the anus.

Sigmoidoscopy is the endoscopic examination of the distal sigmoid colon. This procedure is recommended by many physicians for men over 40 as part of an annual physical examination.

The distal sigmoid colon is not visualized well during radiographic procedures. The procedure may be necessary for individuals complaining of hemorrhoids, constipation, or rectal bleeding. The sigmoidoscope, a rigid tube about 28 cm long, is inserted into the anus after digital dilitation. The patient assumes the knee chest position. This position may be difficult for an elderly or debilitated patient, in which case the patient may assume a side-lying position.

The bowel must be free of stool to permit optical visualization. Patients are instructed to eat a light meal the evening prior to the test and light breakfast the morning of the test. Although specific bowel preparation varies, usually enemas are given or suppositories taken the morning of the test.

Colonoscopy is the direct visualization of the lining of the large intestine with a flexible fiberoptic endoscope (see Fig. 18-2). The patient is positioned on his left side. The right leg is flexed at the knee and extended over the left leg. The endoscope is inserted through the anus and advanced through the large intestine. The physician palpates the patient's abdomen with one hand to aid in the advancement of the colonoscope.

This procedure may be performed for patients with persistent diarrhea or constipation, rectal bleeding, or when the results of other testing have been negative or inconclusive.

ULTRASONOGRAPHY

Ultrasonography is the introduction of a focused beam of high-frequency sound waves into a patient to create echoes that reflect tissue density. The echoes are transmitted to an oscilloscope screen.

The patient will be told to fast 8 to 12 hours before the procedure to reduce bowel gas that can hinder transmission of sound waves. If ultrasound of the gallbladder is to be done, the patient will be ordered to eat a fat-free meal the

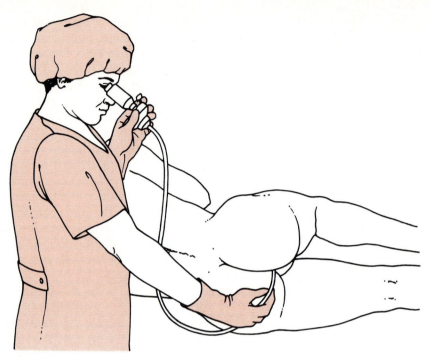

Figure 18-2. *Colonoscopy is used to examine the lining of the large intestine.*

evening before the procedure so bile will accumulate and enhance ultrasonic visualization.

Ultrasonography of the gallbladder is the procedure of choice for distinguishing between obstructive and nonobstructive jaundice. Ultrasound can be used to detect cholelithiasis or cholecystitis when cholecystography proves inconclusive.

The patient has a fat-free dinner the evening prior to the test and then nothing by mouth after midnight. Ultrasound is a noninvasive procedure. The skin over the area to be examined is lubricated with a water-soluble jelly to enhance conduction of the sound waves and reduce friction with the skin surface. A transducer is passed over the lubricated skin in the right upper quadrant. During the procedure, the patient may be given an injection of a drug that stimulates gallbladder contraction. Ultrasound is

less expensive than computerized tomography and introduces no radiation.

Ultrasound of the pancreas consists of high-frequency sound waves transmitted to images on an oscilloscope. Cross sectional images of the pancreas, which detect tissue densities, are produced. This procedure can be used to detect pancreatic carcinoma or pseudocysts of the pancreas. It also can be used to locate the desired insertion site for the needle during tissue biopsy. Although ultrasound can detect structural abnormalities, it is not able to evaluate pancreatic functions.

COMPUTERIZED TOMOGRAPHY

Computerized tomography (CT scan) provides detailed information of tissue densities. It is used in the diagnosis of acute and chronic pan-

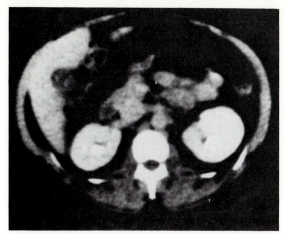

Figure 18-3. *Gallstones as seen on CT scan (Courtesy of the Department of Radiology, Shadyside Hospital, Pittsburgh, PA)*

creatitis, pancreatic cysts, cirrhosis of the liver, ascites, calcium deposits, aneurysms, and pancreatic cancer (see Fig. 18-3). A CT scan of the liver is useful in differentiating between obstructive and nonobstructive jaundice and can distinguish between malignant and benign neoplasms due to its ability to detect variations in tissue density.

The patient must avoid oral intake four hours prior to the study. The patient is placed inside a body scanner that passes radiation impulses through a section of the patient's abdomen. These impulses are picked up by detectors, processed by a computer, reconstructed, and projected to an oscilloscope screen. The three-dimensional image is displayed on the screen as the test is performed. Water soluble contrast dyes administered intravenously may be used to better delineate pancreatic margins.

NUCLEAR MEDICINE

Liver-spleen scanning is used to detect liver disease, evaluate abdominal masses, or evaluate the condition of the liver and spleen after abdominal trauma. A radioactive colloid is injected into the patient. The distribution or "uptake" of the colloid is recorded by a rectilinear scanner or gamma camera. Cold spots are those areas that fail to take up the colloid. Unaffected areas absorb the additional colloid and create a brighter image.

Although most liver-spleen scanning is a static (still) study, flow studies (dynamic scintigraphy) demonstrate the flow of a radionuclide in rapid sequence. Vascularity is detected by this method and this helps to determine metastases, tumors, cysts, and abscesses by identifying their characteristic patterns of uptake.

FUNCTIONAL DISORDERS OF THE GASTROINTESTINAL SYSTEM

ABDOMINAL PAIN

Abdominal pain is often the major or only symptom of gastrointestinal disease. It is important to gather information regarding the onset, duration, location, intensity, and type of pain, and factors that aggravate it or provide relief. Since viscera generally contain few pain receptors, this pain tends to be dull and generalized as compared to superficial pain that probably is more intense and localized. For example, pain resulting from a peptic ulcer may be difficult to distinguish from that resulting from a heart attack or gallbladder disease.

CONSTIPATION

Infrequent bowel movements do not constitute constipation unless the interval between bowel movements is greater than normal for that person. Constipation may result from drying and hardening of the stool as water from the stool is reabsorbed into the wall of the intestinal tract. Ignoring the call to defecate or any factor that decreases an individual's expulsive power can lead to constipation. Inadequate dietary intake of bulk or fiber and a decreased fluid intake can lead to constipation.

DIARRHEA

As a result of severe diarrhea, as much as five to ten liters of fluid can be lost from the GI tract within 24 hours. Patients, particularly infants and the elderly, can become dehydrated in a relatively short period of time. A great deal of sodium and potassium that should have been reabsorbed into the bloodstream is lost in the diarrhea stools. As a result, the patient tends to be acidotic. The number, color, consistency, and odor of the stools are important to note because the character of feces can be significant in determining the cause of the diarrhea.

NAUSEA AND VOMITING

Nausea and vomiting are common indications of gastrointestinal disorders but they are also present in disorders of the other organ systems. Nausea is the subjective feeling that usually precedes vomiting. Persistent vomiting can disturb the patient's acid-base balance. If the vomiting is caused by gastritis, the body must produce increasing amounts of alkaline mucus, which will deplete the blood sodium and may cause acidosis. Vomiting from other causes is more likely to deplete blood hydrogen and cause the patient to become alkalotic.

Vomiting that is not preceded by nausea may be an indication of increased intracranial pressure.

DISORDERS OF THE ORAL CAVITY

STOMATITIS

Stomatitis is an inflammation of the mucous membrane lining of the mouth. This may be the result of infections, vitamin deficiency, trauma to the mouth, or disease elsewhere in the body. Tobacco, alcohol, excessively spicy foods, or chemotherapy administered for the treatment of cancer may also cause stomatitis.

DENTAL CARIES

Diseases of the teeth and gums are prevalent health problems in the United States. Dental caries, or cavities, is related to the consumption of refined carbohydrates. Proper dental hygiene, which includes brushing after meals and flossing, greatly reduces the incidence of dental disease (see Fig. 18-4).

Periodontal disease results from poor dental hygiene, poor nutrition, or malocclusion (improper alignment of the teeth). The gingivae (gums), bone, and other supporting structures of the teeth can be affected. There will be deterioration and loss of bony structure, infection, bleeding, recession of the gums, and loosening of the teeth.

TUMORS OF THE MOUTH

The lips, mouth, and tongue are prone to develop malignant lesions. Cancer of the lip is readily detectable and, consequently, has a high cure rate. A painless ulcer with raised edges or a split in the lip is the first sign. The lesion is usually detected before metastasis has occurred.

Unlike cancer of the lip, cancer of the tongue and floor of the mouth may be undetected. The

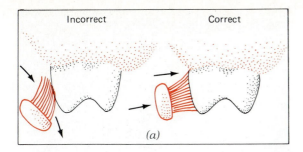

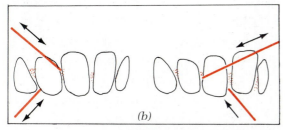

Figure 18-4. *Brushing all surfaces of the teeth and flossing between teeth are important parts of dental care. (a) Bristle ends of the toothbrush slide gently under margin of gingiva (gum). (b) Proper placement of floss for effective cleaning.*

lesions appear hard and plaquelike or as ulcerated areas that do not heal. Because the area is very vascular, a large percentage of patients are found to have metastasis to the neck at the time of diagnosis. Carcinoma of the oral cavity is associated with tobacco use and excessive alcohol consumption.

DISORDERS OF THE STOMACH AND DUODENUM

GASTRITIS

Gastritis can be either an acute or chronic inflammation of the gastric mucosa. In acute gastritis vascular congestion, edema, and degenerative changes occur in the lining of the stomach.

The injury can be caused by chemicals, drugs, or food. Common food sources of gastritis include excess tea and coffee, spices, or foods contaminated with staphylococci.

Signs and symptoms of acute gastritis include epigastric pain, abdominal tenderness, cramping, gas, nausea, and vomiting. Gastrointestinal bleeding is common in patients with gastritis.

Chronic gastritis is seen most often in older women. These patients cannot tolerate spicy or fatty foods. They often complain of **dyspepsia** (dis-pep′se-ah), heartburn, and discomfort after eating large meals. **Hematemesis** (hem″ah-tem′e-sis), vomiting that contains blood, **anorexia** (an″o-rek′se-ah), or lack of appetite, and weight loss are common signs and symptoms.

PEPTIC ULCER DISEASE

Peptic ulcer disease is a break in the mucous lining of the gastrointestinal tract that comes in contact with gastric juice, either in the lining of the stomach or duodenum. Since the term peptic ulcer refers to an ulcer in any part of the GI tract, ulcers are further classified as gastric or duodenal. Not only are the locations of gastric and duodenal ulcers different but the etiology and pathophysiology are different as well. The pain of the peptic ulcer usually occurs one to two hours after meals and is often relieved by eating. Peptic ulcers may be caused by stress. Tension can intensify or prolong the ulcer pain. Periodicity may be another characteristic feature. This occurs when discomfort accompanies digestion over a period of time and is then followed by the complete absence of all symptoms for months or years. Generally, the degree of pain is some indication of the severity of the tissue involvement.

Duodenal ulcers are usually found within 1.5 cm of the pylorus. These patients have a large amount of gastric acid secretion and rapid emptying of their stomachs. Duodenal ulcers occur more frequently than gastric ulcers. Exacerbations of duodenal ulcers frequently occur in the spring and fall.

Gastric ulcers are caused by a break in the peptic epithelium. Evidence strongly suggests a relationship between persons who ingest excessive amounts of salicylates, such as aspirin, and an increased incidence of gastric ulcers. Cigarette smoking is also associated with an increased risk of gastric ulcers. They are not associated with hyperacidity, and the emptying time of the stomach is normal. The regurgitation of bile salts leads to the destruction of the surface mucus of the stomach, and certain drugs such as aspirin and cortisone decrease the mucosal resistance to acid. Alcohol and caffeine increase the secretion of the acids.

The pain experienced by patients with a gastric ulcer usually follows the ingestion of food and is not relieved by food intake. The pain is located in the upper portion of the epigastrium, often localizing to the left of the midline. Vomiting occurs with gastric ulcers more commonly than with uncomplicated duodenal ulcers. Gastric ulcers can become malignant (see Fig. 18-5).

The treatment of peptic ulcers may include medications to reduce the amount of gastric secretion, to neutralize acid, or to protect the mucous barrier of the stomach.

In the treatment of ulcers, bland or ulcer diets have been used extensively in the past. However, now dietary measures are controversial. Some physicians recommend small, frequent meals for patients with ulcer disease. Most physicians agree that foods that increase gastric secretion, foods high in roughage, gas-forming or highly seasoned foods, and smoking should be eliminated.

Complications of peptic ulcer disease include hemorrhage, perforation, and obstruction. Gastrointestinal bleeding can range from occult blood in the stool to vomiting large amounts of bright red blood.

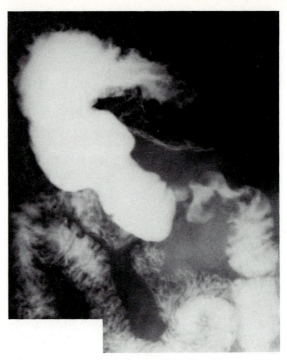

Figure 18-5. Prepyloric ulcer (Courtesy of the Department of Radiology, Shadyside Hospital, Pittsburgh, PA)

Perforation occurs when the ulcer erodes through the gastric wall, often leading to peritonitis. Mortality is high in this condition and surgery, although limited, may be necessary to prevent involvement of other organs.

Damage to the pylorus can lead to obstruction. Obstruction is exhibited by persistent vomiting, which may lead to severe fluid and electrolyte imbalances if not controlled.

DISEASES OF THE LOWER GASTROINTESTINAL TRACT

DIVERTICULAR DISEASE

A **diverticulum** (di″ver-tik′u-lum) of the colon is a blind outpouching of the intestinal mucosa

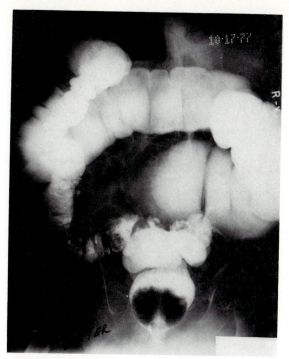

Figure 18-6. Acute diverticulitis. The dark mass in the rectal area is an inflated balloon that helps the patient retain the barium until X-rays are taken. (Courtesy of the Department of Radiology, Shadyside Hospital, Pittsburgh, PA)

forming a sac. When these outpouchings are not inflamed and cause no symptoms, the condition is called diverticulosis. Feces can become trapped in these sacs and, as a consequence, the diverticula can become inflamed and painful. This condition is called diverticulitis (see Fig. 18-6).

Diverticulitis is common in persons over forty years of age and in obese individuals. It usually occurs in the sigmoid colon. In diverticulitis, obstruction, infection, and hemorrhage of the GI tract may occur. The pain associated with diverticulitis is usually a dull pain in the left lower quadrant or midabdominal region and may ra-

diate to the back. Other symptoms are diarrhea, constipation, or alternating episodes of both of these. The patient will have increased flatus, anorexia, and a low-grade fever for a day or two. Exacerbations of the symptoms are noted after a large meal, a large amount of dietary roughage, or alcohol. Diverticulitis is diagnosed by a barium enema, sigmoidoscopy, a white blood cell count, and sedimentation rate.

PERITONITIS

Perforation of a diverticulum can lead to **peritonitis** (per"i-to-ni'tis), an inflammation of the peritoneum. Peritonitis can also be caused by a perforated peptic ulcer or by traumatic rupture of some abdominal organ.

The symptoms of peritonitis include a boardlike, rigid abdomen, pain that increases with motion or pressure to the abdomen, nausea, vomiting, and a low grade fever. The patient often attempts to avoid abdominal movement by shallow breathing.

The peritoneum has the ability to wall-off the infection provided the infection is not massive or the source of the infection does not continue. Normal intestinal movement ceases in the involved segment of the bowel, which helps to localize the infection. Untreated peritonitis, however can result in death.

INFLAMMATORY BOWEL DISEASE

Inflammatory bowel disease afflicts approximately two million Americans. Often, these are young people in the beginning of their adult lives with education, careers, and the raising of families ahead of them. The term **inflammatory bowel disease** is used to include two intestinal disorders: ulcerative colitis and Crohn's disease. These disorders have many similarities but 90% can be differentiated by clinical, radiological, and pathological findings.

Ulcerative Colitis

Ulcerative colitis is an inflammatory disease that usually affects young adults under the age of thirty. The disease usually begins in the rectum and moves upward. Mucosal cells slough away from the surface. Although ulcerations are not an essential part of this disease, they may develop and coalesce until the deep muscular layer of the colon becomes involved. It is a stress-related disease and emotional disturbances can precipitate exacerbations or prolong an attack.

Severe diarrhea is a classic symptom of this disease. Blood loss through the diarrheal stool can lead to anemia. Loss of the absorptive ability of the bowel and the severe diarrhea can lead to serious fluid and electrolyte imbalances.

Toxic megacolon is a medical emergency in which a segment of the diseased colon (usually the transverse colon) becomes extremely dilated. The complete obstruction that accompanies toxic megacolon usually occurs during acute exacerbations. Emergency intervention is necessary.

Individuals diagnosed with ulcerative colitis need to have a biannual sigmoidoscopy and barium enema because these people are predisposed to carcinoma and chronic ulcerative colitis.

Crohn's Disease
(Regional Enteritis)

Symptoms of Crohn's disease are similar to those of ulcerative colitis. These include abdominal pain, diarrhea, vomiting, fever, anal abscess, anorectal fissure fistulas, and weight loss related to nutritional deficits. Crohn's disease is a chronic relapsing disease that may develop in any segment of the alimentary tract from the mouth to the anus. The terminal ileum however, is most commonly affected. "Cobble-stone markings" is the name given to the characteristic edematous, reddish purple segments of the bowel that are interspersed with normal segments of bowel. Where ulcerative colitis usually involves only the distal portion of the large intestine, enteritis frequently involves the entire colon and the distal portion of the ileum, including all layers of the submucosa (transmural). While steatorrhea is common, malignancy rarely occurs. Fistulas frequently form communicating channels from one portion of the intestine to another.

APPENDICITIS

Appendicitis is an inflammation of the appendix characterized by acute abdominal pain that starts in the epigastrium or periumbilical region and progresses to the right lower quadrant. A fecalith (a hardened piece of stool) or fibrous disease of the wall of the bowel may occlude the appendix causing appendicitis. The individual characteristically "guards" this area by lying still and drawing up the right leg to relieve tension on the abdominal muscles. Other signs and symptoms include vomiting, loss of appetite, a low-grade fever, and bad breath. The white blood count is usually slightly elevated.

CANCER OF THE COLON AND RECTUM

Cancer of the lower intestinal tract is the second most frequent cause of death from cancer in the United States. This disease primarily afflicts individuals over fifty years of age and has a 50% cure rate. Risk factors may be familial colon cancer and ulcerative colitis. Other factors include lack of bulk in the diet, high fat diet, and high bacterial counts.

Signs and symptoms include altered bowel patterns, abdominal cramps, pain, and obstruction. Bloody stools, either occult or gross, are indications of moderate to advanced disease. Two-thirds of all colon cancers can be readily seen on a sigmoidoscopic examination. Early detection is important since localized lesions have a high curability rate.

Although carcinoembryonic antigen (CEA) level has previously been used to screen for early colonic cancer, its major value is not believed to be for the management of recurrent or advanced colon cancer. The amount of CEA in the serum clearly indicates the stage of the disease.

The single most important prognostic factor in bowel cancer is the presence and extent of lymph node involvement. Surgery alone or in conjunction with radiation or chemotherapy are the preferred treatments. Surgery may involve removing a large portion of the diseased bowel. This results in a permanent colostomy. Whenever the rectal sphincter becomes involved, a permanent colostomy must be performed.

A colostomy is the surgical opening of a portion of the colon through the abdominal surface. Since the rectal sphincter is no longer functional, stool is diverted through the stoma into a pouch. A temporary colostomy is done to "rest" the bowel for a period of time. Feces are diverted to provide an inflamed or operative area time to heal.

Adjunctive therapies, those used in addition to surgery, include radiation and chemotherapy. Preoperative radiation therapy is aimed at reducing the size of the tumor or killing tumor cells. Postoperative radiation is used to kill any remaining tumor cells in an attempt to prevent the spread of the cancer.

Although chemotherapy has been basically unsuccessful in the treatment of colon cancers, much investigative research is being done in this area. Since no single chemotherapeutic agent has proven effective in the treatment of colon cancer, combinations of drugs are often used.

Anticoagulation therapy with streptokinase has been used to prevent cancer cells from metastasizing distantly. Immunotherapy treatment to enhance function of the immunological system is also being used as an adjunctive therapy.

INTESTINAL OBSTRUCTION

Intestinal obstruction can result from hernias, tumors, severe constipation, or interference with intestinal innervation inhibiting peristalsis. This interference is called paralytic **ileus** (il'e-us) and is a fairly common complication of any abdominal surgery.

Proximal to the obstruction the bowel is distended; whereas distal to the obstruction the bowel is empty. Peristalsis is very forceful proximal to the obstruction and causes severe, intermittent cramps. You can hear these peristaltic waves with a stethoscope. Distal to the obstruction there will be no bowel sounds. The patient will experience severe vomiting, which after a time is foul-smelling. If the obstruction is very low, however, the patient may not vomit. The treatment is the surgical removal of whatever is causing the obstruction.

Surgery is indicated to relieve mechanical obstructions caused by adhesions and hernias. Paralytic ileus, however, may be relieved by intestinal intubation: either a Cantor tube or a Miller-Abbot tube is introduced through the mouth and advanced to the small intestine to remove the contents of the bowel. As the bowel is decompressed, peristalsis returns. These tubes can be used prior to and after abdominal surgery.

HEMORRHOIDS

Congestion in the veins of the rectum can lead to **varicosities** (var-e-kos'i-tes) or hemorrhoids. Constipation, straining at defecation, pregnancy, and a variety of other factors that increase the intraabdominal pressure may contribute to the development of hemorrhoids.

DISORDERS OF THE GALLBLADDER

CHOLELITHIASIS

Cholelithiasis is the presence of gallstones. The two most common symptoms are pain and jaundice. The pain may be constant and intense, starting in the upper midline region and migrating to the right upper quadrant.

Although fatty-food intolerance, flatulence, bloating, and heartburn are characteristic of gallbladder disease, they are not specific for cholelithiasis. The most common treatment for symptomatic patients is a cholecystectomy, the surgical removal of the gallbladder.

CHOLECYSTITIS

Cholecystitis is the inflammation of the gallbladder, which may be either acute or chronic. Acute cholecystitis usually follows impaction of a gallstone in the cystic duct. The gallbladder becomes distended with bile, blood, and pus.

The major symptom of cholecystitis is severe epigastric and subscapular pain or pain in the right upper quadrant. The pain starts suddenly and increases in intensity and peaks after thirty minutes. Nausea and vomiting frequently accompany the pain. Most patients have a low-grade fever and an intolerance to fatty foods. Jaundice may be evident if obstruction is present. Intravenous cholangiography is the preferred diagnostic method since nausea and vomiting may impede use of the oral cholecystogram.

Chronic cholecystitis results from repeated attacks of acute cholecystitis. The ability of the gallbladder to concentrate bile is lost, leading to long-standing dyspepsia, fat intolerance, and flatulence. The treatment is a cholecystectomy after the acute inflammation has subsided.

DISEASES OF THE PANCREAS

PANCREATITIS

Pancreatitis is an inflammation of the pancreas with varying degrees of edema, fat necrosis, and hemorrhage. Chemical inflammation of the pancreas is caused by duct obstruction or increased pancreatic secretion. Acute pancreatitis is frequently found in conjunction with biliary tract disease or alcoholism.

The onset of the disease is characterized by nausea and vomiting, severe left-sided radiating pain, and a boardlike, tender abdomen. Symptoms are generally brought about by ingestion of large quantities of food or alcohol. Hypovolemia can result as the pancreas becomes inflamed and edematous. A large volume of plasma can become trapped in the gland.

Autodigestion is caused by trapped pancreatic enzymes. These enzymes continue digesting within the pancreas and eventually act on other surrounding tissues. Nasogastric suction will inhibit the pancreatic secretions. The patient will not be allowed food or fluids by mouth for several days and so intravenous fluids and electrolytes are given. Antibiotics and analgesics are also given.

Chronic pancreatitis results from repeated attacks of acute pancreatitis. Pancreatic secretions are minimal, leading to malabsorption and steatorrhea (ste"ah-to-re'ah) or fatty stools. Pain may be dull and become severe as acute attacks reoccur. Most patients also have jaundice, hyperglycemia, weight loss, and abdominal distention. Alcoholism is believed to be a major contributing factor in the development of chronic pancreatitis.

DISEASES OF THE LIVER

HEPATITIS

There are three types of viral hepatitis: Type A, Type B, and Type C (or Non-A, Non-B) (see Table 18-1). Distinct viruses have been found to cause Type A and Type B, but both result in similar systemic manifestations. The liver becomes inflamed and tender. The virus of hepatitis A, or infectious hepatitis, is usually transmitted by the fecal-oral route. Ingestion of infected water, milk, or food, particularly raw shellfish, can result in epidemics of hepatitis A. Hepatitis A virus can be found in the feces and other bodily secretions before symptoms are apparent. The incubation period lasts from 15 to 45 days. An infected person is most contagious before symptoms occur, leading to widespread contamination of household members and other close contacts. An exposed individual may be protected from the disease or decrease the severity of the infection by receiving immune serum globulin. Seven to nine days after jaundice occurs, the individual is no longer infectious.

Hepatitis B, serum hepatitis, has a longer incubation period than hepatitis A, lasting from 28 to 160 days. Although hepatitis B is transmitted primarily via the blood, there is evidence of transmission via the semen and respiratory

Table 18-1. Comparison of Types of Viral Hepatitis

Type	Incubation Period and Contamination Source	Signs and Symptoms
A	15 to 45 days Raw shellfish, water, oral contact with fecal matter, rarely blood or body secretions	Fatigue, clay-colored stool, dark yellow urine, right upper quadrant pain, nausea, vomiting, diarrhea, edema of skin and mucous membranes, occasional visceral swelling, cough, sore throat, irritated nasal mucous membrane, fever between 100°F and 104°F, abnormal serum levels of SGOT and SGPT 1 to 2 weeks before jaundice appears, elevated bilirubin and urobilinogen after jaundice appears
B	26 to 160 days Vaginal or anal intercourse, breast milk, saliva, blood, syringes and needles	Low-grade fever, hives or rash, nausea, vomiting, diarrhea, headache, right upper quadrant pain, edema of skin and mucous membranes, occasional visceral swelling, joint pain, elevated SGOT and SGPT 1 to 2 weeks prior to appearance of jaundice, hepatitis B antigen (Australian antigen), symptoms are more severe than Type A possibly leading to massive liver necrosis and death
C	14 to 115 days Blood transfusions, syringes and needles	Mental and physical fatigue, anorexia, nausea, vomiting, diarrhea, headache, right upper quadrant pain from liver distention, hives or rash, joint pain, edema of skin and mucous membranes, elevated SGOT and SGPT 1 to 2 weeks before jaundice appears

secretions. Individuals at risk are health care workers who come into contact with patient's blood, patients who have had multiple blood transfusions or dialysis, drug addicts, dentists, and male homosexuals.

The course of hepatitis B is more virulent than Type A. In this type of hepatitis there may be massive liver destruction, chronic hepatitis, coma, and even death.

The clinical courses of Type A and Type B are similar. The individuals are symptom-free during the incubation period but following this the patient is jaundiced and has clay-colored stools, and dark urine. Pruritis, which is caused by the accumulation of bile in the skin, may precede the jaundice. Other symptoms caused by lack of liver function and infection include fatigue and weakness, anemia, bleeding tendencies, right upper quadrant pain, fever, anorexia, nausea, and vomiting. Profound mental changes or changes in the level of consciousness need to be evaluated closely for the possibility of hepatic coma.

Hepatitis B vaccine has recently become available for individuals at risk. Taken from the serum of carriers, the vaccine is fairly expensive and in limited supply. Immunization must occur prior to exposure to hepatitis B.

Hepatitis C (Non-A, Non-B) is found in individuals who have received multiple blood transfusions. This relatively uncommon form has an incubation period lasting from 14 to 115 days. Recovery from this form is much longer, and these individuals are more prone to develop chronic hepatitis.

The main treatment for hepatitis is rest and diet. The diet for an individual with hepatitis is based on that person's tolerance of specific foods. A sufficient number of calories must be provided for tissue repair. Those individuals who are unable to ingest a sufficient number of calories may need to receive intravenous fluids. Fat and protein intake is not limited unless me-

tabolism of these substances is impaired. Alcohol ingestion and cigarette smoking should be avoided.

Hepatitis caused by alcohol is either an acute or chronic inflammation of the liver. In some cases it is reversible. However, alcoholic hepatitis is the most frequent cause of cirrhosis. Symptoms usually develop after heavy alcohol ingestion. Patients will experience anorexia, nausea, abdominal pain, splenomegaly, hepatomegaly, jaundice, ascites, fever, and encephalopathy. The diagnosis of alcoholic hepatitis is confirmed by a liver biopsy.

Patients are placed on a high carbohydrate diet with high vitamin and folic acid supplements. Intravenous fluids are administered for hydration and to maintain electrolyte balance. Steroids are sometimes administered to decrease the inflammation.

CIRRHOSIS

In cirrhosis of the liver, there is a disruption of the normal flow of blood, bile, and hepatic metabolites leading to the loss of hepatic function. The most common form of cirrhosis, portal cirrhosis, results from chronic alcoholism. The cirrhotic changes are preceded by fatty infiltration of the liver cells. There is abdominal pain, indigestion, and anorexia. The patients fatigue easily, and have frequent infections and general malaise. Jaundice is not generally apparent until the later stages of the disease. **Ascites** (ahsi'tez), an accumulation of fluid in the peritoneal cavity, and edema of the feet and legs are also signs of advanced disease. The liver becomes shrunken and hardened, compressing the blood vessels. The narrowing of the portal venules leads to an increased back pressure in the portal vein and an increased blood pressure in the mesenteric capillaries.

Varicose veins of the esophagus and rectum may develop as a result of this increased pressure in the veins leading to the liver. These varicosities can hemorrhage and the hemorrhages may be complicated by the lack of necessary clotting factors and other blood proteins normally produced by the liver. Surgical ligation may be necessary to control the bleeding. Medical intervention consists of the use of sclerosing drugs, drugs to reduce portal pressure, or the insertion of a tube with a balloon tamponade that constricts esophageal and gastric vessels. The prognosis is generally poor for these patients.

Liver transplant is now considered an alternative intervention for patients with cirrhosis, hepatic malignancy, biliary atresia, and other forms of end-stage liver disease. Immunosuppressive therapy is used to help prevent rejection of the transplanted organ.

POISON

FOOD POISONING

Food poisoning is a particular type of gastritis caused by toxins produced by staphylococci. The illness is not usually caused by eating foods that have "spoiled"; we know that in many parts of the world "aged" or "seasoned" foods are popular and ingested without harm. Pathogenic organisms produce the toxin that causes the illness.

Cooking can destroy the organism but will not eliminate the poison already formed. Foods that are allowed to remain without refrigeration before being cooked are the most dangerous. Seafoods removed from the shell some time before they are eaten, potato salad, creamed chicken, and other creamed or custard dishes are often sources of the problem.

Infections caused by salmonella are associated with ingestion of contaminated eggs and poultry. Recently, eggs cooked "sunny-side up" were identified as a source of salmonella. Also, eating raw eggs, as in eggnog, can cause the illness.

Nausea, vomiting, diarrhea, cramping, and abdominal pain occur from one to six hours after eating the offending food. Although distressing, these symptoms help to remove some of the toxins from the body. The treatment is symptomatic; usually, fluids such as tea, broth, or boiled milk can be tolerated within a short time.

Mushroom poisoning is the most common cause of death from food poisoning. The symptoms are the same as for other types of food poisoning. However, symptoms can be delayed for as much as 24 hours. If the problem is recognized within an hour or so, it may be possible to prevent the absorption by inducing vomiting. Apart from this, the treatment is simply to try to relieve the symptoms. If large amounts of poison are absorbed there is very likely to be shock, confusion, and possibly convulsions.

Botulism (bot'u-lism) is a severe and, fortunately, relatively uncommon type of food poisoning. It is caused by a spore-forming organism. This type of microorganism can develop a thick coat called a spore (spor) which protects the organism from agents that would ordinarily destroy germs. Improper home canning is often the source of this type of food poisoning. The mortality rate from botulism in the United States is about 65%.

INGESTED POISONS

The subject of poisons and the management of cases of poisoning are very complicated because two major unknowns often exist: the sensitivity of the patient to the poisonous substance and the nature of the poison. Of the thousands of Americans who die of accidental poisoning every year, about one-third are children under 5 years of age. Often, it is difficult to determine what the child has ingested. Even when the na-

.ure of the poison is known, a child may be too ill or too frightened to cooperate with attempts to deal with the situation. Parents are very likely overwhelmed with guilt. In many situations, their guilt is not unrealistic because the tragedy might not have happened had they taken proper precautions for the storage of potentially hazardous substances. Clearly, a well disciplined child is likely to be a safe child.

The incidence of fatalities from accidental poisoning has decreased dramatically in recent years due to child-proof packaging and public awareness of poison prevention. The Safety Packaging Law passed in 1974 requires that all prescription drugs, with the exception of nitroglycerin and Isordil, be packaged in safety-seal containers. Parents are advised to keep all medications inaccessible to children. Children should never be told that medication is candy. They may believe it and act accordingly. Many medication poisonings result from children taking medication from medicine cabinets or bedside tables.

Poisoning also results from the ingestion of cleaning compounds by children. Cleaning compounds should always be stored in their original containers, out of reach of children. Dangerous solutions should not be stored in soda-pop bottles or in any container that resembles one ordinarily used for beverages or food.

GENERAL PRINCIPLES FOR THE TREATMENT OF POISONING

In most instances, the unabsorbed poison should be removed as quickly as possible by inducing vomiting or by lavage. You perform lavage by inserting a stomach tube into the nose and on down to the stomach and irrigating the stomach with water or some solution that will inactivate the poison.

It is generally useless to induce vomiting or to lavage if the poison was ingested more than two hours before, unless the victim is in shock, in which case at least some of the poison has probably not been absorbed. Warm mustard or salt water is often recommended to induce vomiting. Although such concoctions are nauseating and will indeed cause vomiting, most children will not swallow such a bad-tasting fluid and you will lose valuable time preparing the concoction. You should give the child a glass of milk or water. Most young children will vomit if they quickly swallow large quantities of fluid. If not, you can gag the child with your finger or by stroking the posterior pharynx with a blunt instrument. To prevent aspiration of the emesis, you should invert the body and support the head. If available, syrup of ipecac (ip′e-kak) in doses of 10 to 15 ml repeated after 15 or 20 minutes will usually induce vomiting. If the ipecac is given and emesis does not occur, lavage is imperative because ipecac is irritating to the stomach and can cause serious problems if absorbed.

In certain situations you should not induce vomiting. If the poison is corrosive (an acid or alkali) it has done enough damage by burning the esophagus when it was swallowed. Clearly, you will compound the damage by causing vomiting. Do not induce vomiting if the victim is unconsious because of the danger of his aspirating the emesis. If the toxic substance is oily, again the danger of aspiration contraindicates inducing vomiting. As discussed in Chapter 16, oil aspiration pneumonia can be very serious.

Neither should you stimulate vomiting if the patient is convulsing, because it will increase the severity of the convulsions. If sedation and measures to control the convulsions are available, you can lavage the patient.

A second general principle to observe in dealing with a patient who has ingested poison, particularly if the unabsorbed poison cannot be removed, is to prevent the absorption of the poison. One or two ounces of olive oil or other vegetable oil by mouth, but not forced, may help delay the absorption of poisons. Demulcents, such as a mixture of flour and water, beaten eggs, or mashed potatoes in water, will not only delay the absorption of the poison but also soothe the irritated mucosa. Administer only limited quantities of these solutions. One cup of the demulcent is sufficient. Excess amounts may open the pyloric valve and allow the poison to pass into the small intestine, where it is much more likely to be absorbed than if it remains in the stomach. Recall that relatively little absorption takes place in the stomach.

Activated charcoal, one or two tablespoons in eight ounces of water, is a potent absorbent and rapidly inactivates many poisons. You can substitute burned toast for activated charcoal, although it is not as effective.

Identify the poison as soon as possible so that specific measures can be taken. Poison Control Centers, which exist in most major U.S. cities, can identify the poisonous ingredient in most household substances. They can also tell you over the telephone what immediate first-aid measures to take until the victim can be brought to a treatment center.

SUMMARY QUESTIONS

1. What preparation is necessary for a patient who is to have X-ray studies of the upper part of his gastrointestinal tract?
2. What preparation is necessary for a patient who is going to have a barium enema?
3. How do gastric and duodenal ulcers differ?
4. Discuss the treatments of peptic ulcers.
5. List several symptoms of cirrhosis of the liver.
6. What is ascites and what causes it?
7. What is cholelithiasis and what is the usual treatment?
8. What causes cholecystitis?
9. Discuss the emergency management of an accidental poisoning.
10. Discuss the causes of the different types of hepatitis.
11. What is a cholecystogram?

KEY TERMS

anorexia
ascites
diverticulum
dyspepsia
dysphagia
hematemesis

ileus
inflammatory bowel disease
occult blood
peritonitis
varicosities

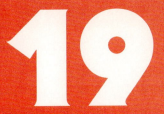

The Urinary System

OBJECTIVES

On completion of this chapter, you will be able to:

1. Describe the structures of the urinary system.
2. Discuss the functions of each part of the nephron unit.
3. List factors influencing urine production.
4. Describe the processes involved in the acidification of urine.
5. Discuss the renal mechanisms that help to maintain normal blood pH.

OVERVIEW

I. KIDNEYS
   A. Cortex
   B. Renal Medulla
   C. Renal Pelvis
II. URETERS
III. URINARY BLADDER
IV. URETHRA
V. URINE FORMATION
   A. Filtration and Selective Reabsorption
   B. Acidification of Urine and Regulation of
      Blood pH
   C. Tubular Secretion
   D. Urine Volume and Concentration
VI. MICTURITION

The organs of the urinary system include the kidneys, ureters, urinary bladder, and urethra. Functions of this system include the elimination of some of the soluble waste products and the regulation of water and electrolyte balance.

In addition to the kidney being an organ of this excretory system, it can cause the production of a hormone that influences the vascular diameter and the amount of sodium in the blood. When the arterial blood pressure falls below normal or there is a decrease in oxygen supply to the kidney, the kidney secretes a substance termed **renin** (re'nin) into the bloodstream. Renin causes the production of a plasma protein, **angiotensin** I (an"ge-o-ten'sin), which is rapidly converted to angiotensin II. Although angiotensin II is in the bloodstream for only one to three minutes, it is a powerful vasoconstrictor. With constriction of the arterioles, blood pressure can return to normal. Angiotensin also causes the adrenal cortex to produce aldosterone, a mineral corticoid, increasing the amount of sodium in the bloodstream and decreasing the blood potassium level.

Certain kidney cells are sensitive to a lack of oxygen and respond by releasing a renal erythropoietic factor. This factor activates a plasma hormone, erythropoietin (e-rith"ro-poi'e-tin), which stimulates the bone marrow to produce and release new erythrocytes.

KIDNEYS

The kidneys are retroperitoneal (behind the peritoneum) on the posterior wall of the abdominal cavity between the level of T12 (twelfth thoracic vertebra) and L3 (third lumbar vertebra). They are about 11 to 12 cm long and 5 to 6 cm wide; they are bean-shaped with their concave border directed toward the midline. The ureters and blood vessels leave and enter from the hilum (hi'lum), which lies in the middle of the concave border. The kidneys are supported by renal fascia (fash'e-ah), the peritoneum, and adipose tissue. With severe weight loss, adipose support may be lacking and the kidneys can become displaced downward; this condition is called **nephroptosis** (nef-rop-to'sis). Nephroptosis can result in stasis of urine and predisposition to renal calculi (kal'ku-li) or kidney stones.

CORTEX

The outer part of the kidney is called the renal **cortex** (kor'tex). On cross section, the cortex has a granular, reddish-brown appearance. This part of the kidney contains most of the structures of the microscopic nephron (nef'ron) units. Most of the work of the kidney is done by the nephron units. You should know the various parts of the nephron units and understand the functions of these structures. Figure 19-1 shows the major anatomical parts of a nephron unit

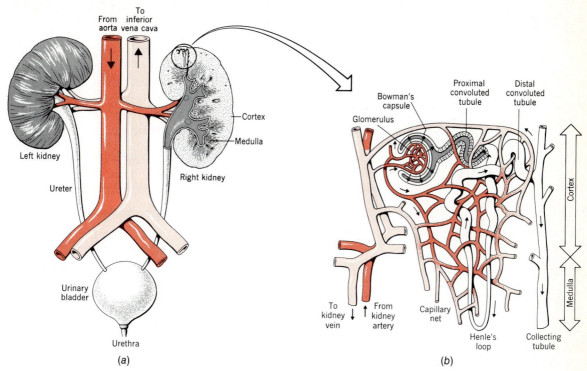

Figure 19-1. *(a) Kidneys, ureters, and bladder, and (b) a nephron unit and related structures. The collecting tubules, which are not microscopic, give the pyramids of the medullary portion of the kidney a striated appearance. As shown, there are some collecting tubules in the cortical portion of the kidney.*

and the related structures. You will find it helpful to refer to this illustration as the functions of the various parts of the nephron and the circulation surrounding it are discussed.

The afferent arteriole, which is derived from the renal artery, leads into a tuft of glomerular (glo-mer′u-lar) capillaries. The blood pressure in these capillaries is normally higher than it is in the capillaries of most other areas of the body. For this reason, a great deal of fluid and crystalline particles are filtered out of the glomerular capillaries into Bowman's capsule. Actually about 100 times the amount of fluid that ultimately will be excreted as urine within 24 hours is filtered out of these glomerular capillaries.

The filtration rate is about 120 ml per minute or 170 liters in 24 hours. Recall that stimulation of the sympathetic nervous system causes vasoconstriction and an increase in blood pressure. This would lead one to believe that the glomerular filtration rate would increase with stimulation of the sympathetic nervous system and that valuable vascular fluid would be lost. Fortunately, this is not the case because with stimulation of the sympathetic nervous system the afferent arteriole is constricted more than the efferent, which results in a decrease in the filtration rate. The glomerular filtrate has the same crystalline composition and pH as does the blood plasma. This fluid contains amino acids, glucose, and electrolytes; however, it does not normally contain blood proteins or blood cells. From the glomerular capillaries, blood flows into a smaller efferent arteriole. Note that here we have blood flowing from an arteriole to a capillary and then to another arteriole, not to a venule. This arrangement is one of the reasons why the blood pressure is so high in these glomerular capillaries. From the efferent arteriole the blood then goes to the peritubular capillaries and finally back to the renal vein. These peritubular capillaries are nutrient to the nephron unit. It is through these peritubular capillaries that much of the glomerular filtrate is returned to the bloodstream.

RENAL MEDULLA

For the most part, the collecting tubules are located in the medullary (med'u-lar"e) portion of the kidney and give the pyramids their striated appearance. In the collecting tubules, depending on the body's need to conserve fluid, varying amounts of water are returned to the bloodstream and the urine becomes more or less concentrated. The specific gravity of normal urine ranges from about 1.010 to 1.030. Ordinarily, the first voiding of the morning will have a higher specific gravity than the urine voided later in the day when the person has consumed fluids.

RENAL PELVIS

The tips of the pyramids are called papillae. The papillae are located within a portion of the renal pelvis called calyces (kal'a-seez). From the collecting tubules the urine then goes into the calyx of the renal pelvis, which has a smooth, yellowish-white appearance. The pelvis merely serves as a basin for the collection of the urine before the urine is passed on to the ureters.

URETERS

The ureters are narrow tubes leading from the kidney to the urinary bladder. The mucous membrane that lines the ureters is continuous with the mucous membrane lining of the urinary bladder and the urethra.

URINARY BLADDER

The urinary bladder is a hollow muscular organ located anterior to the rectum, and in the female it is anterior to the uterus and vagina. A full urinary bladder may rise up into the abdominal cavity and usually can be palpated above the symphysis pubis.

The urinary bladder is lined with mucous membrane. The lining has rugae to allow for expansion. At the inferior and posterior part of the urinary bladder is an area that has no rugae. This area, the trigone (tri'gon), is a triangular structure where urine from the two ureters enters the bladder and urine leaves the bladder to enter the urethra.

URETHRA

The female urethra is about 4 cm long and runs obliquely down and forward from the bladder. It has only an excretory function (see Fig. 21-1).

In the male, the urethra is about 20 cm long and has an S-shaped curve. Normally, one of these curves is straightened out for a man to void or to be catheterized. The male urethra has both an excretory and reproductive function.

Note in Figure 21-6, that from the urinary

bladder the first portion of the male urethra is completely surrounded by the **prostate** (pros'tate) gland. This portion of the urethra is called the prostatic urethra. From the prostatic urethra, urine passes into a short segment called the membranous urethra and then into the cavernous (kav'er-nus) urethra. It is a congestion of blood in these cavernous spaces that causes the erection of the penis.

URINE FORMATION

FILTRATION AND SELECTIVE REABSORPTION

Urine formation begins with the filtration of fluid and crystalline solutes out of the glomerular capillaries into Bowman's capsule. Normally, about 170 liters of fluid are filtered from the glomerular capillaries every 24 hours in an adult male. Since the 24-hour urine output is normally only about 1.5 liters, most of this water will be returned to the bloodstream in the process of urine formation. Many substances, such as glucose, amino acids, and some electrolytes, present in the glomerular filtrate will also be returned to the bloodstream. About 70% of this reabsorption takes place in the proximal convoluted tubules.

The amount of glucose in the glomerular filtrate is the same as in the blood (fasting blood sugar is about 80 to 130 mg/100 ml). Normally, all of this glucose is removed by active transport from the fluid in the proximal tubules and is returned to the bloodstream. The maximum concentration of a substance, such as glucose, that can be returned to the plasma is called the renal threshold. In uncontrolled diabetes mellitus or other conditions in which the blood glucose level is very high, the amount of glucose in

the filtrate may exceed the ability of the kidney tubule cells to reabsorb it. Thus, the glucose will remain in the urine. This is called **glycosuria** (gli-ko-su're-ah). The glucose that remains in the tubular fluid exerts an osmotic pressure, thereby preventing the reabsorption of water causing dehydration and polyuria or increased urinary output.

Normally, all of the amino acids in the glomerular filtrate are reabsorbed by the proximal convoluted tubular cells. With normal kidney function, there is no protein in the urine.

Urea (u-re'ah), a waste product of protein metabolism, is present in the glomerular filtrate. This substance is not actively transported from the tubule and normally will be eliminated in the urine. If the concentration of urea is unusually high, some will pass from the tubule by simple diffusion and be returned to the bloodstream.

The kidney tubular cells reabsorb electrolytes selectively. There will be more reabsorption of an electrolyte when it is present in small amounts in the blood than when it is present in excess amounts. By this process of selective reabsorption, the renal tubules control the concentration of electrolytes in the body fluids. The reabsorption of electrolytes from the glomerular filtrate and their return to the bloodstream, therefore, depend for the most part on the relative concentration of these in the bloodstream. The exception to this is potassium. For the most part, the renal regulatory function as regards potassium is to eliminate it regardless of its blood level.

Some hormones influence the tubular reabsorption of electrolytes. The **parathyroid** (par"-ah-thi'roid) **hormone** increases the reabsorption of calcium ions.

Aldosterone (al-do-ster'on), a hormone from the adrenal cortex, favors the reabsorption of sodium and decreases the potassium reabsorption. Chloride and bicarbonate reabsorption are secondary to that of sodium. For every sodium, a cation, reabsorbed from the tubules, a chloride or bicarbonate anion is also reabsorbed.

The process of selectively reabsorbing solutes from the glomerular filtrate helps maintain the normal electrolyte balance of the body and the delicate blood pH discussed in Chapter 1. The process of producing acid urine from the glomerular filtrate, which has a pH of about 7.4, also helps in the regulation of normal body electrolyte balance and blood pH.

ACIDIFICATION OF URINE AND REGULATION OF BLOOD pH

The acidification of urine is accomplished by the reabsorption of bicarbonate and the conversion of sodium monoamine hydrogen phosphate in the tubular fluid to acid sodium dihydrogen phosphate. Both processes are possible because the kidney tubular cells, as any other cells in the body, produce carbon dioxide and water in the process of their metabolism. The carbon dioxide and water form carbonic acid, which ionizes to form hydrogen and bicarbonate. Because the hydrogen is a cation, it makes an even exchange with the sodium in the tubular fluid. The sodium that enters the tubular cells combines with the bicarbonate and returns to the peritubular capillaries. The hydrogen in the tubular urine increases the acidity of the urine, and the sodium that was saved helps preserve the base pH of the plasma.

By a similar mechanism, base sodium monoamine hydrogen phosphate in the tubular urine is converted to acid phosphate by the exchange of a sodium from the tubular fluid for a hydrogen from the tubular cell.

The kidney also can help maintain the acid-base balance by converting neutral urea to ammonium. Recall that the urea was formed by the liver in the process of the deaminization of proteins. Ordinarily, most of the nitrogenous wastes are eliminated in the form of neutral urea. However, in the presence of acidosis when the kidney is compensating by eliminating more and more acid in the urine, some of the urea will be converted to ammonium (NH_4) to prevent the urine from becoming too acid. This ammonium does not have an ammonia-like odor. However, on standing urine will have an odor because of the decomposition of either urea or ammonium.

Another important aspect of the kidney's role in the regulation of blood pH is that of providing some compensatory mechanisms for acidosis and alkalosis. As discussed in Chapters 1 and 15, disturbances in the delicate blood pH balance can be caused by a variety of conditions.

The mechanisms by which the kidney regulates acid-base balance are slow. Whereas the respiratory responses to alterations in acid-base balance begin almost immediately, the renal response does not begin for several hours after a disturbance in the blood pH has occurred and clinical evidence of the effectiveness of the renal compensation may not be seen for three or four days.

When the blood pH goes below 7.3, the kidney will eliminate more hydrogen and retain more bicarbonate. More nitrogenous wastes will be eliminated in the form of ammonium rather than urea. To compensate for a blood pH over 7.4, the kidney will retain more hydrogen and eliminate increasing amounts of bicarbonate.

TUBULAR SECRETION

In addition to the secretion of urea and ammonium, the tubular cells can secrete other substances such as penicillin, histamine, phenobarbital, hydrogen, potassium, dyes, and **creatinine** (kre-at′i-nin), which is a waste product. Tubular secretion is the basis for a common diagnostic test, the PSP test, used to assess kidney function.

URINE VOLUME AND CONCENTRATION

The volume and concentration of urine is influenced by the quantity of fluid intake and the elimination of fluid waste by other routes such as the sweat glands and intestines. Since the formation of the glomerular filtrate depends on blood pressure, it is clear that an abnormally low blood pressure may be inadequate for the required filtration. Therefore, urine production will be reduced. As a result of this decreased urinary output the vascular volume will not be diminished and therefore to some extent the low blood pressure may be compensated.

The antidiuretic (an"te-di-u-ret'ik) hormone, or ADH, helps regulate both the volume and the concentration of urine. This hormone is released from the posterior pituitary in response to the concentration of solutes in the blood flowing through the hypothalamus. If there has been a decrease in fluid intake and therefore the concentration is high, the hormone is released, increasing the permeability of the distal and collecting tubules, and more water is absorbed and returned to the bloodstream. Less urine is produced, and the concentration of the urine is increased.

Some drugs called **diuretics** (di-u-ret'iks) increase urine volume by decreasing the reabsorption of sodium from the glomerular filtrate. Drugs that increase blood flow to the kidney also have a diuretic effect. Ethyl alcohol inhibits the release of ADH, and therefore more urine is produced.

MICTURITION

Micturition (mik"ter-rish'un) is the reflex act of expelling urine. The stimulus is the stretching of the bladder wall. Normally, this stimulus is the stretching of the wall when approximately 250 to 300 ml of urine has accumulated. Although micturition is a reflex, we develop the ability to control and inhibit the reflex mechanism so that micturition becomes a voluntary act. Micturition can be inhibited voluntarily until about 600 ml of urine has accumulated in the urinary bladder. Micturition can be voluntarily induced by contracting abdominal and pelvic muscles.

SUMMARY QUESTIONS

1. Where are the kidneys located?
2. Name the parts of the nephron unit and discuss the functions of each of these parts.
3. What structures convey urine from the kidney to the urinary bladder?
4. List several factors that influence urine production.
5. Describe the structure of the urinary bladder.
6. Explain the processes involved in the acidification of urine.
7. How do the kidneys help to maintain normal blood pH?

KEY TERMS

aldosterone
angiotensin
cortex
creatinine
diuretics
glycosuria

micturition
nephroptosis
parathyroid hormone
prostate
renin
urea

20

Diseases of the Urinary System

OBJECTIVES

On completion of this chapter, you will be able to:

1. Describe the proper procedures for obtaining several types of urine specimens.
2. List the common abnormal constituents of urine.
3. List blood chemistry studies most commonly done for patients with renal disease.
4. Describe the types of X-ray studies that are commonly done to diagnose diseases of the urinary system.
5. Define hydronephrosis and list possible causes of this condition.
6. List some foods that tend to cause the production of alkaline urine.
7. Describe the signs and symptoms of renal calculi.
8. List the symptoms of cystitis.
9. Define pyelonephritis and list possible causes of this disease.
10. Explain the basic principles of dialysis and tell how these procedures are done.

OVERVIEW

I. DIAGNOSTIC MEASURES
  A. Urine Tests
  B. Blood Tests
  C. X-rays
  D. Other Examinations
II. DISEASES OF THE URINARY SYSTEM
  A. Urinary Obstructions
    1. Strictures
  B. Calculi
  C. Nephroptosis
  D. Tumors
  E. Infections
    1. Cystitis
    2. Pyelonephritis
    3. Glomerulonephritis
    4. Renal Hypertension
    5. Renal Failure
    6. Uremia
III. DIALYSIS
  A. Peritoneal Dialysis
  B. Hemodialysis
IV. KIDNEY TRANSPLANT

In addition to being a major excretory organ of the body, the kidney adjusts the fluid and electrolyte balance of the body and therefore, together with the respiratory system, is of vital importance in maintaining the blood pH. Inasmuch as the kidney also plays an important role in the regulation of blood pressure as well as in the production of red blood cells, it is clear that problems that disrupt kidney function can have some serious consequences. In this chapter, we will consider some of the more common disease processes of the urinary system and the diagnostic measures that are commonly used in conjunction with these problems.

DIAGNOSTIC MEASURES

URINE TESTS

Urinalysis is the examination of urine and is part of any routine physical examination. It is the single most important test used in diagnosing urinary problems. Urine tests are performed ideally on fresh specimens, preferably the first voiding of the day because this sample is most concentrated. All urine samples should be refrigerated as soon as possible after voiding, except those being cultured.

The simple voided specimen is commonly used during any physical examination. However, if urinary tract infection is suspected, the specimen should be obtained by catheterization or a clean-caught midstream sample.

Catheterized Specimens
All equipment used in catheterization must be sterile since there is danger of introducing outside bacteria into the bladder. Necessary supplies include an antiseptic solution for cleansing, cotton balls, a container for the specimen, catheter, lubricant, and gloves. The procedure is normally painless but excess fear and embarrassment can cause tension and discomfort. For this reason, it is important that the procedure is explained to the patient. After the area around the meatus is cleansed, the catheter is inserted through the meatus into the urinary bladder and a sample of about 60 ml of urine is obtained. Even with sterile precautions, this procedure is used only when absolutely necessary.

Clean-Caught Midstream Specimens
This method of obtaining a urine specimen for bacteriologic culture is a reliable alternative to catheterization, since contamination of the urine by organisms residing near the urethral

meatus is avoided. The patient is instructed to expose the urethral orifice and cleanse around the meatus. As the patient voids, the first portion is discarded since this urine washes away any contaminants in the urethra. The midstream portion is collected in a sterile container, and the last portion is discarded.

Appearance and Composition of Urine

Normal, freshly voided urine is clear yellow to golden yellow. Dilute urine is straw-colored and concentrated urine is highly colored. Cloudiness may indicate pus in the urine, and reddish-brown or brown urine may contain blood. Urine color can also be affected by foods or drugs recently ingested.

The concentration of urine or specific gravity is measured with a urinometer. Enough urine to float the urinometer (about 30 ml) is placed in a small cylinder. The reading is taken at the point where the scale touches the surface of the urine. The average range is 1.010 to 1.030. However, concentrations as low as 1.005 or as high as 1.125 are not abnormal. A decreased specific gravity is one of the first indications of renal tubular dysfunction; it is also seen in diabetes insipidus. A high specific gravity is often seen in diabetes mellitus, dehydration, congestive heart failure, and liver disease.

Lab sticks are used to examine the urine for the presence of albumin, blood, glucose, and acetone and to determine the pH of the urine. The lab stick is dipped into the specimen and then compared with a color scale. Normally, urine contains no albumin, blood, acetone, or glucose and the urine pH is acid (see Tables 20-1 and 20-2).

A microscopic examination of urine may be indicated if blood cells are likely to be present. Also, microscopic casts are usually present in tubular renal disease.

Renal Clearance Tests

Clearance tests are done to evaluate the kidney's ability to clear or eliminate urea and creatinine (kre-at'i-nin). Because these substances are removed from the blood by glomerular filtration, a decreased clearance time can reflect a reduced glomerular filtration rate. For this test, the patient voids and discards this urine; the time of voiding is noted. For the next 24 hours all urine is collected and chilled. A measurement is made of the creatinine in these specimens. In addition a blood sample is collected and the plasma creatinine measured.

BLOOD TESTS

When kidney disease is suspected, blood is examined for the amount of blood urea nitrogen (BUN) content. Urea is the main endproduct of protein metabolism and is removed from the blood by the kidneys. Several factors increase the BUN level such as a high-protein diet, use of steroids, stressful situations, fever, and infection. A low-protein diet decreases the BUN level. Normally, the BUN measures 12 to 25 mg per 100 ml of blood. Patients with elevated BUN levels can be mentally confused due to the accumulated waste products remaining in the bloodstream, and this should be explained to their families.

Since the kidneys regulate the electrolyte concentrations of the blood, analysis of the levels of blood sodium, potassium, chloride, calcium, and phosphorus may be helpful in evaluating kidney function.

X-RAYS

Plain Abdominal Film (KUB)

This is an X-ray of the kidneys, ureters, and bladder and is done with no food or drink restriction. It is often the first X-ray done in assessing the urinary system because it notes the

Table 20-1. Composition of Urine in Health and Disease

Normal Range	*Conditions in Which Variations from Normal May Occur*
Volume in 24-hr. 1200–1500 ml (varies greatly with fluid intake)	Increased: diabetes insipidus, absorption of large quantities of edema fluid, diabetes mellitus, certain types of chronic renal disease, tumors of brain and spinal cord, myxedema, acromegaly, tabes dorsalis Decreased: dehydration, diseases that interfere with circulation to kidney, acute renal failure, uremia, acute intestinal obstruction, portal cirrhosis, peritonitis, poisoning by agents that damage kidneys
pH 4.7–8.0	Increased: compensatory phase of alkalosis, vegetable diet Decreased: compensatory phase of acidosis, administration of ammonium chloride or calcium chloride, diet of prunes or cranberries
Specific gravity 1.010–1.020	Increased: dehydration, administration of vasopressin tannate, glycosuria, albuminuria Decreased: diabetes insipidus, chronic nephritis
Urea 20–30 gm	Increased: tissue catabolism, febrile and wasting diseases, absorption of exudates as in suppurative processes Decreased: impaired liver function, myxedema, severe kidney diseases, compensatory phase of acidosis
Uric acid 0.60–0.75 gm	Increased: leukemia, polycythemia vera, liver disease, febrile diseases, eclampsia, absorption of exudates, X-ray therapy Decreased: before attack of gout, but increased during attack
Ammonia 0.5–15.0 gm	Increased: diabetic acidosis, pernicious vomiting of pregnancy, liver damage Decreased: alkalosis, administration of alkalies
Creatinine 0.30–0.45 gm	Increased: typhoid fever, typhus, anemia, tetanus, debilating diseases, renal insufficiency, leukemia, muscular atrophy
Calcium 30–150 mg	Increased: osteitis fibrosis cystica Decreased: tetany
Phosphates 0.9–1.3 gm	Increased: osteitis fibrosa, alkalosis, administration of parathormone
Chlorides 110–250 mEq.	Increased: Addison's disease Decreased: starvation, excessive sweating, vomiting, pneumonia, heart failure, burns, kidney disease
Sodium 43–217 mEq.	Increased: compensatory phase of alkalosis Decreased: compensatory phase of acidosis

17-Ketosteroids
  Men 5–27 mg
  Women 5–15 mg
	Increased: Cushing's syndrome, adrenal malignancy, administration of cortisone, administration of ACTH, ovarian tumors
	
	Decreased: hypopituitarism, pituitary tumors, Addison's disease, myxedema, hepatic disease, chronic debilitating diseases

Aldosterone up to 15 μg	Increased: adrenal malignancy, conditions associated with excessive sodium loss, cardiac failure, nephrosis, hepatic cirrhosis Decreased: Addison's disease, eclampsia

Table 20-1. Composition of Urine in Health and Disease—Con't

Normal Range	Conditions in Which Variations from Normal May Occur

Pressor amines
  Norepinephrine 5–100 μg
  Epinephrine 11.5 μg
	Increased: essential hypertension, pheochromocytoma, severe stress, insulin-induced hypoglycemia

Amylase 8,000–30,000 Wohlgemuth units	Increased: early in acute pancreatitis, perforated duodenal ulcer, stone in common bile duct, carcinoma of the pancreas or bile duct, salivary gland disease Decreased: some liver diseases and some renal diseases

From Shirley R. Burke, *The Composition and Function of Body Fluids* 3rd ed. (St. Louis, Mo.: The C. V. Mosby Co., 1980).

Table 20-2. Abnormal Constituents of Urine

Constituent	Conditions in Which Variations from Normal May Occur
Bence-Jones protein	Multiple myeloma, bone metastases of carcinoma, osteogenic sarcoma, osteomalacia
Albumin	Transient albuminuria may occur during pregnancy or prolonged exposure to cold, or following strenuous exercise; albuminuria present in nephritis, nephrosis, nephrosclerosis, pyelonephritis, amyloidosis, renal calculi, bichloride of mercury poisoning, and sometimes with blood transfusion reactions
Acetone	Diabetes mellitus, eclampsia, starvation, febrile diseases in which carbohydrate intake is limited, pernicious vomiting of pregnancy
Glucose	Unusually high carbohydrate intake, diabetes mellitus
Bilirubin	Obstructive jaundice, hemolytic jaundice, hepatitis, cholangitis
Urobilin and urobilinogen	Hemolytic jaundice, pernicious anemia, hepatitis, eclampsia, portal cirrhosis, lobar pneumonia, malaria
Erythrocytes	Glomerulonephritis, pyelonephritis, tuberculosis of kidneys, tumors of kidney, tumors of ureter and bladder, polycystic kidneys, calculi, hemorrhagic diseases, occasionally with anticoagulant therapy
Leukocytes	Increased in urethritis, prostatitis, cystitis, pyelitis, pyelonephritis (a few leukocytes are found in normal urine)
Casts	Glomerulonephritis, nephrosis, pyelonephritis, febrile diseases, eclampsia, amyloid disease, poisoning by heavy metals

From Shirley R. Burke, *The Composition and Function of Body Fluids* 3rd ed. (St. Louis, Mo.: The C. V. Mosby Co., 1980).

size, shape, and position of the kidneys and re-
veals any calcification in the urinary system.

Intravenous Pyelogram

An intravenous pyelogram is an X-ray examination of the kidney and urinary tract. A radiopaque dye that is injected into a vein will filter

through the kidney and be excreted. During the
test, which usually takes about an hour, films
that reveal the outline of the kidneys, as well as
any stones or tumors, are taken.

In preparation for this test, the patient is
given a laxative the evening before and an
enema the morning of the test to clear the in-

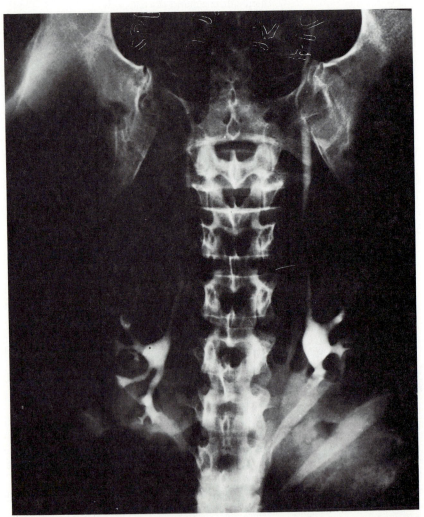

Figure 20-1. *Normal intravenous pyelogram. Note the calyces, renal pelvis, and ureters are clearly visible. (Courtesy of James W. Lecky, M.D.,
University of Pittsburgh)*

testinal tract of feces or gas that might decrease visualization of the kidneys, ureters, and bladder. No food or fluids are allowed for at least 8 hours before the test so that the dye used for the examination will be concentrated. Because the dye contains iodine, the patient should be questioned about allergies and a skin test for iodine allergy may be done prior to the procedure. During the examination, it is normal to feel a flushing or burning sensation and to experience a salty or metallic taste following the dye injection. Figure 20-1 shows a normal intravenous pyelogram.

Following the test, it is important for the patient to take fluids liberally to flush any remaining dye from the urinary tract and to overcome the dehydration.

Retrograde Pyelogram

The retrograde (ret"ro-grade) pyelogram is similar to the intravenous test. The patient has the same preparation; however, a sedative is usually ordered prior to the test. The dye will be injected directly into the pelvis of the kidney through ureteral catheters. These catheters are inserted through a **cystoscope** (sis-to'skope).

OTHER EXAMINATIONS

Cystoscopy

Cystoscopy is a procedure that allows the examiner to see directly into the urinary bladder through a small metal or flexible scope. Through this instrument the operator can obtain specimens for a biopsy, urine specimens from each kidney, or perform a retrograde pyelogram (see Fig. 20-2). Before the examination the patient should drink liberal amounts of fluid so that adequate urine will be available for the specimens. The procedure is usually performed under local anesthesia. However, if general anesthesia is used, intravenous fluids must be given.

The patient is placed in a **lithotomy** (lith-

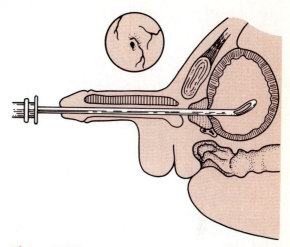

Figure 20-2. *A cystoscope being introduced into a male bladder. Appearance of normal ureteral opening as seen through a cystoscope. (From Miller, P.L., "Assessment of Urinary Function." Phipps, W.J., Long, B.C., and Woods, N.F. (Eds.), Medical-Surgical Nursing, 2nd ed. St. Louis: The C.V. Mosby Co., 1983)*

ot'o-me) position (feet or legs up in stirrups). Aseptic technique is maintained throughout the procedure. The flexible cystoscope (see Fig. 20-3) is lubricated and inserted into the urethra. After the urine is removed, the bladder is irrigated with warm sterile fluid to remove any material that might interfere with visualization.

Following the examination, the patient should drink extra fluids to dilute the urine and lessen the irritation of the urinary tract lining. Voiding is normally accompanied by a burning sensation for a day or two, and some **hematuria** (he-mah-tu're-ah) (blood in the urine) is to be expected.

Ultrasound

Ultrasonic examination of the abdomen is an important diagnostic tool in investigating urinary tract disorders. Ultrasonography is a technique in which ultrasonic or high-frequency

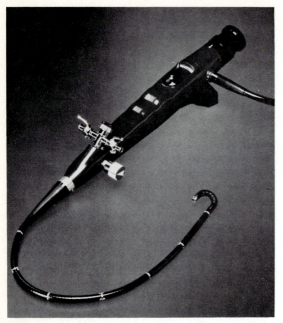

Figure 20-3. *A flexible cystoscope (Courtesy CITCON ACMT, Stamford, CT)*

waves are directed into body tissues. These waves strike tissues of varying density, and some of the sound waves are reflected back as echoes. These are displayed on a screen and show the tissue being examined. The test is painless, safe, and requires no preparation other than an explanation.

DISEASES OF THE URINARY SYSTEM

URINARY OBSTRUCTIONS

Obstructions can occur at any point in the urinary tract and can be caused by strictures, tumors, stones, spasms of the ureter, cysts, or a kink in the ureter. Regardless of the cause, ob-

struction can result in kidney damage if not corrected.

When the urine cannot pass the obstruction, it causes back pressure on the structures above the blockage. For example, if a stone is lodged in a ureter, distention or swelling of the ureter, called hydroureter (hi″dro-u-re′ter), occurs (see Fig. 20-4). If the stone is not passed or removed, it can lead to **hydronephrosis** (hi″dro-ne-fro′sis). The pressure of the urine in the pelvis of the kidney compresses vital portions of the kidney and blood vessels. This condition can result in permanent kidney damage.

The treatment is first to establish free flow of urine and then remove the obstruction. The ur-

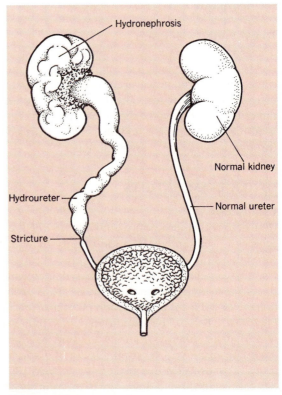

Figure 20-4. *Hydroureter and hydronephrosis resulting from a ureteral stricture*

ine may be drained by a ureteral catheter or it may be necessary to insert a tube into the kidney pelvis through a skin incision. This procedure is called a **nephrostomy**

Strictures

Strictures are bands of fibrous tissue that narrow the lumen of the ureter or urethra. They can be caused by infections or injury or from congenital abnormalities. Symptoms include a slow stream of urine, burning, frequency, urine retention, and difficulty voiding. Treatment involves dilating or stretching the tract with instruments and catheters. The procedure is painful and may have to be repeated several times. There will be some hematuria after the treatments and voiding will be uncomfortable for several days. If dilation is not successful, surgery must be performed to cut the bands of scar tissue or possibly remove the constricted area and insert a graft.

CALCULI

Calculi are stonelike formations. They may be found anywhere from the kidney to the urinary bladder and can vary in size from small granular deposits like gravel or sand to bladder stones the size of an orange. Normally the crystalline substances in the urine remain in solution. However, if the urine is alkaline, stones can form. Cereals and meats favor acidity of urine and, although most fruits and vegetables favor alkalinity, cranberry juice is quite helpful in making the urine more acid. Other factors that can lead to stone formation are infection, urinary stasis, prolonged bed rest or inactivity, osteoporosis, parathyroid disease, and low estrogen levels.

Symptoms depend on the location of the stone and the degree of obstruction. Frequently there is hematuria because of the abrasive action of the stone as urine is passed. When a stone lodges in the ureter, there is sharp stabbing pain due to muscle spasms in the ureter. The pain radiates from the kidney area down to the genitalia. Medication to relieve the pain is needed.

About 90% of the stones pass spontaneously. Since these stones are very small, the urine should be strained. Unless the patient is vomiting, extra fluids should be taken to assist in flushing the stone out of the tract. For large stones that cannot pass, it will be necessary to do lithotripsy (lith′o-trip″se). In this procedure, the stones are crushed with sound waves while the patient is under water. Once the stones are crushed they can be passed.

It is important to determine the composition of the stone because a major part of the treatment is based on limiting certain foods that make up the main ingredient of the stone. Citrus fruits and carbonated beverages may have to be eliminated from the diet as they favor alkaline urine formation.

NEPHROPTOSIS

Since the kidneys are supported by fat pads rather than ligaments, they may drop slightly as a result of a large weight loss. This is **nephroptosis** (nef-rop-to′sis), which is often referred to as a "dropped kidney" or a "floating kidney."

Usually, the only symptom is an ache in the flank area, and this is relieved by bed rest with the hips elevated. A kidney belt may be used to help keep the kidney in the normal position. In severe cases, the ureter may become kinked and impair urine flow. Sharp pain, nausea and vomiting, and at times chills and fever can result. Surgery may be needed to suture the kidney to adjacent structures for support and to straighten the ureter and provide adequate drainage.

TUMORS

Tumors of the kidney or urinary bladder are usually first evidenced by painless hematuria.

Often, cytological examination of the urine will reveal tumor cells. Most kidney tumors are malignant and spread early to other areas. Treatment is surgery combined with radiation and chemotherapy.

The most common site of cancer in the urinary tract is the bladder. This cancer occurs more often in men than women. A cystoscopy and biopsy confirms the cell type, the size of the tumor, and the depth of tissue involved. Surgery is done to resect the tumor or it may be necessary to completely remove the bladder. If the bladder is removed, the urine must be permanently diverted into the intestinal tract or through the abdominal wall to an opening in the skin, which will require an external device for urine collection. Adjustments to such changes are difficult and much support is needed.

A Wilms' tumor is a solid tumor that occurs during childhood. The child has an abdominal mass. Other signs and symptoms include pain, hematuria, fever, anorexia, nausea, and vomiting. There also may be hypertension. Treatment includes surgery, chemotherapy, and radiation.

INFECTIONS

Cystitis

Cystitis (sis-ti′tis) is an inflammation of the urinary bladder. Women are affected more often than are men because the urethra is shorter and organisms can more easily enter the bladder. Signs and symptoms include frequency, burning, urgency (a feeling of needing to void although the bladder is not full), and cloudy urine due to the presence of bacteria. If the infection is severe, there may be chills, fever, nausea, and vomiting as well as abdominal or low back pain. Occasionally, a patient may have no symptoms at all.

Treatment hinges on discovering the causative organism so that appropriate antibiotics can be used. It is important to continue these medicines for at least 7 to 10 days even though the symptoms may subside earlier. Fluids are forced and analgesics are given. Warm baths are often helpful in relieving the discomfort. Unfortunately, cystitis frequently recurs and may become chronic. Hygiene is most important, so patients are instructed to shower rather than take tub baths. Alkaline bubble baths are particularly likely to cause recurrence of the infection because of the bath water entering the bladder. Patients should be told to cleanse the perineal area from front to back after each bowel movement and to drink liberal amounts of fluids and void every 2 to 3 hours during the day.

Pyelonephritis

Pyelonephritis (pi″el-o-ne-fri′tis) is an infection of the kidney and the renal pelvis. It can be either acute or chronic. The acute disease may result from an infection elsewhere in the body. Chronic pyelonephritis develops if treatment of acute pyelonephritis is not successful. In chronic cases, the kidneys become scarred and almost useless.

Symptoms include chills and fever, flank pain, pyuria, nausea, and vomiting. Bed rest is necessary and fluids are encouraged to dilute the urine. Medication is used to acidify the urine and a culture is done to identify the causative organism. Then the appropriate antibiotic is given.

Glomerulonephritis

Glomerulonephritis (glom-er″u-lo-ne-fri′tis) is a kidney infection characterized by inflammation of the glomeruli. It can be either acute or chronic. Acute glomerulonephritis frequently follows a "strep" throat by two or three weeks. In chronic glomerulonephritis, the kidneys shrink and become full of fibrous tissue.

The disease may be so mild that there are no symptoms. In more severe cases, symptoms include headache, fatigue, facial edema, and flank pain. This progresses to decreased urine output, headaches, hypertension, and visual disturbances. The urine contains blood and albumin and the patient becomes anemic. Eventually, as the kidneys cease to function, the patient becomes comatose.

Treatment is mainly symptomatic. During acute stages, the patient is on bed rest and is given a low-sodium, high-carbohydrate diet. Protein intake may be restricted. If there is a residual streptococcal infection, penicillin is given. Patients, especially those with chronic glomerulonephritis, must avoid exposure to infections.

Renal Hypertension

Many conditions that damage the kidneys can cause renal hypertension. Kidney infections, particularly if the renal arteries are constricted, can elevate the blood pressure.

An ischemic kidney secretes large amounts of renin, which leads to the formation of angiotensin. This causes vasoconstriction, increased peripheral resistance, and often leads to severe hypertension.

Renal Failure

Renal failure is either acute or chronic. Acute failure may be caused by a decrease in blood volume due to hemorrhage or severe burns, an incompatible blood transfusion, crush injury to a limb, acute glomerulonephritis, or tubular obstruction. There will be oliguria. The urine is dark and contains protein and blood. There is an elevated BUN and an increase in the blood potassium, which leads to metabolic acidosis and coma. If the patient survives, large quantities of urine are passed because the kidneys cannot conserve electrolytes or water. This dehydration and electrolyte imbalance can be life threatening.

Chronic renal failure can be caused by glomerulonephritis, lupus erythematosus, or chronic obstruction. The patient will have an elevated BUN, blood potassium, and be acidotic. In chronic renal failure the kidneys cannot concentrate or dilute and the urine has a fixed specific gravity of 1.010.

Uremia

When sufficient renal function is lost, there will be multiple organ systems disturbances. Patients with uremia have weight loss, dyspnea, muscle weakness, fatigue, anorexia, nausea and vomiting, tetany, neuropathy, itching, pericarditis, and convulsions. They may have a "uremic frost" on their face. This is a white granular secretion from the sweat glands. These salts can be irritating to the skin.

DIALYSIS

Dialysis (di-al'is-is) is the diffusion of crystalline particles through a semipermeable membrane, passing from the area of higher concentration to lower. When a patient has a marked decrease in renal function, repeated dialysis treatments may be necessary to remove the waste products from the bloodstream and restore electrolyte balance. Dialysis helps maintain the patient's life until kidney function is restored. It cannot cure renal failure but, rather, merely approximates some renal functions. In dialysis, the patient uses either a machine equipped with a semipermeable filtering membrane or his own peritoneal membrane to cleanse the blood.

PERITONEAL DIALYSIS

In peritoneal dialysis, sterile dialyzing fluid is introduced into the peritoneal cavity at intervals. The large surface area of the peritoneum acts as the diffusing membrane, with blood supplied by the peritoneal blood vessels. A special silicone catheter can be implanted in the patient's abdominal wall, thus providing a permanent access to the peritoneal cavity for repeated treatments (see Fig. 20-5).

After the dialyzing solution has remained in the peritoneal cavity for 15 to 30 minutes, it is allowed to drain out. This procedure is repeated, with fresh solution instilled until the blood chemistry levels improve. The time involved is usually 12 to 36 hours depending on the severity of the patient's condition. Patients with chronic renal disease can learn to do their own treatments at home, allowing them to resume most normal activities.

Continuous ambulatory peritoneal dialysis (CAPD) involves continuous contact of the dialysate and peritoneal membrane. Through a permanent peritoneal catheter, the patient exchanges two liters of dialysate four or five times

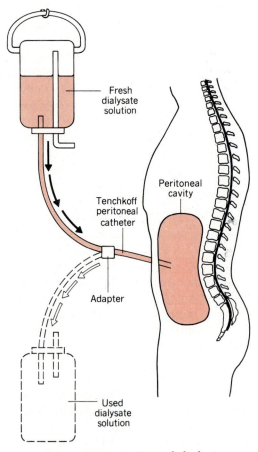

Fresh dialysate solution

Peritoneal cavity

Tenchkoff peritoneal catheter

Adapter

Used dialysate solution

Figure 20-5. Peritoneal dialysis.

a day. The exchange takes about 20 minutes. For someone who is away from home for several hours a day, the fresh dialysate is worn in a plastic bag around the waist. When it is time for the exchange, the dialysate in the peritoneal cavity is drained off by gravity into the toilet. Then the plastic bag is hung on a hook so the fluid will be drained into the peritoneal cavity.

HEMODIALYSIS

In **hemodialysis** a sheet of cellophane or a plastic capillary tube serves as the semipermeable membrane in the dialyzer machine; plastic tubing carries the blood from the body to the membrane. The renal failure patient must usually have dialysis two or three times per week. If the

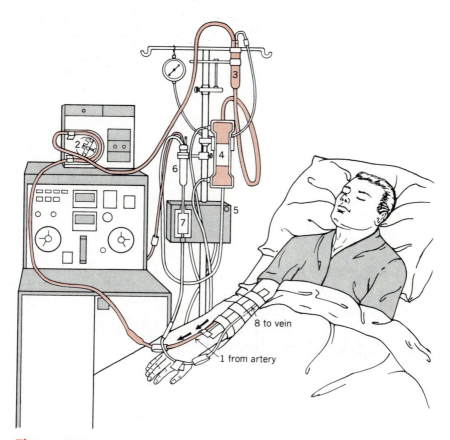

Figure 20-6. Hemodialysis. (1) Blood leaves the body via an artery. (2) Arterial blood passes through the blood pump. (3) Blood is filtered to remove any clots. (4) Blood passes through the dialyzer. (5) Blood passes into the venous blood line. (6) Blood is filtered to remove any clots. (7) Blood flows through air detector. (8) Blood returns to the patient through the venous blood line.

patient is not hospitalized, the treatments can be done at a dialysis clinic or the patient can do them at home.

Many types of artificial kidney machines are used for hemodialysis but they all operate on the same principles. A cannula is placed in a peripheral artery (see Fig. 20-6). The cannula is connected to the machine that contains the dialyzing fluid. As blood flows from the patient through the dialyzer, electrolytes or other crystalline particles that are more concentrated in the patient's blood than in the dialyzing fluid diffuse from the blood into the fluid. Purified blood is then returned to a peripheral vein. Time varies but averages six to eight hours per treatment. With some of the newer hemodialysis equipment, the treatment can be completed in three to four hours.

Diet is very important and very restricted. Protein foods as well as those containing sodium and potassium are limited. The resulting unpalatable meals, plus living with thirst from a restricted fluid intake, add to a regimented and complicated life that can be very demoralizing to the patient as well as to the family.

In addition to maintaining patients who suffer from chronic renal disease, hemodialysis is used to help people who have taken overdoses of diffusible drugs, such as barbiturates or other sedatives. Dialysis helps clear the drug from the bloodstream.

KIDNEY TRANSPLANT

One solution for a patient with very limited renal function is to have a healthy kidney transplanted into his body. The kidney must be from a compatible donor, preferably a near blood relative, since such tissues are less likely to be rejected. Drugs to suppress the patient's immune system are given to help prevent rejection of the new kidney. The immune-suppressing drugs will cause the patient to be very susceptible to infection and so precautions must be taken to prevent exposure. In case of rejection, the patient must return to dialysis therapy.

SUMMARY QUESTIONS

1. What is the proper procedure for obtaining a clean-caught urine specimen?
2. What are several abnormal constituents of urine?
3. What blood chemistry studies are most often done for patients with kidney disease?
4. How does an intravenous pyelogram differ from a retrograde pyelogram?
5. What is hydronephrosis and what might cause it?
6. What symptoms does a patient with renal calculi have?
7. What foods tend to cause alkaline urine?
8. List the symptoms of cystitis.
9. What is pyelonephritis and what might cause it?
10. How does dialysis work?

KEY TERMS

cystitis   hydronephrosis
cystoscope   lithotomy
dialysis   nephroptosis
hematuria   nephrostomy
hemodialysis   pyelonephritis

21

The Reproductive Systems

OBJECTIVES

On completion of this chapter, you will be able to:

1. Describe the structure of the female reproductive organs and their functions.
2. List the phases of the menstrual cycle.
3. Describe the structure of the male reproductive organs and their functions.
4. Explain the functions and the sources of the male and female sex hormones.
5. Discuss the formation and maturation of the oocytes and sperm.
6. List factors necessary for fertility.
7. Discuss several patterns of genetic transmission of human traits.
8. List in sequence all of the structures through which the sperm must travel from the place of sperm formation until fertilization occurs.
9. Describe the period of embryo development.
10. Describe the stages of labor.

OVERVIEW

I. FEMALE REPRODUCTIVE SYSTEM
   A. Internal Organs
      1. Ovaries
      2. Oviducts
      3. Uterus
         a. The Menstrual Cycle
         b. Menarche and Menopause
      4. Vagina
   B. External Organs
      1. Mons Pubis
      2. Labia
      3. Clitoris
      4. Vestibule
      5. Perineum
   C. Mammary Glands
II. MALE REPRODUCTIVE SYSTEM
   A. Testes
   B. Excretory Ducts
      1. Epididymis
      2. Vas Deferens
      3. Ejaculatory Ducts
      4. Urethra
   C. Accessory Structures
      1. Scrotum
      2. Spermatic Cords
      3. Seminal Vesicles
      4. Prostatic Gland
      5. Cowper's Glands (Bulbourethral Glands)
      6. Penis
   D. Semen
III. PHYSIOLOGY OF REPRODUCTION
   A. Fertilization and Pregnancy
   B. Parturition
IV. FERTILITY
V. CONTRACEPTION

VI. GENETICS
   A. Modes of Inheritance
      1. Dominant Inheritance
      2. Recessive Inheritance
      3. Codominance
      4. Sex-Linked Inheritance
      5. Polygenetic Inheritance
      6. Intermediate Inheritance
      7. Tissue Cultures
   B. Expression of Hereditary Traits

The ability to reproduce is one of the characteristics of living matter. Reproduction may be the simple process of cellular division described in Chapter 4. In this type of reproduction, the division of one parent cell results in the production of two identical daughter cells. In higher forms of life, a new individual is produced only by the union of a female sex cell, or ovum (o'vum), and a male sex cell, or spermatozoa (sper"mah-to-zo'ah). In this chapter, we shall study the organs concerned with the formation of human male and female sex cells and the route through which these cells can unite.

FEMALE REPRODUCTIVE SYSTEM

INTERNAL ORGANS

Ovaries

The ovaries (o'vah-res) are almond-shaped organs about 3 cm long, 2 cm wide, and 1 cm deep (1.5 x 0.75 x 0.5 inches). They are located lateral to the uterus (u'ter-us) near the sides of the pelvis (see Fig. 21-1). The ovaries are attached to the posterior surface of the broad ligaments that extend from the sides of the uterus across the pelvis to the pelvic wall and floor (see Fig. 21-2).

The outer surface of the ovaries is germinal epithelium. Beneath the germinal epithelium is connective tissue in which the ovarian follicles are formed. Each follicle contains one germ cell,

Kathleen B. Gaberson contributed the sections on the physiology of reproduction, fertility and contraception.

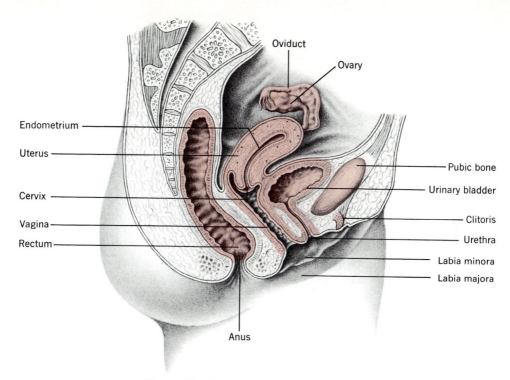

Figure 21-1. *Female pelvis, lateral view*

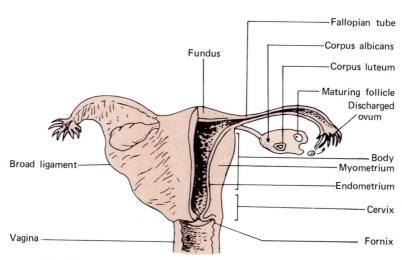

Figure 21-2. *Female reproductive organs, posterior view*

or **oocyte** (o′o-site). During the childbearing years of a woman's life, usually only one follicle matures each month (except during pregnancy, when none mature). The mature follicle can be seen bulging from the surface of the ovary and will rupture and release a mature oocyte. This process is called **ovulation** (ov-u-la′shun) and usually occurs 14 days before the menstrual period.

The mature oocyte has 23 chromosomes; 22 of these are regular autosomal chromosomes, which are nonsex-determining chromosomes, and one is an X chromosome or sex cell. The chromosomes contain genes that will help determine the hereditary characteristics of the child in the event that the egg is fertilized. The immature oocyte contains 46 chromosomes, as do other cells of our body. However, during the maturation of the oocyte, the chromosomes undergo a reduction division resulting in only half the original number of chromosomes. (Review meiosis in Chapter 4.)

The follicles also produce a hormone, **estrogen** (es′tro-jen). Estrogen is essential for the normal development of the female reproductive organs and the development and maintenance of the secondary sex characteristics of the female (distribution of body hair, development of the breasts, and characteristic female body build).

At the site where the follicle has ruptured, the **corpus luteum** (lu′te-um) develops. It produces **progesterone** (pro-jes′ter-on) and estrogen. The progesterone is essential for the preparation of the lining of the uterus to receive the fertilized egg. Under the influence of progesterone, the lining of the uterus increases in thickness. If the egg is not fertilized, the corpus luteum remains for about two weeks and then is replaced with a white scar called the corpus albicans (al′bi-kanz). If pregnancy occurs, the corpus luteum continues to develop, and ovulation and menstruation cease. Late in pregnancy, the progesterone promotes the development of the secretory tissue of the breasts.

Relaxin is a hormone produced by the corpus luteum during pregnancy. This hormone softens the cervix for dilatation, inhibits uterine motility, and softens the pelvic ligaments and joints. During pregnancy, the corpus luteum also produces a hormone called inhibin, which inhibits the secretion of the follicle-stimulating hormone.

The follicle-stimulating hormone (FSH) from the anterior pituitary causes the maturation of the ovarian follicle and, as a consequence, the production of estrogen. Increased blood levels of estrogen inhibit the production of FSH and stimulate pituitary production of the luteinizing (lu′te-in-i″zing) hormone (LH). This luteinizing hormone causes ovulation and the formation of the corpus luteum. LH is responsible for the production and secretion of progesterone and some estrogen by the corpus luteum following ovulation.

Oviducts

The oviducts (o′vi-dukts), or **fallopian** (fah-lo′pe-an) **tubes**, are located in the upper folds of the broad ligaments and are attached to the upper part of the uterus (see Fig. 21-2). Each tube, which is about 10 cm long, opens into the pelvic cavity near the ovary. The tubes have a serous covering under which is found smooth muscle and a ciliated mucous membrane lining. The movement of the cilia and peristaltic contractions carry the ovum toward the uterus. The ends of the tubes have a fringe of fingerlike processes called fimbriae (fim′bre-ah).

The function of the uterine tubes is to convey the ovum toward the uterus. Fertilization usually occurs in the outer one-third of the tube.

Uterus

The uterus is located in the pelvic cavity between the urinary bladder and the rectum. It is a hollow, muscular, pearshaped organ. During the childbearing years of a woman's life, it is about 7.5 cm long, 5 cm wide, and 2.5 cm thick. During pregnancy, obviously, it greatly increases in size. The fundus of the uterus is the upper convex portion just above the entrance of the tubes. The body is the central portion, and the cervix is the lower necklike portion (see Fig. 21-2).

The external surface of the fundus and body of the uterus is serous membrane. The **myometrium** (mi-o-met′re-um) or muscle of the uterus is composed of an interlacing of longitudinal, circular, and spiral muscular fibers. The myometrium is capable of the powerful contractions necessary for the normal birth of an infant. The uterus is lined with mucous membrane called the **endometrium** (en-do-

met′re-um). In the nonpregnant woman, the thickness of the endometrium varies during the menstrual cycle; it is thickest just before the menstrual period (see Fig. 21-3).

The ligaments of the uterus give it some support. However, its main support is provided by the pelvic muscles.

The broad ligaments that extend laterally from the uterus to the pelvis and pelvic floor enclose the tubes, round ligaments, blood vessels, and nerves. Two round ligaments pass from the lateral angles of the uterus below the entrance of the tubes and extend toward the sides of the pelvis, out the inguinal canals, and

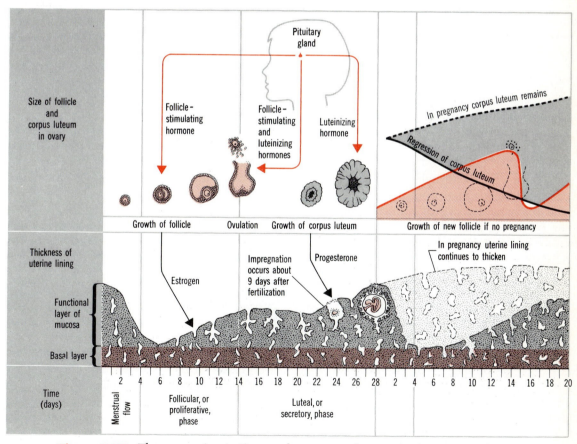

Figure 21-3. *The approximate time and sequence of events in the menstrual cycle*

then into the labia majora and mons pubis. One anterior ligament extends from the uterus to the urinary bladder. A posterior ligament extends from the uterus to the rectum. The uterosacral (u″ter-o-sak′ral) ligament extends from the posterior part of the cervix on either side to the sacrum.

Normally, these ligaments hold the uterus in a position in which the fundus tilts forward over the urinary bladder and the cervix points downward and back (see Fig. 21-1). A full urinary bladder tilts the fundus of the uterus backward. For this reason, the bladder should be emptied prior to a gynecological examination.

The function of the uterus is to retain the fertilized egg during its growth and development. It sustains the growing fetus. During the birth process, it also produces powerful contractions to expel the mature infant.

The Menstrual Cycle The endometrium undergoes cyclic changes at intervals of about 25 to 35 days from puberty to menopause, except during pregnancy and **lactation** (lak-ta′shun). A typical cycle has three broad phases: menstrual, follicular, and luteal (see Fig. 21-3).

1) During the menstrual phase, there is a discharge of bloody fluid from the uterine cavity. This discharge consists of epithelial cells from the superficial layer of the endometrium, mucus, fluid, and about 25 to 65 ml of blood. The flow lasts from four to six days, until the entire superficial layer of epithelium has degenerated and the endometrium is very thin.

2) The follicular or preovulatory phase is associated with the developing ovarian follicle and the production of estrogen. Early in this phase, FSH is the dominant pituitary hormone. However, for the production of estrogen both FSH and LH are necessary. Under the influence of estrogen, there is a regeneration of the superficial layer of endometrium. The estrogen level increases and, on about the thirteenth day of a 28-day cycle, there is a shift in the FSH-LH mixture. FSH is inhibited, LH secretion is greatly increased, and ovulation occurs.

3) The luteal or postovulatory phase follows ovulation. The corpus luteum develops and secretes progesterone. Estrogen is also produced by the luteal cells but progesterone causes the final preparation of the endometrium to receive a fertilized ovum. The superficial endometrium becomes thick and vascular. Progesterone also affects the mammary glands and helps regulate the secretion of the gonadotropins (FSH and LH) from the anterior pituitary.

If fertilization does not occur, the corpus luteum degenerates and becomes the corpus albicans (al′bih-kanz), a small white scar. The estrogen and progesterone production decline and menstruation occurs as the endometrium is deprived of the hormonal stimulation. If the ovum is fertilized and implanted in the uterus, the corpus luteum continues to secrete progesterone for about 3 months. During this period, the embryonic tissues produce a hormone, chorionic (ko-re-on′ik) gonadotropin (go-nad″o-tro′pin), which is similar to LH. The chorionic gonadotropin serves to maintain the corpus luteum until the embryonic tissue is capable of producing progesterone and estrogen.

Menarche and Menopause Secondary sex characteristics, such as the development of breast tissue, growth of body hair, and a general rounding of the female body, occur at puberty between the ages of 10 and 14. At this time the ovarian follicles also begin development, and there is a maturation of the uterus and vaginal mucosa. Puberty terminates with **menarche** (men-ar′ke), the first menstrual period. The average age at menarche is 12 to 14 years, but it can range from 10 to 18 years.

The early menstrual cycles are often irregular, and sometimes ovulation does not occur. With the hormonal changes taking place during puberty and shortly thereafter, this period is sometimes a particularly stressful stage.

Between the ages of 45 and 50, the ovaries gradually fail to respond to the stimulation of the pituitary hormones and there is a cessation of menstruation, or menopause. The ovaries, uterus, vaginal mucosa, external genitalia, and breasts atrophy. Even though the menstrual periods have ceased, the ovaries may continue to produce ova for several more months. Eventually, the ovaries no longer produce ova or secrete hormones, and the period of possible childbearing is over.

There may be hot flashes, headache, and occasionally emotional instability associated with this change of life. Estrogen therapy is sometimes helpful in relieving these symptoms of menopause.

Vagina

The vagina is located behind the urinary bladder and urethra. It is anterior to the rectum. This musculomembranous tube extends down and forward from the uterus to the vulva (external genitalia). The lining of the vagina is mucous membrane arranged in many folds, or rugae. Mucus produced by this lining provides lubrication and has a low pH unfavorable to the growth of most bacteria. Some lubricating fluid is also produced by Bartholin's glands located on either side of the vaginal orifice. The hymen is a fold of connective tissue that may partially close the external orifice of the vagina.

The fornix (for'niks) is a recessed area around the cervix. The posterior fornix is more recessed than the anterior fornix. It is through this posterior fornix that a small incision can be made to insert an endoscope to view the pelvic cavity.

The functions of the vagina are to serve as a passageway for menstrual flow, to receive the erect penis during sexual intercourse, and to serve as the birth canal.

EXTERNAL ORGANS

Mons Pubis

The mons pubis or mons veneris is a rounded eminence, or protuberance, anterior to the symphysis pubis. It is a fat pad covered over with skin and hair.

Labia

The labia majora are large longitudinal folds of skin and fatty tissue extending from the mons to the anus. The labia minora are smaller cutaneous folds between the labia majora. These folds meet anteriorly to form the prepuce (pre'pus) (see Fig. 21-4).

Clitoris

The clitoris (kli'to-ris) is a small body of erectile tissue analogous to the male penis. The clitoris becomes markedly distended during sexual activity.

Vestibule

The vestibule is the space between the labia minora. The urethral and vaginal openings are located in the vestibule, as are Bartholin's glands, located on either side of the vaginal opening. These glands secrete lubricating fluid.

Perineum

Strictly speaking, the **perineum** (per-i-ne'um) is the entire external surface of the pelvic floor from the pubis to the coccygeal region. In obstetrical practice, however, it is only the area between the vagina and the anus that is called the perineum.

MAMMARY GLANDS

The mammary glands, or breasts, are located anterior to the pectoralis major between the second and sixth ribs. These compound glands are lateral to the sternum and extend over to the axilla. The nipples, located just above the fifth

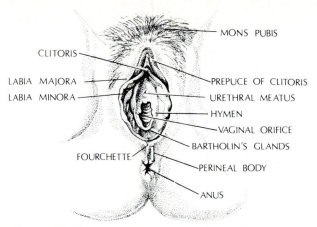

Figure 21-4. *External female genitalia (From Hill, P.,
and Humphrey, P.,* Human Growth and Development
Throughout Life: A Nursing Perspective. *New York:
John Wiley & Sons, Inc., 1982)*

rib, are smooth muscle tissue covered over with
a pigmented area called the areola (ar-e′o-lah)
(see Fig. 21-5).

Only slight changes in the mammary tissue
take place from infancy until the approach of
puberty. After the onset of the menses, there are
changes in the developing mammary glands
with each period. In the premenstrual phase,
vascular engorgement and an increase in the
glands take place. During the postmenstrual
phase, the glands regress and remain in an inactive stage until the next premenstrual phase.

After the second month of pregnancy, a visible enlargement of the breasts and increased
pigmentation of the nipples takes place. For the
first three days after the birth of the infant, the
breasts produce colostrum (ko-los′trum), a
small amount of thin yellowish fluid. The secretion of true milk begins on the third or fourth
day and continues through the nursing period.
Prolactin, a pituitary hormone, stimulates the
production of milk, and oxytocin, also from the
pituitary, favors the release of the milk from the
breasts.

MALE REPRODUCTIVE SYSTEM

In our study of the male reproductive system,
we shall follow the same general pattern as with
the study of the female reproductive system.
First, we shall consider the place of the sex-cell
formation, and then the route to the outside of
the body and the accessory organs along this
route.

TESTES

The male testes correspond to the female ovaries. The testes are located in the scrotum. These
organs are oval structures enclosed in a fibrous
capsule. Inside the testes are lobules that contain the seminiferous (se-mi-nif′er-us) tubules
with germinal cells to produce the spermatozoa.
These tubules open into the epididymis (ep-e-
did′e-mis) (see Fig. 21-6).

In fetal life, the testes are formed in the abdomen, near the kidneys. As the fetus grows,
the testes move downward through the inguinal

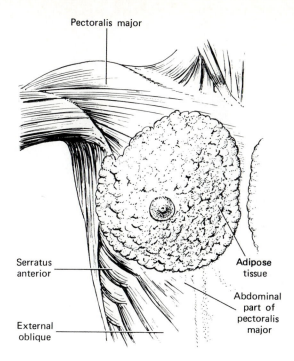

Pectoralis major

Serratus
anterior

External
oblique

Adipose
tissue

Abdominal
part of
pectoralis
major

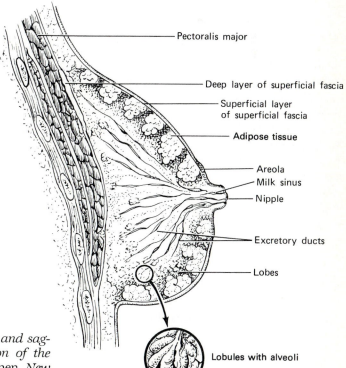

Pectoralis major

Deep layer of superficial fascia

Superficial layer
of superficial fascia

Adipose tissue

Areola

Milk sinus

Nipple

Excretory ducts

Lobes

Lobules with alveoli

Figure 21-5. *Frontal view (upper left) and sagittal view (lower right) of cross section of the breast (From Sloane, E.,* Biology of Women. *New York: John Wiley & Sons, Inc., 1980)*

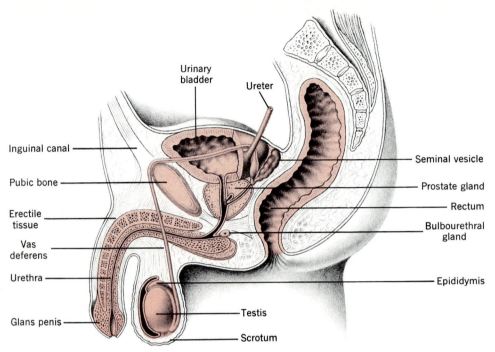

Figure 21-6. Male reproductive organs

canal and usually enter the scrotum a month or two before birth. The descent of the testes into the scrotum is important to the proper functioning of these glands. Spermatogenesis, the formation of the male sex cells, can occur only at temperatures lower than those within the abdominal cavity. For this reason, if the testes do not descend into the scrotum, where the temperature is approximately two degrees Centigrade below the internal body temperature, sterility will result. Failure of the testes to descend from the abdomen is called **cryptorchidism** (krip-tor'kid-izm).

The follicle-stimulating hormone from the anterior pituitary gland causes spermatogenesis. Beginning at the time of puberty, approximately 300,000,000 sperm are produced each day. The sperm is about 0.06 mm long and resembles a

tadpole with a head, short body, and a long motile tail. The tail contains adenosine triphosphate (ATP), which causes lashing movements that aid the motility of the sperm. With advancing age there is some decline in the production of sperm, but apparently sperm continue to be produced throughout a man's lifetime.

Like the mature ovum, the mature sperm has 23 chromosomes. The immature spermatocyte has 46 chromosomes, of which one is an X chromosome and one a Y chromosome. When the reduction division takes place forming the mature sperm, the Y, or male, chromosome passes to one of the sperm and the X chromosome passes to the other. If an ovum is fertilized by a sperm with an X chromosome, the combination leads to the formation of a female. The combination of a sperm containing a Y chromosome with an ovum creates an XY pattern and causes the development of a male.

In addition to the production of sperm, the testes produce a male hormone, **testosterone** (tes-tos'ter-on). This hormone is essential for the development and maintenance of the male secondary sex characteristics such as growth of hair on the face and body, an increase in skeletal muscle mass, and the growth of the larynx that causes the deeper pitch of the male voice. Unfortunately, the precise action of the testosterone on spermatogenesis is not known. However, in the absence of testosterone sperm will not develop. In addition to testosterone the testes also produce inhibin to decrease the production of FSH.

Testosterone is produced in response to the luteinizing hormone or interstitial cell-stimulating hormone from the pituitary, and pituitary FSH causes the maturation of the sperm. The production of these pituitary hormones in the male begins at about the age of 10 to 14.

EXCRETORY DUCTS

Epididymis
The epididymis is an elongated, triangular structure located at the upper and posterior part of each testis. It receives the immature sperm from the tubules and the maturation of the male sex cells is completed here (see Fig. 21-6). The sperm are stored in the epididymis until ejaculation, when they enter the vas deferens (vas' def'er-ens).

Vas Deferens
The vas deferens is a muscular tube about 48 cm long. It leads, one from each epididymis, up through the inguinal canal into the pelvic cavity, crosses to the inferior surface of the urinary bladder, and unites with the ducts of the sem-

inal vesicles to form the ejaculatory ducts (e-jak'u-lah-to-re ducts).

Ejaculatory Ducts
The ejaculatory ducts are two short tubes that descend through the prostatic gland and empty into the prostatic portion of the urethra (see Fig. 21-6).

Urethra
The male urethra has both excretory and reproductive functions. The urethra in the male is an S-shaped tube about 20 cm long and leads from the urinary bladder to the external opening. It has three portions: the prostatic, membranous, and cavernous.

ACCESSORY STRUCTURES

Scrotum
The scrotum is a pouch of thin, dark skin continuous with the skin of the groin and perineum. There are smooth muscles in the walls of the scrotum that function to regulate the temperature within the structures where the sperm are being formed and stored. When it is cold, these smooth muscles contract and bring the testes and epididymis closer to the warmth of the body. When it is hot, the muscles relax so that the sperm being formed and stored can be kept at an optimum temperature.

Spermatic Cords
The spermatic cords extend from the testes through the inguinal canal and terminate at the internal inguinal ring. These cords contain the vas deferens and also the blood vessels and nerves for the testes and epididymis.

Seminal Vesicles
The seminal (sem'i-nal) vesicles are two membranous pouches directly behind the urinary bladder. They produce a thick alkaline secretion

that aids in the motility of the sperm. The viscous secretions of the seminal vesicles contain fructose and prostaglandins (pros-tah-glan' dinz). The fructose is a source of energy for the sperm, and the prostaglandins facilitate ejaculation and stimulate uterine contractions thus helping the sperm to move to the uterine tubes where fertilization takes place.

Prostatic Gland

The prostate lies directly below the urinary bladder and surrounds the prostatic portion of the urethra. It secretes a milky alkaline fluid to aid in the motility of the sperm and to neutralize the acidity of the urethra.

Cowper's Glands (Bulbourethral Glands)

Cowper's glands are two small glands just below the prostate on either side of the membranous urethra. Just before the sperm reach this point in the pathway, they secrete a small amount of alkaline mucus to lubricate and alkanize the distal portion of the urethra.

Penis

The penis, which is suspended from the front and sides of the pubic arch, is composed of three cylindrical masses of cavernous (erectile) tissue. The spaces in this cavernous tissue become congested with blood during sexual activity and cause an erection. The epididymis and vas deferens contract forcing sperm into the urethra. Contraction of the seminal vesicles and muscles surrounding the prostate expel fluids from these glands. Rhythmic contractions of the muscle surrounding the erectile tissue cause **ejaculation**, (e-jak"u-la'shun) or the release of semen from the urethra.

SEMEN

Semen contains the secretions of the above glands and the sperm. Each milliliter of semen contains about 90,000,000 sperm. Normally there are about two to six ml of fluid with each ejaculation. Semen has a pH of 7.35 to 7.5 giving the sperm protection against the acidity of the pathway.

PHYSIOLOGY OF REPRODUCTION

In the female, primary oocytes are formed during prenatal life, undergo the first reduction division by the time of birth, and remain dormant until puberty. Many oocytes have degenerated by this time; those remaining will gradually mature throughout the reproductive years. The mature oocyte is about 0.1 mm in diameter.

Spermatogenesis begins with the onset of puberty and continues throughout adult life. Sperm are continuously produced in the seminiferous tubules and stored in the epididymis and vas deferens. After they are deposited in the vagina, a process called **insemination** (in-sem" i-na'shun), they may live as long as 48 hours.

FERTILIZATION AND PREGNANCY

Fertilization is the union of ovum and sperm. Fertilization usually takes place in the outer one-third of the fallopian tube shortly after ovulation and insemination. Although fertilization usually occurs as a result of sexual intercourse, it can sometimes be achieved by artificial insemination using seminal fluid from the male partner or a donor.

The sperm penetrates the ovum by releasing an enzyme, hyaluronidase (hi"ah-lu-ron'i-das), that makes the surface of the ovum more permeable. As the sperm enters the ovum, the nuclei fuse, and the process of fertilization is complete. The resulting cell, the zygote (zi'got) has 46 chromosomes and all the potentials of the new individual: sex, size, hair color, eye color, and so on.

Within hours, the zygote begins mitotic cell divisions, soon becoming a fluid-filled ball of cells. As these early cell divisions occur, the zygote travels along the fallopian tube, reaching the uterus in about three days. After three to four days in the uterus, the zygote implants itself in the uterine lining. Thus, about seven days elapse between fertilization and implantation.

From implantation until the end of the eighth week after fertilization, the developing organism is called an embryo. This is the period of organogenesis, or differentiation of cells into specific organs and parts. After the beginning of the ninth week, the organism is called a fetus and undergoes further growth and development until delivery. By the twentieth week, the mother is usually aware of fetal movements (quickening), and fetal heart sounds can be heard through a stethoscope placed on the mother's abdomen. Figure 21-7 shows various stages in the development of the embryo and fetus.

The fetus is nourished by the placenta (plah-

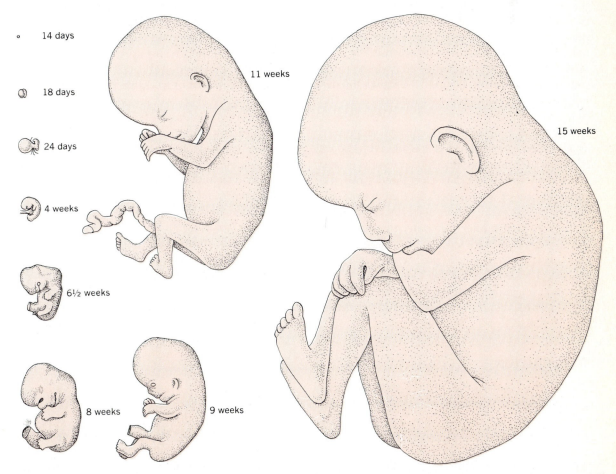

14 days

18 days

24 days

4 weeks

6½ weeks

8 weeks

9 weeks

11 weeks

15 weeks

Figure 21-7. *Changes in the body size of the embryo and fetus during development in the uterus (all figures natural size)*

sen'tah), a disclike organ formed by a union of fetal and maternal tissues. The placenta serves as a nutritive and excretory organ for the fetus, and also secretes estrogen, progesterone, chorionic gonadotropin, and chorionic somatomammotropin. The umbilical cord connects the fetus and the placenta. It contains two arteries that carry blood to the placenta and one vein carrying blood to the fetus. The maternal and fetal blood supplies are not connected in any way.

The fetus is surrounded by two thin, opaque membranes covering the fetal surface of the placenta. The amnion (am'ne-on) forms a fluid-filled sac around the fetus. The outermost membrane, the chorion (ko-re-on'), is initially covered with villi that penetrate the endometrium to form the placenta. Figure 21-8 shows the development of the fetal membranes and the placenta.

In clinical practice, the length of pregnancy or gestation (jes-ta'shun) is considered to be 40 weeks or 10 lunar months (28 days each) or 280 days. This time period is calculated from the date of onset of the mother's last menstrual period. Although conception does not occur until about two weeks after this date, the last menstrual period is used to calculate the expected date of delivery, since the precise date of fertilization usually cannot be determined. The length of pregnancy is divided into three **trimesters** (tri-mes'ters) of approximately three months each.

PARTURITION

Parturition (par-tu-rish'un), or the process of giving birth, is accomplished by rhythmic involuntary uterine contractions. These contractions (often called labor pains) increase in frequency, duration, and intensity, and gradually cause the cervix to dilate (open). Then, accompanied by voluntary abdominal muscle contrac-

tions (bearing down or pushing), the uterine contractions expel the fetus and placenta.

The first stage of labor begins with dilation of the cervix. Usually the fetal membranes (bag of water) rupture at this time and amniotic fluid escapes through the vagina. When the cervix is fully dilated (about 10 cm in diameter), the second stage begins with the descent of the fetus through the pelvis and ends with the delivery of the baby (see Fig. 21-9). The umbilical cord is clamped and cut, and the placenta is then delivered (the third stage of labor).

The infant should be observed carefully to determine management priorities. An Apgar scoring method is frequently used in this assessment. Heart rate, respiratory effort, muscle tone, reflex irritability, and color are observed at one and five minutes after birth and given scores of 0, 1, or 2, with a perfect total score being 10 for an infant with a heart rate of over 100, good respirations, active and well flexed muscles, vigorous cry, and a completely pink body, hands, and feet.

Following childbirth, the mother's reproductive organs must return to near their original size, shape, and position. This process, called involution, takes about six weeks. Immediately after delivery, the fundus of the uterus can be palpated at about the level of the umbilicus. It gradually decreases in size due to uterine contractions. Breastfeeding assists in this process by causing the release of pituitary oxytocin, which stimulates uterine contractions.

FERTILITY

Fertility is the ability to conceive and bear a child. This capacity depends on the normal structure and functioning of the reproductive organs, as well as on favorable conditions at the time of insemination.

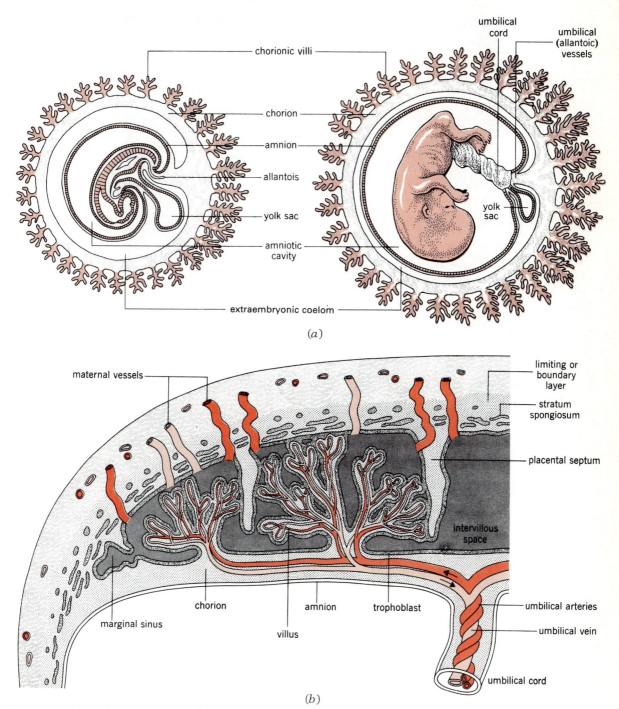

Figure 21-8. *(a) Development of the fetal membranes and (b) placental circulation. Through the placenta, the fetus gets nourishment and excretes wastes.*

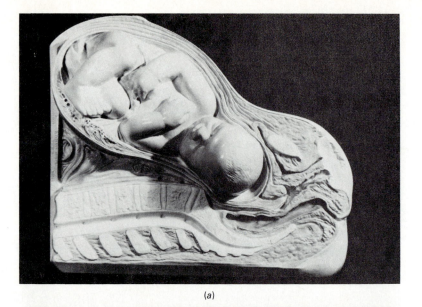

(a)

(b)

Figure 21-9. *(a) Position of the baby just prior to the first stage of labor (dilatation of the cervix and rupture of the amnionic sac), and (b) second stage of labor, the delivery of the infant (Dickinson-Beiskie Models. Courtesy of Cleveland Health Education Museum)*

Appropriate timing of insemination in relation to ovulation is important. The ovum remains viable no more than 24 hours after ovulation, and the sperm can survive in the female reproductive tract up to 48 hours. Thus, fertilization is usually possible only within a 72-hour time period surrounding ovulation.

The adequacy of the sperm to fertilize the ovum is affected by their number and motility. A sperm count of at least 20 million per ml (normal is about 90 million per ml) of semen, with at least 50% highly motile sperm is thought to be adequate.

The characteristics of cervical and vaginal secretions can facilitate or inhibit fertilization. Normally, these secretions are acid, and the semen must have a high enough pH to allow the sperm to survive in this environment. Changes in the quality of cervical mucus can affect fertility. During most of the menstrual cycle, the mucus is thick and viscous, but around the time of ovulation it becomes clear, watery, and more alkaline, facilitating the passage of the sperm.

Depending on the cause, infertile couples may be able to conceive through artificial insemination or in vitro (in ve'tro) fertilization.

If the male partner's sperm count is low or motility is poor, artificial insemination may be attempted with a semen specimen pooled from several samples collected from him. A couple may decide to use donor sperm either alone or mixed with the male partner's sperm. However, this procedure usually involves complicated legal and ethical issues.

In vitro fertilization may be attempted when a woman's fallopian tubes are blocked or absent. Ovulation is stimulated with hormones, and the ova are removed from mature follicles through a laparoscope (lap'ah-ro-skop''). The ova are fertilized in a tissue culture with the male partner's sperm. After several cell divisions, several fertilized ova are transferred to the uterus where one or more implant, and embryonic development continues.

CONTRACEPTION

There are many methods of preventing conception, but their effectiveness varies considerably. Ideally, the method used should be esthetically acceptable to both partners, simple to use, inexpensive, and without permanent effects (unless this is desired).

The most effective contraceptive methods work by preventing ovulation (oral contraceptive pills), preventing implantation (intrauterine devices or IUDs), or providing a barrier to the passage of the sperm (condom or diaphragm with spermicidal cream or jelly, or vaginal contraceptive sponge impregnated with spermicide). Fertility awareness methods use various ways of determining time of ovulation so that intercourse can be avoided during this period. Such methods employ the calendar (rhythm) method or observation of changes in cervical mucus characteristics and basal body temperature (CM-BBT). These techniques are somewhat less effective than the oral contraceptive, IUD, and barrier methods but are safe and inexpensive.

Permanent sterilization can usually be accomplished by tubal **ligation** (li-ga'shun), the blocking or cutting of the fallopian tubes, and vasectomy (vas-ek'to-me), surgical resection of a segment of each vas deferens. The use of vasectomy valves can make this a reversible procedure. A tubal ligation can sometimes be surgically reversed. But because this procedure is not always successful, a tubal ligation should be done only when permanent sterilization is desired.

Information concerning contraceptive methods and devices and instructions for their use can be obtained from local Planned Parenthood Associations.

GENETICS

How you appear is referred to as your **phenotype** (fe′no-tipe), and your genetic makeup is your **genotype** (jen′o-tipe). The genotype includes the genes for traits that are expressed (height, eye color, intelligence, and so on) and for some unexpressed inherited traits (although unexpressed in one individual, these can be passed on to the offspring who may express them). Mendel, the father of genetics, considered a single gene to be responsible for a single trait, but we now know that many genes can be involved in the production of a single trait and that one gene can affect more than one trait. Although we do not know how many genes an individual has, it is estimated to be about 50,000.

Genes are located on the chromosomes of the cell. Reviewing the process of cell reproduction, recall that in the formation of the sex cells, sperm and ova, the number of chromosomes is reduced from 46 to 23. The process in which the cytoplasm of these cells is divided and the number of chromosomes reduced by half is called meiosis or reduction division (see Fig. 21-10). The united ovum and sperm result in a cell with the full complement of 46 chromosomes, half contributed by the mother and half by the father.

Genes, like chromosomes, are in pairs known as alleles (a-lelz′). Allelic genes from father and mother are situated on the same spot on the two members of the same pair of chromosomes and are concerned with the same trait. A person can be **homozygous** (ho-mo-zi′gus), that is, having received the same gene for a trait from each parent, or can be **heterozygous** (het″er-o-zi′gus) if each parent has contributed a different type of gene for a particular trait. It is the genes that are inherited, not the traits.

MODES OF INHERITANCE

Dominant Inheritance

Simple dominance is the expression of one contrasting gene over another for the same trait. Each individual who expresses a trait transmitted by a dominant gene has a parent who expresses the same trait. The gene can come from either parent and can be expressed in a child of either sex.

If one parent has the dominant gene, two out of four children normally will inherit this gene, and, although the condition is heterozygous, they will show the trait. The other two children who did not receive the dominant gene will not express the trait. This is not to say that if there are four children from this marriage that two and only two will receive the dominant gene. With each pregnancy, the chances of receiving the gene are the same, two in four.

Recessive Inheritance

With recessive inheritance, the trait is only expressed in homozygous individuals. For parents who are heterozygous for a recessive gene and therefore do not express the trait, there is only one in four chances of their offspring inheriting and expressing the recessive gene. Although three out of four of their offspring will normally inherit the gene, two of these three will be heterozygous, and the trait will be unexpressed.

In the next generation, if the mate of one of these heterozygous offspring does not carry the recessive gene, there is no chance of its expression in their children. There is, however, one chance in four that their offspring will be a carrier of the recessive gene.

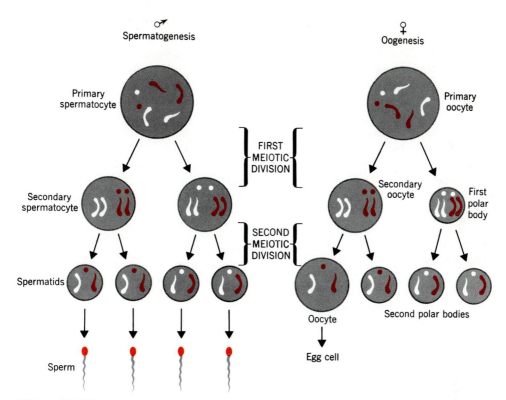

Figure 21-10. *Spermatogenesis and oogenesis. A primary spermatocyte produces four sperm, but only one egg results from meiosis of a primary oocyte. The polar bodies are functionless.*

Codominance

With codominance, the genes have equal expression. Blood types for type A blood and type B blood are codominant. Both A and B types are dominant over type O. If a person who is homozygous for type A mates with a person who is homozygous for type B, the offspring will have type AB blood. If, however, these parents are phenotype for A and B types but their genotypes are different (i.e., they have a recessive gene for one of the other blood types), the offspring will not necessarily have type AB blood.

Sex-Linked Inheritance

The X and the Y chromosomes not only determine the sex of the offspring but also carry additional nonsexual genes called sex-linked genes. The Y chromosome is very small and carries few genes. In a male, a sex-linked gene on the upper part of the X chromosome has no pair for it on the short Y chromosome, and therefore this genetic trait will be expressed. Because the female with two X chromosomes will have another gene to pair with, the trait may not be expressed. It will be expressed if it is a dominant gene or if she has received the same recessive gene from both her mother and her father. Whether expressed or not, the sex-linked gene can be transmitted from the mother to her offspring.

The criteria for determining characteristics that are transmitted by sex-linked inheritance are: (1) they are expressed more frequently in males, (2) the traits are transmitted from an affected male through his daughters to half of the daughters' sons, (3) they are not transmitted directly from father to son, (4) the gene may be transmitted from father to daughter and mother to son, but if it is recessive it is only apparent in the male.

Polygenetic Inheritance

A polygene is a gene that individually exerts little effect on phenotype but together with other genes controls a quantitative trait such as height, weight, or skin pigmentation. Polygenetic inheritance differs from the classical patterns of inheritance discussed above in that averages rather than discrete values are the consideration for individuals. The concept of polygenetic inheritance, therefore, is statistical in nature.

The transmission of polygenetic traits depends on the cumulative action of several genes, each of which contributes a small proportion of the total effect. Qualities relevant to human nutrition, time required to reach maturity, and life expectancy are a few examples of human characteristics dependent on multiple genes. Since environmental factors clearly influence these traits, great efforts are made to identify and control these as completely as possible so that the genetic component can be measured and subjected to statistical treatment.

Because of the practical significance of information of this type, it is not surprising that in recent years almost all genetic experimental projects involve quantitative or polygenetic inheritance.

Intermediate Inheritance

When both genes of an allelic pair are about equally expressed, the inheritance is intermediate. Sickle cell disease is an example. An individual who has inherited a sickle cell gene from both his mother and father will have sickle cell anemia, whereas an individual who has inherited only one defective gene generally does not have the disease. An analysis of the hemoglobin of the latter individual shows about equal proportions of normal hemoglobin and sickle hemoglobin. This is intermediate inheritance of hemoglobin.

Tissue Cultures

Geneticists can do tissue cultures to study genes. Cells that grow and divide regularly are the easiest to culture. At the present time, we cannot culture nerve or muscle tissues. Cells from young donors live longer than cells from older individuals. Most cells have contact inhibition that causes them to stop growing when they come in contact with other cells. Cancer cells do not have contact inhibition and, apparently, grow indefinitely.

EXPRESSION OF HEREDITARY TRAITS

Regardless of the pattern by which the hereditary material is transmitted, a trait is not always expressed at birth. The expression of a genetic trait may be delayed for years. Sex-linked hereditary baldness does not usually appear for 25 or 30 years, but hemophilia, also sex-linked, is apparent at birth. Albinism (al'bin-izm), an abnormal whiteness of the skin and hair, is an example of a recessive inheritance evident at birth. Muscular dystrophy, also a recessive trait, does not appear for 10 to 15 years.

Penetrance is the frequency with which a heritable trait is manifested by individuals carrying the gene or genes for this trait. A dominant gene with complete penetrance is expressed by all who carry it. A dominant gene with 80% penetrance is not expressed in 20% of the people who carry it. Homozygous recessive genes can also have reduced penetrance.

Whether a hereditary trait is expressed or not may in some instances depend on environmental factors. For example, some types of allergy are hereditary, but the allergic response depends on exposure to the allergen. The interaction between genes and particular environmental situations is becoming an important factor in industrial hygiene and health education. At the present time, there are some 3,000 occupational disorders involving a combination of environmental factors and genetic makeup.

Ecogenetics, a relatively new branch of genetics, is the study of the gene-environment interaction. Perhaps 10% to 20% of all cancers are linked to the workplace. Approximately 150 chemicals used in industry are thought to have toxic effects on the nervous systems of individuals with a particular genetic makeup. These chemicals may cause behavioral changes and cognitive defects. Ecogenetics evaluates these health risks and seeks to protect individuals who are susceptible to these hazards in the workplace.

Like other new scientific undertakings, ecogenetics faces controversy, ethical and otherwise. For example, should industry do genetic screening on prospective employees, or spend enormous sums of money making the work environment safer for a small fraction of the workers? Also, would the screening be considered discriminatory?

There are inherited variations in sensitivity in response to drugs. An example of this is the metabolism of isoniazid, used primarily in the treatment of tuberculosis. Some persons inactivate the drug rapidly, some do so slowly, depending on gene combinations.

Apparently, some behaviors are inherited, for example the birthing behavior of salmon and the building of particular types of nests by birds. Geneticists are currently constructing a genome map that will plot some inherited human behaviors. The federal government has allotted three billion dollars and fifteen years for this project, which started in 1990.

There seems little doubt that within the next few years we will be able to do prenatal screening early in pregnancy (in the first 20 weeks) for such lethal hereditary diseases as cystic fibrosis, muscular dystrophy, and Huntington's chorea. Although it has been suspected that there might be some hereditary factors involved, it is only recently that the specific defective genes involved in multiple sclerosis, juvenile-onset diabetes, chronic hepatitis, and lupus have been identified. Geneticists are also now able to identify people who are highly susceptible to emphysema, certain types of arthritis, arteriosclerosis, high blood pressure, allergies, peptic ulcers, lymphomas, and several types of leukemia.

Genetic engineering is not new and should not be feared. For many years, some dairy farmers have bred cows that produce milk with a high butterfat content. Other farmers raise cows that produce large amounts of milk with a low butterfat content. Our pedigree dogs and cats are bred so they have unique appearances and characteristics. Even the Thanksgiving turkey now has more white meat compared to the turkey our great-grandmothers prepared.

Recently, grain crops that produce their own nitrogen to avoid using fertilizers and seed corn with its own pesticide are being studied.

In the field of health, we now have Humulin, human insulin, which is less expensive than insulin from cattle. Also, allergies to Humulin do not exist. Genetic engineering has made available the human growth hormone for the treatment of dwarfism and a blood-clotting factor for the treatment of hemophilia. Also, genetic research has produced vaccines for several diseases that were once fatal.

SUMMARY QUESTIONS

1. Where are the oocytes formed?
2. Where are the sperm formed?
3. List the hormones produced by the ovary and discuss the functions of these hormones.
4. What hormone is responsible for the male secondary sex characteristics and what causes the production of this hormone?
5. Describe the structure of the uterus.
6. Where does the fertilization of the oocyte usually take place?
7. List some factors that can cause infertility.
8. Which ovarian hormone dominates before ovulation?
9. What causes this hormone to be produced?
10. What is the function of the smooth muscle of the scrotum?
11. Where is the epididymis located and what is the function of this structure?
12. What is the function of the vas deferens?
13. Where is the prostate located and what is its function?
14. List some contraceptive methods and describe how they work.
15. What causes the erection of the penis?
16. List the phases of the menstrual cycle.
17. In terms of genetics, what is the difference between simple dominance and codominance?
18. How are sex-linked hereditary characteristics transmitted?
19. List in sequence all of the structures through which the sperm must travel from the place of sperm formation until fertilization occurs.
20. Describe the period of embryo development.
21. Describe the stages of labor.

KEY TERMS

corpus luteum
cryptorchidism
ejaculation
endometrium
estrogen
fallopian tubes
genotype
heterozygous
homozygous
insemination
lactation

ligation
menarche
myometrium
oocyte
ovulation
parturition
perineum
phenotype
progesterone
testosterone
trimesters

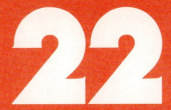

22

Diseases of the Reproductive Systems

OBJECTIVES

On completion of this chapter, you will be able to:

1. Explain how fertility tests are done.
2. Discuss how gynecological examinations are done.
3. Define some menstrual disorders.
4. Explain the different types of abortions.
5. Discuss the problems that might be associated with labor and delivery.
6. Discuss diseases of the prostate and describe their treatment.
7. Explain how venereal diseases are diagnosed and treated.
8. Define AIDS and list the people most likely to become its victims.
9. Discuss diseases due to chromosomal abnormalities and mutations.
10. List the symptoms of Down syndrome.
11. State at what age the symptoms of Huntington's chorea first appear.

OVERVIEW

I. DIAGNOSTIC PROCEDURES
   A. Tests to Determine Causes of Infertility
   B. Tests to Confirm Pregnancy
   C. Gynecological Examination
      1. Cervical Biopsy
      2. Culdoscopy
      3. Colposcopy
      4. Dilatation and Curettage (D and C)
   D. Diagnosis of Breast Tumors
   E. Venereal Disease Examination
   F. Examination of the Unborn Child
      1. Amniocentesis
      2. Chorionic Villi Sampling
      3. Sonography
      4. Abdominal Electrocardiography
      5. Direct Monitoring of the Fetal Heart

II. DISORDERS OF THE FEMALE
REPRODUCTIVE SYSTEM
   A. Disorders of Menstruation
      1. Dysmenorrhea
      2. Amenorrhea
      3. Menorrhagia
      4. Metrorrhagia
   B. Abortions
      1. Spontaneous Abortion
      2. Threatened Abortion
      3. Incomplete Abortion
      4. Missed Abortion
      5. Induced Abortion
   C. Ectopic Pregnancy
   D. Complications of Pregnancy
      1. Toxemia
      2. Infections
      3. Thrombophlebitis
   E. Problems Associated with Labor and
Delivery
      1. Prolonged Labor
      2. Placental Abruption

This chapter was written by Judith A. DePalma and Kathleen B. Gaberson.

      3. Placenta Previa
      4. Postpartum Hemorrhage
      5. Puerperal Infection
   F. Tumors
      1. Endometriosis
      2. Ovarian Tumors
      3. Uterine Tumors
      4. Cancer of the Uterus
   G. Infections
      1. Pelvic Inflammatory Disease
      2. Vaginitis
   H. Uterine Displacements
   I. Vaginal Fistulas
   J. Diseases of the Breasts
      1. Cystic Mastitis
      2. Benign Tumors
      3. Breast Malignancies
      4. Breast Abscess

III. DISEASES OF THE MALE
REPRODUCTIVE SYSTEM
   A. Benign Prostatic Hypertrophy
   B. Cancer of the Prostate
   C. Cancer of the Testes
   D. Infections
      1. Orchitis
      2. Epididymitis
      3. Prostatitis

IV. VENEREAL DISEASES
   A. Gonorrhea
   B. Syphilis
   C. Genital Herpes
   D. AIDS

V. INHERITED DISEASES
   A. Chromosomal Abnormalities
      1. Klinefelter's Syndrome
      2. Turner's Syndrome
      3. Trisomy of Sex Chromosomes
      4. Trisomy-21 or Down Syndrome
      5. Cancer
   B. Diseases Due to Mutations
      1. Autosomal Recessive Mutations
      2. Autosomal Dominant Mutations
      3. Sex-Linked Mutants
   C. Polygenic Inheritance

Although the main problems resulting from disease processes of most organ systems directly affect the functioning of the system, some of the diseases of the reproductive systems do not decrease the patient's fertility. In this chapter, we will consider problems concerned with fertility and other types of problems related to the organs of the reproductive systems. A brief discussion of some more common genetic diseases is also included.

DIAGNOSTIC PROCEDURES

TESTS TO DETERMINE CAUSES OF INFERTILITY

Infertility is the inability to conceive within one year despite adequate sexual contact without contraceptive use. Causes of infertility can be attributed to male factors (40%–50%), female factors (40%–50%), and unknown factors (no detectable problem in either mate) (10%–20%).

An evaluation of a couple's fertility usually begins with the simplest laboratory test, a microscopic examination of a semen specimen. For this test, the man is asked to produce a specimen by ejaculation into a container after two or three days of sexual abstinence. The specimen should be kept at room temperature and delivered to the laboratory within an hour or two.

In addition to the sperm count, the specimen is examined for motility of the sperm and any abnormality in shape. A low sperm count with high motility is a more favorable finding than a high count with poor motility.

The first step in diagnosing possible causes of infertility in the female is to confirm that she ovulates regularly. Blood tests may be done to determine the progesterone level; if ovulation does not occur, progesterone is not being produced. A biopsy of endometrial tissue taken late

in the menstrual cycle may also confirm if ovulation has occurred. Secretory changes in the endometrium indicate that the corpus luteum is functioning.

A woman may determine the time of ovulation by taking daily measurements of her basal body temperature (BBT). The temperature should be taken each morning before any activity. A slight drop in body temperature will occur just before ovulation, followed by a sharp rise in temperature at the time of ovulation. A woman will need at least a six-months record in order to determine the amount of her temperature fluctuations. Figure 22-1 shows a basal body temperature record.

Evaluation of cervical mucus may provide evidence of ovarian hormone activity. The cervical mucus is examined for cyclic changes that facilitate sperm penetration. Ordinarily the mucus is viscous and acid. At the time of ovulation the mucus is watery and more alkaline. Cervical mucus may also be evaluated 8 to 24 hours after sexual intercourse. This postcoital (post-ko′i-tal) test examines a sample of cervical mucus to determine if it contains motile sperm.

If the woman is ovulating, tests to determine if the fallopian tubes are patent (open) may be done. The Rubin test is a procedure by which carbon dioxide is injected through a cannula into the uterus and fallopian tubes and into the pelvic cavity. If one or both tubes are patent, only the normal amount of pressure will be needed to force the gas through the tubes. As the gas escapes into the pelvic cavity, the patient will experience pain referred to her shoulder as a result of diaphragmatic irritation. This pain is temporary and will subside as the gas is absorbed. Assuming a knee-chest position for a short time after the Rubin test may help prevent discomfort. In some cases, the Rubin test may actually clear an obstruction from the tube.

A more accurate test of tubal patency is the hysterosalpingogram (his″ter-o-sal-ping′o-gram). A radiopaque dye is injected into the

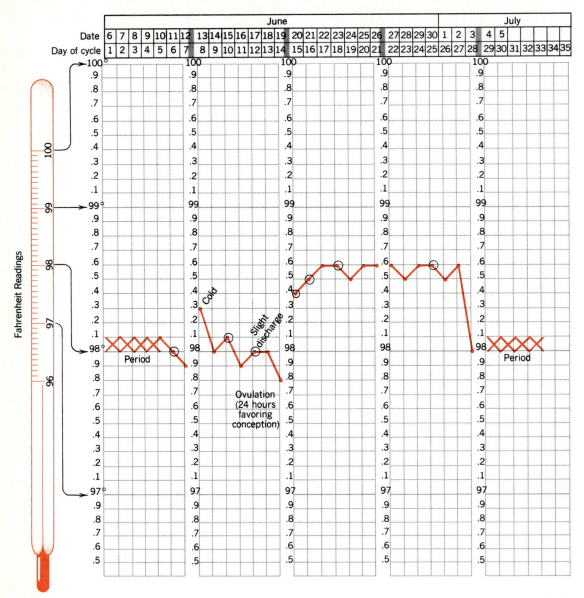

Figure 22-1. *The basal temperature chart (Courtesy of Philips Roxane Laboratories, Inc., Columbus, OH)*

uterine cavity so that the uterus and tubes can be visualized on X-ray and fluoroscopy. If the tubes are patent, the dye will distend the uterus and tubes and spill out into the pelvic cavity. This test causes discomfort similar to that of the Rubin test. It does expose the patient to pelvic radiation, but it can provide information about the site of an abnormality and can also clear an obstruction from the tube. Figure 22-2 shows an X-ray of a hysterosalpingogram.

An ultrasound pelvic examination can be used to visualize ovarian changes associated with ovulation and to identify abnormalities such as ovarian cysts or tubal kinking. A full bladder is required for this examination so that the reproductive organs are pushed upward for better visualization.

A more invasive procedure, the laparoscopic examination, may be used to diagnose and sometimes correct problems that interfere with fertility. This procedure usually requires a general anesthetic. The laparoscope, an instrument with a small telescope, is inserted through an incision in the abdominal wall. The abdominal wall is lifted off the pelvic and abdominal organs by introducing carbon dioxide gas into the peritoneal cavity. Procedures such as ovarian biopsy, aspiration of cysts, or removing adhesions may be performed through the laparoscope. After the procedure, the woman may have shoulder pain similar to that commonly experienced after the Rubin test.

TESTS TO CONFIRM PREGNANCY

Tests for diagnosis of pregnancy are based on the fact that human chorionic gonadotropin (HCG) is produced by the placenta and excreted into the maternal bloodstream; it is then filtered into the mother's urine. HCG is present in the blood serum 8 to 10 days after fertilization and can be detected in the urine 10 to 14 days after the first missed menstrual period. In biologic tests for pregnancy, such as the Friedman and Aschheim-Zondek tests, urine is injected into a laboratory animal. If HCG is present, there will be changes in the reproductive tract of the animal. Newer pregnancy tests use immunologic methods to detect the presence of HCG in blood or urine. These tests are based on the fact that HCG is an antigen, and it can be detected by serum containing antibodies specific for this antigen. The radioimmunoassay (RIA) for HCG can be used to diagnose pregnancy as early as five days before the first missed menstrual period.

Urine for pregnancy testing should be the first morning specimen. This voiding is likely to contain a sufficient concentration of HCG to permit accurate testing. Most immunologic tests take from 20 seconds to two hours to obtain results; the RIA takes about 24 hours. Kits for self-testing are available.

An ultrasound examination can diagnose pregnancy by detecting the presence of a gestational sac in the uterus as early as the sixth week.

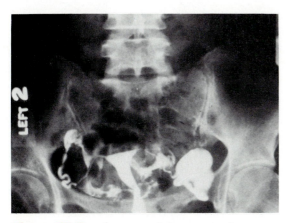

Figure 22-2. A hysterosalpingogram showing a normal left side and normal uterus. On the right side there is a hydrosalpinx. (Courtesy of Magee-Women's Hospital, Pittsburgh, PA)

GYNECOLOGICAL EXAMINATION

To prepare for a gynecologic examination, a patient should be instructed not to douche prior to the examination and to empty her bladder. If the examiner is a man, the patient may feel more comfortable if a woman assistant is present.

The most common position for a gynecological examination is the lithotomy position. The patient should be draped with a sheet over her knees and upper body, with the perineum exposed. Although the vagina is not sterile, the equipment used must be sterilized between patient uses to avoid the spread of infectious organisms.

The examiner inspects and palpates the abdomen and breasts, and inspects the external genitalia for signs of irritation or abnormal vaginal discharge. In order to see the cervix and the

vaginal mucosa, a speculum as shown in Figure 22-3b is inserted to separate the vaginal walls. With the speculum in place, vaginal and cervical smears can be obtained to diagnose various conditions. The **Papanicolaou** (pap"ah-nik'o-lao) **test** or pap test is a cytological examination of cervical secretions to detect abnormal cells that suggest malignancy. If a pap test is to be performed, the vaginal speculum should only be lubricated with water to prevent interference with the cytological examination. The pap smear slide is sprayed with a chemical fixative before it is delivered to the laboratory. If the results of the pap test are positive or questionable, the patient should have a cervical biopsy, culdoscopy (kul-dos'ko-pe), colposcopy (kolpo'scop-e), or dilatation and curettage (kur"ehtazh') done.

After the speculum is removed, the examiner does a bimanual examination by inserting one

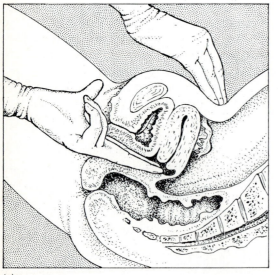
(a)

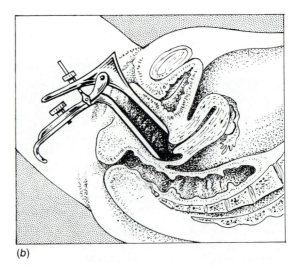
(b)

Figure 22-3. (a) Position of the hands in a bimanual pelvic examination. (b) Lateral view of the speculum in position. (From Sloane, E., Biology of Women. *New York: John Wiley & Sons, Inc., 1980)*

or two fingers of a gloved hand into the vagina and palpating the abdomen with the other hand (see Fig. 22-3a). Between the two hands, the size, shape, and position of the reproductive organs can be determined.

Cervical Biopsy

A cervical biopsy can be performed as an outpatient procedure in a doctor's office or clinic. Although the patient may experience some discomfort, this procedure is not painful because the cervix does not have pain receptors. The specimen, properly labeled, is sent to the laboratory immersed in a fixative solution. If the patient has had vaginal packing inserted, she should be instructed not to remove it for 24 hours. Some vaginal discharge and slight bleeding may occur for a few days following the procedure. If bleeding is excessive, the patient should be examined by the doctor. Because of the danger of infection, the patient should not use tampons, douche, or have sexual intercourse for about a week after the biopsy.

Culdoscopy

For a culdoscopic examination, the patient assumes a knee-chest position as shown in Figure 22-4. The culdoscope is inserted into the vagina and through a small incision in the posterior fornix. The pelvic viscera can be directly visualized.

Colposcopy

Colposcopy is an office or clinic procedure that uses an intense light and a magnifying lens to allow detailed inspection of the cervix. The patient is positioned as for a vaginal exam, and a speculum is inserted to separate the vaginal walls. The colposcope (kol'po-skop) shows areas of abnormal tissue that can be biopsied for further study. Some cervical lesions may be treated with laser vaporization or cryosurgery (kri"o-

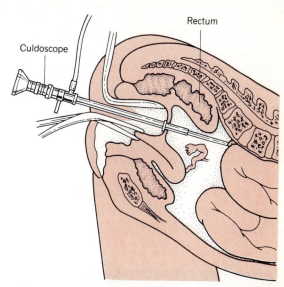

Figure 22-4. A culdoscopic examination (From Barber, J.M., Stokes, L.G., and Billings, D.M., Adult and Child Care, *2nd ed. St. Louis: The C.V. Mosby Co., 1977)*

ser'jer-e), which is the application of extreme cold to destroy the abnormal cells.

Dilatation and Curettage (D and C)

Dilatation, or enlargement of the cervical os (mouth) with dilators, permits curettage, or scraping, of the endometrium with an instrument called a curette to obtain tissue samples for laboratory examination. The D and C usually requires a general anesthetic. Following the surgery, the patient usually experiences little or no discomfort but may have a vaginal discharge for a few days.

DIAGNOSIS OF BREAST TUMORS

In **mammography** (mam-og'rah-fe), X-ray films of the breast are taken from various angles. This technique can detect breast lesions too small to be palpated by the woman or her health care provider. The accuracy of mammography is generally higher in older women whose breast tissue is not as glandular and dense (see Fig. 22-5).

Thermography (ther-mog'rah-fe) detects changes in the blood circulation of breast tissue by infrared photography. There will be increased heat in areas of increased blood supply indicating the possible presence of a tumor. A positive thermogram is not specific for cancer, and not all cancers cause increased skin temperature. Therefore, this technique is less effective than mammography.

VENEREAL DISEASE EXAMINATION

Examinations used to detect venereal or sexually transmitted diseases include microscopic examinations of patient secretions and serologic tests. Gonorrhea can be diagnosed by bacteriological culture of the Neisseria gonococcus from vaginal or urethral secretions. Serology tests, such as the Wasserman or Kahn tests, are used to diagnose syphilis from a serum sample. These tests are based on antigen-antibody reactions and can result in false positives in patients who have collagen diseases or who have recently been immunized. If central nervous system involve-

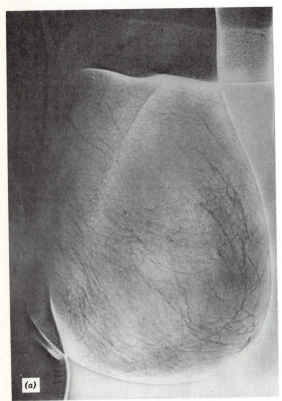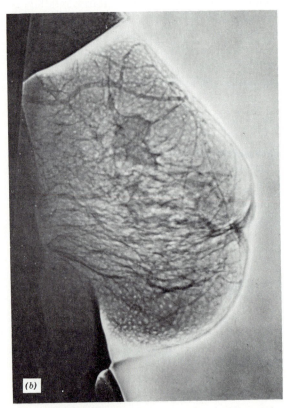

Figure 22-5. *Mammogram showing (a) a normal breast and (b) a lesion in the upper part of the breast (Courtesy of Elizabeth A. Patterson, M.D.)*

ment is suspected, the cerebrospinal fluid can also be tested. Herpes genitalis (Herpes type II), cytomegalovirus, and chlamydia trachomatis (klah-mid′e-ah trah″ko-mah′tis) can be diagnosed by cytological examinations of secretions from the cervix or suspicious lesions. Immunologic tests of blood serum are used to diagnose **Acquired Immune Deficiency Syndrome** (AIDS), a fatal disease caused by a virus that destroys the immune system. The human immunodeficiency virus (HIV), also diagnosed by immunologic tests, is transmitted through sexual contact or exchange of certain body fluids. Also, the fetus can be infected during pregnancy. In fact, maternal infections with sexually transmitted organisms may result in fetal illness, abnormal development, or even death. The importance of early diagnosis and treatment cannot be overemphasized.

EXAMINATIONS OF THE UNBORN CHILD

Amniocentesis

Amniocentesis (am″ne-o-sen-te′sis) can be performed as early as the twelfth week of pregnancy. After locating the position of the fetus and placenta by **sonography** (so-nog′rah-fe), the doctor inserts a sterile needle through the mother's abdomen into the amniotic sac. Less than one ounce of fluid is withdrawn and examined. Amniotic fluid analysis can be performed to determine the maturity of the fetal lung tissue, the degree of Rh immunization (maternal-fetal Rh incompatibility), the level of alpha-fetoprotein (al″fah-fe″to-pro′ten) for diagnosis of brain and spinal cord defects, and to detect signs of fetal distress. By examining the chromosomal structures of fetal cells and enzyme components in the amniotic fluid, a geneticist can identify the presence of several kinds of genetic or metabolic defects in the fetus. The sex of the fetus can also be determined, which can assist in the diagnosis of sex-linked disor-

ders, but this procedure is not routinely done to satisfy the parents' curiosity.

The potential risks of amniocentesis include spontaneous abortion, fetal injury, infection, and premature labor. Although this procedure is not recommended for routine use in pregnancy, it is considered a safe diagnostic procedure when family history or parental age suggest a potential problem.

Chorionic Villi Sampling

Chorionic villi (ko″re-on′ik vil′i) sampling involves removing a small piece of the fetal portion of the placenta for diagnosis of a genetic disorder in the fetus. The tissue sample is taken through a cannula (kan′u-lah) inserted through the cervical canal, guided through ultrasound. This procedure can be done as early as the eighth week of pregnancy. Potential complications include spontaneous abortion, infection, and injury to the fetus or placenta. These risks are usually outweighed by the benefits of early diagnosis when there is a family history of a genetic disorder.

Sonography

With sonography, it is possible to safely obtain an image of the fetus within the uterus. Prior to the development of this technique, an image could be seen only by means of X-ray studies, which, because of the potential damage from radiation, are now used only in extreme cases.

Sonography employs sound waves to produce a two-dimensional image of the fetus, which is projected on the screen of an oscilloscope and can be photographed for future reference (see Fig. 22-6). After covering the mother's abdomen with a conducting jelly, a transmitting device called a transducer is placed on the abdominal skin. Electrical current is then introduced to cause the transducer to emit sound waves as it is moved back and forth across the abdomen.

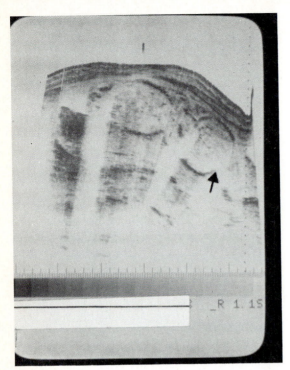

Figure 22-6. A sonogram showing a 26-week-old fetus. The arrow points to the fetal head. (Courtesy of Magee-Women's Hospital, Pittsburgh, PA)

These waves traverse the abdominal cavity and reverberate echoes from the various organs. The echoes pass back through the transducer and register as bright dots on the oscilloscope screen to form an image of the fetus.

Sonography is frequently used to measure the size of the fetal skull (biparietal diameter) for assessment of gestational age, especially if the date of the mother's last menstrual period is unknown or uncertain. It can also be used to diagnose the presence of a pregnancy as early as six weeks after the last menstrual period, iden-

tify a multiple pregnancy, locate the placenta before amniocentesis, diagnose certain placental abnormalities, and detect intrauterine fetal death by lack of mitral valve activity.

Abdominal Electrocardiography

In the past, the only techniques available for monitoring the fetal heart rate were phonocardiography, an application of a microphone to the mother's abdomen to pick up the fetal heart sounds, or Doppler ultrasound, which uses a small transducer to direct a sound beam to the fetal heart so that its beat comes back in the form of an echo. The effectiveness of these methods is limited due to the presence of abdominal noise and to fetal movement that makes location of the heartbeat difficult.

In abdominal electrocardiography, two small electrodes are placed on the mother's abdomen, one to record her heart rate and the other to monitor the heart rate of the fetus. The strength of the mother's uterine contractions can also be monitored by a pressure transducer, and the effect of these contractions on the fetal heart rate can be observed.

Direct Monitoring of the Fetal Heart

In high-risk labors, once the cervix has begun to dilate and the fetal membranes have ruptured, a catheter can be passed through the cervix and into the uterine cavity to record intrauterine pressure, and a small electrode can be affixed to an accessible part of the fetus to monitor heart rate. The normal fetal heart rate is 120 to 160 beats per minute, fluctuating within this range in response to uterine contractions during labor. If the expected pattern of fluctuation does not occur, the fetus may be suffering from lack of oxygen caused by insufficient blood flow through the placenta, and immediate delivery may be indicated.

DISORDERS OF THE FEMALE REPRODUCTIVE SYSTEM

DISORDERS OF MENSTRUATION

Dysmenorrhea

Painful menstruation is called **dysmenorrhea** (dis″men-o-re′ah). Most cases of dysmenorrhea have no identifiable organic cause. However, the patient with severe or chronic discomfort should be examined by a gynecologist so that possible pathology can be discovered and treated. For example, malposition of the uterus, which can cause dysmenorrhea, can be surgically corrected.

Many theories have been advanced about the causes of dysmenorrhea. Recently, it has been suggested that an overproduction of prostaglandins, a group of naturally occurring substances in menstrual blood as well as in other body tissues, might stimulate uterine muscle spasm causing dysmenorrhea. Medications that inhibit the production of these hormones may help to alleviate the discomfort. Motrin and Ponstel act as antiprostaglandins.

If there is no organic cause for the dysmenorrhea, application of heat to the lower abdomen, rest, exercise, or use of a mild analgesic such as aspirin may give symptomatic relief.

Amenorrhea

The absence of menstrual flow is called **amenorrhea** (ah-men-o-re′ah). This condition is normal during pregnancy, after menopause, and often during lactation. However, it can also be caused by endocrine disturbances, chronic wasting diseases (such as starvation and tuberculosis), and psychological factors. Occasionally, women who discontinue the use of the contraceptive pill experience a temporary amenorrhea, and those who exercise excessively may also cease their menstrual function.

Menorrhagia

Menorrhagia (men-o-ra′je-ah), or excessive bleeding, at the time of normal menstruation, can be caused by endocrine imbalances and psychological factors. It may also result from ovarian or uterine tumors, especially **fibroid** (fi′broid) tumors, and inflammatory diseases of the pelvic organs. It is difficult to determine how much menstrual flow is experienced; a rough estimate can be made from the number of pads or tampons needed per day.

Metrorrhagia

Bleeding or spotting between periods or after menopause is called metrorrhagia (me-tro-ra′je-ah). The causes include the same conditions involved in menorrhagia; however, a common cause of metrorrhagia is carcinoma (cancer) of the cervix. The amount of bleeding is not related to the seriousness of the underlying condition; therefore, even when she experiences only slight spotting,. the woman should have a complete gynecologic examination.

ABORTIONS

Abortion is the termination of a pregnancy before the fetus is **viable** (vi′ah-bl). Gestational age and weight of the fetus are usually used to define viability. Medical and legal definitions of viability may vary. However, a gestational age of 20 to 24 weeks and a fetal weight of 500 to 600 grams are the usual standards. After this time and until the time of a full-term delivery, the expulsion of the fetus is called a premature birth. Abortion can occur spontaneously (commonly referred to as a miscarriage) or be induced.

Spontaneous Abortion

Spontaneous abortions are most often associated with an abnormal development of the embryo or fetus. Of known pregnancies, one in six terminates in spontaneous abortion. Many more spontaneous abortions occur before the pregnancy is diagnosed or suspected. Maternal disease may also cause an abortion, but physical trauma or emotional shock are rarely the cause.

Threatened Abortion

Slight bleeding during pregnancy, with or without cramping, may indicate that an abortion is likely to occur. Sometimes the symptoms subside within several days and the pregnancy continues. Continued bleeding, stronger uterine cramps, and dilatation of the cervix indicate that progression to an inevitable abortion has occurred, and any attempt to maintain the pregnancy is useless. In most instances, the death of the embryo or fetus has occurred several weeks before the first symptoms, and there is no way to change the ultimate course by bed rest or hormone treatment.

Incomplete Abortion

In this instance, some of the products of the pregnancy are expelled and some are retained. The retention of a portion of the placenta or membranes can result in continued bleeding and infection. For this reason, all expelled tissues must be examined by a physician, who can determine if the abortion was complete. If it is an incomplete abortion, the woman may need a D and C to remove the retained parts.

Missed Abortion

A missed abortion is one in which the fetus has died but is not expelled. It may be retained for several months, requiring the use of medication to induce uterine contractions to expel the fetus and other products of conception. If this procedure fails, the fetus can be removed surgically.

Most doctors prefer to have labor start naturally or be induced medically rather than do a D and C because the cervix and uterine wall are soft at this time and there is danger of a perforation.

Induced Abortion

It is legally possible to perform an abortion if the woman does not feel that she is physically, emotionally, or financially able to bear and raise the child. Although in many cases abortion may be a desirable solution to such problems, it is not a sensible substitute for the use of an effective contraceptive method.

If the pregnancy might endanger the mother's physical or mental health, or if it seems certain that the baby will have serious defects, a therapeutic abortion may be performed. The decision to terminate a pregnancy for these reasons is made jointly by the patient and the physician.

ECTOPIC PREGNANCY

In an ectopic pregnancy, the fertilized ovum is implanted outside the uterine cavity. The most common ectopic site is the fallopian tube. Because the tube has so little room for expansion, the growing embryo and placenta will rupture the tube. The woman will experience severe abdominal pain and show signs of shock due to the profuse intraabdominal bleeding.

This is an emergency situation requiring immediate salpingectomy (sal-pin-jek'to-me), surgical removal of the tube.

COMPLICATIONS OF PREGNANCY

Toxemia

Toxemia (tok-se'me-ah) of pregnancy is a condition characterized by high blood pressure during the last several months of gestation. The early stages of this condition are characterized not only by an elevation of blood pressure but also edema, proteinuria, and headache. This cluster of signs and symptoms is known as pre-eclampsia. In severe cases, this condition may progress to eclampsia (e-klamp′se-ah), which involves convulsions and coma and can result in death.

Good prenatal health supervision is necessary to detect the earliest signs of toxemia and treat the condition so that it does not progress. Bed rest is often prescribed for the elevated blood pressure, and this treatment alone can be very effective in arresting the progress of the condition. Good prenatal nutrition, including adequate protein intake, is thought to reduce the frequency of toxemia.

Infections

Urinary tract infections are common during pregnancy due to the pressure of the enlarging uterus on the structures of the urinary tract. Cystitis (infection of the urinary bladder) is characterized by urinary frequency, urgency, and burning. A most serious complication is pyelonephritis, which can lead to premature labor. Pyelonephritis is characterized by fever and flank pain. If a urinary tract infection is suspected, the urine should be cultured and an appropriate antibiotic prescribed.

Thrombophlebitis

Thrombophlebitis (throm″bo-fle-bi′tis) is an inflammation of a vein that can lead to clot formation within the vein. Symptoms include fever as well as pain over the affected vein. In femoral thrombophlebitis, the affected leg is warmer than the other and swollen. The skin may be reddened, and dorsiflexion of the foot while the leg is extended may cause calf pain.

Treatment includes bed rest with elevation of the leg. The affected leg should not be massaged as this might cause the clot to be dislodged and travel to the pulmonary circulation. Anticoagulants may be prescribed to prevent further clot formation, although this is somewhat risky during pregnancy; it can cause intrauterine bleeding and interfere with fetal oxygenation.

PROBLEMS ASSOCIATED WITH LABOR AND DELIVERY

Prolonged Labor

Labor that lasts over 24 hours is classified as prolonged labor. Prolonged labor increases the risk of postpartum shock, hemorrhage, and fetal death. The most common causes of prolonged labor are uterine inertia (weak, poorly coordinated uterine contractions), cephalopelvic disproportion (a disparity between the size of the fetus and the space available for its passage through the mother's pelvis), and abnormal fetal position. It may be possible to rotate the fetus so that it can be delivered normally.

Frequently, a **cesarean** (se-za′re-an) **delivery** is necessary to terminate a prolonged labor. This procedure involves an incision into the mother's abdomen and uterus and removal of the baby and placenta.

Placental Abruption

The placenta normally separates from the uterus only after the birth of the baby. The premature separation of the placenta, called abruptio placenta is a leading cause of fetal death. The separation is accompanied by severe abdominal pain and bleeding, which may or may not be apparent from the vagina. Fetal heart sounds may be absent or slow and irregular. Immediate delivery is indicated to save the life of the fetus. This is usually accomplished by rupture of the membranes and use of a drug to stimulate uterine contractions. A cesarean delivery may be indicated.

Placenta Previa

The fertilized ovum normally implants high on the uterine wall. Implantation low in the uterus or covering the cervix results in placenta previa.

The main symptom of placenta previa is painless vaginal bleeding late in pregnancy. This condition is hazardous to the mother because of the hemorrhage and to the fetus because of hypoxia resulting from decreased placental circulation. If bed rest does not stop the bleeding, the condition is usually treated by inducing labor, if the cervix is not completely covered, or by performing a cesarean delivery.

Postpartum Hemorrhage

Postpartum hemorrhage is a leading cause of maternal death. The most common cause of hemorrhage in the first few hours following delivery is uterine atony; after this time, the usual cause is retained placental tissue. In most cases, this bleeding can be stopped by giving ergotrate, a drug that stimulates uterine contractions. If this procedure is ineffective, curettage must be performed.

Puerperal Infection

Although infections following childbirth are not common today, they can be very serious if the organisms enter the bloodstream and cause a generalized sepsis. Possible causes of puerperal infections include prolonged rupture of the fetal membranes before delivery, delivery of the baby under unsterile conditions, and postpartum thrombophlebitis.

TUMORS

Endometriosis

In **endometriosis** (en″do-me-tre-o′sis), there are implants of endometrial tissue outside the uterine cavity. These implants can be found on the ovaries or fallopian tubes or on other abdominal organs. This tissue responds to the same hormonal stimulation as does the endometrium in the uterus, but, because there is no outlet for the menstrual flow, patients often experience severe dysmenorrhea, and adhesions can develop within the pelvic cavity.

This condition can sometimes be successfully treated with hormones that keep the woman in a nonbleeding phase of her menstrual cycle for a prolonged period of time. Pregnancy can achieve the same result. However, severe cases of endometriosis are often associated with infertility.

Ovarian Tumors

Cysts are the most common tumors of the ovaries. Often women with ovarian cysts have no symptoms and no treatment is required. Occasionally, the cysts must be removed surgically if they are pressing on other structures and causing discomfort. Some cysts can cause problems of infertility. Other ovarian tumors can have masculinizing effects due to the production of androgen hormones. These effects can include atrophy of breast tissue, hirsutism (her′su-tism) (excess body and facial hair), and sterility.

Cancer of the ovary is very dangerous because it is difficult to detect until the tumor has spread to other organs. Regular gynecologic examinations may help to detect ovarian tumors before they metastasize, but the prognosis in any case is not encouraging. Surgery is the treatment of choice, and chemotherapy is often used to improve the patient's chances.

Uterine Tumors

Fibroid tumors of the uterus are benign growths in the muscle layer. These tumors vary greatly in size and may be single or multiple. Often women with fibroids have no symptoms. However, menorrhagia is the most common symptom. If the tumor is large, the woman may experience symptoms related to pressure on other organs such as the bladder or rectum. In such cases, surgical removal of the tumor or the uterus may be indicated.

Cancer of the Uterus

The most common malignancy of the female reproductive tract is carcinoma of the cervix. Any spotting or abnormal bleeding should be thoroughly investigated because these may be signs of malignant cell growth. Cure is possible only if the disease is diagnosed before it has spread. The importance of routine examinations and pap tests cannot be overemphasized. Cancer of the cervix can be treated surgically in conjunction with radiation and/or chemotherapy.

INFECTIONS

Pelvic Inflammatory Disease

Inflammation of the organs of the pelvis may result when pathogens enter these structures through the vagina, the lymphatics, or the bloodstream. Symptoms include a foul vaginal discharge, backache, and abdominal and pelvic pain in addition to fever and other common signs of infection. Gonorrhea is a common cause of pelvic inflammatory disease.

Treatment includes bed rest, antibiotics, and warm sitz baths. Tampons should not be used as they obstruct the flow of the discharge. Because adhesions can block the fallopian tubes, pelvic inflammatory disease may result in infertility.

Vaginitis

The normal acidity of the vaginal secretions provides a natural defense against most organisms. However, a variety of pathogens can infect the vagina. The most common organisms are a protozoa, Trichomonas vaginalis (trik″o-mo′nas vaj″in-a′lis), and a fungus, Candida albicans (kan′di-dah al′bi-kanz).

Both of these organisms cause a vaginal discharge called leukorrhea (lu-ko-re′ah). The discharge is irritating and causes severe itching. Often the urinary meatus is affected causing frequency and burning on urination.

Treatment involves medications specific to these organisms, usually in the form of vaginal suppositories. Flagyl is an oral medication specific for trichomonas, but it cannot be taken during pregnancy because it is harmful to the fetus. Usually the patient should avoid douching because she may reinfect herself with unsterile equipment.

In menopausal vaginitis, the atrophied vaginal membrane is easily traumatized and infected. Pruritus (itching) and vaginal discharge occur, and intercourse can be painful. Estrogens in the oral form and vaginal cream are used to treat this condition.

UTERINE DISPLACEMENTS

The uterus may be displaced backward, which is called retroversion (ret″ro-ver′zhun), or bent forward at an acute angle (antiflexion). Sometimes no symptoms occur; however, frequently the displacement causes dysmenorrhea. If the displacement causes severe discomfort, surgery may be necessary to move the uterus into a more natural position (see Fig. 22-7).

When the muscles of the pelvic floor are weakened, the uterus may herniate downward. This condition is called a prolapsed uterus. Symptoms include backache, fatigue, and pelvic pain. The woman may experience stress incontinence (a little urine seeps out when she coughs).

Often a rectocele (rek′to-sel) or cystocele (sis′to-sel) occurs when the uterus is prolapsed. A rectocele is a protrusion of a part of the rectum into the vagina, and a cystocele is a protrusion of the urinary bladder into the vagina.

Surgical repair of the prolapsed uterus and of a rectocele or cystocele is a relatively simple procedure. Generally, even women of advanced age tolerate the surgery quite well. If, however, the woman is a poor surgical risk, the displacement can be reduced by inserting into the vagina a

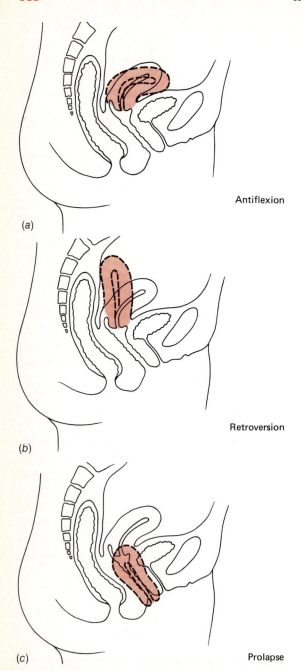

(a)   Antiflexion

(b)   Retroversion

(c)   Prolapse

Figure 22-7. Dotted lines showing uterine displacements in (a) antiflexion, (b) retroversion, and (c) prolapse

pessary, which holds the uterus in a more normal position. If a pessary is used it should be removed, cleaned, and replaced about every six weeks.

VAGINAL FISTULAS

An opening between the urinary bladder and the vagina is called a vesicovaginal fistula (ves″e-ko vaj′i-nal fis′tu-lah); between the rectum and the vagina it is called rectovaginal fistula. These fistulas may be congenital or develop as a result of an obstetric or surgical injury. The most common cause, however, is breakdown of tissue due to cancer. Symptoms are most distressing, as the vagina is constantly being irritated by urine or feces.

Although surgery may help correct vaginal fistulas, it can only be done when inflammation and edema have been controlled. Unfortunately, surgery is not always successful.

DISEASES OF THE BREASTS

Cystic Mastitis

Cystic mastitis (mas-ti′tis) is characterized by lumps in the breasts. There may be tenderness of the breasts, especially a few days before the menstrual period. Often a well fitted brassiere is all that is necessary to relieve the symptoms. In the case of multiple cystic disease, surgery may be necessary.

Benign Tumors

Fibroadenoma (fi″bro-ad-e-no′mah) is a type of benign tumor of the breast. It is less common than are cystic diseases. The fibroadenoma is removed surgically.

Breast Malignancies

Cancer of the breast is the most common type of malignancy in women. Although the disease can occur at any age, it is the leading cause of death among women between the ages of 40 to 44 in the United States. Successful treatment depends on early detection. From the local American Cancer Society office or your doctor, you can obtain a pamphlet that gives directions for self-examination of the breasts. Medical assistants can also give a woman instructions on how to do this simple examination. Routine monthly breast self examinations are the most valuable aid in detecting an abnormal lump in the breast. Annual mammography is recommended for all women over age 50, after an initial screening mammogram between the ages of 35 and 40.

Treatment usually includes surgery to remove the tumor alone (lumpectomy), the tumor and part of the breast (segmental resection), or the entire breast with primary lymphatic drainage (mastectomy). Radiation therapy may be used before surgery to reduce the size of the tumor. Radiation, chemotherapy, and/or hormonal therapy may be administered for advanced or inoperable cancers or after surgery to improve the prognosis.

Following a mastectomy, the patient may be bothered by edema of the arm on the affected side, because the axillary lymphatics have been removed. Exercises help in reducing the edema and are important in helping the woman regain full range of motion of the arm. "Exercises After Mastectomy: A Patient Guide," a pamphlet published by the American Cancer Society, is available at local Cancer Society offices. It describes exercises to be done following a mastectomy.

Breast Abscess

Abscesses of the breast occur most frequently following pregnancy. A localized abscess can be incised and drained. Antibiotics and warm compresses may also be helpful.

DISEASES OF THE MALE REPRODUCTIVE SYSTEM

BENIGN PROSTATIC HYPERTROPHY

Prostatic enlargement, called benign prostatic hypertrophy or hyperplasia (BPH), is one of the more common afflictions of middle-aged males. Half of the men over 50 years of age and 75% of the men over 70 experience some symptoms of prostate enlargement.

As the prostate enlarges, the surrounding capsule hinders it from expanding outward; the swelling presses inward, squeezing the bladder neck and the urethra. The process is usually slow, with the symptoms increasing over many months. These symptoms include frequency of urination, nocturia, urgency, hesitancy, and a weak urinary stream with a dribbly finish. As the prostate continues to grow, it can extend upward into the bladder, forming a pouch that retains urine. This pouch is not emptied during urination, and the residual urine decomposes, favors growth of bacteria, and leads to cystitis.

BPH is usually treated by surgically removing part or all of the prostate. The simplest and most common surgical procedure is a transurethral resection of the prostate. In this procedure there is no incision from the outside. A cystoscope is inserted into the bladder and pieces of the enlarged gland are removed with a cutting edge (see Fig. 22-8). Electric cauterization minimizes the bleeding from the vascular prostate and the excised tissue is flushed out with irrigating fluid.

Following the surgery, a foley catheter is in place with continuous irrigation to flush clots that might obstruct the flow of urine from the bladder. The urine should change in color from red to light pink within 24 hours. The patient usually has this surgery under a spinal anesthetic. Perineal exercises are taught to help re-

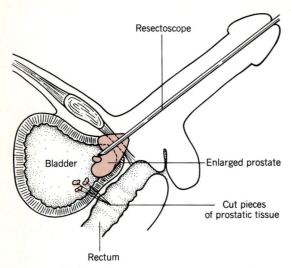

Figure 22-8. A transurethral resection being done for benign prostatic hypertrophy

gain urinary control following removal of the catheter. Following discharge from the hospital, the patient should continue to force fluids for several weeks, and avoid straining at stool and strenuous exercise. Sexual activity may be resumed in six to eight weeks.

For some patients, it may be necessary to do more extensive surgery. With a suprapubic prostatectomy or a retropubic prostatectomy there is a low abdominal incision. Postoperative care must then also include wound care.

CANCER OF THE PROSTATE

Cancer of the prostate is the second most common cancer and the third most common cause of cancer deaths in men. The disease is uncommon in men before the age of 50. Unfortunately, there are few early symptoms. If the tumor is large enough there will be obstruction of urine

flow. Prostatic cancer commonly metastasizes to the lymph nodes, pelvis, and lower spine.

Most prostate gland cancers can be detected by a rectal examination before symptoms appear. Therefore, every male over the age of 40 should have yearly rectal examinations. Early detection increases the probability of successful treatment. If the tumor is contained within the capsule of the prostate, a radical perineal prostatectomy is usually the treatment of choice. Urinary and sexual dysfunctions may result after radical prostate surgery.

If the tumor has spread, medical treatment may be the choice with hormone (estrogen) therapy to alleviate the symptoms temporarily. A bilateral orchiectomy (removal of both testicles) and radiation therapy may also be done.

CANCER OF THE TESTES

Cancer of the testes is the second most common malignancy in men between the ages of 25 and 34, and the frequency is increasing. If it is detected and treated early, there is an excellent chance of cure. Regular testicular self-examination is recommended after a bath or shower when the scrotum is relaxed. Any lumps, swelling, or tenderness should be reported to a physician.

Symptoms of cancer of the testes include a lump or swelling, a heaviness in the scrotum, a dull ache in the lower abdomen, and pain in the scrotum. Surgical treatment, an orchiectomy, consists of removal of the spermatic cord, the contents of the inguinal canal, and the testis. Surgery may be followed with radiation or chemotherapy.

INFECTIONS

Orchitis
Orchitis (or-ki'tis) is an inflammation of the testis. Most cases occur as complications of

mumps in adolescent boys and men but may also accompany syphilis, gonorrhea, or any acute infection. Orchitis can also be caused by injury. The testis is swollen and painful. There is often fever and nausea. The treatment is antibiotics and bed rest with the scrotum elevated and supported by an ice bag. Bilateral orchitis may lead to infertility.

A **hydrocele**, a collection of fluid in the scrotum, frequently occurs with orchitis. The fluid can be removed by aspiration, but the condition tends to recur.

Epididymitis

Epididymitis (ep″i-did″i-mi′tis) is an inflammation of the epididymis usually descending from an infected prostate or urinary tract. It can also develop as a complication of gonorrhea or from catheterization. Symptoms are similar to those of orchitis. Antibiotics, bed rest with the scrotum elevated, and a large fluid intake are usually ordered.

Prostatitis

Infections of the prostate may be acute or chronic and can be caused by a variety of pathogens that reach the prostate via the blood or lymph stream or directly through the urethra.

Chronic prostatitis occurs most commonly between the ages of 30 and 50. However, it can and does occur in all ages from puberty on. This infection is very common and may be present for years without producing symptoms.

Symptoms include pain in both inguinal regions and usually a mild pain in the testicles. There is usually a low backache, burning and frequent urination, and urethral discharge. Pus and blood cells may be found in the urine.

Treatment is usually antibiotics for 30 days, forcing fluids, rest, and local application of heat with sitz baths. Prostatic massage can be done but not during the acute attack.

VENEREAL DISEASES

Venereal diseases are infectious diseases transmitted from one person to another during intimate contact or sexual intercourse. It is estimated that in the United States there are anywhere from two to three million cases annually.

Genital herpes is one of the most common sexually transmitted diseases today and it is considered very serious because it has no known cure. Gonorrhea and syphilis are also serious public health problems. AIDS has recently appeared and has a high mortality rate.

GONORRHEA

Gonorrhea is caused by the gonococcus, a gram-negative diplococcus. It is also known as "clap" or "GC." The highest incidence occurs in persons 20 to 24 years of age, with the next highest incidence in those 15 to 19 years old. Symptoms appear in 3 days to 4 weeks after contact. Early symptoms are pain and burning on urination followed by urinary frequency. Urethral discharge develops and becomes yellow or brown, purulent, and profuse. Even without treatment these early symptoms subside in a short time. Unfortunately, this does not mean that the disease has disappeared.

Culture of the urethral discharge confirms the causative organism in men. Women may develop purulent vaginal discharge and aching in the lower abdomen.

If untreated, the infection can move up into a woman's uterus and fallopian tubes and into a man's epididymis, prostate, and seminal vesicles. Infections result in adhesions that can cause sterility. Even more dangerous is septicemia caused by the infection entering the bloodstream. Endocarditis and arthritis can also occur.

The mucous membranes of the eyes are very susceptible to gonorrheal infections, and an infected pregnant woman may pass gonorrhea to her baby's eyes during the birth process. The law in most states requires that the eyes of newborns be treated with silver nitrate or antibiotic drops to prevent gonorrheal eye infections.

Gonococcal infections are very sensitive to most antibiotics, and at least 90% of patients promptly respond to appropriate medications given in adequate dosages. Procaine penicillin, tetracycline, or probenecid may be used. Follow-up cultures should be done 3 to 7 days after completing treatment. Most infections that recur after treatment are due to reinfections, since no immunity results from having had the disease. All cases must be reported to local health departments and all sexual contacts of the patient within the last 30 days need to get treatment.

SYPHILIS

Syphilis is caused by Treponema pallidum (trep″o-ne′mah pal′i-dum), a distinctive spirochete that gains entrance through skin or mucous membrane during sexual intercourse. "Lues," "bad blood," or "pox" are other names for syphilis. The disease occurs three times more often in males than in females, with most cases found in those 25 to 29 years of age. Congenital syphilis is transmitted through the placenta of an infected mother to the fetus.

In the primary stage a painless lesion called a **chancre** (shang′ker) develops at the site of inoculation. Most chancres occur on the genitals, but they can develop on other areas of the body such as the lips, tongue, hands, rectum, or nipples. Without treatment the ulcer will heal spontaneously but slowly. In women this chancre may be inside the vagina and be completely unnoticed.

Secondary syphilis appears within six months after the chancre has healed, usually about six weeks after the initial infection. At this stage the serology blood tests become positive. Symptoms are extremely variable and include early flulike symptoms, generalized lymph node swelling, and eruptions on the skin and mucous membranes. The rash is usually painless, nonitchy, and symmetrical, favoring the palms of the hands and soles of the feet.

In the latent phase the patient feels well and has no symptoms. Blood tests will be positive because the spirochetes are still present in the body.

The final stage is characterized by involvement of one or more body systems and may be terminal. Cardiovascular problems, skin lesions, central nervous system problems, and chronic inflammation of the bones and joints may occur, because the unchecked spirochete can invade every cell of the body.

Because other penile lesions resemble the chancre of syphilis, all penile ulcers are considered syphilitic until proven otherwise. Finding the spirochete in serous discharges from the chancre is positive identification. Treatment of choice is the administration of benzathine penicillin G. Follow-up is very important and patients should be seen at 3-, 6-, and 12-month intervals after treatment. The disease can be completely cured. Syphilis is a disease that must be reported to the local health department. It is important that sexual contacts be identified, and an anonymous form is used to facilitate this.

GENITAL HERPES

Herpes genitalis (genital herpes simplex) is an acute, self-limited, and usually localized disease with no known cure. It is usually due to herpes virus Type II. Type I herpes is associated with infections occurring above the waist and Type II with those below the waist.

Symptoms usually appear within 3 to 7 days after exposure. There is a burning sensation and local tender lymph nodes, followed by multiple swollen and itchy blisters. Systemic symptoms include fever, headache, chills, and generalized lymph node swelling. Urination may be painful. The blisters rupture quickly and cause shallow, painful ulcers. This exudate is very contagious. These primary lesions normally last 3 to 6 weeks and heal without scarring, but they tend to recur spontaneously throughout the person's life, usually in the same place.

An unborn child of a mother with active genital herpes can contract the disease during vaginal delivery. Since there is presently no reliable or consistent cure, many measures are used. Comfort measures are advocated as is the need to keep the infected area clean. Sexual intercourse should be avoided if lesions are present to avoid spreading the infection.

AIDS

AIDS refers to acquired immune deficiency syndrome and has been identified by the U.S. Public Health Service as its number one priority. The disease was first reported in the United States in 1978. From 1981 to 1985, 12,000 cases of AIDS were identified, resulting in 5,000 deaths.

AIDS is caused by a retrovirus (HTLV-3) and is transmitted through sexual contact and exposure to infected blood products. Therefore, the people most at risk to develop AIDS are people with numerous sexual partners, intravenous drug users, people who require frequent blood transfusions (hemophiliacs), and the fetus of an infected mother. The incubation period ranges from 5 months to 5 years.

Symptoms include sudden weight loss, severe fatigue, fever, watery diarrhea, and night sweats. The presence of a persistent infection may lead to the diagnosis of AIDS.

The function of the T cells in the immune system is disrupted. With the decrease in the function of the immune system, opportunistic infections and neoplasms are likely to develop. The most common disorders are Pneumocystis carinni pneumonia and Kaposi's sarcoma of the skin and mucous membrane.

Health personnel are advised to utilize Universal Precautions to avoid any exposure to blood or other body fluids of AIDS patients. This means blood samples must be taken while health care workers are gloved and all precautions must be taken to prevent spillage of blood. Frequent handwashing is advised and careful disposal of used needles and intravenous catheters.

Experimental treatments include interferon a virus-fighting compound, and Interleukin-2 (IL-2), a chemical that can improve the immune response. Test tube experiments have shown that IL-2 restores the function of T cells, a crucial part of the immune system.

INHERITED DISEASES

CHROMOSOMAL ABNORMALITIES

To better understand how an abnormal number of chromosomes can occur, review the discussion of meiosis in Chapter 4.

Klinefelter's Syndrome
In men with Klinefelter's syndrome there is an additional sex chromosome, XXY. The testes are small, there is infertility, eunuchoid features, and the breasts may be enlarged. Mental deficiency commonly occurs.

Turner's Syndrome
This condition involves the loss of an entire chromosome, which is called monosomy (mon'o-so"me). The single X chromosome is often written as XO. These individuals appear to be fe-

male, but at puberty no secondary sex characteristics develop and there is no menstruation.

Trisomy of Sex Chromosomes
When there are three chromosomes of a kind instead of the normal two it is called **trisomy** (tri'so"me). Nearly all such cases involve sex chromosomes, and the most commonly recognized involve either triple X or triple X-Y complexes.

Trisomy-21 or Down Syndrome
In Down syndrome there are three 21 chromosomes instead of two. This trait occurs in about one birth in 500 or 600 with the greatest proportion coming from mothers who are over 40 years of age. Most genetic defects as well as congenital abnormalities are more common in babies born to older parents (either mother or father).

Down syndrome is often referred to as Mongolism. Its victims are mentally retarded, have mongoloid (slanted) eyes, hyperextensibility of finger joints, and other physical malformations.

Cancer
Cancer occurs whenever the genes that code for normal cell growth are sabotaged and rearranged. Researchers studying human chromosomes, the rod-shaped bodies that carry the genes, have found that in tumor cells taken from cancer patients the chromosomes are almost always broken and scrambled. Particular rearrangements consistently show up in certain cancers. These defects include translocations, associated mostly with leukemias and lymphomas, deletions or missing pieces, which occur in solid tumors such as are found in kidney and lung cancer, and extra chromosomes, which are linked to various other tumors. Such findings involve "fragile sites," points where chromosomes often break. Many of these fragile sites are inherited.

DISEASES DUE TO MUTATIONS
A change or mutation in the structure of a gene can cause a functional disturbance somewhere in the body. Since genes are in pairs, the expression of a genetic trait can depend on whether the mutant gene is dominant or recessive. Dominant genes are expressed whether the arrangement is homozygous or heterozygous. When the mutant gene is recessive, it is not expressed unless it is homozygous. Even though a person with a mutant recessive gene is not affected, the genetic defect can be passed on to this person's children.

Mutations can occur on the genes of either autosomal or sex chromosomes. Since the gene complex is such a delicately balanced system, the majority of new mutations are harmful or even lethal. Some environmental mutagenic agents are certain drugs, some smog particles, irradiation, and viral infections. Most chemical carcinogens are also mutagenic. Mutations can be spontaneous, seeming to occur without cause.

Autosomal Recessive Mutations
This type of disorder represents the larger number of hereditary diseases and occurs in the infants of unsuspecting, unaffected parents. Several disorders characterized by serious metabolic errors are transmitted by autosomal recessive genes. Lipoidosis (lip-oi-do'sis) is a disorder of fat metabolism, galactosemia (gah-lak"to-se'me-ah) involves errors in carbohydrate metabolism, and PKU or **phenylketonuria** (fen"il-ke-to-nu're-ah) results in improper metabolism of an essential amino acid. Some forms can be treated with dietary measures if recognized early.

Cystic fibrosis, which affects most or all of the exocrine glands, is transmitted by an autosomal recessive mutant. In this condition, there are serious lung problems similar to those of bronchitis, pneumonia, and asthma as well as gastrointestinal problems such as chronic diarrhea and intolerance of milk. In cases that are recognized early, diet therapy and a pulmonary hygiene regimen can relieve the patient's symptoms.

Autosomal Dominant Mutations

Many different abnormalities of hemoglobin are transmitted by this type of mutant as are polyps of the colon and multiple neurofibromas. Another result is Huntington's chorea (ko-re′ah), a degenerative disease of the cerebral cortex (especially the frontal cortex) and the basal ganglia. Symptoms include mental deterioration, speech disturbances, and irregular involuntary movements (chorea). As the disease progresses, walking becomes impossible, swallowing difficult, and there are severe mental disturbances. It is unique among hereditary diseases for its late onset (average age of 37 years). This is tragic, because the symptoms do not appear until well after the affected individual has had an opportunity to pass the trait on to an offspring.

Sex-Linked Mutants

The hemophilias, or bleeder's diseases, are examples of this type of hereditary disease. Severe bleeding can occur with slight trauma because the individual's blood lacks an essential clotting factor. Almost all affected individuals are males; their mothers and some of their sisters are carriers but are asymptomatic. The missing blood factor is used to treat the hemophiliac's bleeding.

Muscular dystrophy also depends on a sex-linked recessive gene. One-half of the male children of a carrier mother can be expected to be normal, since the possibility of their being homozygous for a sex-linked recessive gene is remote. The disease is characterized by progressive weakening and wasting of the skeletal or voluntary muscles and first appears at about the age of 10 to 14. Muscular deterioration progresses rapidly during the early teen years with these children usually becoming crippled and paralyzed by their late teens. Parents and siblings of the affected person are advised to seek genetic counseling.

POLYGENIC INHERITANCE

A large number of diseases tend to occur within families, but no chromosomal abnormality has been identified. Diabetes mellitus, some types of hypertension, and arthritis are examples of very common diseases that can be due to combinations of genes, the interactions among genes and gene products, and gene interactions with the environment. Variations in resistance to infection may also be a polygenic trait.

SUMMARY QUESTIONS

1. Discuss some of the tests that determine the cause of infertility.
2. How is a patient prepared for a gynecological examination?
3. Differentiate between amenorrhea, menorrhagia, metrorrhagia, and dysmenorrhea.
4. During what time of pregnancy is a spontaneous abortion most likely to occur?
5. What is an incomplete abortion?
6. What is a placenta previa and what are the signs and symptoms?
7. What is the most common cause of postpartum hemorrhage?

8. What are the signs and symptoms of benign prostatic hypertrophy?

9. Discuss the surgical procedure used to treat BPH.

10. What method is recommended for early detection of cancer of the testes?

11. How is gonorrhea treated?

12. Discuss the symptoms that occur during the various stages of syphilis.

13. What are the symptoms of genital herpes?

14. What is AIDS and who is most likely to contract it?

15. What are the symptoms of Down syndrome?

16. At about what age do the symptoms of Huntington's chorea appear?

17. Discuss diseases due to chromosomal abnormalities and mutations.

18. For what purpose is a Papanicolaou test done?

19. Discuss some problems that might be associated with labor and delivery.

20. How are venereal diseases diagnosed?

KEY TERMS

Acquired Immune Deficiency Syndrome

amenorrhea

amniocentesis

cesarean delivery

chancre

dysmenorrhea

endometriosis

epididymitis

fibroid

hydrocele

mammography

orchitis

Papanicolaou test

phenylketonuria

sonography

thrombophlebitis

toxemia

trisomy

viable

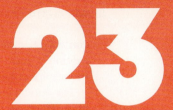

23

The Endocrine System

OBJECTIVES

On completion of this chapter, you will be able to:

1. Discuss the functions of the hormones secreted by the pituitary.
2. With respect to the endocrine system, explain what is meant by the negative feedback mechanism.
3. Tell what factors oppose the action of insulin.
4. Explain how blood calcium levels are regulated.
5. Discuss the functions of the thymus.
6. Name the three main classifications of hormones produced by the adrenal cortex and explain their actions.
7. Compare the actions of epinephrine and norepinephrine.
8. Discuss the actions of the hormones produced by the pancreas.
9. List the local hormones and give examples of their actions.
10. Discuss hormonal responses to stressful situations.

OVERVIEW

I. PITUITARY GLAND
   A. Adenohypophysis
     1. Thyrotropic Hormone
     2. Adrenocorticotropic Hormone
     3. Gonadotropic Hormones
     4. Somatotropic Hormone (Growth Hormone)
     5. Melanocyte-Stimulating Hormone
     6. Beta-Lipotropin
   B. Neurohypophysis
     1. Antidiuretic Hormone (ADH)
     2. Oxytocin
II. HYPOTHALAMUS
III. PINEAL GLAND
IV. THYROID
   A. Thyroxin and Triiodothyronine
   B. Calcitonin
V. PARATHYROID GLANDS
VI. THYMUS
VII. ADRENAL GLANDS
   A. Adrenal Cortex
     1. Glucocorticoids
     2. Mineralocorticoids
     3. Sex Hormones
   B. Adrenal Medulla
VIII. PANCREAS
IX. KIDNEY
X. GONADS
XI. PLACENTA
XII. LOCAL HORMONES
XIII. PROSTAGLANDINS
XIV. STRESS
   A. Factors Determining the Degree of Response to Stress
   B. Alarm and Resistance

The endocrine system works together with the nervous system in regulating and integrating the body processes. The chemical regulating mechanisms are much slower in action than nerve control but the hormones (meaning "to set in motion") have a more sustained action. Hormones are either proteins or steroid compounds.

The endocrine glands are ductless glands that pour their secretions directly into the bloodstream. These secretions flow throughout the entire circulation to affect cells and organs in far different parts of the body (see Fig. 23-1).

In addition, exocrine glands have ducts that allow their secretions to flow into a body cavity or onto the surface of the body. Sweat glands are exocrine glands.

In general, there are two mechanisms by which the hormones act. The steroid hormones from the adrenal cortex, ovaries, and testes enter the cytoplasm of the target cells and bind with a protein receptor. This complex enters the nucleus and activates genes to form proteins that will do the job of the hormone. Other hormones bring specific messages to their target cells. The hormone is called the first messenger and, to give its message, the hormone must attach to a receptor site on the cell membrane. This attachment increases the activity of adenyl cyclase (ad'e-nil si'klas), an enzyme that causes ATP to be converted to cyclic AMP (adenosine monophosphate) in the cell. The cyclic AMP acts as the second messenger, performing the specific function according to the message indicated by the hormone.

PITUITARY GLAND

The pituitary (pi-tu'i-tar-e) gland is located in the sella turcica and is attached to the hypothalamus by a stalk. The anterior lobe of the pituitary is called the adenohypophysis (ad"e-no-hi-pof'is-is). Although it has no direct nerve connections with the hypothalamus, it is under its control. This control is maintained by means of blood neurohumors (nu'ro-hu'mors) that circulate in the bloodstream between the hypo-

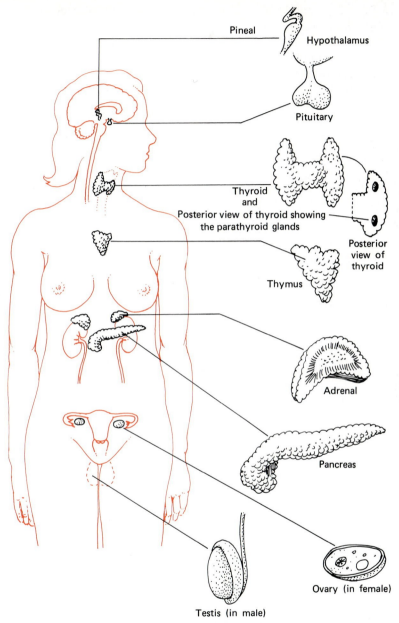

Figure 23-1. *General locations of major endocrine glands*

thalamus and the adenohypophysis. The posterior pituitary is also under the control of the hypothalamus but this control is by way of nerve connections. The posterior pituitary is called the neurohypophysis (nu"ro-hi-pof'is-is) (see Fig. 23-2).

ADENOHYPOPHYSIS

Most of the hormones produced by the adenohypophysis are secreted in response to substances from the hypothalamus called releasing factors (RF). These releasing factors are specific

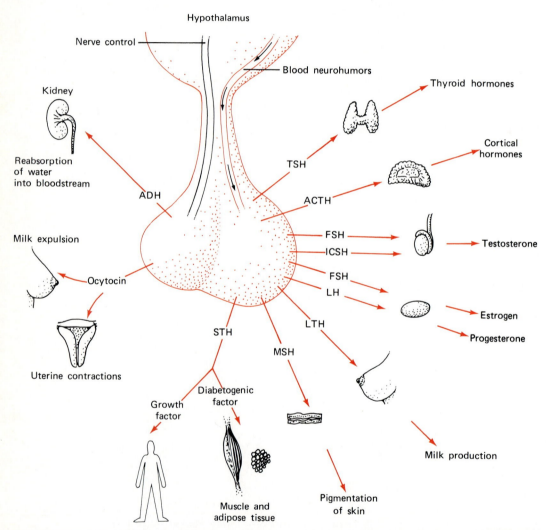

Figure 23-2. *Hypothalamic control of the anterior and posterior lobes of the pituitary and the hormones released by the pituitary*

for the particular hormone to be released. No releasing factor for the luteotropic hormone has been identified. However, there is a luteotropic inhibitory factor to inhibit secretion of the luteotropic hormone. In the absence of the luteotropic inhibiting factor, the adenohypophysis secretes the luteotropic hormone continually.

The function of some hormones of the adenohypophysis (the tropic hormones, meaning "stimulative") is to cause some other endocrine glands to secrete hormones. The increased secretion of hormones from the target gland in most instances causes a decrease in the secretion of the tropic hormone from the adenohypophysis. This mechanism is called negative feedback. Essentially, it operates like a furnace thermostat. When the room temperature is lower than the thermostat setting, the furnace turns on; once the temperature is high enough, the furnace turns off.

Thyrotropic Hormone

The **thyrotropic** (thi″ro-tro′pic) **hormone** (or thyroid-stimulating hormone, TSH) from the adenohypophysis stimulates the growth and some of the secretory activity of the thyroid gland. Increased secretions of thyroxin from the thyroid cause a decrease in the production of the thyrotropic hormone.

With exposure to severe cold, increased amounts of thyrotropic hormone will be produced. In three or four weeks the thyroid gradually enlarges and thyroxin secretions increase. The basal metabolic rate can be increased 20 to 30%, thereby producing more body heat.

Adrenocorticotropic Hormone

ACTH or the adrenocorticotropic (ad-re″no-kor″te-ko-trop′ik) hormone causes the adrenal cortex to secrete some of its hormones, chiefly the **glucocorticoids** (gloo″ko-kor′te-koids). Although many other hormones are produced by the adrenal cortex, it is high blood levels of glucocorticoids that ordinarily decrease the production of ACTH. This particular negative feedback mechanism, however, does not operate if the individual is experiencing great stress, since the glucocorticoids help prepare the individual to cope with emergency situations.

Gonadotropic Hormones

These hormones are concerned with the maturation and secretions of the gonads or sex glands. In the male, the follicle-stimulating hormone (FSH) causes the maturation of the sperm. In the female, it stimulates the development of the ovarian follicles and causes the ovaries to produce estrogen.

The luteinizing hormone (LH) in the female causes ovulation and stimulates the formation of the corpus luteum and the secretion of progesterone and some estrogen by the corpus luteum. This hormone, called the interstitial cell-stimulating hormone (ICSH), in the male stimulates the secretion of testosterone.

Estrogen, progesterone, and testosterone inhibit the production of these gonadotropic hormones.

During pregnancy, the lactogenic hormone promotes the breast development that makes possible milk secretion after delivery. In addition to its effect on milk secretion, the lactogenic hormone works with the luteinizing hormone in maintaining the corpus luteum in the postovulatory or premenstrual phase of each menstrual cycle and during the first six months of pregnancy. Because of this supportive role, the lactogenic hormone is also called the luteotropic hormone (LTH).

Somatotropic Hormone (Growth Hormone)

The **somatotropic** (so-mat″o-trop′ik) **hormone** (from the Greek soma, meaning "body") has a growth factor that stimulates the growth of bone, muscle, and organs. Normally, its level is high in infants, but by the age of 4 it is at the adult level. The growth factor stimulates protein anabolism, increases fat catabolism, and decreases glucose catabolism. It tends to cause cells to shift from glucose catabolism to fat catabolism for their energy supplies.

The other part of the somatotropic hormone is the diabetogenic (di"ah-bet"o-jen'ik) factor, which reduces peripheral glucose uptake by muscle and fatty tissue thereby increasing the blood sugar. It is an insulin antagonist. However, it stimulates the release of insulin from the pancreas.

Melanocyte-Stimulating Hormone (MSH)

The **melanocyte** (me"lan'no-site)-**stimulating hormone** may be responsible for normal pigmentation. The chemical structure of MSH is similar to ACTH. Both of these hormones, under certain circumstances, can cause increased pigmentation of the skin. The darkening of the face, nipples, and to a lesser extent the genitalia during pregnancy are caused by the high levels of estrogen and progesterone, which are also called "darkening hormones."

Beta-Lipotropin

Beta-lipotropin is a protein that enzymes from the pituitary gland can break down into hormones having a variety of psychological and behavioral effects. These hormones are known as **endorphins** (en-dor'finz) and **enkephalins** (en-kef'ah-linz). Beta-endorphin has a powerful analgesic effect and has been shown to reduce depression and anxiety in mentally disturbed individuals. Alpha-endorphin also has an analgesic and tranquilizing effect. Gamma-endorphin produces violence, increased irritability, and an increased sensitivity to pain. The enkephalins appear to be the body's natural pain relievers. They also appear to improve memory and induce pleasure.

NEUROHYPOPHYSIS

The hormones released by the neurohypophysis are actually made by the hypothalamus and are merely stored in the neurohypophysis until the hypothalamus causes their release into the bloodstream.

Antidiuretic Hormone (ADH)

The **antidiuretic** (an"te-di-u-ret'ik) **hormone** (ADH) works mainly on the collecting tubules of the kidney to increase their permeability and cause reabsorption of water back into the bloodstream. Normally the stimulus for the release of ADH is any condition that causes dehydration. With an increased fluid intake there will be a decrease in the production of ADH. Release of ADH is inhibited by alcohol and promoted by nicotine, barbiturates, and estrogen.

Vasopressin (vas-o-pres'in) is another name for ADH. This can be misleading as it suggests that the hormone causes vasoconstriction and elevates the blood pressure. Normal physiological levels of the hormone produce little if any vasoconstriction. However, a pharmacological preparation, pitressin, in large doses will cause vasoconstriction.

Recent studies suggest that in some unknown way this hormone functions to assist in learning and memory. It is hoped that ADH or some synthetic preparation of it may be useful in the treatment of senility.

Oxytocin

Oxytocin (ok-se-to'sin) also has a mild antidiuretic effect. However, its main actions are the expulsion of milk from the lactating breasts and causing uterine contractions after the delivery of an infant. Frequently, mothers who are breastfeeding their babies have uterine contractions (afterpains) for the first couple of weeks following delivery when the infant is nursing. These contractions are helpful in returning the uterus to its normal nonpregnant size and position in the pelvis.

HYPOTHALAMUS

In addition to ADH and oxytocin, the hypothalamus also produces **somatostatin** (so-mat″o-sta′tin). This hormone inhibits the secretion of the growth hormone by the anterior pituitary and some of the secretions of the intestinal mucosa. It also inhibits pancreatic hormones, insulin, and glucagon. Somatostatin is distributed throughout the central nervous system and has been shown to influence the transmission of nerve impulses.

Gastrin and **cholecystokinin** (ko-le-sis″to-kin′in) are also probably produced by the hypothalamus as well as by the duodenal mucosa. Whether they produce the same effects on the digestive tract as those produced by the duodenal mucosa is not clear.

PINEAL GLAND

The pineal (pin′e-al) gland, formerly called the "pineal body," was thought to do nothing other than act as a radiological landmark because it calcifies soon after puberty. Even now what its function is in the human is somewhat controversial. It is located just posterior to the third ventricle in the brain.

Research evidence seems to support the idea that the pineal may regulate cyclic phenomena in the body. One of its hormones, **melatonin** (mel″ah-ton′in), appears to follow a diurnal (day-night) cycle. Its production rises in the evening and through the night and drops to a low around noon. This hormone inhibits luteinizing hormone secretion and ovarian function.

Serotonin (ser″o-ton′in) from the pineal appears to oppose extremes in vascular diameter in the brain. For example, if there is too much vasoconstriction in the cerebral vessels, serotonin causes these vessels to dilate. Serotonin levels in humans are highest at noon and lowest at midnight.

Glomerulotropin (glo-mer″u-lo-tro′pin) produced by the pineal gland stimulates the secretion of adrenal aldosterone.

THYROID

The thyroid gland has two lobes that are lateral to the trachea just below the larynx. These lobes are connected by an isthmus (see Fig. 23-3). The thyroid is influenced by TSH from the anterior pituitary.

THYROXIN AND TRIIODOTHYRONINE

Thyroxin (thi-rok′sin) or T4 and triiodothyronine (tri″i-o″do-thi′ro-nine) or T3 perform essentially the same functions. However the action of thyroxin is longer lasting and less intense than that of T3. Each of these hormones increases metabolism. Both are secreted in response to TSH, and increasing blood levels of thyroxin and triiodothyroxin cause a negative feedback.

Thyroxin is the most abundant of these two hormones. It is essential for normal growth and development—mental, physical, and sexual.

CALCITONIN

The thyroid also produces **calcitonin** (kal″se-ton′in). This hormone lowers the calcium level in the blood by favoring the activity of the obsteoblasts and osteocytes, which deposit the calcium in the bones. Calcitonin causes a decrease in the absorption of calcium from the gastrointestinal tract and an increase in the urinary

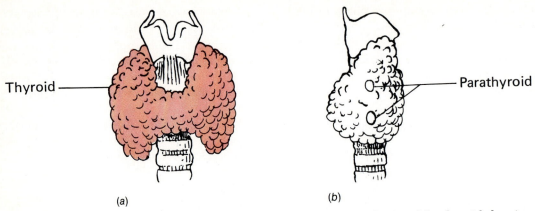

Thyroid

Parathyroid

(a)   (b)

Figure 23-3. (a) Anterior view of the thyroid gland, and (b) lateral view of the thyroid showing the parathyroid glands

excretion of calcium. Calcitonin also inhibits parathormone, which functions to withdraw calcium from the bone and elevates the calcium levels in the blood. The stimulus for the production of calcitonin by the thyroid is an excess of calcium in the blood.

increases the absorption of both phosphate and magnesium from the intestinal tract. The net result is an increase in the blood calcium level and a decrease in the amount of phosphate in the blood.

PARATHYROID GLANDS

The four parathyroid glands are found behind the thyroid and in the same capsule with the thyroid. Each of these glands measures approximately 6 x 3 x 1 mm. They produce **parathormone** (par-ah-thor′mon), which works together with calcitonin in regulating the calcium level in the blood.

The function of parathormone is to increase the calcium level in the blood by causing calcium to be withdrawn from the bone and by increasing the absorption of calcium by the intestinal tract. Parathormone decreases the phosphate level in the blood by stimulating the kidneys to eliminate phosphate in the urine. It also

THYMUS

The thymus (thi′mus) gland has both endocrine and lymphatic functions. It is found inferior to the thyroid at about the level of the bifurcation of the trachea. It is conspicuously large in the infant and during puberty it reaches its maximum size. After puberty it is replaced by fat and connective tissue. By the time the person reaches maturity, the gland has atrophied.

In the child, the thymus consists primarily of lymphocytes. In fact, in the fetus it is the only source of lymphocytes. It produces a mold for other organs (spleen and lymph nodes) to produce lymphocytes. The thymus produces **thymosin** (thi′moh-sin), a hormone that enables lymphocytes to develop into "T" cells (thymus-dependent lymphocytes), which mediate the cellular immune response. These T cells have the ability to destroy antigens.

Several other hormones have recently been isolated from the thymus; their actions are under investigation.

ADRENAL GLANDS

The adrenal glands are small triangular bodies located at the upper pole of each kidney. They have an abundant blood supply. The outer yellow portion is called the adrenal cortex and the inner gray portion is the adrenal medulla (see Fig. 23-4).

ADRENAL CORTEX

Many of the hormones from the adrenal cortex are essential to life. Circulating levels of these hormones vary over a 24-hour period. For a person on an ordinary schedule, maximum secretions occur between 2 AM and 8 AM; secretions are lowest in the late evening.

These hormones are grouped into three classes: glucocorticoids, which are concerned with metabolism of foodstuffs and the preservation of our carbohydrate reserves in stressful situations; mineralocorticoids, which are essential to the fluid and electrolyte balance of the body; and sex hormones. All are steroids.

Glucocorticoids

There are several different glucocorticoids. Cortisol or hydrocortisone is the most abundant glu-

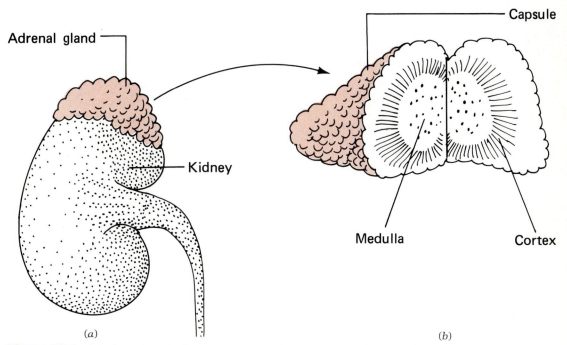

Figure 23-4. (a) The adrenal gland superior to the kidney. (b) The internal cortical and medullary portions are shown on the right.

cocorticoid. Cortisone and corticosterone also function as glucocorticoids. These hormones are produced in response to pituitary ACTH; however, the primary stimulus that initiates glucocorticoid secretion is stress, which includes almost any type of damage to the body as well as intense emotions. Under ordinary circumstances, the glucocorticoids provide the negative feedback mechanism for ACTH. However, this is overridden if the stress is severe.

In general, glucocorticoids help the body cope with stressful situations, primarily by preserving the carbohydrate reserves. Specifically, some of the functions of the glucocorticoids are as follows:

1. The concentration of glucose in the blood is increased as a result of cortisol depressing the utilization of glucose by most tissues and forcing them to use fat for fuel. The glucocorticoids also cause gluconeogenesis, the production of glucose from noncarbohydrate sources, like fat and protein. Although the blood sugar is increased, the glucocorticoids antagonize insulin. This can result in hyperglycemia. However, the action preserves the glucose for use by neurons that do not require insulin to utilize glucose. Under ordinary circumstances glucose is the only fuel that can be used by nerve tissue.

2. Glucocorticoids increase the amount of amino acids in the extracellular fluid. These proteins are moved out of tissue cells, primarily muscle, and transported to the liver where they are synthesized into new proteins, such as enzymes needed for metabolic reactions. If the body's fuel sources are low, the liver can convert these amino acids into glucose. In patients on prolonged steroid therapy this action can result in spindly arms and legs, tissue wasting, and a negative nitrogen balance.

3. Fat from fat depots is mobilized by the glucocorticoids, and there is an increased use of

fat for energy and other purposes. The cells are forced to shift from carbohydrates to fats for their fuel supplies. Unless the fats are used immediately, there is a possibility of their concentration in the extracellular fluid causing acidosis. This mobilization of fat can promote deposition of fat in the face ("moon face") and shoulders ("buffalo hump") in patients on prolonged steroid therapy.

4. Glucocorticoids are antiinflammatory in that they decrease vascular permeability so that fluid does not leak out and swelling is suppressed. They decrease the activity of the fibroblasts (fi'bro-blasts) that form scar tissue. For this reason, patients who have been on long-term steroid therapy may have poor wound healing.

5. These hormones increase gastric acidity. This fact, together with their antiinflammatory action, explains why prolonged steroid therapy can cause gastric ulcers.

6. Glucocorticoids are antiallergenic. Patients who suffer severe allergy may benefit from cortisone preparations that suppress T cells.

7. Blood vessels are sensitized to vasopressor substances by the glucocorticoids. The release of these hormones at the time of serious injury helps to limit the degree of shock that usually occurs with severe trauma.

8. The glucocorticoids increase neural excitability and give a person a general feeling of wellbeing.

Mineralocorticoids

Although several mineral corticoids are produced by the adrenal cortex, the main one is **aldosterone** (al-dos'ter-on). Mineralocorticoids act primarily on the kidney tubules but also to some extent on sweat and salivary glands. They cause the conservation of sodium and elimination of potassium. As do the glucocorticoids, these hormones help the body cope with stressful situations. Under stress, mineralocorticoids help preserve the fluid and electrolyte balance.

Mineralocorticoids are produced mainly in response to the amount of sodium and potassium in the bloodstream. A decrease in the amount of sodium in the blood or an increase in the amount of potassium will cause an increased production of aldosterone by the adrenal cortex. Glomerulotropin from the pineal gland and a plasma hormone, angiotensin, are tropic hormones for aldosterone.

Aldosterone production is also increased in the presence of hemorrhage. The aldosterone helps to correct the condition by increasing the quantity of sodium chloride and water in the extracellular fluid and ultimately increasing the volume of fluid in the circulation.

Sex Hormones

In both males and females, the adrenal cortex produces physiologically significant amounts of male hormones (androgens) and insignificant amounts of female hormones (estrogens). These androgens do not have strong masculinizing properties, except for testosterone, but the cortex secretes only small amounts of this. In the female, apparently the androgens are important for sexual behavior.

ADRENAL MEDULLA

The hormones from the adrenal medulla are not essential to life; however, they are important in our fight and flight responses. These hormones, called **catecholamines** (kat′e-kol″a-mines), are norepinephrine and epinephrine. About 80% of the medulla's secretion is epinephrine. Both do essentially the same thing as does the sympathetic nervous system (discussed in Chapter 9); However, the action of the hormones is of greater duration than neural stimulation.

The actions of norepinephrine dominate in anger, and those of epinephrine dominate in fear. Norepinephrine is a much more powerful vasoconstrictor than epinephrine and, therefore, elevates the blood pressure more. It does little if anything to increase the activity of the central nervous system. If you consider these two facts, the norepinephrine secreted in anger obviously does not help you think through the situation, and, indeed, it may raise the blood pressure to dangerously high levels. On the other hand, the actions of epinephrine secreted in fear are helpful in preparing you to cope with the danger.

PANCREAS

Because it has both an exocrine portion and an endocrine portion, the pancreas is actually a heterocrine (het′er-o-krin) gland. It is found in the abdominal cavity inferior to the stomach. The head of the pancreas is surrounded by the curve of the duodenum and the tail extends over to the spleen (see Fig. 23-5).

The tissue of pancreas that produces the hormones is called the islets of Langerhans. Four kinds of cells have been identified in the islets: (1) A cells, which produce glucagon; (2) B cells, which produce insulin; (3) D cells, which produce somatostatin; and (4) F cells, which produce pancreatic polypeptide (PP). Most of the islet cells are B cells.

Glucagon helps in the conversion of glycogen to glucose and raises the blood sugar. Glucagon production is controlled by the level of the blood sugar. When the blood sugar drops, the secretion of glucagon is stimulated; when it rises, the secretion of glucagon is suppressed. Because glucagon increases the blood sugar, it stimulates the production of insulin by the pancreas.

Insulin from the B cells lowers the blood sugar. Factors that stimulate the release of insulin by the pancreas are high levels of blood sugar and the growth hormone. Glucose also

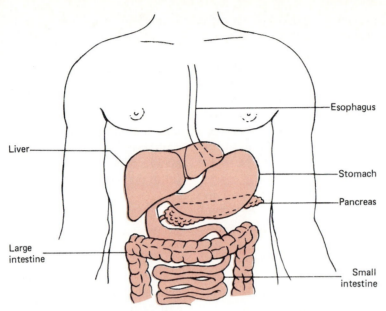

Esophagus

Liver

Stomach

Pancreas

Large
intestine

Small
intestine

Figure 23-5. *Pancreas and surrounding viscera*

stimulates insulin synthesis, but this process is relatively slow. Normally, you require about 50 units of insulin per day and you store a five-day supply. Insulin is degraded by the liver and to a lesser extent by the kidney. Half the circulating insulin is degraded in about 10 to 25 minutes. Insulin is antagonized by epinephrine, the glucocorticoids, the diabetogenic factor, thyroxin, and glucagon. Like glucagon, insulin is primarily regulated by the level of blood sugar. When the blood sugar level increases, the secretion of insulin is stimulated. When the blood sugar level drops, the secretion of insulin is suppressed.

There are several mechanisms by which insulin lowers the blood sugar. It favors the storage of glucose in the form of glucogen, decreases gluconeogenesis, and increases cell utilization of glucose.

Somatostatin, which is a growth hormone-inhibiting hormone, is the same hormone produced by the hypothalamus. It is also produced

by some cells of the digestive tract. The function of somatostatin is to suppress the release of other hormones from the pancreas and the hormones of the digestive tract. Somatostatin also reduces the rate at which triglycerides are absorbed from the intestine after a fatty meal. The pancreatic polypeptide inhibits the release of digestive secretions of the pancreas.

KIDNEY

In addition to its excretory function, the kidney has an endocrine function in the regulation of blood pressure and the production of red blood cells.

The renal cortex, particularly if it is ischemic, produces the hormone **renin** (ren′in). In the bloodstream renin (actually an enzyme) converts a plasma protein into **angiotensin** (an″je-o-ten′sin). The angiotensin is a powerful vaso-constrictor elevating the blood pressure. Angi-otensin is also a tropic hormone for aldosterone.

Renal erythropoietin (er-ith″ro-po-e′tin) acti-vates the blood protein erythropoietin, which stimulates the production of erythrocytes.

GONADS

The gonads are the sex glands. These glands pro-duce hormones that are essential to the normal functioning of the male and female reproductive systems. Chapter 21 discussed the sex hormones in greater detail. In the female, the ovaries pro-duce estrogen, progesterone, and relaxin. In the male, the testes produce testosterone.

PLACENTA

In addition to providing for the exchange of nu-trients and wastes between the mother and the fetus, the placenta also has some endocrine functions. The hormones produced by the pla-centa are **human chorionic gonadotropin**, chorionic growth hormone-prolactin, thyroid-stimulating hormone, **estrogen**, and **proges-terone**. The estrogen and progesterone have the same functions as in the nonpregnant state. However, in addition, the progesterone helps to maintain pregnancy.

The human chorionic gonadotropin (HCG) stimulates the ovary to continue its production of hormones, and it is also the hormone on which most pregnancy tests are based. The cho-rionic growth hormone-prolactin and the thy-roid-stimulating hormone have effects similar to their counterparts in the pituitary gland.

LOCAL HORMONES

Some hormones affect cells in the vicinity of the tissues secreting the hormone. For this reason, they are called local or tissue hormones. These hormones, although usually produced near their target cells, are carried in the bloodstream as are the hormones produced by endocrine glands.

Several of these hormones are produced by the organs of digestion and influence the motility and secretions of the gastrointestinal tract. The stomach (as well as the hypothalamus) pro-duces gastrin to cause the production of gastric juice. The duodenum produces secretin and CCK-PZ (cholecystokinin-pancreozyme). Both of these hormones are produced in response to the presence of acid chyme. Secretin causes the pan-creas to release sodium bicarbonate to alkalinize the intestinal contents. CCK-PZ causes the gall-bladder to release bile and the pancreas to re-lease its digestive enzymes into the duodenum.

Vasoactive intestinal peptide (VIP) stimulates the intestinal secretion of electrolytes by the in-testinal mucosa, and villikinin stimulates the motility of the villi in the intestine. Enterocrinin causes the production of digestive juices by the small intestine. Enterogastrin inhibits digestive secretions and the motility of the gastrointes-tinal tract. All of these hormones are produced by the mucosa of the small intestine.

PROSTAGLANDINS

Prostaglandins behave like hormones but their actions are very rapid and they cannot travel in the bloodstream for any significant distance be-cause they are so rapidly metabolized and in-activated. There are three classes of prostaglan-dins: prostaglandin A (PGA), prostaglandin E

(PGE), and prostaglandin F (PGF). All have been isolated and identified from a wide variety of tissues including the brain, lungs, kidneys, testes, eyes, and thymus. It may be that all cells produce some prostaglandin.

PGA has a digitalis-like effect and lowers the blood pressure. How PGA reduces the blood pressure is not clear. However, it probably involves relaxation of the smooth muscle fibers of the blood vessels.

In response to PGE there is bronchial dilatation. It also functions as a sedative and a nasal decongestant, reduces the stomach secretions, particularly hydrochloric acid, and dilates blood vessels. This prostaglandin regulates platelet aggregation and prevents clot formation. PGE also plays a role in certain systemic manifestations of inflammation such as fever. It may be that aspirin and other antiinflammatory agents used to lower fever function by inhibiting PGE synthesis.

PGF in some ways is an antagonist of PGE. It constricts blood vessels and the bronchial passageways. Both PGE and PGF cause uterine contractions and dilatation of the cervix. PGF compounds cause regression of the corpus luteum and, in the male, they facilitate ejaculation and sperm motility.

STRESS

We all have preconceived ideas about what "stress" means. In this discussion, however, we are concerned with the response of the body to adapt to some situation. It is not necessarily bad. For example, investigations have shown that a certain amount of stress is necessary in infancy and childhood for the development of normal adaptive ability to cope with the events of everyday life. Although the stressor can be a serious trauma or illness, it can also be a won-

derful party, an interesting challenge, or one's wedding. Dr. Hans Selye, who originated the concept of physiological stress in the 1930s, makes a distinction between stress that is productive and stress that is harmful. The former he called eustress; the latter he called distress. Regardless of the nature of the stress agent, or stressor, whether it acts on the personality of the individual involved, traumatizes body cells, or alters established living patterns of the individual, the body's responses to the stress are the same.

Extensive investigations have revealed in specific, observable changes caused by stress that has been induced by a variety of means. These changes are adrenal hypertrophy, atrophy of the thymus, and small bleeding lesions in the lining of the stomach and duodenum. Dr. Selye called these responses the general adaptation syndrome.

There are three distinct stages in the response to stress. The initial phase is called the alarm stage; the hypothalamus is activated, and the body's defenses are called into action. This is followed by the stage of resistance or adaptation. This occurs when the body has been successful through the alarm reaction in adjusting to the effects of the stressor and there is no need for any further response to the stress. During the resistance stage, the body repairs the damages of the stressor. Finally, if there is prolonged or severe stress, the ability to adapt may be lost and this leads to the stage of exhaustion or death.

In the preceding chapters of this text, we have been predominantly concerned with the uniqueness of particular disease processes. The chest X-ray of a patient with fractured ribs is different from that of a patient with pneumonia. However, both patients have much in common. They both experience stress.

It is therefore appropriate that we now consider what is common to all disease processes:

stress. Much of this involves homeostasis—the adaptive mechanisms of the body functioning to maintain equilibrium. Ironically, the more the body is able to change, the better able it is to stay the same: the stability and equilibrium of an individual depend greatly on the rapidity and efficiency with which change can be accomplished. The ability to adapt or to change determines the ease or disease of the individual. The skill and knowledge with which the stressed person's helpers support the appropriate body defense mechanisms may spell the difference between recovery or exhaustion.

FACTORS DETERMINING THE DEGREE OF RESPONSE TO STRESS

Obviously, the intensity of the stress has something to do with the response. However, this is not the only factor nor is it necessarily the major factor. How the individual perceives the situation is of great importance. Probably none of you considers your last flu shot a particularly stressful situation, yet the injections you received when you were three or four years old evoked quite different reactions. At that time, you had no idea why the usually kind adults suddenly held you down and stuck needles into you. You naturally responded to the situation in the way appropriate to how you perceived it. The reactions of an elderly patient with impaired sight and hearing in a strange hospital setting and being attended by strangers may be another example of how faulty perception of a situation may evoke responses that seem inappropriate. In *A Midsummer Night's Dream* Shakespeare explains this point beautifully: "—or in the night with some imagined fear how easy a bush a bear both appear."

Age is another factor that influences the degree of reaction to stress. Generally speaking, the younger the individual the greater the response and the more likely the individual will be able to adapt. Observe the resiliency of the healthy youth. He undergoes much turmoil during the process of his adaptation to stress. Remember we are talking about nonspecific causes of stress by a specific syndrome. The delight of the four-year-old on Christmas morning when he sees all of the wonderful gifts is probably no greater than that of his grandmother, but the observable reactions are quite different. If the stress agent is a disease—for example, an infection—the vital signs of the four-year-old will change markedly, whereas the vital signs of an aged individual with a similar infection change very little. The aged are not able to change as much or as rapidly; as a result, their stability—their lives—may be sacrificed.

Previous exposure to the same or similar stressors tends to decrease some of an individual's body responses, and at the same time equips the person to deal more effectively with the stress situation. During some of the early studies of stress, investigators exposed rats to thermal stress. They were placed in cold environments but not cold enough to be a threat to their lives. On subsequent occasions, they were exposed to colder and colder temperatures. Finally, the rats who were so conditioned were dipped in cold water and confined to even lower temperatures. Simultaneously, rats that had not been conditioned to the stress of lower and lower temperatures were subjected to the same wet, cold environment. The rats who had the previous exposure to the thermal stress survived the experiment, but those who had not had the previous exposure died. The investigators found on examination that there was considerable adrenal hypertrophy in the conditioned rats but none in the rats who had not been conditioned to the stress and were unable to adapt to it.

Perhaps this previous-exposure aspect of determining the degree of response helps to explain some of the amazing accounts of escape by prisoners of war. When an opportunity to escape arose, prisoners who had been kept on near starvation rations, tortured, poorly clothed, and caged in most unsanitary quarters were able to accomplish astonishing feats that one would assume could be done only by a person in the peak of physical condition.

Undoubtedly, other factors influence the degree of response to stress. What is important is the realization that response is a composite of many factors. Some factors you can do little about in your efforts to help the stressed individual, but the fact that you are giving them some thought may increase your sensitivity to their needs.

ALARM AND RESISTANCE

In considering some of the specific aspects of the alarm and resistance phases of stress, it is well to remember that the causes of stress are nonspecific but the responses are the same regardless of the cause of the stress. The degree of response that will occur depends on many things.

Initially, a decrease in the blood sugar level occurs because glucose is being used for the energy needed to meet the emergency. Energy needs of the body are paramount in the process of adapting to the stress situation. Glucocorticoids will be released from the adrenal cortex and cause gluconeogenesis, thus increasing the blood sugar level. The glucocorticoids antagonize insulin and force muscle and most body tissues to use fats for fuel. This preferentially saves the glucose for use by the brain. Glucose is the only fuel the healthy brain can use. Brain cells do not need insulin in order to use glucose. Normally, an increased production of glucocorticoids will function as a negative feedback mechanism and depress the pituitary production of ACTH, but stress depresses this negative feedback, and the glucocorticoids are produced in quantities greatly above their ordinary levels.

Also in response to the initial low blood sugar level, glucagon is released to cause the liver to convert glycogen to glucose, thereby further increasing the blood sugar level.

Early in the stress situation, sodium and water are lost from the vascular compartment, lowering the blood pressure. There is likely to be some degree of shock. Many compensatory mechanisms help the stressed individual resist this shock.

There will be a decrease in capillary filtration of fluid into the interstitial spaces of the peripheral body tissues, which will save the remaining vascular volume to supply vital organs, heart, and brain. The relatively greater colloidal osmotic pressure in the peripheral capillaries will help to pull interstitial fluid back into the capillaries, thereby increasing the circulatory volume at the expense of the peripheral tissues whose nutrition is less vital in this emergency than that of the heart and brain.

The resulting dehydration of the peripheral tissues stimulates the pituitary release of ADH. This hormone causes a decreased urinary output and the conservation of fluid. Mineralocorticoids, chiefly aldosterone, are released to effect the kidney conservation of sodium and water. To compensate further for the lowered blood pressure, the kidney produces renin, which enters the plasma and causes the production of the hormone angiotensin, a powerful vasoconstrictor, which helps elevate the blood pressure.

Epinephrine and norepinephrine from the adrenal medulla also help elevate the blood pressure by causing vasoconstriction. The increased levels of glucocorticoids sensitize the blood vessels to all of the vasopressor substances. Serotonin from the pineal opposes the vasoconstriction in the vessels of the brain.

Initially, there will be an increase in the blood potassium. High levels of blood potassium depress cardiac action, which will also contribute to the shock picture of stress. Under the influence of aldosterone from the adrenal cortex, the normal kidney will compensate by excreting the excess potassium.

There will also be an increased white blood cell count in the initial phase. This increase may be due to the manufacture and release of new white blood cells and these cells will probably be immature cells (bands or metamyelocytes) that are not capable of phagocytizing bacteria if the nature of the stress is infection, and they are not capable of removing the tissue debris that results from trauma. To compensate, the antiinflammatory glucocorticoids are produced, and the atrophy of the thymus and other lymphatic tissues will depress the production of these white blood cells. If the increase in the number of circulating white blood cells is due to the release of splenic stores of mature white cells that can be helpful, then the proinflammatory mineralocorticoids will favor the actions of these white blood cells.

The neural response to a threatening situation is the fight or flight response mediated by the sympathetic nervous system. The widespread actions of the sympathetic nervous system are intended to help the body cope with the threat by physical combat or escape.

Our society, however, does not generally approve of these methods of dealing with the aggravations of daily life. Considering the fact that the sympathetic nervous system equips a person to deal with fear and anger in one way, and society expects a different type of behavior, it is not surprising that many psychosomatic illnesses, such as those evidenced by increased skeletal muscle tone (chronic, functional low back pain or a stiff neck) or essential hypertension, may have a fairly sound physiological basis. You might think about the implications of this on the health of an individual whose life situation is dominated by either fear or anger. In *Die Fledermaus*, Johann Strauss wrote, "Happy (and healthy) is he who forgets what cannot be altered."

SUMMARY QUESTIONS

1. Name the hormones secreted by the neurohypophysis and discuss the actions of these hormones.
2. What gland produces calcitonin and what is its function?
3. What hormones oppose the action of insulin?
4. List the hormones produced by the adenohypophysis and discuss the functions of each.
5. Name the three main classifications of hormones produced by the adrenal cortex.
6. What hormones are produced by the thyroid gland and what are the actions of these hormones?
7. What is the function of parathormone?
8. Compare the actions of epinephrine with those of norepinephrine.
9. Under stressful situations, what hormones are primarily concerned with preserving our carbohydrate reserves?
10. Under stressful circumstances, what hormones are primarily concerned with maintaining our normal fluid and electrolyte balance?
11. With respect to the endocrine glands, what is meant by the negative feedback mechanism?
12. Discuss the functions of the thymus.

13. What gland produces glucagon and what is the function of this hormone?

14. List the local hormones and give examples of their actions.

15. Discuss hormonal responses to stressful situations.

16. How is the blood calcium level regulated?

17. Why do the glucocorticoids antagonize insulin and favor an increased blood sugar?

18. How do the kidneys help compensate for the shock of stress?

19. Discuss the ways in which the blood sugar becomes elevated in a stress situation.

KEY TERMS

aldosterone

angiotensin

antidiuretic hormone

calcitonin

catecholamines

cholecystokinin

endorphins

enkephalins

estrogen

gastrin

glomerulotropin

glucocorticoids

human chorionic gonadotropin

melanocyte-stimulating hormone

melatonin

oxytocin

parathormone

progesterone

prostaglandins

renin

serotonin

somatostatin

somatotropic hormone

thymosin

thyrotropic hormone

thyroxin

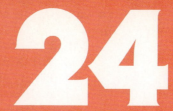

Diseases of the Endocrine System

OBJECTIVES

On completion of this chapter, you will be able to:

1. List the common diagnostic tests used in the evaluation and management of a patient with an endocrine dysfunction.
2. Describe three thyroid disorders.
3. Compare and contrast diabetes mellitus and diabetes insipidus.
4. Describe symptoms associated with adrenocortical insufficiency and an excess production of cortisol.
5. Discuss three common health problems frequently associated with obesity.

OVERVIEW

I. DIAGNOSTIC TESTS
   A. Hormone Radioimmunoassay
   B. Stimulation and Suppression Tests
   C. Twenty-four-hour Urine Specimens
   D. Tests for Diseases of the Thyroid
     1. Blood Tests
     2. Thyroid Scans
     3. Thyroid Ultrasonography
     4. Congenital Hypothyroidism Screening
   E. Tests for Diseases of the Parathyroid Glands
   F. Tests for Diabetes Mellitus
     1. Urine Examinations
     2. Fasting Blood Sugar
     3. Two- and Five-Hour Oral Glucose Tolerance Tests
   G. Tests for Adrenal Disorders
     1. Plasma Cortisol and Cortrosyn Tests
     2. Dexamethasone Suppression Tests
     3. Urine and Serum Potassium
     4. Serum Aldosterone and ACTH
     5. Plasma Catecholamines
   H. Tests for Pituitary Disorders
     1. Water Deprivation Tests
     2. Growth Hormone
II. HYPERTHYROIDISM
III. HYPOTHYROIDISM
IV. HYPERPARATHYROIDISM
V. HYPOPARATHYROIDISM
VI. DIABETES MELLITUS
   A. Insulin-Dependent Diabetes Mellitus
   B. Non-Insulin-Dependent Diabetes Mellitus
   C. Complications of Diabetes Mellitus
VII. ADDISON'S DISEASE
VIII. CUSHING'S SYNDROME
IX. PHEOCHROMOCYTOMA
X. PITUITARY GLAND DISORDERS
   A. Hyposecretion of the Growth Hormone
   B. Hypersecretion of the Growth Hormone
XI. POSTERIOR PITUITARY HYPOSECRETION
XII. OBESITY

Since the function of the endocrine system is to assist the nervous system in the regulation of body processes, it is not surprising to find that pathology of this system will result in the disruption of many different body functions. While studying these disease processes, keep in mind the normal interdependence of different endocrine glands. This concept helps to explain some of the widespread and seemingly unrelated signs and symptoms characteristic of many endocrine disorders.

DIAGNOSTIC TESTS

Since the endocrine system affects so many body functions, tests for diseases of other organ systems are often used in diagnosing endocrine problems. Chemical analysis of the blood is usually ordered to ascertain the stability of blood electrolytes, particularly sodium, potassium, and calcium. Renal function tests are helpful in determining the ability of the kidney to concentrate and dilute urine and thus maintain water balance.

HORMONE RADIOIMMUNOASSAY

Of the tests that are specific for endocrine problems, those that determine the quantity of a hor-

This chapter was written by Judith A. DePalma.

mone in the bloodstream are particularly valuable. These tests can be done by means of hormone radioimmunoassay methods. These blood examinations are helpful in the initial diagnosis of an endocrine disease and in determining the patient's response to treatment.

STIMULATION AND SUPPRESSION TESTS

These tests help establish whether the disease process is within an endocrine gland or is the result of some abnormal pituitary influence on an otherwise healthy target gland. After the blood level of the hormone from the gland in question has been established, the patient is given a medicine that normally will influence its production. Urine and blood specimens are then analyzed to determine the response.

TWENTY-FOUR-HOUR URINE SPECIMENS

Since the activity of endocrine glands fluctuates during a 24-hour period, an analysis of the total quantity of urine produced over this period is often helpful. The first urine voided in the morning is discarded and the time of this voiding is recorded. All urine voided from that time until the last voiding at the end of the 24-hour period is collected for analysis. Table 20-1 indicates some of the disease processes that might be evidenced by abnormal 24-hour urine specimens.

TESTS FOR DISEASES OF THE THYROID

Blood Tests
Blood levels of L-thyroxin (T4), triiodothyronine (T3), thyroxin-binding globulin (TBG), and thyroid-stimulating hormone (TSH) are helpful in assessing thyroid function. In hyperthyroidism, the blood levels of these will be increased, and they will be decreased in hypothyroidism.

Thyroid Scans
Thyroid scanning is done by giving the patient radioactive iodine, I^{131}, either orally or intravenously, and then a scintillation camera is used to produce a pattern representing the size of the thyroid and the pattern representing the uptake of I^{131}. If the iodine was given orally, the examination will be done 24 hours later. However, if given intravenously, the examination can be done 30 minutes later. In hyperthyroidism, the scan will show an increased iodine uptake, which will appear gray or black, and the image will be larger than normal. In hypothyroidism there will be a decreased iodine uptake, which will be white on the scan, and the image will be smaller than the normal thyroid.

A Thyroid Radioactive Iodine Uptake Test is similar but in this instance the scan is done 2, 6, and 24 hours after an oral administration of the I^{131}. In hypothyroidism and subacute thyroidism there is a decreased I^{131} uptake, and there will be an increased uptake in hyperthyroidism and iodine-deficient goiter.

Thyroid Ultrasonography
A sonogram can help discriminate between a cystic thyroid or a solid mass. The ultrasound beam easily passes through the fluid-filled cyst and produces a detailed image. A tumor is solid, and the ultrasound wave will project an image without clearly defined borders.

Ultrasonography is often used if the patient is pregnant, breastfeeding, or allergic to iodine and therefore cannot take the radioisotope necessary for a scan or uptake test.

Congenital Hypothyroidism Screening
Thyroid function and phenylketonuria (PKU) studies are performed on newborns. For the PKU test to be effective, the newborn must have ingested milk for four full days. A heelstick is done and blood is placed on a special filter paper for T_4, TSH, and PKU evaluation. Urine testing is

usually done on the infant's first well-baby examination at six weeks of age.

TESTS FOR DISEASES OF THE PARATHYROID GLANDS

Blood examinations for calcium, phosphate, parathyroid hormone, and alkaline phosphatase are helpful in assessing parathyroid function. Normal serum calcium is 8.5 to 10.5 mg/dl, phosphate is 2.5 to 4.5 mg/dl, normal parathyroid hormone levels are 20 to 70 µl Eq/ml, and alkaline phosphatase is 1.5 to 4 Bodansky units/dl. In hyperparathyroidism, the serum calcium, alkaline phosphatase, and parathyroid hormone are elevated, and the phosphate will be decreased. In hypoparathyroidism there are lower than normal levels of the parathyroid hormone and calcium but higher than normal levels of serum phosphate.

TESTS FOR DIABETES MELLITUS

Urine Examinations

There will be glucose and **acetone** (as'e-ton) in the urine of a patient with untreated or poorly controlled diabetes mellitus.

Fasting Blood Sugar

A fasting patient with uncontrolled diabetes mellitus will have a considerably higher level of glucose in the blood than the normal of 70 to 120 mg/100 ml. With a value of above 130 mg/100 ml under fasting conditions, diabetes mellitus may be present. However, the analysis should be repeated in order to confirm the diagnosis.

Two- and Five-Hour Oral Glucose Tolerance Tests

For oral glucose tolerance tests, a fasting blood sugar is measured and the urine examined for glucose and acetone and then the patient is given a 150–300 gm oral carbohydrate drink.

Blood and urine specimens are collected at intervals of one half, 1, and 2 hours. If the five-hour test is being done, three additional hourly blood and urine specimens will be collected. These tests will establish the level at which glucose spills over into the urine, usually 160–180 mg/100 ml. Some patients have higher or lower renal thresholds for glucose in the urine. In order to interpret urine tests it is important to know the renal threshold for the individual patient. Two hours after receiving the loading dose of carbohydrate, the blood sugar should be within normal limits. Levels above 120 mg/100 ml should be investigated further.

TESTS FOR ADRENAL DISORDERS

Plasma Cortisol and Cortrosyn Tests

Plasma cortisol normally peaks between 6 AM and 8 AM and so radioimmunoassay tests for plasma cortisol are done at this time. Normal cortisol blood levels are between 7 and 28 mcg/dl. Stress, illness, and certain drugs may falsely elevate the plasma cortisol levels. Low levels of plasma cortisol suggest Addison's disease. People with Cushing's syndrome often have normal plasma cortisol levels in the morning but do not exhibit decline during the day.

Dexamethasone Suppression Tests

This test may be used as a screening procedure for a patient suspected of having Cushing's syndrome. At midnight the patient is given the dexamethasone and then a plasma cortisol level is drawn at 8 AM. Normal plasma cortisol levels should be less than 5 µl/100 ml.

Urine and Serum Potassium

These tests are helpful in diagnosing aldosteronism. In this condition there will be high urine potassium levels and low serum levels of potassium. Normal urine potassium levels are less than 20 mEq in 24 hours and serum potassium levels are 3.8 to 5 mEq/liter.

Serum Aldosterone and ACTH

There will be high aldosterone levels in aldosteronism, kidney disease, liver cirrhosis, pregnancy, or congestive heart failure. There are lower than normal levels of aldosterone in Addison's disease.

The plasma level of ACTH will be elevated in Cushing's syndrome and lower than normal in Addison's disease. The specimen for this radioimmunoassay should be drawn early in the morning. Normal ACTH level is 120 pg/ml.

Normal serum aldosterone after the patient has been lying down for at least two hours is between 3 and 11 ng/dl. After the patient has been upright for two hours the values will have increased to between 5 and 22 ng/dl.

Plasma Catecholamines

For at least two days before these tests, the patient should avoid foods such as cheese, wine, beer, cocoa, coffee, tea, avocados, and bananas. The patient should not smoke for twenty four hours before the blood is drawn and should not have anything to eat or drink twelve hours prior to the test.

A blood sample is drawn while the patient is lying down between 6 AM and 8 AM and a second specimen is taken ten minutes later while the patient is standing. The supine value for epinephrine is 110 pg/ml and for norepinephrine is 70 to 750 pg/ml. The standing value for epinephrine is 140 pg/ml and 200 to 1,700 pg/ml for norepinephrine. Values will be elevated in patients with pheochromocytoma.

TESTS FOR PITUITARY DISORDERS

Water Deprivation Tests

Several tests may be used to assess levels of antidiuretic hormone (ADH) and assist in the diagnosis of diabetes insipidus (in-sip'i-dus). These tests include the Mosenthal test, the Fishberg test, and the 14- and 8-hour deprivation tests. Each test involves the withholding of fluid intake over a period of time. The urine osmolarity and serum osmolarity is checked as well as any changes in the person's weight.

Growth Hormone

Blood specimens for this test are drawn between 6 AM and 8 AM when the blood levels of the growth hormone are the highest. Drugs that may influence growth hormone include arginine, levodopa, insulin, beta blockers, estrogens, phenothiazines, and corticosteroids.

High levels of growth hormone occur in acromegaly and gigantism and low levels in pituitary dwarfism. The normal blood level in adults is 0 to 8 ng/ml and in children is 0 to 10 ng/ml.

HYPERTHYROIDISM

Hyperthyroidism is a clinical state resulting from an excess of thyroid hormone. There are several disorders that can result in signs and symptoms consistent with hyperthyroidism.

There are nodular goiters that will not only result in increased blood levels of T_3 and T_4 but also cause an enlargement of the thyroid. Graves' disease is an autoimmune disease with a production of abnormal immunoglobulins, which have activity similar to the thyroid-stimulating hormone.

Patients with hyperthyroidism have a marked increase in their metabolic rate. They are nervous, have diarrhea, heart palpitations, and weight loss despite an increased appetite and food intake. They frequently complain of insomnia, heat intolerance, and fatigue. They may have an enlarged thyroid and **exophthalmos** (ek″sof-thal′mus), an abnormal protrusion of the eyeball (see Fig. 24-1).

The therapy is directed toward reducing the output of the thyroid hormone. Antithyroid medications or radioactive iodine are used successfully for most patients. Occasionally surgery may be necessary.

HYPOTHYROIDISM

Hypothyroidism and low levels of thyroid hormone lower the body's metabolic rate. These patients experience extreme fatigue, cold intoler-

ance, weight gain, constipation, dry skin, and may even notice memory loss. Most hypothyroid adults have **myxedema** (mik-se-de′mah), a nonpitting edema around their eyes, feet, and hands (see Fig. 24-2). The tongue is often edematous and may protrude slightly. Edema of the vocal cords may cause hoarseness. These patients usually respond quickly to the administration of the deficient thyroid hormone.

Congenital absence or atrophy of the thyroid gland in infancy causes **cretinism** (kre′tin-izm). In this condition, physical and mental development is retarded. With early recognition and treatment, normal physical growth may be possible (see Fig. 24-3).

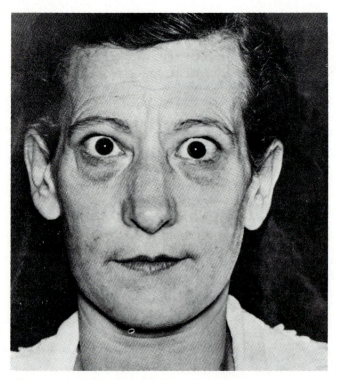

Figure 24-1. *Graves' disease with exophthalmos (From DeGroot, The Thyroid and Its Diseases, 4th ed. New York: John Wiley & Sons, Inc., 1975)*

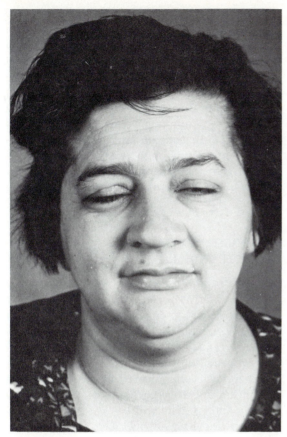

Figure 24-2. *Myxedema (Courtesy of Mercy Hospital, Pittsburgh, PA)*

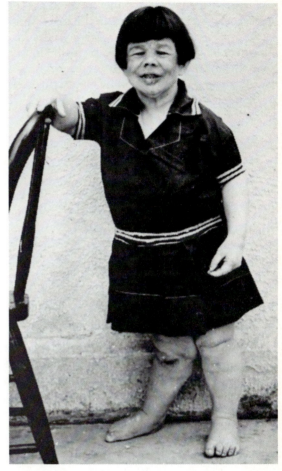

Figure 24-3. *Cretinism. This woman is 42 years old, weighs 38 kg, and is 125 cm tall. (From Chaffee, E.E., and Lytle, I.M., Basic Physiology and Anatomy, 4th ed. Philadelphia: J.B. Lippincott, Co., 1980)*

HYPERPARATHYROIDISM

Patients with primary **hyperparathyroidism** frequently complain of muscle weakness and wasting, depression, memory loss, inability to concentrate, and personality changes. Elevated parathyroid hormone levels may be associated with peptic ulcers, kidney stones, and hypertension. The recommended treatment is surgery.

HYPOPARATHYROIDISM

A deficiency of parathyroid hormone may occur after neck surgery if the parathyroid gland is damaged or removed; it can also develop in

Addison's disease. The patient will have low blood calcium levels and tetany or severe muscle spasms. Prompt treatment must be given so that severe reactions such as convulsions can be prevented. Calcium gluconate is given intravenously. Large doses of vitamin D and calcium salts are started orally as soon as possible.

DIABETES MELLITUS

Diabetes mellitus is a chronic endocrine disorder that affects the metabolism of carbohydrates, fats, and proteins. The number of people who develop diabetes mellitus is increasing by 6% each year.

INSULIN-DEPENDENT DIABETES MELLITUS

Insulin-dependent diabetes mellitus (IDDM) accounts for 10 to 20% of all cases of diabetes. Its peak incidence occurs in children between the ages of 10 to 14. The onset of this condition is abrupt. The patients with insulin-dependent diabetes mellitus have increased thirst, increased appetite, and increased urination. They will have a sudden weight loss and complain of dehydration and fatigue. Their blood sugar levels are elevated and there will be glucose and ketones in their urine. The patient usually develops this type of diabetes before the age of 35. These patients will need insulin injections.

NON-INSULIN-DEPENDENT DIABETES MELLITUS

Non - insulin - dependent diabetes mellitus (NIDDM) accounts for 80 to 90% of all cases of diabetes and increases with age. A patient with non-insulin-dependent diabetes mellitus usually comes to the doctor complaining of fatigue, weight gain, blurred vision, and numbness and tingling of the feet and legs. These patients also have increased thirst, increased appetite, and increased urination. The onset is usually gradual after the age of 40. Obesity, heredity, and a sedentary life style are associated with the occurrence of NIDDM.

Diet, exercise, and oral hypoglycemic agents alone or in combination can be used to treat NIDDM. Oral agents are not insulin. They control hyperglycemia by increasing the insulin secreted from the pancreatic islet cells or by increasing the sensitivity of the body's cells to insulin.

COMPLICATIONS OF DIABETES MELLITUS

Hypoglycemia or low blood sugar is caused by a sudden increase in exercise without sufficient food intake or an increase in insulin or oral agents (see Table 24-1). Patients are weak, irritable, nervous, and trembling. They are apprehensive and have palpitations and dizziness. Their speech is often slurred and they are unable to concentrate. This condition can progress very rapidly and patients will become comatose unless they are given some form of sugar.

Hyperglycemia or high blood sugar is caused by not taking the prescribed insulin or oral agents, noncompliance with prescribed diet, infection, or physiological or emotional stress. Hyperglycemia can lead to ketoacidosis, which usually has a rather slow onset and does not progress as rapidly as does hypoglycemia. Signs and symptoms include frequent and increased urination, headache, visual changes, dry skin, thirst, hunger, fruity odor to the breath, high blood sugar level, and glucose and ketones in the urine. The patient becomes increasingly drowsy and unconsciousness may develop with prolonged hyperglycemia.

Long-term complications of diabetes mellitus are related to the changes that occur in the

Table 24-1. A Comparison of Diabetic Coma and Insulin Reaction

	Diabetic Coma	*Insulin Reaction (Hypoglycemia)*
Cause	Infection	Excessive insulin
	Insufficient insulin	Too little food
	Dietary indiscretion	Unusual exercise
	Stress	
Symptoms	Slow onset, hours to days	Sudden onset, within minutes
	Dry, hot, flushed skin	Pale, moist, cool skin
	Drowsy to comatose	Blurred vision
	Rapid shallow respirations (Kussmaul's)	Trembling
	Fruity odor to breath	Anxiety, incoherent speech
	Thirsty	Possible convulsions and unconsciousness
	May vomit	Hunger
	Sugar and acetone in urine	Second urine specimen free of sugar and acetone (first specimen unreliable)
Treatment	Give regular insulin	Give high carbohydrate foods, by mouth or intravenous glucose solutions
	Hydrate by giving fluids either by mouth or intravenously	Determine and treat the cause of the reaction, usually by means of reinforced health teaching
	Frequently test glucose level in blood and urine	
	Maintain patent airway	
	Determine and treat the cause of the coma	

blood vessels and nerves over time. These complications include retinopathy, which may lead to blindness; nephropathy, which may lead to renal failure; and neuropathies, which may lead to sensory loss, impaired digestion, and poor bladder tone. Vascular changes and sensory loss in the lower extremities result in poor healing. Therefore, foot care is an important aspect of care for a person with diabetes.

ADDISON'S DISEASE

Addison's disease is a rare condition resulting from adrenocortical insufficiency. The onset of the disease is insidious or acute but both can be life threatening because the adrenocorticoid hormones are necessary for life.

Blood potassium levels rise owing to the lack of aldosterone. This causes weakness, numbness and tingling, confusion, paralysis, ECG changes, and irregular heart rate, which may progress to cardiac standstill. These patients have postural hypotension, hypoglycemia, and may experience dizziness or fainting. Patients with Addison's disease also complain of fatigue, muscle pain, nausea, vomiting, abdominal pain, and increased skin pigmentation.

The treatment consists of administration of a glucocorticoid and a mineralocorticoid. Any physiologic stress such as infection, surgery, injury, or emotional upset can increase the need for hormone replacement.

CUSHING'S SYNDROME

Cushing's syndrome is caused by increased production of cortisol by the adrenal cortex. It may be due to a pituitary dysfunction, tumors, or a prolonged prescribed therapy of cortisol or similar drugs. Due to changes in fat metabolism, body weight increases and abnormal deposition of fat produces the moon face (see Fig. 24-4) and buffalo hump characteristics. The patients also have hypertension, increased bruising, hy-

perglycemia, muscle weakness, poor wound healing, and a tendency to develop osteoporosis and kidney stones.

The treatment for Cushing's syndrome owing to a tumor is surgery, chemotherapy, or radiotherapy. If the adrenal glands are totally or partially removed, the patient is treated to prevent symptoms of Addison's disease. Pituitary tumors can usually be radiated successfully. Patients with Cushing's syndrome are sometimes given metyrapone, which inhibits the final step in cortisol synthesis.

PHEOCHROMOCYTOMA

Pheochromocytoma (fe″o-kro″mo-si-to′mah) is a tumor of the sympatheticoadrenal system, most frequently in the adrenal medulla. Small tumors produce norepinephrine and large tumors secrete both norepinephrine and epinephrine. The most common manifestation of pheochromocytoma is sustained hypertension. Patients complain of a sudden onset of intermittent symptoms of headache, sweating, fear, nervousness, and heart palpitations. Their blood pressures are intermittently elevated. The treatment is the surgical removal of the tumor.

PITUITARY GLAND DISORDERS

HYPOSECRETION OF THE GROWTH HORMONE

Dwarfism is an uncommon condition occurring before puberty caused by pituitary malfunction and resulting in the lack of the growth hormone. X-rays of long bones demonstrate early closure of the epiphyseal cartilages. The treatment consists of replacement hormones.

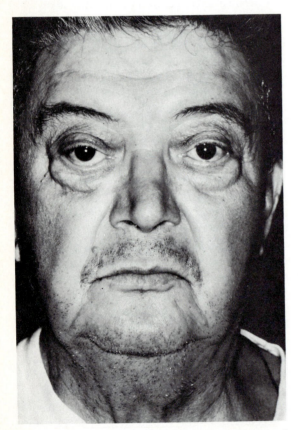

Figure 24-4. Cushing's disease. Note the facial edema. (Courtesy of Mercy Hospital, Pittsburgh, PA)

HYPERSECRETION OF THE GROWTH HORMONE

Giantism is due to an excess of the growth hormone in childhood producing an overgrowth of bone and soft tissue. The usual cause is an adenoma of the anterior pituitary and the treatment is usually radiation of the tumor.

Acromegaly occurs in adulthood and is caused by a pituitary tumor that produces an excess of the growth hormone. The onset is insidious. There is enlargement of the facial features, head, hands, and feet (see Fig. 24-5). Treatment is usually radiation of the pituitary gland.

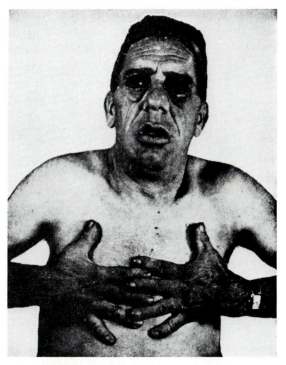

Figure 24-5. *Acromegaly. A lantern-shaped lower jaw and unusually large hands and feet are typical of this disease. (From Chaffee, E.E., and Lytle, I.M., Basic Physiology and Anatomy, 4th ed. Philadelphia: J.B. Lippincott, Co., 1980)*

POSTERIOR PITUITARY HYPOSECRETION

Diabetes insipidus is due to a lack of the antidiuretic hormone (ADH), caused by a tumor, head trauma, or cranial surgery. These patients have excess urination and extreme thirst. The treatment is the administration of vasopressin by injection or a synthetic vasopressin taken nasally.

OBESITY

Obesity is defined as weight that is 20% over the recommended weight for that person's height on a standard chart. It is important to consider an individual's frame size and muscular development because muscle weighs more than fat tissue. Obesity affects 25 to 45% of adults over age 30 years according to the U.S. Public Health Service. People from lower socioeconomic groups and women are more commonly obese.

Dr. George Bray, a noted authority on obesity and weight loss, lists six causes of obesity: genetics, endocrine function, hypothalamic obesity, certain drugs that promote weight gain, physical inactivity, and a diet high in fat and protein.

Recent research in this field has been directed toward finding out why slender people seem to be able to use fuel more efficiently. This approach has led to the discovery that in some cases of obesity, the patient has a deficiency of ATPase, and therefore muscle work is inefficient and requires more fuel.

Endocrine disorders linked to obesity are hypothyroidism, insulin-dependent diabetes mellitus, Cushing's syndrome, and polycystic ovary diseases. Inasmuch as some prostaglandins prevent the normal breakdown of body fat, it may be that an excess of this hormone also is related to obesity, particularly in people who are not able to lose weight even though their caloric intake is low. Treatment of endocrine related obesity begins with management of the underlying condition. Other important aspects of the treatment involve behavior modification, a low calorie diet calculated on an individual basis, and exercise. Only rarely should drugs to curb the appetite or surgical intervention be used to achieve and maintain desired body weight. The most important aspect of the treatment of obesity is patient motivation and compliance.

Obese patients are more likely to have impaired glucose tolerance, high lipid levels, high insulin levels, decreased daily rhythm changes in plasma growth hormone, and an increase in the number and size of fat cells. Obesity predisposes an individual to an increased risk of atherosclerotic disease affecting the heart, brain, and kidneys. Gallstones, hypertension, fatty liver, and some types of cancer are also correlated with obesity. The usual cause of non-insulin-dependent diabetes mellitus is obesity because the number of insulin receptors on body cells is reduced owing to increased body mass.

In 1983, the Metropolitan Life Insurance Company revised their height and weight charts for the first time since 1959. The charts are based on information obtained from studying 4.2 million people followed by 25 insurance companies for over 20 years. The heights and desirable weights are those ranges at which individuals live the longest (see Table 24-2). The

Table 24-2. 1983 Metropolitan Life Height and Weight Tables

Men					Women				
Height		Small Frame	Medium Frame	Large Frame	Height		Small Frame	Medium Frame	Large Frame
Feet	Inches				Feet	Inches			
5	2	128–134	131–141	138–150	4	10	102–111	109–121	118–131
5	3	130–136	133–143	140–153	4	11	103–113	111–123	120–134
5	4	132–138	135–145	142–156	5	0	104–115	113–126	122–137
5	5	134–140	137–148	144–160	5	1	106–118	115–129	125–140
5	6	136–142	139–151	146–164	5	2	108–121	118–132	128–143
5	7	138–145	142–154	149–168	5	3	111–124	121–135	131–147
5	8	140–148	145–157	152–172	5	4	114–127	124–138	134–151
5	9	142–151	148–160	155–176	5	5	117–130	127–141	137–155
5	10	144–154	151–163	158–180	5	6	120–133	130–144	140–159
5	11	146–157	154–166	161–184	5	7	123–136	133–147	143–163
6	0	149–160	157–170	164–188	5	8	126–139	136–150	146–167
6	1	152–164	160–174	168–192	5	9	129–142	139–153	149–170
6	2	155–168	164–178	172–197	5	10	132–145	142–156	152–173
6	3	158–172	167–182	176–202	5	11	135–148	145–159	155–176
6	4	162–176	171–187	181–207	6	0	138–151	148–162	158–179

Weights of ages 25–59 based on lowest mortality. Weight in pounds according to frame (in indoor clothing weighing 5 lbs for men and 3 lbs for women; shoes with 1″ heels).

Source of basic data: 1979 Build Study, Society of Actuaries and Association of Life Insurance Medical Directors of America, 1980.

American Heart Association has suggested, however, that people continue to follow the stricter 1959 guidelines and avoid weight gain. Their statement refers to the increase in desirable weight for height on the new charts by as much as 10 to 15 pounds.

SUMMARY QUESTIONS

1. List 10 diagnostic tests used in the management of a patient with endocrine dysfunction.
2. Discuss three thyroid disorders.
3. Compare and contrast diabetes mellitus and diabetes insipidus.
4. What are the signs and symptoms of adrenal cortical insufficiency?
5. Discuss the problems associated with an excess production of cortisol.
6. Discuss common health problems associated with obesity.

KEY TERMS

acetone
cretinism
diabetes insipidus
diabetes mellitus
exophthalmos

hyperparathyroidism
hyperthyroidism
hypothyroidism
myxedema
pheochromocytoma

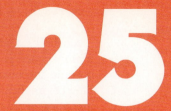

Aging

OBJECTIVES

On completion of this chapter, you will be able to:

1. Describe the changes that aging brings about in each of the body systems.
2. Explain why elderly people are more prone to respiratory infections than young adults.
3. Describe some techniques that may be helpful in giving health instructions to an elderly patient.

OVERVIEW

I. THEORIES OF AGING

II. LONGEVITY

III. CONSEQUENCES OF AGING
   A. Skin
   B. Nervous System
   C. Circulatory System
   D. Respiratory System
   E. Gastrointestinal System
   F. Musculoskeletal System
   G. Urinary System
   H. Reproductive Systems
   I. Endocrine System

IV. AGE-ASSOCIATED DISEASES

Although for centuries people have been interested in aging (or, perhaps to be more accurate, delaying or preventing the aging process), there was not a great deal of systematic research in this field until the end of World War II. The quantity of literature published on **gerontology** (jer-on-tol′o-je), the study of old age, between 1950 and 1960 exceeded that produced in the preceding 100 years. Since then, interest and research in the field have expanded rapidly, and there is reason to believe that efforts to find solutions to some of the problems of aging are likely to continue.

What a relatively short time ago was a technical question for workers in a biochemistry laboratory has now become an issue with important political, economic, and psychosocial concerns. The elderly are now the fastest growing population in the United States. Part of this of course may be due to the decline in the birth rate in recent years. However, probably more important is the fact that we are living longer. Since we are living longer, it is important that we learn how to enjoy our added years.

Mortality and life tables that once were mainly concerns of the insurance industry have become important considerations in the planning of practically every aspect of our lives. The influence of this change in the composition of the population on areas such as housing design, recreation facilities, job training, and health care is particularly noteworthy.

Just as a change in one body system affects the well-being of the entire person, so does a change in a segment of society affect the total society. As discussed in Chapter 3, all aspects of our environment—physical, social, psychological, and spiritual—influence our health.

THEORIES OF AGING

Genetic transmission of longevity can be demonstrated in lower animals, but since the human environment cannot be experimentally controlled, the extent of this influence on the human population is difficult to demonstrate. Most authorities would agree that there is a genetically determined upper limit to the human life span and that environmental factors provide important physical determinants of longevity.

There is evidence that with lifelong cellular divisions, successive mutations occur that adversely affect organ functions. A special elaboration of this mutation theory of aging is an autoimmune theory. This links the basic aging process with age-related diseases. It is believed that the accumulation of somatic mutations stimulates the production of autoantibodies causing widespread cellular injury, degenerative diseases, and a decline in the immune response.

Some theorize that ionizing radiation may be responsible for the physical changes observed in the aging process. Radiation can cause mutations and cellular damage.

Another point of view relates aging specifically to changes in connective tissue. This is called the collagen theory because the chief protein of connective tissue is collagen. Aging changes in collagen result in the loss of elasticity and in increased stiffness not unlike the changes characteristic of aging blood vessels, joints, and some other organs.

Hormone research has produced several clues that suggest that aging is a process induced by hormonal action. If some hormone or group of hormones is responsible, aging can be genetic since the release of all hormones is programmed by genes as is all other cellular activity. Recently, much research attention has been given to the hormone thymosin. If this proves fruitful, the autoimmune theory will also be strengthened.

That aging is caused by somatic mutations is supported by the fact that researchers have found a greater incidence of chromosomal abnormalities in the cells of older mice than in the cells of young mice. Perhaps also supporting this theory is the high incidence of congenital abnormalities in children born to older parents. Obviously, no single theory proposed to date adequately explains the set of events that we call the aging process. Probably several processes mutually interacting produce the many different time-dependent changes called aging.

All of the theories agree that with aging there are cellular changes. Cellular energy is reduced. There is a decrease in cellular metabolism, particularly of protein synthesis necessary for enzyme production and tissue repair. Eventually there is cell death.

Different types of cells have different life spans. Those of the central nervous system do not reproduce and seem to drop out randomly, but in general, functioning neurons last about the expected 70 or 80 years. White blood cells and cells of the lining of the gastrointestinal tract have a life span of only a few days and do reproduce. Red blood cells circulate and con-

tinue to carry oxygen and carbon dioxide for three or four months. Clearly the life expectancy of different types of cells differs greatly. The amazing fact is that their life spans are somehow programmed in synchrony. The teeth of mammals are not reproduced. Yet the mechanical wearing away of the teeth of herbivorous mammals, for example, horses and mice, proceeds at such a rate that the teeth last about as long as the rest of the animal. The synchrony of different aging changes may be a function of the physiological interdependence of the various organ systems.

LONGEVITY

Obviously, the quality of medical care should have some influence on our longevity. However, it probably does not affect it as much as was once thought. What is probably more important is our life style. Mormon and Seventh Day Adventists have substantially longer survival rates than does the average American male.

Marital status is a significant factor in determining longevity. Married people, on the average, have life expectancies of as much as five years longer than single people. Single people live longer than those who are divorced, and widowed people have the shortest average life span. The significance of these statistics may be changing because of the increasing number of unmarried people living together on a long-term basis. Their longevity may approach that of married people. Another factor involved in the analysis of life spans of married and unmarried people has been revealed in a study of Catholic nuns and monks. The nuns live 2.2 years longer than other unmarried women and the monks live 1.2 years longer than other unmarried men.

Society's values and our own estimate of our personal worth may well have something to do with our longevity. They certainly influence the way we age. We have all known people who seemed to age before their time. They are not happy people and have a very limited number of interests. These people also find it very difficult to change their established ways of doing things. As the number of people in this "senior citizen" population increases, their political and economic power increases, and the contributions of this group to society gain more attention and respect. Grandmothers have always been valued as babysitters by both the children and their parents, but it is only relatively recently that grandfathers' contributions have been applauded. Programs such as SCORE (Service Corps of Retired Executives) recognize the value of many years of experience and call upon retired people to help new businesses or rehabilitate failing businesses. The value of status of this sort in prolonging life should not be underestimated.

Perhaps another indicator of society's value of a particular group is evidenced in what it expects of that group. At any age there are certain implied expectations, whether justified or not. We all recall how annoyed we were when our parents told us we were too young to do something or other. Could it be that maturity and understanding are solely a function of the passage of time or indeed that a matter of time endows us with such valuable assets? Perhaps we should be a bit careful about the comments that we often make to healthy, interesting, attractive older people, such as "You don't look 70!" Isn't that really saying that age 70 is a pretty sad and worthless time of life? It seems unlikely that the risks and rewards are no less beyond our three score and ten than are those of a child. Maturity and understanding are not merely dependent on the passage of time.

Since human beings are problem-solving creatures, perhaps our ability to solve problems (or our inability) may well be an important factor in our longevity or at least in the enjoyment of our lives. In recent years we have been hearing a great deal about the problems of aging. The problems people have at age seventy are probably no different than those of younger people. What is different is the resources one has to cope with the problems. We have all known elderly people who very much wanted to continue to be independent and stay in their own homes, but in the interest of safety their children insisted they go to a nursing home. Obviously, in many instances this may be the best and only solution; however, it is a major decision and must be weighed carefully. If we ask our young people to go to war and die for our freedom and independence, it is not surprising that many elderly people are willing to risk life and limb to live independently.

The dependency of aging is different from other types of dependency in that it occurs after years of independence and it is irreversible. These facts make it very difficult to accept, and anything we can do to help our elderly people cope with this will probably make their lives happier, if not longer.

The social sciences offer us at least two theories on how to manage some of the problems of our later years. One approach is to replace each of our losses. For example, when you retire, replace your job with a hobby or volunteer work. Replace your friends who have moved to the sun belt or died with new friends. The other approach favors a gradual withdrawal. Slow down and try to match your diminishing abilities with more limited goals. Do not seek out new friends to replace those you have lost. The essence of this approach is not to push the individual into useless activity when that person has decided to "sit it out."

Ellen J. Langer, professor of psychology at Harvard, has done some interesting studies concerned with the care of the elderly. Her research suggests that many elderly people die prematurely as a result of mental stagnation. When the care givers make greater intellectual demands on the elderly, some of the "irreversible" by-products of aging such as arthritis, memory loss, hearing impairment, and depression are reversed.

Dr. Langer had two groups of retirees suffering from arthritis play word games. She gave the control group familiar sayings, like "A bird in the hand is worth two in the bush," to explain. The other group was given different versions of the same sayings, like "A bird in the bush is worth two in the hand." After two weeks, the experimental group with the doctored versions of the sayings reported their arthritis was less uncomfortable and their spirits were lifted. The sedimentation rates (used as an index of the amount of infection) of the experimental group were lowered. The control group's sedimentation rate was unchanged. Langer reports in the follow-up study of these subjects, done three years later, that 87.5% of the experimental group was still alive versus 62.5% of the control group.

In another study, she had the individuals participate in a twenty-minute session each morning and evening. They were to select a controversial subject and argue the side that was contrary to their own belief. After three weeks, the elderly subjects' blood pressures were lower, they felt younger, happier, and more in control of their lives.

It appears that when the care givers create for the elderly a world without challenges, without surprises, without responsibility, they are creating a dull, uninteresting world.

CONSEQUENCES OF AGING

When we consider the consequences of the aging of the various body systems, we find an important common thread—aging systems have a de-creased ability to adapt. The developmental, or maturing process, on the other hand, is characterized by increasing effectiveness of the adaptive mechanisms. In addition, the higher the level of the organism and the more interdependent the systems, units, and subunits of which it is composed, the more striking will be the progressive interference with function. Small changes in the structure of a unit can lead to big changes in performance. The more highly integrated the functions of the structures involved, the more vulnerable they are to the artillery of time. A striking example of this is the aging of vision. Recall how complex and beautifully interdependent the processes are that produce perfect vision: refraction, accommodation, convergence, and pupillary action. Aging changes visual ability well before the ravages of time may become evident in the other body tissues.

While we can state with some certainty the age at which a child will walk, talk, and accomplish many other skills, we cannot predict when an adult will become "old" and demonstrate the changes that will be discussed in this chapter. We all age at our own rates.

We shall now take a system-by-system approach to the process of aging and explore the changes in each system. In doing this, however, we must not lose sight of the fact that the human body functions as a whole, not just as a group of isolated systems.

SKIN

Changes in the skin of the aging person are most obvious and are a direct result of cell catabolism, decreased protein synthesis, and decreased available energy. The skin is dry and the hair loses its luster. The hair becomes gray and later white due to a reduction in pigment. The density of the hair follicles decreases markedly in the elderly. There is a decline in the rate of growth of the nails, and they are more prone to splitting. The elderly perspire much less than young adults. Cells that once produced lubricants have been lost or have decreased their functional abilities. Wrinkled and characteristically thin skin is also a result of cell catabolism.

NERVOUS SYSTEM

In the central nervous system, total brain weight is decreased one-sixth or more in the aged. In women this decline occurs around the age of 60 to 70, about ten years earlier than it does in men. This may be due to the fact that the female brain peaks a decade earlier, at 18 to 20 years of age.

A decline in intelligence in the elderly is so widely accepted that many intelligence tests are corrected for age. There is, however, a greater decline in motor performance ability than in verbal ability.

Convolutional atrophy may be generalized but is most conspicuous in the frontal lobes, where the neurons are assigned the most complex thought processes. The fallout seems to occur in strips, suggesting some relationship to vascular dysfunction. Here, as elsewhere, vascular changes accelerate and accentuate the cellular loss. Recall that it is on the vascular system that cells depend for the supplies and for the removal of the products of cellular metabolism.

The more intricate the task and the more judgment demanded for it, the greater the deficit in the aged. Generally, animals with organic brain disease perform simple tasks as well as do intact animals.

In the aged person, input and output are tightly coupled. Thus, an error made once or twice during the process of learning a new skill is difficult to eliminate. The old person needs continuous reassurance and information to proceed with the task. This information may be hard to come by because vision and hearing may be defective. In addition, the information giver may unfortunately be impatient with the elderly learner.

Most of the delay in performing tasks is due to pauses between successive acts rather than to the slowing of the acts themselves. At any age it takes longer to plan an action than to perform it. This planning takes progressively longer with age. A sequence of acts broken down into a series of individual ones with pauses between is also characteristic of interference with proprioceptive and cerebellar systems.

In general, what the novelist Henry James called "sagacity," or the ability to cope with life, deteriorates with age later than the mental abilities required to perform tasks. Apparently, the reason is that experience and wisdom continue to grow for a time after speed, memory, learning ability, and simple reasoning begin to fail.

Much has been written about the loss of recent memory in the elderly while their memory of past events seems to remain crystal clear. Whether this phenomenon is physiological or psychological (although it is difficult to separate the two) is not clear. Perhaps the events of yesteryear are more worth remembering than the day-to-day lives of many aged people.

To explore some possible physiological bases for the loss of short-term memory with retention of long-term memory, we need to consider where these two types of memories are stored. Apparently, the specific area for short-term memory is in the anterior part of the temporal lobe of the brain. New memories that will become long term are stored with other memories of the same type and, presumably, in unique areas of the brain. This suggests neuron losses in the specific short-term area will result in damage to most short-term memory while the long-term memories connected with similar types of memories and stored in different parts of the brain are not as vulnerable to neuron losses in a specific area.

As mentioned, there is a decrease in brain

weight in elderly people. A number of specialists in neurology and psychiatry relate the capacity to remember with the decrease in brain weight. In men, there is a decrease in brain weight of about 10% at age 80 and 20% at age 90. In women, there is a similar loss. However, this loss begins about a decade earlier, at 60 to 70 years of age.

Postmortem studies on persons who were apparently mentally competent at death showed that a 6% brain weight loss is associated with mild to moderate memory loss, over 12% with moderate memory loss, and 20% with severe memory loss.

People with more education and those in white collar and professional occupations usually exhibit better memory in old age than those with less education and with lower occupational status. People who continue to work at their occupations in later life and those who do comparable volunteer activities after retirement have better recall than those who retire and fail to maintain interest in challenging activities.

Degeneration of the fibrils of the nerve fibers in the brain is not a constant feature of aging. However, it is a characteristic of some diseases like Alzheimer's disease, which occurs in later years. Neurofibrillar degeneration and senile plaques in brain cells both are more common in women than they are in men.

The deteriorating aspects of the central nervous system, and the consequences of this deterioration, obviously have something to do with the original equipment of the individual. If one has had an IQ of 140 or 150, a loss of 10 or 15 points is not going to make as inadequate an elder as a similar loss would in an individual whose original IQ was 90 or 100. Unattractive personality traits are likely to become more obvious. The youthful coping mechanisms to cover up negative features do not operate as effectively—in essence, we become who we really are.

Another aspect of the aging of the nervous system that is interrelated with the other body systems is the marked decrease in the range of vital signs exhibited by the elderly. In disease, the elderly do not respond with great changes in body temperature, pulse rate, respirations, and blood pressure. Indeed, a fever of one or two degrees in an elderly patient may indicate a much more serious illness than does a fever of three or four degrees in a child.

The elderly have a decreased sensitivity to pain, which might be responsible for the fact that some serious health problems are not reported. Reflexes such as knee jerk and ankle jerk are markedly diminished or absent.

There is a decrease in all sensory perception. Most people expect vision and hearing to diminish with time, and they do. Diminution in smell and taste affect appetite and perhaps nutrition. The decline in touch sensitivity does not appear to be very critical to well being, but the sensation of touch is a part of a person's capacity to adapt to the environment.

CIRCULATORY SYSTEM

Some authorities attribute most, if not all, of the consequences of aging to circulatory changes. As has been mentioned, because human body cells depend on the circulatory system for supplies, this hypothesis has some validity. However, were this dependence the entire story, other living organisms that do not have circulatory systems would not age, and they do.

Some of the main changes that take place in the human circulatory structures as they age include increased rigidity of the heart valves, thickening and roughening of the auricular endocardium, and atrophy of the apical portion of the left ventricle. The arteries harden, and the lining of these vessels becomes roughened. Destruction of the elastic tissue in the blood vessel walls takes place, and perfusion of blood through the circulatory system becomes more dependent on the force of systole. Diastolic pressure increases because peripheral resistance increases. There is a decrease in cardiac output and a decreased pulse rate.

In the hemopoietic system, the total volume of red bone marrow decreases. However, no abnormality occurs in the blood cell counts of the aged.

RESPIRATORY SYSTEM

Changes in the lungs that are strictly due to aging are less well defined than are those in most other tissues because these structures are more exposed to environmental factors such as air pollution. The major changes that are related to aging are probably an increased susceptibility to respiratory infections and a decline in the efficiency of the bronchoeliminating system. These changes are due to the atrophy of columnar epithelium and the mucous glands of the lining of the bronchi.

Most elderly individuals, even in health, are dehydrated. This causes the mucus to thicken, decreasing its effectiveness in cleaning the respiratory tract. Thick mucus is difficult to eliminate and can provide nutrition for resident bacteria thereby increasing their virulence.

Sclerosis of the bronchi and supportive tissues interferes with normal respiratory movements and causes a decrease in vital capacity. Certain deteriorations in the cardiovascular system also adversely affect the pulmonary system. Decreased perfusion and ventilation are both due to an increase in the anatomical dead space (the prealveolar respiratory tract structures) in the aged individual and to the loss of functioning alveoli and pulmonary capillaries.

GASTROINTESTINAL SYSTEM

Some of the changes in the gastrointestinal system of the aged are similar to the changes that occur in the mucous membrane lining of the respiratory tract. These are particularly apparent in the mouth. The mouth is dry, and parotitis (infection of the parotid glands) may be associated with the decrease in saliva production. A dry mouth also causes a diminished sense of taste which will influence other digestive processes. It is common for the elderly to complain that food does not taste as good as it once did. Good mouth care can help reduce the problems related to this aspect of aging.

Atrophic changes in the glands of the stomach occur that may lead to achlorhydria and atrophic gastritis. The resulting indigestion will increase the nutritional problems of the elderly. There is a decrease in the liver's ability to metabolize certain drugs. Therefore, drug dosages for chronic ailments often need adjustment.

A decrease in protein synthesis causes a loss of muscle tone and predisposes the elderly to intestinal obstruction from hernia or from scarring adhesions or diverticula. Hiatal hernias are particularly common. These diseases are not much different in the elderly than they are in a young adult. However, fluid and electrolyte losses and toxic absorption associated with intestinal obstruction are more likely to be fatal in the elderly who may already be debilitated. Pulmonary aspiration of vomitus in the elderly is more dangerous than it is in a youthful patient because of respiratory changes that we have already discussed.

Bowel atony (lack of muscle tone) may be responsible for chronic constipation in many elderly individuals. In addition to this, the elderly have a decreased sense of thirst and as a consequence are likely to be dehydrated. These factors will lead to hardening of the feces and constipation.

MUSCULOSKELETAL SYSTEM

Osteoarthritis is so common in the elderly that it might be regarded as physiological. There is destruction of the articular cartilages and a decrease in the ability of the cartilage to function as a cushion. Articular cartilage is at a great disadvantage, with regard to healing, because cartilage normally has little blood supply.

Osteoporosis, which is an imbalance between bone formation and reabsorptions, leads to diminution in bone density. Elderly individuals are more prone to fractures than are the young because of this change in the osseous tissue.

Skeletal muscles decrease in mass and strength. Fatigue and increased flaccidity (lack of tone) of skeletal muscle is common. Impaired muscle coordination as well as other changes that occur in the musculoskeletal system may account for the increased incidence of accidents in older persons.

URINARY SYSTEM

The urinary system undergoes aging changes similar to those of the other body systems. Probably about 50% of the nephron units are lost in people over the age of 60. There is a decrease in the glomerular filtration rate.

Although kidney disease in the aged has no particularly unique feature, clearly the aged individual is not as well equipped to cope with any additional kidney dysfunction.

Loss of sphincter tone in postmenopausal women is a frequent cause of stress incontinence. In men, loss of smooth muscle tone in the bladder and enlargement of the prostatic gland may predispose to retention of urine.

REPRODUCTIVE SYSTEMS

In the elderly female, there is obvious atrophy of the reproductive organs, and the ovaries no longer produce hormones. (Menopause was discussed in Chapter 21). In the male, there is little change in the production of testosterone until well after the sixth decade. By the eighth decade,

it has fallen to 40% of the circulating level in middle-aged men. Spermatogenesis may decrease. Prostatic hypertrophy, discussed in Chapter 22, is a frequent occurrence in men past middle age.

Infants of older parents are more likely to have congenital defects than are the children of younger parents. This increase in the incidence of birth defects seems to be progressive. However, the statistical evidence suggests the onset is with parents in their third decade.

ENDOCRINE SYSTEM

Impairment of the adrenal cortex function has been suggested by researchers as a cause of senescence (aging). Reviewing the functions of two of the main groups of adrenal cortical hormones, you should recall that the glucocorticoids provide the fuel and issue repair supplies, which the body needs to cope with emergency situations, and the mineralocorticoids function to preserve the normal fluid and electrolyte balance. Considering this, the adrenal atrophy of aging certainly reduces the individual's ability to cope and to adapt.

AGE-ASSOCIATED DISEASES

Although aging is not a disease, morbidity does increase with age, and there are diseases that are age associated. These are diseases in which aging increases susceptibility and the likelihood of a fatal outcome. Young people, even infants, may suffer these diseases but they occur with greater frequency in the elderly. In the United States, the major age-associated diseases are cancer, heart disease, atherosclerosis, stroke, diabetes, arthritis, osteoporosis, and senile dementia or mental deterioration.

Most disease processes in the elderly tend to be more of a chronic nature than similar diseases in a young patient. Both the objective and subjective indications of any disease and even life-threatening pathology are less obvious in the elderly patient. Because of these factors, as well as the characteristics of aging, some special skills are needed by those providing health care for the elderly.

SUMMARY QUESTIONS

1. What skeletal changes take place with aging?
2. Describe the changes that aging brings about in the cardiovascular system.
3. What factors predispose the elderly to chronic constipation?
4. Why are elderly people more prone to respiratory infections than young adults?
5. Discuss some of the consequences of adrenal atrophy.
6. Describe the structural and functional changes that aging brings about in the nervous system.
7. What factors should you keep in mind when giving health instructions to an elderly patient?

KEY TERMS

gerontology
osteoarthritis
osteoporosis

Appendix A

COMMON MEDICAL PREFIXES AND SUFFIXES

a absent or deficient
adeno glandular
algia pain
an absent or deficient
arthro pertaining to joints
brachio arm
cysto bladder
dynia pain
dys difficult or painful
ecto exterior
ectomy surgical removal
emia pertaining to a condition of the blood
endo interior
entero pertaining to the intestines
gastro pertaining to the stomach
hema pertaining to blood
hemo pertaining to blood
hydro pertaining to water
hyper above or having a greater concentration
hypo below or having a lesser concentration
inter between
intra within
itis inflammation

mal disorder
meno pertaining to menstruation
meta after or changing
myo muscle
nephro pertaining to the kidney
neuro pertaining to nerve
oma tumor
osis abnormal condition or process
osteo pertaining to bone
para beside or beyond
pathy abnormality
peri around
phlebo pertaining to vein or veins
phobia abnormal fear
pneumo pertaining to air, lung, or breathing
psycho mental
ptosis falling or drooping
pyo pus
stomy surgical opening
sub under
super over
tomy surgical cutting
uria contained within the urine

Appendix B

MEDICAL ABBREVIATIONS

aa of each
a.c. before meals
A/G albumin globulin ratio
b.i.d. twice a day
BMR basal metabolic rate
BP blood pressure
BUN blood urea nitrogen
CBC complete blood count
cc cubic centimeter(s)
cm centimeter(s)
CNS central nervous system
CSF cerebrospinal fluid
CVP central venous pressure
D and C dilatation and curettage
dr dram
ECG or EKG electrocardiogram
EEG electroencephalogram
G.I. gastrointestinal
gm gram
gr grain
gtt. drop(s)
Hg mercury
Ht hematocrit

Hgb hemoglobin
h.s. at bedtime
I.M. intramuscular
I.P.P.B. intermittent positive pressure breathing
I.V. intravenous
kg kilogram
mEq milliequivalent
mg milligram
ml milliliter
oz ounce
PBI protein-bound iodine
p.c. after meals
pCO$_2$ partial pressure of carbon dioxide
pO$_2$ partial pressure of oxygen
p.r.n. as needed
q.d. every day
q.h. every hour
q.i.d. four times a day
q.s. sufficient quantity
sp. gr. specific gravity
stat immediately
t.i.d. three times a day

Appendix C

WEIGHTS, MEASURES, AND EQUIVALENTS

Apothecaries' System
Weight
1 dram (3–) = 60 grains (gr)
1 ounce (3–) = 480 grains
= 8 drams
1 pound (lb) = 16 ounces
Volume
1 fluid dram = 60 minims (m)
1 fluid ounce = 8 drams
1 pint (pt) = 16 ounces
1 quart (qt) = 2 pints

Metric System
Weight
1 gram (gm) = 1,000 milligrams (mg)
1 kilogram (kg) = 1,000 grams
Volume
1 liter = 1,000 cubic centimeters (cc)

APPROXIMATE EQUIVALENTS

Household, Metric, and Apothecaries'		
1 teaspoon (tsp)	= 4 cc	= 1 fluid dram
1 tablespoon (tbsp)	= 15 cc	= 1/2 ounce
1 teacup	= 120 cc	= 4 fluid ounces
1 tumbler	= 240 cc	= 8 fluid ounces

Weights			
Metric	*Apothecaries'*	*Metric*	*Apothecaries'*
0.4 mg = 1/150 grain		30 mg = 1/2 grain	
0.6 mg = 1/100 grain		60 mg = 1 grain	
1.0 mg = 1/60 grain		1 gm = 15 grains	
10.0 mg = 1/6 grain		15 gm = 4 drams	
15.0 mg = 1/4 grain		30 gm = 1 ounce	

Pounds to Kilograms Conversion

1 lb = 0.4536 kg 1 kg = 2.2 lb

lb	kg
5	2.3
10	4.5
20	9.1
30	13.6
40	18.1
50	22.7
60	27.2
70	31.7
80	36.3
90	40.8
100	45.5
110	49.9
120	54.4
130	58.9
140	63.5
150	68.0
160	72.6
170	77.1
180	81.6
190	86.2
200	90.7
210	95.3
220	99.5
230	104.3

- To convert kilograms to pounds:
  Multiply weight in kilograms by 2.2
- To convert pounds to kilograms:
  Divide weight in pounds by 2.2

Linear Measures

1 millimeter (mm) =	0.04 inch (in)
1 centimeter (cm) =	0.4 inch
1 decimeter (dm) =	4.0 inches
1 meter (m) =	39.37 inches
1 inch =	2.54 centimeters
1 foot =	30.48 centimeters

- To convert centimeters to inches:
  Divide length in centimeters by 2.54
- To convert inches to centimeters:
  Multiply length in inches by 2.54

Celsius (Centigrade) Fahrenheit Equivalents			
Celsius	Fahrenheit	Celsius	Fahrenheit
36.0	96.8	39.0	102.2
36.5	97.7	39.5	103.1
37.0	98.6	40.0	104.0
37.5	99.5	40.5	104.9
38.0	100.4	41.0	105.8
38.5	101.3	41.5	106.7

- To convert degrees Fahrenheit to degrees Centigrade:
  Subtract 32, then multiply by 5/9
- To convert degrees Centigrade to degrees Fahrenheit:
  Multiply by 9/5 then add 32

Appendix D

SUGGESTED READINGS

American Health Care Association Journal
American Journal of Diseases of Children
American Journal of Occupational Therapy
American Journal of Public Health
American Review of Respiratory Diseases
Canadian Journal of Medical Technology
Choices in Respiratory Management
Community Mental Health Journal
Diagnostic Imaging
Emergency Medicine
Food Technology
Geriatrics
Heart and Lung
Journal of Allied Health
Journal of Gerontology
Journal of Medical Technology
Journal of Nuclear Medicine
Journal of Nutritional Education
Journal of Pharmacy Technology

Journal of Practical Nursing
Journal of the American Dietetic Association
Journal of the American Medical Record
    Association
Journal of Ultrasound in Medicine
Laboratory Medicine
Nutrition News
Nutrition Today
Patient Care
Physical Therapy
Public Health Report
Radiologic Technology
Respiratory Care
Respiratory Therapy
Scientific American
Surgical Technology
Topics in Health Records Management
Ultrasound in Medicine and Biology
Your Life and Health

Glossary

This glossary is not intended to be a substitute for a dictionary. The author recommends that students have access to *Dorland's Medical Dictionary*, 26th ed., W. B. Saunders Company, Philadelphia: 1981.

Vowels and consonants have their usual English sounds. A vowel followed by a consonant in the same syllable is pronounced short, as *dom* in abdominal (ab-dom′i-nal), and a vowel not followed by a consonant is pronounced long, as *do* in abdomen (ab-do′men).

Abduction (ab-duk′shun). Moving an extremity away from the midline.

Abortion (ah-bor′shun). The expulsion or removal of the embryo or fetus from the uterus any time before the twenty-eighth week of pregnancy, either by natural or artificially induced means.

Abrasion (ah-bra′zhun). The scraping away of superficial layers of skin; a brush burn.

Abscess (ab′ses). Localized collection of pus.

Accommodation (ah-kom-o-da′shun). Power of the lens of the eye to focus.

Acetabulum (as-e-tab′u-lum). Cup-shaped cavity on the lateral surface of the innominate bone.

Acetone (as′e-ton). A colorless liquid (dimethylketone) having a characteristic odor. Acetone may be present in the urine of patients with diabetes mellitus.

Acetylcholine (as″e-tul-ko′lin). A chemical mediator of nerve impulses.

Achlorhydria (ah-klor-hi′dre-ah). Absence of hydrochloric acid in the stomach.

Acidosis (as-e-do′sis). An abnormally high amount of acid in the bloodstream or a decrease in the amount of base.

Acquired Immune Deficiency Syndrome (AIDS). A fatal disease caused by a virus that destroys the immune system.

Acromegaly (ak-ro-meg′ah-le). An enlargement of the bones of the face and extremities caused by an excess of growth hormone.

ACTH (adrenocorticotropic hormone). A pituitary hormone that stimulates the release of some of the hormones from the adrenal gland.

Acute (ah-kut′). Sudden, severe, or sharp.

Addison's disease. A disease resulting from a decreased function of the adrenal glands.

Adduction (ah-duk′shun). Moving an extremity toward the midline.

Adenohypophysis (ad″e-no-hi-pof′us-is). Anterior pituitary.

Adenoids (ad′en-oidz). Hypertrophy of the pharyngeal tonsil.

Adenoma (ad′e-no′mah). A benign epithelial tumor.

Adenosine triphosphate (ah-den″o-sin-tri-fos′fat) (**ATP**). A high-energy compound of the cell.

ADH (antidiuretic hormone). A pituitary hormone that causes the conservation of fluid by the kidney.

Adhesions (ad-he′zhuns). Scar tissue binding together tissues that are not normally joined.

Adipose (ad′e-pos).   Fat or fatty tissue.

Adrenergic (ad-ren-er′jek).   Pertaining to the sympathetic nervous system.

Aerobe (a′er-ob).   An organism that requires oxygen.

Afferent (af′er-ent).   A structure such as a nerve or blood vessel leading from the periphery to the center.

Agglutinate (ah-gloo″ti-nate).   A clumping together.

Albuminuria (al″bu-mi-nu′re-ah).   The presence of protein or albumin in the urine.

Aldosterone (al-dos′ter-on).   A hormone from the adrenal gland that causes the conservation of sodium and elimination of potassium.

Alkali (al′kah-li).   A soluble base; any chemical that neutralizes acid.

Alkalosis (al-kah-lo′sis).   Increased bicarbonate content of the blood.

Allergen (al′er-jen).   An antigen that produces an allergy.

Allergy (al′er-je).   A hypersensitivity to an allergen.

Alveolus (al-ve′ol-us).   A small space or cavity such as the air sacks of the lungs.

Amenorrhea (am-en-or-e′ah).   Absence of menses.

Amino acid (am-e″no as′id).   The basic structure of protein.

Amniocentesis (am-ne-o-sin-te′sis).   The removal of a sample of amniotic fluid from the amniotic sac surrounding a fetus.

Amniotic fluid (am-ne-ot′ik floo′id).   Fluid within the amniotic sac surrounding the fetus.

Amniotic sac (am-ne-ot′ik sac).   A sac in which a growing fetus is contained within the uterus. Sometimes called the "bag of water."

Amphiarthrotic (am-fe-ar-thro′tik) *joints*.   An articulation permitting little movements.

Amylase (am′il-as).   Any starch-digesting enzyme.

Anabolism (a-nab′o-lizm).   Constructive metabolism.

Anaerobe (an-a′er-ob).   An organism that does not require oxygen.

Analgesic (an″al-je′zik).   A drug used to relieve pain.

Anaphylaxis (an″ah-fi-lak′sis).   A severe allergic reaction.

Anastomosis (ah-nas-to-mo′sis).   The joining together of structures.

Androgen (an′dro-jen).   A male hormone.

Anemia (ah-ne′me-ah).   A condition in which the blood is deficient in quality or quantity.

Anesthetic (an-es-thet′ik).   An agent used to produce insensibility to pain.

Aneurysm (an′u-rizm).   A bulging or weakness in a blood vessel wall.

Angina pectoris (an-ji′nah pek′tur-is).   Spasmodic pain in the chest.

Angiogram (an′je-o-gram).   An X-ray procedure used for visualization of blood vessels.

Angiotensin (an-je-o-ten′sin).   A plasma hormone that causes vasoconstriction.

Anion (an′i-on).   A negative ion.

Anorexia (an-o-rek′se-ah).   Loss of appetite.

Anoxia (an-ok′se-ah).   Lack of oxygen.

Antagonist (an-tag′o-nist).   One that acts in opposition to another; for example, a muscle or a drug.

Anthelmintic (an-thel-min′tic).   A remedy for worms.

Antiarrhythmic (an′te-ah-rith′mik).   A drug used to treat cardiac dysrhythmias or irregularities of the heart beat.

Antibody (an′te-body).   A substance produced in the body that protects against specific infectious diseases.

Anticholinergic (an″te-ko″lin-er′jik).   A drug that blocks the passage of impulses through the parasympathetic nerves.

Anticoagulant (an″te-ko-ag′u-lant). A drug that decreases blood clotting.

Anticonvulsant (an″te-kon-vul′sant). A drug used to treat convulsions.

Antidiuretic hormone (an′te-di″u-ret′ik). A hormone from the posterior pituitary that causes suppression of urine.

Antiemetic (an″te-e-met′ik). A drug used to relieve nausea and vomiting.

Antigen (an′te-jen). An agent that provokes the production of antibodies in the body.

Antihistamine (an″te-his′tah-min). A drug used to counteract the effects of histamine, commonly used in the treatment of allergy.

Antimetabolites (an″te-meh-tab′o-lits). Drugs used in the treatment of cancer to decrease cellular division.

Antipyretic (an″te-pi-ret′ik). A drug used to reduce fever.

Antiseptic (an-te-sep′tik). An agent that inhibits microorganisms.

Antispasmodic (an″te-spaz-mod′ik). A drug used to decrease muscle tone and contractions.

Antitoxin (an-te-tok′sin). An antibody that neutralizes a toxin.

Anuria (an-u′re-ah). Lack of urine production.

Aphasia (ah-fa′ze-ah). Inability to speak.

Apnea (ap′ne-ah). A transient cessation of breathing.

Apneustic center. A part of the respiratory centers in the pons that prolongs inspiration.

Aqueous humor (a′kwe-us hu′mor). Clear fluid found in the anterior and posterior chambers of the eye.

Arachnoid (ah-rak′noid). Delicate weblike middle meninges covering the brain and spinal cord.

Arrhythmia (ah-rith′me-ah). An irregularity of heartbeat.

Arteriole (ar-te′re-ol). Microscopic artery.

Arteriosclerosis (ar-te″re-o-skle-ro′sis). Hardening of the arteries owing to deposits of fatty plaques in the lining of the arteries.

Artificial insemination. The deposit of seminal fluid in the vagina or cervix by artificial means.

Ascites (ah-si′tez). An abnormal collection of fluid in the peritoneal cavity.

Aseptic (ah-sep′tik). Sterile; free of microorganisms.

Asthma (az′mah). Paroxysmal (episodic) dyspnea caused by constriction of the bronchioles.

Astigmatism (ah-stig′mah-tizm). Visual defect owing to an imperfect curvature of the refractive surfaces of the eye.

Atelectasis (at-e-lek′tah-sis). Incomplete expansion of the lungs at birth or the collapse of an adult lung.

Atherosclerosis (ath″er-o-skle-ro′sis). A form of arteriosclerosis in which cholesterol and lipoid material form within the inner media of the arteries.

Atlas (at′las). The first cervical vertebra.

ATP (adenosine triphosphate). A high-energy compound of the cell.

Atrioventricular (a″tre-o-ven-trik″u-lar) **(AV) block.** A disturbance in the conduction of impulses across the AV node.

Atrophy (at′ro-fe). Diminution in size.

Auscultation (aws-kul-ta′shun). Listening for sounds in the body.

Autoclave (aw′to-klav). A device that sterilizes by steam under pressure.

Autosome (aw′to-som). Any chromosome not related to sex.

Avitaminosis (a-vi-tah-min-o′sis). Vitamin deficiency.

Axilla (ak-sil′ah). The armpit.

Axon (ak′son). The efferent fiber of a nerve cell.

Bacillus (bah-sil′us). A rod-shaped microorganism.

Bacteremia (bak-ter-e′me-ah). The presence of bacteria in the blood.

Bacteria (bak-te′re-ah). Microbes or germs.

Bacteriostatic (bak-ter″e-o-stat′ik). An agent that halts the growth of bacteria.

Barbiturate (bar-bit′u-rat). A drug used as a sedative or a sleeping pill.

Basal ganglia (ba′sal gang′gle-ah). Deep lying masses of gray matter in the brain.

Base (bas). A chemical that furnishes OH⁻ ions.

Bell's Palsy. A condition resulting from injury to the facial nerve causing weakness or paralysis of the muscles of facial expression on the affected side.

Benign (be-nin′). Harmless; not malignant.

Bifurcation (bi-fur-ka′shun). The division of a structure, such as the branching of a large artery into two smaller arteries.

Bilateral (bi-lat′er-al). Affecting both sides.

Biopsy (bi′op-se). The removal of a specimen of tissue for examination.

Bleeding time. The duration of the bleeding that follows a finger puncture, normally about one to three minutes.

Blepharitis (blef-ah-ri′tis). Inflammation of the eyelid.

Brachial (bra′ke-al). The region beween the elbow and the shoulder.

Bradycardia (brad-e-kar′de-ah). An abnormally slow pulse.

Bronchi (brong′ki). Major air passageways in the lungs.

Bronchiectasis (brong-ke-ek′tah-sis). A chronic pulmonary disease characterized by a widening of the air passageways.

Bronchitis (brong-ki′tis). Inflammation of the bronchi.

Bronchogram (brong′ko-gram). An X-ray examination of the lungs that allows the bronchi and bronchioles to be visualized.

Bronchopneumonia (brong″ko-nu-mo′ne-ah). Inflammation of the lungs.

Bronchoscopy (brong-kos′ko-pe). An examination used to visualize directly the bronchus.

Buffer (buf′er). An agent that resists a change in pH.

Bursa (bur′sah). A fluid-filled sac, usually lined with a synovial membrane.

Calcification (kal″se-fi-ka′shun). A process by which tissue becomes hardened by deposits of calcium salts within its substance.

Calcitonin (kal′se-ton′in). A hormone from the thyroid gland that favors the deposition of calcium into bone.

Calculus (kal′ku-lus). A stonelike formation, usually composed of mineral salts.

Calorie (kal′o-re). A unit of heat. The amount of heat required to raise the temperature of 1 kg of water 1°C.

Calyx (ka′liks). A recess of the pelvis of the kidney.

Cannula (kan′u-lah). A small tube for insertion into a body cavity.

Canthus (kan′thus). The angle formed by the meeting of the upper and lower eyelids.

Cantor tube. A hollow tube used to remove fluids and gas from the small intestines.

Capillary (kap′i-lar-e). A minute vessel that connects an arteriole and venule.

Carbaminohemoglobin (kar-bam″in-o-hem-o-glo′bin). A combination of carbon dioxide and hemoglobin, one of the forms in which carbon dioxide exists in the blood.

Carbohydrate (kar-bo-hi′drat). A class of organic compounds containing starches and sugars.

Carbon dioxide (car′bon di-ok′sid). A gas formed in the body through oxidation of foodstuffs.

Carbon monoxide (car′bon mon-ok′sid). A

poisonous gas formed by incomplete burning of carbon.

Carbuncle (kar′bung-kl).   An inflammation of subcutaneous tissue, terminating in sloughing and suppuration.

Carcinoma (kar-si-no′mah).   A malignant growth of epithelial tissue.

Cardiac catheterization (kar′de-ak kath″e-ter-i-za′shun).   A procedure in which a tube is passed through a vein or artery into the heart.

Cardiac output (kar′de-ak out′put).   The amount of blood pumped per minute by one ventricle (normally about 5 liters per minute in a resting subject).

Catabolism (ka″tab′o-lizm).   The phase of metabolism involving the breakdown of substances and the production of energy.

Catalyst (kat′ah-list).   An agent that alters the speed of a chemical reaction but itself remains unchanged in the process.

Cataract (kat′ah-rakt).   An opacity or clouding of the crystalline lens of the eye.

Catecholamines (kat-e-kol′a-menz).   Hormones produced by the adrenal medulla.

Catheterize (kath′e-ter-ize).   The introduction of a hollow tube into a body cavity, such as the urinary bladder, to draw off fluid.

Cation (kat′i-on).   A positive ion, such as sodium or potassium.

Cellulitis (cel-u-li′tis).   Inflammation of cellular tissue, especially subcutaneous tissue.

Centrosome (sen′tro-som).   A cytoplasmic organelle that is active in cellular division.

Cerebrovascular (ser-e-bro-vas′ku-lar) **accident (CVA).**   Pathology of a blood vessel in the brain; either a rupture of a vessel or an occlusion of the vessel with a blood clot.

Cerumen (se-ru′men).   Waxlike material found in the external meatus of the ear; earwax.

Cervix (ser′viks).   Neck.

Cesarean delivery (se-za′re-an).   Delivery of an infant through a surgical incision in the mother's abdominal wall and uterus.

Chalazion (kah-la′ze-on).   An infection of a meibomian gland in the upper lid of the eye.

Chancre (shang′ker).   Primary sore of syphilis.

Chemotherapy (ke-mo-ther′ah-pe).   Treatment of a disease by means of administering chemicals.

Chiasm (ki′azm).   A crossing.

Chlamydia trachomatis (klah-mid′e-ah trah″ko-mah′tis).   A bacterial infection of the genital tract or eye.

Cholecystectomy (ko″le-sis-tek′to-me).   The surgical removal of the gall bladder.

Cholecystitis (ko″le-sis-ti′tis).   An infection of the gall bladder.

Cholecystogram (ko″le-sis′to-gram).   An X-ray procedure used to visualize the gall bladder.

Cholecystokinin (ko″le-sis-to-kin′in).   A hormone secreted by the small intestine to stimulate contraction of the gallbladder and secretion of pancreatic enzymes.

Cholelithiasis (ko″le-lith′i-ah-sis).   Gall stones.

Cholinergic (ko-lin-er′jik).   Pertaining to the parasympathetic nervous system.

Cholinesterase (ko-lin-es′ter-as).   The enzyme that inactivates acetylcholine.

Chromosome (kro′mo-som).   A rod-shaped body that appears in the nucleus of a cell at the time of cellular division.

Chronic (kron′ik).   Persistent or prolonged.

Chyle (kil).   Milky fluid taken up by the lacteals in the small intestines.

Cilia (sil′e-ah).   Microscopic hairlike projections on the free surface of some columnar cells.

Circumcision (ser-kum-sizh′un).   The surgical removal of the foreskin or a part of it.

Cirrhosis (cir-o′sis).   Hardening of an organ.

Claudication (klaw-de-ka′shun). Calf pain when walking up a grade or upstairs.

Coagulate (ko-ag′u-lat). To congeal or clot.

Coarctation (ko″ark-ta′shun). A stricture or narrowing of the lumen of a blood vessel.

Cocci (kok′si). Spherical-shaped type of microorganism.

Colitis (ko-li′tis). Inflammation of the large bowel.

Collagen (kol′ah-jen). A protein of the skin and connective tissue.

Collateral circulation (ko-lat′er-al ser-ku-la′shun). An alternative blood supply.

Colloid (kol′oid). A gelatinous substance; a particle that is held in suspension instead of being dissolved.

Colostomy (ko-los′to-me). A surgical procedure to form an artificial opening into the large bowel.

Colposcope (kol′po-skop). An instrument using intense light and magnification to show areas of abnormal tissue in the cervix.

Colposcopy (kol-po′skop-e). An examination of the cervix using magnification to allow detailed inspection of tissue.

Computerized tomography (to-mog′rah-fe). An examination that differentiates tissue and structures by density, and provides a three-dimensional look at the structures.

Conception (kon-sep′shun). Fertilization of an ovum.

Concha (kong′kah). A structure resembling a shell in shape.

Concussion (kon-kush′un). A violent shock or jar, or the condition resulting from such an injury.

Condyle (kon′dil). A rounded articular surface at the end of a bone.

Congenital (kon-jen′i-tal). Existing at or before birth.

Conjunctiva (kon-junk-ti′vah). The tissue lining the inner surface of the eyelid.

Conjunctivitis (kon-junk-te-vi′tis). Inflammation of the conjunctiva.

Contaminate (kon-tam′in-ate). To soil or to make inferior by contact or mixture.

Contraception (kon-trah-sep′shun). The prevention of conception; birth control.

Contracture (kon-trak′tur). A shortening or distortion like that resulting from shrinkage of muscles or from scar formation.

Contusion (kon-too′zhun). Injury to a body part without a break in the skin.

Convolution (kon-vo-lu′shun). An elevated part of the surface of the brain.

Convulsion (kon-vul′shun). Violent, uncoordinated, involuntary contractions of muscles.

Cornea (kor′ne-ah). Transparent outer surface of the eyeball.

Coronal (ko-ro′nal). Being in a plane parallel to the long axis of the body dividing it into front and back portions.

Coronary occlusion (kor′o-na-re ok-klu′zhun). The blockage of a blood vessel supplying the heart.

Coronary thrombosis (kor′o-na-re throm-bo′sis). A clot in a blood vessel supplying the heart.

Cor pulmonale (kor pul-mon-al′e). Right sided heart enlargement.

Corpus luteum (kor′pus loo′te-um). A yellow mass in the ovary formed after the rupture of a Graafian follicle.

Cortex (kor′teks). The outer part of an organ.

Cortisone (kor′te-son). A hormone produced by the adrenal cortex. A drug used in the treatment of many diseases, particularly allergies and chronic inflammatory diseases.

Cranial (kra′ne-al). Referring to the skull.

Craniotomy (kra-ne-ot′o-me). A surgical opening of the cranium.

Creatinine. A waste product resulting from the breakdown of phosphocreatine, a high energy compound present in active cells.

Crepitation. A crackling sound made by the rubbing together of the ends of fractured bones. Also, the sensation produced by palpating tissues that contain air.

Cretinism (kre'tin-izm). A chronic condition owing to a congenital lack of thyroxin.

Cryosurgery (cri"o-ser'jer-e). The application of extreme cold to destroy abnormal cells.

Cryptorchidism (krip-tor'kid-izm). Undescended testis.

Crystalloid (kris'tal-oid). A substance that will pass readily through body membranes when in solution.

Culdoscopy (kul-dos'ko-pe). A visual examination of the organs of the female pelvic cavity through a small incision in the pouch of Douglas.

Cutaneous (ku-ta'ne-us). Referring to the skin.

Cyanosis (si-ah-no'sis). A bluish or dusky discoloration of the mucous membranes and skin owing to insufficient oxygen in the blood.

Cyst (sist). A sac, especially one that contains a liquid or a semisolid.

Cystitis (sis-ti'tis). Inflammation of the urinary bladder.

Cystocele (sis'to-sel). A hernial protrusion of the urinary bladder.

Cystoscopy (sis-tos'ko-pe). A visual examination of the interior of the urinary bladder.

Cytology (si"tol'o-je). The study of cells.

Cytoplasm (si'to-plazm). The protoplasm of a cell excluding that of the nucleus.

Deamination (de-am-in-i-za'shun). The removal of an amino group from an amino acid.

Decongestant (de-kon-jest'ant). A type of medication, such as nose drops, used to relieve congestion of mucus.

Decubital (de-ku'be-tal) **ulcers.** Pressure sores or bed sores.

Defecation (def-e-ka'shun). Elimination of wastes from the intestine.

Dehydration (de-hi-dra'shun). Deficiency of body water.

Delusion (de-lu'zhun). A false belief that is contrary to the evidence.

Demulcent (de-mul'sent). A soothing, bland substance used to treat inflamed or abraded surfaces.

Demyelinating (de-mi'e-lin-at-ing). Destroying or losing the myelin sheath of nerves.

Dendrite (den'drit). A process of a neuron that carries impulses toward the cell body.

Dermatitis (der-mah-ti'tis). Inflammation of the skin.

Dermis (der'mis). The true skin.

Desquamation (des-kwah-ma'shun). Peeling of the skin.

Dextrose (deks'tros). Glucose, a monosaccharide.

Diabetes insipidus (di-ah-be'tes in-sip'i-dus). A disease caused by a deficiency of the antidiuretic hormone, ADH.

Diabetes mellitus (di-ah-be'tes mel'i-tus). A metabolic disorder in which carbohydrates are poorly oxidized.

Dialysis (di-al'is-is). The separation of crystalloids and colloids by means of a semipermeable membrane.

Diaphoresis (di"ah-fo-re'sis). Excessive perspiration.

Diaphragm (di'ah-fram). The muscular sheath between the thorax and abdomen.

Diaphysis (di-af'is-is). The shaft of a long bone.

Diarthrotic (di-ar-thro'tik) **joints.** A freely movable joint.

Diastole (di-as'to-le). The relaxation of the heart between contractions.

Diencephalon (di-en-sef'ah-lon). The portion of the brain between the cerebrum and the midbrain.

Diffusion (de-fu′zhun). The spreading out of particles from an area of greater concentration to an area of lesser concentration.

Digitalis (dij-e-tal′is). A drug used to increase the efficiency of the heartbeat.

Diplococci (dip-lo-kok′si). Spherical-shaped microorganisms that occur in pairs.

Disaccharide (di-sak′ah-rid). A sugar with two simple sugar molecules.

Disinfectant (dis-in-fek′tant). An agent that kills some pathogens.

Distal (dis′tal). Farther from the body or from the origin of a part.

Diuresis (di-u-re′sis). Increased urine production.

Diuretic (di-u-ret′ik). A drug used to cause diuresis.

Diverticulum (di-ver-tik′u-lum). A pouch leading from a main cavity or tube.

DNA (deoxyribonucleic acid). A spiral-shaped molecule that contains the hereditary material of the cell.

Dorsal (dor′sal). The posterior aspect or back of the body or organ.

Dorsiflexion (dor-se-flek′shun). Flexion or bending the foot toward the leg.

Droplet infection (drop′let in-fek′shun). Transmission of pathogenic microorganisms via minute particles of sputum.

Duodenum (du-o-de′num). The first portion of the small intestine (12 fingerbreadths in length).

Dura mater (du′rah ma′ter). The outermost meninges covering the brain and spinal cord.

Dynorphin (di-nor′fin). A chemical with morphinelike actions produced by the brain in response to severe, acute pain.

Dysfunction (dis-funk′shun). Disturbed or abnormal function of an organ.

Dysmenorrhea (dis″men-o-re′ah). Painful menstruation.

Dyspepsia (dis-pep′se-ah). Impairment of the power or function of digestion.

Dysphagia (dis-fa′je-ah). Difficulty swallowing.

Dyspnea (disp′ne-ah). Labored breathing.

Dysrhythmia (dis″rith′me-ah). Irregular heartbeat.

Dystrophy (dis′tro-fe). Faulty or defective nutrition.

Dysuria (dis-u′re-ah). Difficult or painful urination.

Ecchymosis (ek-e-mo′sis). A bruise; a discoloration of the skin caused by extravasation of blood.

Echocardiogram (ek″o-kar′de-o-gram). A recording of the position and motion of the heart walls obtained from beams of ultrasonic waves directed through the chest wall.

Ectopic (ek-top′ik). Out of place.

Eczema (ek′ze-mah). A skin disease characterized by patches of vesicles and crusts.

Edema (e-de′mah). An abnormal collection of fluid in the intercellular tissue spaces.

Efferent (ef′er-ent). Leading from some central structure toward the periphery.

Effusion (ef-u′zhun). The escape of fluid into a space such as the pleural cavity.

Ejaculation (e-jak-u-la′shun). The expulsion of semen.

Electrocardiogram (e-lek″tro-kar′de-o-gram) (**ECG**). A graphic recording of the electric current produced by the contractions of the heart.

Electroencephalogram (e-lek″tro-en-sef′ah-lo-gram) (**EEG**). A graphic recording of the electrical currents produced by brain action.

Electrolyte (e-lek′tro-lit). A solution, such as a salt solution, that can conduct electricity.

Electromyogram (e-lek″tro-mi′o-gram). A graphic recording of the electrical currents produced by skeletal muscle.

Element (el′e-ment). A substance composed of like atoms.

Embolus (em′bo-lus). A blood clot moving in the bloodstream.

Embryo (em′bre-o). The fetus before the end of the second month of intrauterine life.

Emesis (em′es-is). An act of vomiting.

Emetic (e-met′ik). A drug used to induce vomiting.

Emphysema (em-fi-se′mah). A chronic lung disease usually characterized by greatly distended alveoli.

Empyema (em-pi-e′mah). Pus in the pleural cavity.

Emulsion (e-mul′shun). A colloidal system of one liquid dispersed in another.

Encephalitis (en″sef-ah-li′tis). Inflammation of the brain.

Endocarditis (en″do-kar-di′tis). Inflammation of the lining of the heart.

Endocardium (en-do-kar′de-um). The lining of the heart.

Endocrine (en′do-krin) **glands.** Ductless glands that produce hormones.

Endogenous (en-doj′e-nus). Originating within the body.

Endolymph (en′do-limf). The fluid contained in the membranous labyrinth of the inner ear.

Endometriosis (en-do-me-tre-o′sis). A disease caused by the presence of endometrial tissue outside the uterus.

Endometrium (en-do-me′tre-um). The lining of the uterus.

Endoplasmic reticulum (en′do-plaz-mik re-tik′u-lum). Microscopic tubular structures used for the transport of substances through cells.

Endorphins (en-dor′finz). Substances produced by the brain and having a morphine-like action.

Endoscope (en′do-skop). An instrument used to inspect the interior of a body cavity such as the stomach.

Endothelium (en-do-the′le-um). A type of tissue such as that lining blood vessels.

Enkephalin (en-kef′a-lin). A chemical mediator for neural messages within the brain.

Enzyme (en′zim). An organic catalyst.

Eosinophil (e-o-sin′o-fil). A type of white blood cell.

Epicardium. The outermost layer of the heart; also the visceral layer of the pericardium.

Epicondylitis (ep-i-kon″di-li′tis). Inflammation of the epicondyle or of tissues adjoining the humeral epicondyle.

Epidermis (ep-e-der′mis). The outer layer of skin.

Epididymitis (ep″i-did″i-mi′tis). Inflammation of the epididymis.

Epigastric (ep-e-gas′trik). In an abdominal region located medial to the hypochondric regions.

Epiglottis (ep-e-glot′is). A leaf-shaped cartilage that covers the entrance to the larynx during the act of swallowing.

Epilepsy (ep′e-lep-se). A disease characterized by seizures or "fits."

Epinephrine (ep-e-nef′rin). A hormone produced by the adrenal medulla and sympathetic nerve tissue.

Epiphysis (e-pif′is-is). The ends of long bones.

Epistaxis (ep-e-stak′sis). Nosebleed.

Epithelial (ep-e-the′le-al) **tissue.** A type of tissue that protects underlying structures, secretes fluids, and absorbs substances needed by the body.

Erythema (er-e-the′mah). An unusual redness of the skin.

Erythrocyte (e-rith′ro-sit). A red blood cell.

Eschar (es′kar). A slough produced by burning; a crust.

Esophagoscopy (e-sof-ah-gos′ko-pe). The visual examination of the esophagus.

Esophagus (e-sof′ah-gus). The canal extending from the pharnyx to the stomach.

Estrogen (es'tro-jen).   A female hormone.

Etiology (e-te-ol'o-je).   Study of the cause of disease.

Euphoria (u-fo're-ah).   An exaggerated feeling of well being.

Eustachian tube (u-sta'ke-an).   The canal extending from the throat to the middle ear.

Evisceration (e-vis-er-a'shun).   The protrusion of internal organs through a wound.

Evoked responses or potentials.   Tests that measure the electrical activity in specific sensory pathways in response to external stimuli.

Exacerbation (eg-sas-er-ba'shun).   An increase in the severity or intensity of the symptoms.

Excoriation (eks-ko-re-a'shun).   An area where the skin has been scraped away or chafed.

Exocrine (ek'so-krin) *glands.*   Glands with ducts, such as sweat glands.

Exocytosis (ek"so-si-to'sis).   Discharge from the cell of particles too large to diffuse through the cell wall.

Exogenous (eks-oj'e-nus).   Originating outside of the body.

Exophthalmos (ek-sof-thal'mos).   Abnormal protrusion of the eyeball.

Extension (eks-ten'shun).   The increasing or straightening of the angle at a joint.

Extrasystole (eks-trah-sis'to-le).   A premature contraction of the heart; a type of cardiac arrhythmia.

Exudate (eks'u-dat).   A substance thrown out; pus or serous fluid.

Fallopian (fah-lo'pe-an) *tubes.*   Oviducts; tubes leading from the ovaries to the lateral aspect of the uterus.

Fascia (fash'e-ah).   A sheet of fibrous tissue that covers muscles and certain other organs.

Feces (fe'sez).   Excrement from the bowels.

Fetus (fe'tus).   The unborn infant.

Fibrillation (fi-bre-la'shun).   A type of cardiac arrhythmia.

Fibrin (fi'brin).   Protein threads that form the framework of a clot.

Fibrinogen (fi-brin'o-jen).   A protein of the blood plasma.

Fibroid (fi'broid).   A benign type of tumor of the uterus.

Fibrosis (fi-bro'sis).   The formation of fibrous or scar tissue.

Filtration (fil-tra'shun).   A process by which water and dissolved substances are pushed through a permeable membrane from areas of high pressure to areas of lower pressure.

Fissure (fish'ur).   A cleft or groove.

Fistula (fis'tu-lah).   A deep ulcer or abnormal passage often leading from a hollow organ to the body surface.

Flaccid (flak'sid).   Poor muscle tone; lax and soft.

Flatus (fla'tus).   Gas or air in the stomach or intestines.

Flexion (flek'shun).   Decreasing the angle at a joint; for example, bending the elbow.

Flora (flo'rah).   Plant life; the bacterial content of the intestine.

Fluoroscope (floo-o'ro-skop).   A machine used to examine internal organs visually and to observe the movement and contour of the organs.

Foley catheter (fo'li kath'e-ter).   A tube used for the continuous drainage of urine.

Follicle (fol'e-kl).   A small sac containing a secretion.

Fomite (fo'mit).   A contaminated object.

Fontanel (fon-tah-nel').   A membranous spot in an infant's skull.

Foramen (fo-ra'men).   An opening or hole.

Fossa (fos'ah).   A shallow or hollow place in a bone.

Frontal (fron'tal).   A region of the forehead;

or a plane that divides the body into front and back portions.

Fundus (fun'dus).   A round base or part of a hollow organ most remote from its mouth.

Fungus (fun'gus).   A mold.

Furuncle (fu'rung-kl).   A boil.

Gamete (gam'et).   Sex cell.

Gamma globulin (gam'ah glob'u-lin).   A blood fraction that carries antibodies.

Gamma rays (gam'ah raz).   One of three types of rays emitted by radioactive substances.

Ganglion (gang'le-on).   A collection of nerve cells.

Gangrene (gan'gren).   Death of tissue.

Gastrectomy (gas-trek'to-me).   The surgical removal of a part or all of the stomach.

Gastrin (gas'trin).   A hormone produced by the stomach to stimulate the secretions of the stomach.

Gastritis (gas-tri'tis).   An inflammation of the lining of the stomach.

Gavage (gah-vahzh').   Feeding by means of a stomach tube.

Gene (jen).   A hereditary unit of the chromosome.

Genetics (je-net'iks).   The study of heredity.

Genotype   oc   makeup   of an organism.

Germicide (jer'me-sid).   An agent that kills germs.

Gerontology (jer"on-tol'o-je).   A study of the problems of aging.

Gingivitis (jin-je-vi'tis).   Inflammation of the gums.

Glaucoma (glaw-ko'mah).   An eye disease characterized by increased intraocular pressure and impaired vision or blindness.

Glomerulotropin (glo-mer"u-lo-tro'pin).   A hormone produced by the pineal to stimulate the secretion of aldosterone.

Glomerulus (glo-mer'u-lus).   A coiled mass of blood capillaries within Bowman's capsule of the kidney.

Glucagon (gloo'ka-gon).   A hormone produced by the pancreas.

Glucocorticoid (gloo"ko-kor'te-koid).   A group of hormones produced by the adrenal cortex.

Gluconeogenesis (gloo"ko-ne-o-jen'e-sis).   The manufacture of glucose by the body from noncarbohydrate materials.

Glucose (gloo'kos).   A simple sugar, a monosaccharide.

Glycogen (gli'ko-jen).   Animal starch, the storage form of glucose.

Glycogenesis (gli"ko-jen'e-sis).   The formation of glycogen from glucose.

Glycogenolysis (gli"ko-jen-o'li-sis).   The breakdown of glycogen to release glucose.

Glycolysis (gli-kol'is-is).   The anaerobic breakdown of glucose to pyruvic acid.

Glycosuria (gli-ko-su're-ah).   Glucose in the urine.

Golgi (gol'je) **complex.**   A cytoplasmic organelle concerned with the export of substances manufactured by the cell.

Gonad (gon'ad).   Sex gland.

Gonadotropin (gon-ad-o-tro'pin).   A hormone from the anterior pituitary that stimulates the sex glands.

Gonorrhea (gon-o-re'ah).   A common venereal disease.

Gout (gowt).   A metabolic disease characterized by excess amounts of uric acid in the blood and painful swollen joints.

Graafian follicle (graf'e-an fol'e-kl).   A structure in the ovary where the ovum is formed.

Gram.   A unit of weight in the metric system.

Gram negative.   Taking the counterstain when stained according to Gram's method.

Guillain-Barré (Gil-an Bar'a) **syndrome.**   Inflammation and demyelination in the peripheral nerves with ascending polyneuropathy.

Gynecologist (gin-e-kol'o-jist). A specialist in diseases of women.

Gyrus (ji'rus). A convolution of the cerebral cortex; an upfold of the surface of the brain.

Half-life. The time required for a given mass of a radioactive element to lose half of its radioactivity.

Hallucination (hah-lu"sin-a'shun). Hearing, seeing, or feeling things that do not exist.

Haversian (ha-ver'se-an) **system.** Concentric lamellae surrounding a canal in compact bone.

Hematemesis (hem-at-em'e-sis). Bloody vomitus.

Hematinic (hem-ah-tin'ik). A type of drug used to treat diseases of the blood.

Hematocrit (hem-ah'to-krit). The proportion of the volume of blood occupied by the cells.

Hematology (hem-ah-tol'o-je). The study of the blood.

Hematoma (hem-ah-to'ma). A swelling that contains blood.

Hematuria (hem-ah-tu're-ah). Blood in the urine.

Hemiplegia (hem-e-ple'je-ah). Paralysis of one side of the body.

Hemodialysis (he"mo-di-al'is-is). A procedure to remove waste or other toxic substances from the blood that cannot be eliminated by the kidney.

Hemoglobin (he-mo-glo'bin). Oxygen-carrying substance of the red blood cells.

Hemolysis (he-mol'is-is). Destruction of red blood cells.

Hemophilia (he-mo-fil'e-ah). A sex-linked, hereditary blood disease characterized by an increased bleeding tendency.

Hemopoiesis (he-mo-poi-e'sis). Formation of blood cells and platelets.

Hemoptysis (he-mop'tis-is). Bloody sputum.

Hemorrhoids (hem'o-roids). Varicose veins in the walls of the anus.

Hemostasis (he-mo-ta'sis). Stopping the flow of blood.

Hemostat (he'mo-stat). An instrument or clamp used to stop bleeding.

Heparin (hep'ah-rin). An anticoagulant.

Hepatitis (hep-ah-ti'tis). An infectious disease of the liver.

Hernia (her'ne-ah). A protrusion of a loop or part of an organ through a weakness in the muscle wall.

Herpes (her'pez) **simplex.** A virus infection characterized by blisters on the skin and mucous membrane.

Heterosome (het'er-o-som). An accessory chromosome.

Heterozygous (het"er-o-zi'gus). The genes of a pair of alleles that are not the same.

Hirsutism (her'sut-ism). Abnormal hairiness.

Histamine (his'tah-min). A drug or a substance produced by body cells that causes vasodilatation.

Histology (his-tol'o-je). The study of tissues.

HNP (herniated nucleus pulposus). A slipped disc, usually in the lumbar region of the spine.

Hodgkin's disease. A malignant disease characterized by swelling of the lymph glands.

Homeostasis (ho-me-o-ta'sis). A mechanism by which the internal environment of the body tends to return to normal whenever it is disturbed.

Homozygous (ho-mo-zi'gus). The genes of a pair of alleles that are the same.

Hordeolum (hor-de'o-lum). A sty.

Hormone (hor'mon). A chemical produced by an endocrine gland.

Human chorionic gonadotropin (ko-ri-on'ik go-nad-o-trop'in). A hormone produced by the placenta which has an action similar to the luteinizing hormone and maintains the corpus luteum during pregnancy.

Human immunodeficiency virus (HIV). A virus transmitted through sexual contact or the exchange of certain body fluids that causes Acquired Immune Deficiency Syndrome (AIDS).

Hydrocele (hi′dro-sel). An abnormal accumulation of fluid in the sac surrounding the testes.

Hydrocephalus (hi-dro-sef′ah-lus). A condition characterized by an increased amount of cerebrospinal fluid and a dilation of the cerebral ventricles.

Hydrocortisone (hi-dro-kor′te-son). A hormone produced by the adrenal cortex; a drug used to treat allergies and chronic inflammatory diseases.

Hydrolysis (hi-drol′is-is). A chemical reaction involving water.

Hydronephrosis (hi″dro-ne-fro′sis). An abnormal collection of urine in the pelvis of the kidney.

Hydrotherapy (hi-dro-ther′ah-pe). The use of water in treating disease.

Hyperemia (hi-per-e′me-ah). An excess of blood in any part of the body.

Hyperglycemia (hi″per-gli-se′me-ah). Excess sugar in the blood.

Hyperkalemia (hi″per-ka-le′me-ah). Excess potassium in the blood.

Hypernatremia (hi-per-nah-tre′me-ah). Excess sodium in the blood.

Hyperopia (hi-per-o′pe-ah). Farsightedness.

Hyperparathyroidism (hi″per-par″a-thi′roid-ism). Excess activity of the parathyroid glands.

Hyperplasia (hi-per-pla′ze-ah). An increase in the number of cells.

Hyperpnea (hi-perp-ne′ah). Abnormally rapid breathing.

Hypertension (hi-per-ten′shun). High blood pressure.

Hyperthyroidism (hi-per-thi′roid-izm). Overactivity of the thyroid gland.

Hypertonic (hi-per-ton′ik). A solution that has a greater osmotic pressure than another solute with which it is compared.

Hypertrophy (hi-per′tro-fe). Overgrowth.

Hyperventilation (hi-per-ven-ti-la′shun). Rapid breathing.

Hypervolemia (hi″per-vol-e′me-ah). Abnormally high blood volume.

Hypnotic (hip-not′ik). A drug used to induce sleep.

Hypochondriac (hi-po-kon′dre-ak). Concerning the regions of the abdomen lateral to the epigastric region; a person with a morbid anxiety about health.

Hypogastric (hi-po-gas′trik). Under the stomach; the region of the abdomen inferior to the umbilical region.

Hypoglycemia (hi-po-gli-se′me-ah). Abnormally low blood sugar.

Hypokalemia (hi″po-ka-le′me-ah). Deficiency of potassium in the blood.

Hyponatremia (hi-po-nah-tre′me-ah). Deficiency of sodium in the blood.

Hypotension (hi-po-ten′shun). Low blood pressure.

Hypothalamus (hi-po-thal′ah-mus). A part of the brain concerned with the regulation of many visceral functions, temperature, water balance, and pituitary hormones.

Hypothyroidism (hi′po-thi′roid-izm). Deficiency of thyroid activity.

Hypotonic (hi′po-ton-ik). A solution having less osmotic pressure than one with which it is compared.

Hypovolemia (hi″po-vo-le′me-ah). A decreased amount of vascular volume.

Hysterectomy (his-ter-ek′to-me). The surgical removal of the uterus.

Iatrogenic (i″at-ro-jen′ik). Caused by the physician or other health workers.

Idiopathic (id-e-o-path′ik).   Of unknown cause.

Idiosyncrasy (id″e-o-sin′krah-se).   A peculiar sensitivity to some drug or other agent.

Ileostomy (il-e-os′to-me).   An artificial opening into the ileum.

Ileus (il′e-us).   Obstruction of the bowel, usually as a result of inhibition of nerve impulses necessary to the maintenance of normal peristalsis.

Illusion (i-lu′zhun).   A misinterpretation of a sensory impression.

Immunity (e-mu′ni-te).   The ability of the body to resist an infection.

Impetigo (im-pe-ti′go).   A contagious infection of the skin.

Incontinence (in-kon′ti-nens).   Inability to hold urine or feces.

Incubation period (in-ku-ba′shun pe′ri-od).   The time betwen the entrance of the pathogen and the first manifestation of infection.

Induration (in′du-ra′shun).   Hardening.

Infarct (in′farkt).   An area of necrosis owing to lack of blood supply.

Inferior (in-fe′re-or).   Lower.

Inflammation (in-flah-ma′shun).   A response of the tissues to injury. The signs of inflammation are pain, heat, redness, and swelling.

Inflammatory bowel disease.   Inflammation of the large intestine, includes Crohn's disease and ulcerative colitis.

Infrared (in-frah-red′).   Electromagnetic waves that provide intensive dry heat.

Inguinal (ing′gwi-nal).   The region of the groin.

Inorganic (in-or-gan′ik).   A chemical compound not containing both hydrogen and carbon; not associated with living things.

Insemination (in-sem-i-na′shun).   Fertilization of an ovum by a sperm.

Insulin (in′su-lin).   A hormone produced by the pancreas; also a drug used to lower the blood sugar.

Integument (in-teg′u-ment).   The skin.

Intercellular (in-ter-sel′u-lar).   Between the cells.

Intercostal (in-ter-kos′tal).   Between the ribs.

Interferon (in-ter-fer′on).   A substance produced by virus-infected cells that helps to prevent the infection of other cells.

Internal capsule.   White matter tracts lateral to the thalamus in the brain.

Interstitial (in-ter-stish′al).   Lying between; the spaces between the cells; intercellular.

Intervertebral disc (in-ter-ver′te-bral disk).   A cartilagenous structure between each pair of vertebrae.

Intracellular (in-trah-sel′u-lar).   Within the cell.

Intracranial (in-trah-kra′ne-al).   Within the cranium.

Intracranial pressure, increased.   Cranial contents (brain, blood, and cerebrospinal fluid) are contained within a non-expandable skull and therefore any increase in the volume of one component will result in an increase in intracranial pressure.

Intraocular (in-trah-ok′u-lar).   Within the eye.

Intravenous (in-trah-ve′nus).   Within a vein, often meaning an injection into a vein.

In vitro (in ve′tro) *fertilization.*   The process of uniting ova with sperm in a tissue culture.

Involution (in-vo-lu′shun).   The return of an enlarged organ to its normal size, such as the uterus following the birth of the infant.

Ion (i′on).   A charged particle.

Ionization (i″on-i-za′shun).   A dissociation of a substance in solution into ions.

Iris (i′ris).   The colored circular muscle of the eye behind the cornea.

Irradiation (ir-ra″de-a′shun).   Exposure to

any form of radiant energy, such as X-ray or radioisotopes.

Ischemia (is-ke′me-ah).   Decreased blood supply.

Isotonic (i-so-ton′ik).   Solutions that have the same concentration or number of particles.

Isotopes (i′so-tops).   Elements that have the same atomic number but differ in their atomic weights.

Jaundice (jawn′dis).   A yellow discoloration of the skin.

Jejunum (je-ju′num).   The second portion of the small intestine.

Ketones (ke′tons).   Organic compounds containing the carboxyl (CO) group; acetone or ketone bodies.

Ketosis (ke-to′sis).   A disturbance of the acid-base balance of the body.

Kyphosis (ki-fo′sis).   Hunchback.

Laceration (las-er-a′shun).   A wound caused by tearing.

Lacrimal (lak′re-mal) **glands**.   Glands that produce tears.

Lactase (lak′tas).   An enzyme that acts on lactose.

Lactation (lak-ta′shun).   The act and time of the production of milk by the breasts.

Lacteals (lak′te-als).   Lymph vessels in the small intestine.

Lactic acid (lak′tik a′cid).   A waste product produced by active cells.

Lactose (lak′tos).   A disaccharide sugar present in milk.

Laparoscope (lap′ah-ro-skop″).   An instrument with a small telescope inserted through an incision in the abdominal wall to view abdominal and pelvic organs.

Lateral (lat′er-al).   Toward the side.

Lesion (le′zhun).   Any pathological or traumatic change in a tissue.

Leukemia (lu-ke′me-ah).   A disease of the blood-forming organs resulting in an overproduction of white blood cells.

Leukocyte (lu′ko-sit).   White blood cell.

Leukocytosis (lu″ko-si-to′sis).   An increased number of white blood cells.

Leukopenia (lu-ko-pe′ne-ah).   A reduction in the number of white blood cells.

Levin tube (le′vin tube).   A type of stomach tube used to gavage (tube feed) or to remove by suction the contents of the stomach.

Lidocaine (li′do-kan).   A local anesthetic agent.

Ligament (lig′ah-ment).   A fibrous band of tissue that connects bones or supports viscera.

Ligation (li-ga′shun).   The application of a tie around a vessel or hollow tube, such as the uterine tubes.

Lipase (lip′as).   A fat-splitting enzyme.

Lipid (lip′id).   A fatty substance.

Lithiasis (lith-i′ah-sis).   Stone formation.

Lithotomy (lith-ot′o-me).   The surgical removal of a stone; a common position for a gynecologic examination.

Lordosis (lor-do′sis).   Curvature of the spine with a forward convexity.

Lumbar (lum′bar).   Pertaining to the loin.

Lumbar puncture.   A procedure used to withdraw cerebrospinal fluid.

Lumpectomy.   Surgical removal of only the breast tumor.

Lymphocyte (lim′fo-sit).   A type of white blood cell.

Lysosome (li′so-som).   A cytoplasmic organelle.

Lysozyme (li′so-zim).   An antibacterial enzyme in saliva and tears.

Maceration (mas-er-a'shun). Softening of a solid by soaking.

Macule (mak'ul). A small discolored spot on the skin that is not elevated.

Magnetic resonance imaging (MRI). A type of imaging that does not use radiation. It images the brain and spinal cord for areas of necrosis, ischemia, malignancies, degenerative diseases, and tumors.

Malaise (mal-az'). A generalized discomfort or sick feeling.

Malignant (mah-lig'nant). Usually pertaining to cancer or other life-threatening conditions.

Maltase (mawl'tas). An enzyme that converts maltose into glucose.

Mammary (mam'er-e). Pertaining to the breasts.

Mammography (mah-mog'rah-fe). X-ray of the mammary gland.

MAO inhibitor. A drug, such as an amphetamine, that inhibits monamine oxidase.

Mastectomy (mas-tek'to-me). The surgical removal of a breast.

Mastitis (mas-ti'tis). Inflammation of the breasts.

Mastoiditis (mas-toid-i'tis). Infection of the mastoid sinuses.

Matrix (ma'triks). Intercellular material.

Meatus (me-a'tus). Passageway.

Mediastinum (me″de-as-ti′num). The space in the middle of the thorax.

Medulla (me-dul'ah). The central part of a gland or organ.

Meiosis (mi-o'sis). Cellular division in which the chromosome number is halved; also called reduction division.

Melanin (mel'ah-nin). A dark pigment in the skin and hair.

Melanocyte (mel-ah'no-sit) *stimulating hormone* (**MSH**). Hormone responsible for normal pigmentation.

Melanoma (mel-ah-no'mah). A malignant tumor of the skin.

Melatonin (mel″ah-to′nin). A hormone formed by the pineal which influences skin pigmentation; probably inactive in humans.

Menarche (men'ar-ke). Onset of menstruation.

Meninges (me-nin'jez). The coverings of the brain and spinal cord.

Meningitis (men-in-ji'tis). Inflammation of the meninges.

Menopause (men'o-pawz). The cessation of menstruation at the end of the reproductive period of life.

Menorrhagia (men-o-ra'je-ah). Profuse menstrual flow.

Mesentery (mes'en-ter-e). The tissue that anchors the intestine to the posterior abdominal wall.

Metabolism (me-tab'o-lizm). The chemical processes of life.

Metastasis (me-tas'tah-sis). The transfer of a disease from one part of the body to another.

Metrorrhagia (me-tro-ra'je-ah). Abnormal bleeding from the uterus during the intermenstrual period.

Microfilament (mi″kro-fil′ah-ment). A cellular organelle involved in maintaining cell shape and motility.

Microtubule (mi″kro-tu′bul). A cellular organelle involved in maintaining cell shape and motility.

Micturition (mik-tu-rish'un). The passage of urine.

Midsagittal (mid-saj'i-tal). A plane dividing the body or an organ into right and left halves.

Mitochondria (mit-o-kon'dre-ah). A cytoplasmic organelle that produces the cellular energy.

Mitosis (mi-to'sis). Cellular division by means of which two daughter cells receive the same number of chromosomes as the parent cell.

Monamine oxidase (mon-am'in ok'si-das). An enzyme that breaks down some neurotransmitters.

Mononucleosis (mon″o-nu-kle-o'sis). An infectious disease characterized by fever, malaise, and swelling of the lymph nodes.

Monosaccharide (mon-o-sak'ah-rid). A simple sugar, such as glucose.

Monosomy (mon″o-so'me). Existence in a cell of only one instead of the normal pair of a particular chromosome.

Mucous membrane (mu'kus mem'bran). A type of membrane that lines body cavities that open to the outside of the body.

Mucus (mu'kus). A secretion produced by mucous membranes.

Multiple sclerosis (mul'ti-pl skle-ro'sis). A progressive disease of the nervous system.

Muscular dystrophy (mus'ku-lar dis'tro-fe). A progressive disease characterized by wasting of the voluntary muscles.

Mutation (mu-ta'shun). An inheritable altered gene.

Myasthenia gravis (mi-as-the'ne-ah grah'vis). A disease characterized by progressive paralysis of muscles without any sensory disturbance.

Myelin (mi'el-in). A fatty covering around certain nerve fibers.

Myelogram (mi'e-lo-gram). An X-ray of the spinal cord after injection of a contrast medium into the subarachnoid space.

Myocardial infarction (mi″o-kar'de-al in-fark'shun). A localized area of ischemic necrosis in the heart muscle.

Myocardium (mi-o-kar'de-um). The heart muscle.

Myoma (mi-o'mah). A muscle tumor.

Myometrium (mi″o-me'tre-um). Muscle of the uterus.

Myopia (mi-o'pe-ah). Nearsightedness.

Myositis (mi-o-si'tis). Inflammation of muscle tissue.

Myositis ossificans (mi-o-si'tis os'e-fi-kanz). A disease in which calcium salts are deposited in muscle tissue.

Myringotomy (mi″ring-got'o-me). Incision of the tympanic membrane.

Myxedema (mik-se-de'mah). A disease caused by a deficiency of thyroid hormones.

Naline (na'len). A narcotic antagonist.

Narcotics (nar-kot'iks). Drugs that produce sleep and relieve pain.

Necrosis (ne-kro'sis). Death of tissue.

Neoplasm (ne'o-plazm). A new growth such as a tumor.

Nephrectomy (nef-rek'to-me). The surgical removal of a kidney.

Nephritis (ne-fri'tis). Inflammation of the kidney.

Nephron (nef'ron). A microscopic functional unit of the kidney.

Nephroptosis (nef-rop-to'sis). A downward displacement of the kidney.

Nephrosis (ne-fro'sis). A kidney disease.

Nephrostomy (ne-fros'to-me). A surgical procedure involving the placing of a tube into the pelvis of the kidney for drainage purposes.

Neuralgia (nu-ral'jah). Pain extending along the course of one or more nerves.

Neurilemma (nu-re-lem'ah). A covering around certain nerve fibers.

Neuritis (nu-ri'tis). Inflammation of nerve tissue.

Neurodermatitis (nu″ro-der-mah-ti'tis). A chronic skin disease owing to a nervous disorder.

Neuroglia (nu-rog'le-ah). Supporting tissue around neurons.

Neuron (nu'ron). A nerve cell.

Neurosis (nu-ro'sis). A psychic or mental illness usually characterized by anxiety and difficulties in adjusting to new or stressful situations.

Neutrons (nu'tronz).   Uncharged particles of matter existing in atoms.

Nevus (ne'vus).   A mole or birth mark.

Nocturia (nok-tu're-ah).   Excessive urination at night.

Norepinephrine (nor"ep-e-nef'rin).   A hormone produced by the adrenal medulla and sympathetic nerve tissue.

Normal saline.   A 0.85% solution of sodium chloride.

Nucleus (nu"kle-us).   The central part of a cell containing the hereditary material of the cell.

Obesity (o-bes'i-te).   The condition of being overweight.

Obstetrics (ob-stet'riks).   Medical specialty that deals with pregnancy and childbirth.

Occipital (ok-sip'i-tal).   Pertaining to the base of the skull.

Occlusion (o-klu'zhun).   A blockage.

Occult (o-kult').   Hidden.

Olfactory (ol-fak'to-re).   Pertaining to the sense of smell.

Oligemia (ol-e-ge'me-ah).   A deficiency in the volume of blood.

Omentum (o-men'tum).   A fold of peritoneum attached to the stomach.

Oocyte (o'o-sit).   An immature ovum.

Oophorectomy (o"of-o-rek'to-me).   The surgical removal of an ovary.

Ophthalmoscope (of-thal'mo-skop).   An instrument used to examine the interior of the eye.

Optic disc (op'tik disk).   The origin of the optic nerve, or the "blind spot."

Orchitis (or-ki'tis).   Inflammation of the testes.

Organic (or-gan'ik).   Pertaining to living matter.

Orifice (or'i-fis).   The entrance or outlet of a body cavity.

Orthopedics (or-tho-pe'diks).   A medical specialty that deals with disorders of the skeletal system.

Orthostatic   hypotension   (or"tho-stat'ic hi'po-ten'shun).   Low blood pressure when in a standing position.

Osmosis (os-mo'sis).   The passage of water through a semipermeable membrane from areas of lesser concentration to areas of higher concentration.

Osseous (os'e-us).   Pertaining to bony tissue.

Ossification (os"e-fi-ka'shun).   Bone formation.

Osteoarthritis (os"te-o-ar-thri'tis).   Degenerative joint disease with hypertrophy of bone and synovial membrane.

Osteoarthropathy (os"ti-o-ar-throp'ah-the).   Any disease of the bones or joints.

Osteoblast (os'te-o-blast).   A bone-building cell.

Osteoclast (os'te-o-klast).   A cell that causes the absorption of bone.

Osteocyte (os'te-o-sit").   An osteoblast that has become embedded within the bone matrix.

Osteomyelitis (os"te-o-mi-e-li'tis).   Infection of bone.

Osteoporosis (os"te-o-po-ro'sis).   A disease in which there is a decrease in bone density.

Otitis media (o-ti'tis me'de-ah).   An infection of the middle ear.

Otosclerosis (o"to-skle-ro'sis).   The formation of spongy bone in the capsule of the labyrinth of the ear.

Ovulation (o-vu-la'shun).   The release of a mature ovum from the ovary.

Oxidation (ok-si-da'shun).   Loss of electrons.

Oxyhemoglobin   (ok"si-he'mo-glo"bin).   Hemoglobin charged with oxygen.

Oxytocin (ok"si-to'sin).   A hormone from the posterior pituitary which stimulates uterine contractions and milk ejection.

Palliative (pal′e-a-tiv). Treatment to remove the symptoms but not affecting the cause of the symptoms.

Palpation (pal-pa′shun). Examination of the body by means of feeling with the hand.

Pancreatitis (pan″kre-ah-ti′tis). Inflammation of the pancreas.

Papanicolaou (pap″ah-nik′o-la-o) **test.** Cytological examination of cervical secretions to detect abnormal cells that suggest malignancy.

Papillae (pah-pil′e). Small, nipple-shaped elevations.

Papilledema (pap-i-le-de′mah). Edema around the optic disc.

Papule (pap′ul). A small, raised lesion.

Paracentesis (par-ah-sen-te′sis). The removal of fluid from the peritoneal cavity.

Paraplegia (par-ah-ple′je-ah). Paralysis of the lower extremities.

Parasite (par′ah-sit). A plant or animal that feeds on another plant or animal.

Parasympathetic (par″ah-sim-pah-thet′ik). Pertaining to autonomic nerves that originate in the lower part of the brain and the sacral portion of the cord.

Parathormone (par″ah-thor′mon). A parathyroid hormone that increases blood calcium by withdrawing calcium from the bone and increases intestinal absorption of calcium.

Parathyroid (par-ah-thi′roid) **glands.** Four small endocrine glands located on the posterior surface of the thyroid.

Parathyroid hormone. A hormone secreted by the parathyroid gland to increase the blood calcium.

Parietal (pah-ri′e-tal). Pertaining to the body wall; also the region of the head posterior to the frontal region and anterior to the occipital region.

Parkinson's disease. A progressive disease of the central nervous system characterized by stiffness, slowed movements, and rhythmic, fine tremors of resting muscles.

Paronychia (par-o-nik′e-ah). An infected hangnail.

Parotid (pah-rot′id) **glands.** Saliva-producing glands in the back of the mouth.

Parturition (par-tu-rish′un). The birth of an infant.

Passive immunization (pas′iv im-un-i-za′shun). The injection of a serum to provide temporary protection from a specific infectious disease.

Pasteurization (pas″tur-i-za′shun). Destruction of pathogens by use of moderate heat.

Pathogen (path′o-jen). A disease-producing microbe.

Pathogenic (path′o-jen′ik). Anything that causes disease.

Pathology (pah-thol′o-je). A branch of medicine concerned with the structural and functional changes caused by disease.

Pectoral (pek′to-rol). Pertaining to the breast or chest.

Pediatrics (pe-di-at′riks). A medical specialty that deals with diseases of children.

Pediculosis (pe-dik-u-lo′sis). Infestation of lice.

Pellagra (pel-lag′rah). A vitamin-deficiency disease.

Pelvimetry (pel-vim′e-tre). Measurement of the dimensions and capacity of the pelvis.

Percussion (per-kush′un). A diagnostic procedure in which a part is struck with short, sharp blows to aid in determining the condition of the parts beneath by the sound obtained.

Perfusion (per-fu′zhun). A liquid pouring over or through something.

Pericarditis (per″e-kar-di′tis). Inflammation of the sac that surrounds the heart.

Pericardium (per-e-kar′de-um). The membranous sac containing the heart.

Perineum (per-i-ne′um). The anatomic region at the lower end of the trunk between the thighs.

Periosteum (per-e-os'te-um). The outer covering of bone.

Peripheral (peh-rif'er-al). Away from center.

Peristalsis (per-e-stal'sis). Contractions of smooth muscle causing a wavelike motion.

Peritoneum (per"i-to-ne'um). A serous membrane that surrounds the abdominal organs and lines the abdominal cavity.

Peritonitis (per"i-to-ni'tis). Inflammation of the peritoneum.

Petechiae (pe-te'ke-ah). Small hemorrhagic areas.

pH. A measure of acidity or alkalinity equal to the logarithm of the reciprocal of the amount of hydrogen ion (in grams) in a liter of solution.

Phagocytosis (fag"o-si-to'sis). The engulfing and destruction of bacteria and other foreign particles by white blood cells and other cells of the reticuloendothelial system.

Pharyngitis (far-in-ji'tis). Inflammation of the pharynx.

Pharynx (far'inks). The part of the alimentary canal that connects the mouth and esophagus.

Phenotype (fe'no-tip). The organism's physical appearance.

Phenylketonuria (fe'nol-ke"ti-nu're-ah). An inborn error of metabolism that results in mental retardation, light pigmentation, eczema and neurological manifestations unless treated.

Pheochromocytoma (fe-o-kro"mo-si-to'mah). An adrenal tumor.

Phlebitis (fle-bi'tis). Inflammation of veins.

Phlebotomy (fle-bot'o-me). Inserting a needle into a vein.

Phonocardiogram (fo"no-kar'de-o-gram). A graphic recording of sounds produced by the heart.

Pia mater (pi'ah ma'ter). The innermost membrane of the meninges.

Pigmentation (pig-men-ta'shun). The coloration or discoloration of a part.

Pilonidal cyst (pi-lo-ni'dal sist). A sac containing hairs usually located at the base of the spine.

Pineal (pin'e-al). An endocrine gland located posterior to the third ventricle in the brain.

Pinocytosis (pi"no-si-to'sis). A mechanism by which cells ingest extracellular fluid and its contents.

Pitocin (pi-to'sin). A drug used to induce uterine contractions during and after childbirth.

Pituitary (pi-tu'i-tar-e). An endocrine gland located at the base of the brain.

Placebo (plah-se'bo). A substance that has no pharmacological action, which is given to satisfy a patient's desire for drug treatment. It is also used as a control in scientific medical experiments.

Placenta (plah-sen'tah). The nutrient and excretory organ of the fetus.

Plasma (plaz'mah). The fluid portion of the circulating blood.

Platelet (plat'let). One of the formed particles of the blood that is important in clot formation.

Pleura (ploor'ah). The serous membrane that surrounds the lungs.

Pleurisy (ploor'i-se). Inflammation of the pleura.

Plexus (plek'sus). A network of nerves or blood vessels.

Pneumococcus (nu-mo-kok'us). A type of microorganism.

Pneumoconiosis (nu"mo-ko"ne-o'sis). A lung disease due to permanent deposition of large amounts of particulate matter in the lung.

Pneumoencephalogram (nu"mo-en-sef'ah-lo-gram). A radiographic examination of the fluid-containing structures of the brain.

Pneumonectomy (nu-mo-nek'to-me). The surgical removal of a lung.

Pneumonia (nu-mo'ne-ah). An infectious disease of the lungs.

Pneumothorax (nu"mo-tho'raks). Air in the pleural cavity.

Polyarthritis (pol"e-ar-thri'tis). Inflammation of several joints.

Polydipsia (pol-e-dip'se-ah). Excessive thirst.

Polyuria (pol-e-u're-ah). A greatly increased urinary output.

Postcoital (post-ko'i-tal) **test.** Examination of a sample of cervical mucus after intercourse to determine if it contains motile sperm.

Posterior (pos-te're-or). Situated behind or toward the rear.

Prenatal (pre-na'tal). The period of life before birth.

Presbyopia (pres-be-o'pe-ah). A type of far-sightedness that comes with advancing years.

Pressor (pres'or). A substance used to increase the blood pressure.

Procaine (pro'kan). A local anesthetic.

Proctoscopy (prok-tos'ko-pe). A visual inspection of the rectum.

Progesterone (pro-jes'ter-on). A female hormone.

Prognosis (prog-no'sis). An opinion of the probable outcome of a disease or injury.

Prolapse (pro-laps'). An abnormal downward displacement of an organ.

Pronation (pro-na'shun). Turning the palm downward.

Prophylaxis (pro-fi-lak'sis). The prevention of disease.

Proprioceptor (pro"pre-o-sep'tor). End organ of a sensory nerve fiber located in muscles and joints.

Prostaglandins (pros"ta-glan'dinz). A group of hormones produced by many body tissues.

Prostate (pros'tat). A gland in the male, located below the bladder and encircling the urethra.

Prosthesis (pros'the-sis). An artificial replacement for a part of the body that has been lost.

Protein (pro'ten). A large molecule composed of amino acids.

Proton (pro'ton). A positively charged particle of the atomic nucleus.

Proximal (prok'si-mal). Closest to the point of attachment or origin.

Pruritus (proo-ri'tis). Itching.

Psoriasis (so-ri'ah-sis). A chronic skin disorder.

Psychogenic (si-ko-jen'ik). Caused by emotional factors.

Psychoneurosis (si"ko-nu-ro'sis). A mental illness produced by conflicts in the unconscious mind.

Psychosis (si-ko'sis). A severe form of mental illness in which the patient may have hallucinations and personality changes.

Psychosomatic (si"ko-so-mat'ik). Concerning a type of illness in which thought processes may disturb organic functions.

Ptosis (to'sis). A drooping or a prolapse of a part.

Pulmonary (pul'mo-na-re). Pertaining to the lungs.

Purpura (pur'pu-rah). A disease characterized by the formation of purple patches on the skin and mucous membranes owing to subcutaneous bleeding.

Pus. A product of inflammation consisting of fluid, white cells, and bacteria.

Pustule (pus'tul). A small elevation filled with pus.

Pyelitis (pi-e-li'tis). Inflammation of the pelvis of the kidney.

Pyelogram (pi′el-o-gram). An X-ray of the ureter and kidney, especially showing the pelvis of the kidney.

Pyelonephritis (pi″el-o-ne-fri′tis). An inflammation of the kidney and its pelvis.

Pyelonephrosis (pi″el-o-ne-fro′sis). Any disease of the kidney and its pelvis.

Pylorus (pi-lo′rus). The valve between the stomach and the duodenum.

Pyogenic (pi-o-jen′ik). Producing pus.

Pyorrhea (pi-o-re′ah). An infection of the gums.

Pyruvic (pi-voo′vik) *acids.* Two acids formed when the glucose molecule is broken down to produce energy.

Pyuria (pi-u′re-ah). Pus in the urine.

Quadriplegia (kwod-re-ple′je-ah). Paralysis of all four extremities.

Radiation (ra-de-a′shun). The emission of radiant energy.

Radical (rad′e-kal). A group of two or more elements that act as a unit.

Radioactivity (ra″de-o-ak-tiv′i-te). The spontaneous emission of alpha, beta, and/or gamma rays.

Radioimmunoassay (ra″de-o-im-u-no-as′a). An immunologic test used to measure small amounts of specific antibodies, hormones, or drugs.

Radioisotope (ra″de-o-i′so-top). A radioactive element often used as a tracer in the body since it can be detected and followed by the radioactivity emitted.

Radiopaque (ra-de-o-pak′). Not readily penetrated by X-rays.

Rale (rahl). An abnormal respiratory sound usually associated with fluid in the air passages.

Rectocele (rek′to-sel). A protrusion of part of the rectum.

Refraction (re-frak′shun). Deviation of light rays as they pass from one transparent medium to another; also the testing of eyesight for abnormalities of the lens or cornea.

Remission (re-mish′un). Disappearance of the symptoms of a disease.

Renal (re′nal). Pertaining to the kidney.

Renin (re′nin). An enzyme produced by the kidney in response to ischemia.

Resuscitation (re-sus″i-ta′shun). The restoration to life or consciousness.

Reticuloendothelial (re-tik″u-lo-en-do-the′le-al) *system.* Tissue of the spleen, lymph nodes, liver, and bone marrow engaged in phagocytosis.

Retina (ret′i-nah). The innermost coat of the eyeball which contains the end organs of vision.

Retroperitoneal (re″tro-per-i-to-ne′al). Behind the peritoneum.

Rheumatic (ru-mat′ik) *fever.* A systemic inflammatory disease that may damage the heart valves.

Rheumatoid arthritis (ru′mah-toid ar-thri′tis). An inflammatory disease of connective tissue characterized by remissions and exacerbations of pain and stiffness of the joints.

Rh factor. A substance in the red blood cells important in the typing of blood for transfusions and in obstetrical care.

Rhinitis (ri-ni′tis). Swelling of the mucous membranes of the nose and an increased production of nasal mucus.

Ribosome (ri′bo-som). Cytoplasmic organelles lining the endoplasmic reticulum and concerned with protein synthesis.

RNA (ribonucleic acid). Molecules within the cells that carry the genetic pattern from DNA to the cells being newly formed.

Roentgenogram (rent-gen′o-gram). X-ray.

Rugae (roo′gi). Folds inside some of the hollow organs, such as the stomach and urinary bladder.

Sacroiliac (sa-kro-il′e-ak). The joint between the sacrum and the ilium.

Sagittal (saj′i-tal). Pertaining to a plane that divides the body into right and left portions.

Salicylate (sal-i′sil-at). A class of drugs used to relieve pain and reduce fever; aspirin is a salicylate.

Salpingitis (sal-pin-ji′tis). Inflammation of the ovarian tubes.

Scabies (ska′bez). A skin disease caused by a mite that bores beneath the surface of the skin.

Schlemm (shlem), ***canal of.*** A canal for the drainage of aqueous humor from the chambers of the eye.

Sclera (skle′rah). The outer coat of the eyeball.

Scleroderma (skle-ro-der′mah). A disease characterized by smooth, hard, and tight skin. Other organs such as the lungs, heart, and muscles may also become hardened.

Sclerosis (skle-ro′sis). Hardening.

Scoliosis (sko-le-o′sis). A lateral curvature of the spine.

Scurvy (skur′ve). A disease caused by a deficiency of vitamin C and characterized by bleeding tendencies.

Sebaceous (se-ba′shus) ***glands.*** Glands that secrete sebum, an oily substance that helps to keep the skin soft.

Seborrhea (seb-o-re′ah). An excessive secretion of sebum from the sebaceous glands.

Sebum (se′bum). The secretion of sebaceous glands.

Secretin (se-kre′tin). An intestinal hormone that stimulates the pancreas to produce sodium bicarbonate.

Segmental resection. Surgical removal of a breast tumor and part of the breast.

Sella turcica (sel′ah tur′si-kah). A part of the sphenoid bone that contains the pituitary gland.

Semen (se′men). A white fluid produced by the male sex organs that serves as a vehicle for sperm.

Sepsis (sep′sis). Poisoning by bacteria.

Septicemia (sep-ti-se′me-ah). Blood poisoning.

Serology (se-rol′o-je). The study of blood serum.

Serosanguineous (se″ro-sang-gwin′e-us). Pertaining to or containing both serum and blood.

Serotonin (ser″o-to′nin). A hormone produced by the pineal gland and also found in the platelets.

Serous (se′rus) ***membrane.*** A type of membrane that lines the closed cavities of the body.

Serum (se′rum). Plasma minus fibrinogen.

Sigmoidoscopy (sig-moid-os′ko-pe). A visual examination of the sigmoid.

Sign. An objective manifestation of disease.

Silicosis (sil″i-ko′sis). A respiratory disease caused by the inhalation of stone, sand, or splint.

Solute (sol′ut). That which is dissolved in the solvent.

Somatostatin (so″mah-to-stat′in). A hormone produced by the hypothalamus to inhibit the secretion of the growth hormone.

Somatotropic hormone (growth hormone) (so-mah-to-trop′ik). A hormone produced by the anterior pituitary to stimulate growth of bone, muscle and organs.

Sonography (son-o′gra-fe). Using sound waves to produce a two-dimensional image of a fetus.

Sordes (sor'dez). Dark-brown foul matter that collects on the lips and teeth in the absence of good oral hygiene.

Spastic (spas'tik). Involuntary muscle spasms.

Sphincter (sfingk'ter). A muscle that closes an orifice.

Sphygmomanometer (sfig"mo-mah-nom'e-ter). An instrument used to measure blood pressure.

Spinous process (spi'nus pros'es). A more or less pointed projection of a bone.

Spirochete (spi'ro-ket). A spiral-shaped microorganism.

Spirometry (spi-rom'e-tre). A measurement of air inhaled and expired.

Spirometer (spi-rom'et-er). An instrument for determining the volume of expired air.

Splenectomy (sple-nek'to-me). The surgical removal of the spleen.

Staphylococcus (staf"i-lo-kok'us). A ball-shaped microorganism that grows in clusters.

Stasis (sta'sis). A stoppage of the flow of any body fluid.

Status asthmaticus (sta'tus az-mah'ti-kus). An asthmatic crisis; a sudden intense and continuous attack.

Stenosis (ste-no'sis). A narrowing.

Sterilization (ster"i-li-za'shun). A process by which materials are made free of microorganisms; also, a procedure that makes an individual incapable of reproduction.

Steroid (ste'roid). A type of hormone such as those produced by the reproductive glands and some of the hormones produced by the adrenal glands; a chemical compound containing a carbon ring of alcohols.

Stethoscope (steth'o-skop). An instrument used to listen to sounds produced within the body.

Strabismus (strah-biz'mus). The condition of being cross-eyed.

Streptococcus (strep-to-kok'us). A ball-shaped microorganism that grows in chains or in pairs.

Stricture (strik'tur). A narrowing of a passageway.

Sty (sti). Inflammation of a sebaceous gland of the eyelid.

Subarachnoid (sub-ah-rak'noid). Beneath the arachnoid or middle covering of the brain and spinal cord.

Subcutaneous (sub-ku-ta'ne-us). Beneath the skin.

Subdural. Beneath the dura or outer covering of the brain and spinal cord.

Subluxation (sub-luk-sa'shun). An incomplete or partial dislocation of a joint.

Sucrase (su'kras). An enzyme that converts sucrose to glucose and fructose.

Sudoriferous (su-dor-if'er-us) **glands.** Sweat glands.

Supination (su-pi-na'shun). Turning the palm upward.

Suprarenal (su-prah-re'nal). Above the kidney; another name for the adrenal glands.

Surfactant (sur'fakt-ant). A secretion that reduces the surface tension of the alveoli of the lungs.

Suture (su'tur). Material used for sewing up a wound; the joints between the bones of the skull.

Symbiosis (sim-bi-o'sis). The living together or close association of two dissimilar organisms.

Sympathetic nerves. The fibers of the autonomic nervous system, which originate in the thoracic and lumbar regions of the spinal cord.

Symphysis pubis (sim'fi-sis pu'bis). The place where the pubic bones join together.

Symptom (simp'tum). Subjective evidence of

disease; something the patient feels but cannot be seen, heard, or felt by another person.

Synapse (sin′aps).   The microscopic gap between one neuron and the next.

Synarthrotic (sin-arth-ro′tik) ***joints.***   An immovable joint.

Syndrome (sin′drom).   A set of signs and symptoms.

Synovial (si-no′ve-al) ***membrane.***   A type of membrane found surrounding the freely movable joints such as the knee.

Systole (sis′to-le).   The contraction of the heart.

Tachycardia (tak-e-kar′de-ah).   Abnormally rapid pulse.

T cells.   Lymphocytes involved in delayed immunity.

Tendon (ten′dun).   White, fibrous connective tissue that connects muscles to bones.

Testes (tes′tes).   The male reproductive glands that produce sperm and the male hormone, testosterone.

Testosterone (tes-tos′te-ron).   A male sex hormone.

Tetany (tet′ah-ne).   Muscle twitching and cramps caused by hypocalcemia.

Thalamus (thal′ah-mus).   A part of the brain that serves as the relay station for sensory impulses to the higher centers of the cerebrum.

Therapy (ther′ah-pe).   Treatment.

Thoracentesis (tho″rah-sen-te′sis).   A procedure used to remove fluid from the pleural cavity.

Thoracotomy (tho-rah-kot′o-me).   An artificial opening into the chest usually for the purpose of drainage of fluid.

Thorax (tho′raks).   Pertaining to the chest.

Thrombocyte (throm′bo-sit).   One type of formed particle of the blood; one of the blood elements concerned with blood clotting.

Thrombocytopenia(throm″bo-si-to-pe′ne-ah).   A blood disease in which there is a reduction in the number of thrombocytes or platelets.

Thrombophlebitis (throm″bo-fle-bi′tis).   Inflammation of veins and clot formation within the affected veins.

Thrombus (throm′bus).   A stationary blood clot within a vessel.

Thymosin (thi′mo-sin).   A humoral factor secreted by the thymus promoting growth of peripheral lymphatic tissue.

Thymus (thi′mus).   An organ that has both lymphatic and endocrine functions and is located in the thoracic cavity.

Thyroid (thi′roid).   An endocrine gland producing hormones that influence metabolism and blood calcium levels.

Thyrotropic hormone (thi″ro-trop′ik) ***(TSH).***   A pituitary hormone that stimulates the thyroid gland.

Thyroxin (thi-rok′sin).   A hormone produced by the thyroid.

Tidal air.   The volume of air inspired or expired during quiet breathing.

Tonometer (to-nom′e-ter).   An instrument used to measure intraocular pressure.

Torticollis (tor-te-kal′is).   Wry neck; abnormal contraction of cervical muscles producing an unnatural position of the head.

Toxemia (toks-e′me-ah).   A general intoxication owing to the absorption of bacterial products. The condition may also occur in pregnancy for reasons not presently understood.

Toxicity (toks-is′i-te).   The quality of being poisonous.

Toxin (tok′sin).   A poison.

Trachea (tra′ke-ah).   The windpipe.

Tracheostomy (tra-ke-ost′o-me).   An artificial opening into the trachea.

Trachoma (trah-ko′mah).   A serious infectious disease of the conjunctiva and cornea.

Trauma (trau′mah).   Any type of injury.

Traumatic pneumothorax (trau-mat′ik nu″ mo-tho′raks).   Air in the pleural space as a result of trauma.

Tremor (trem′or).   Involuntary shaking or trembling.

Trichomonas vaginalis (tri-kom′o-nas vaj″in-al′is).   A parasitic infection of the vagina.

Trimester (tri-mes′ter).   A period of three months; one-third of pregnancy.

Trisomy (tri′so-me).   Existence in a cell of three of a particular chromosome instead of the normal pair.

Trochanter (tro-kan′ter).   Large, bony processes on the upper end of the femur where certain muscles are attached.

Tubercle (tu′ber-kl).   A small, rounded projection of a bone where muscles are attached; small, rounded nodules produced by the bacillus of tuberculosis.

Tuberosity (tu-ber-os′i-te).   A large, roughened projection of bone where muscles are attached.

Tumor (tu′mor).   Any swelling or new growth.

Tympanic (tim-pan′ik) *membrane.*   Ear drum.

Ulcer (ul′ser).   An open lesion.

Ulnar (ul′nar).   Pertaining to blood vessels, nerves, or one of the bones of the forearm.

Ultraviolet (ul-trah-vi′o-let) *light.*   Electromagnetic radiation.

Umbilicus (um-bi-li′kus).   The navel.

Unilateral (u-ne-lat′er-al).   Occurring on only one side of the body.

Urea (u-re′ah).   A nitrogenous substance that is one of the end products of protein digestion.

Uremia (u-re′me-ah).   A condition in which there is an excess accumulation of waste products in the bloodstream that should normally be eliminated by the kidneys.

Ureter (u′re-ter).   The tube leading from the kidney to the urinary bladder.

Urethra (u-re′thrah).   The tube leading from the urinary bladder to the outside of the body.

Urinalysis (u-ri-nal′is-is).   An examination of the urine.

Urology (u-rol′o-je).   A medical specialty that deals with disorders of the urinary system.

Urticaria (ur-ti-ca′re-ah).   Hives.

Uterus (u′ter-us).   The womb.

Vaccine (vak-sen′).   A preparation made from a killed or weakened pathogen.

Varices (var′i-sez).   Enlarged and tortuous veins.

Varicosity (var″i-kos′i-te).   Being varicose, as in a vein.

Vasoconstriction (vas″o-kon-strik′shun).   A decrease in the caliber of blood vessels.

Vasodilatation (vas″o-di-la-ta′shun).   An increase in the diameter of blood vessels, particularly the peripheral arterioles; also called vasodilation.

Vasomotor (vas-o-mo′tor).   Presiding over the expansion or contraction of blood vessels.

Vasopressin (vas-o-pres′in).   A hormone of the posterior pituitary that stimulates the absorption of water from the tubules of the kidney.

Vasospasm (vas′o-spazm).   Spasm of the blood vessels, decreasing the caliber of the vessels.

Ventral (ven′tral).   Pertaining to the anterior surface of the body or of an organ.

Vernix caseosa (ver'niks ka-se-o'sah). A white, cheesy substance that covers the skin of the fetus and newborn infant.

Vertebral (ver'te-bral) **canal.** The canal that contains the spinal cord.

Vertigo (ver'te-go). Dizziness.

Vesicle (ves'e-kal). A blister.

Viable (vi'ah-bl). Capable of living.

Virulence (vir'u-lens). The relative infectiousness of a microorganism.

Virus (vi'rus). An ultramicroscopic parasite.

Viscera (vis'er-ah). Internal organs.

Visceral (vis'er-al). Pertaining to the internal organs.

Vital (vi'tal) **capacity.** The amount of air that can forcibly be expelled after the largest possible inhalation.

Vitreous humor (vit're-us hu'mr). A clear jellylike substance that fills the eye posterior to the lens.

Xanthochromic (zan-tho-kro'mik). A yellow color.

Zygote (zi'got). The fertilized ovum.

Index

Abdomen
blood supply to, *266*
venous blood return and,
267–68
Abdominal
aorta, 57
cavity, 57
muscles,
deep, *138*
wall, *138*
pain, gastrointestinal disorders
and, 373
Abortions, types of, 443–44
Abrasion, described, 40
Abscesses, breast, 449
Accutanen, acne and, 84
Acetylcholine, 125, 168
Achlorhydria, 43
Acid-fast bacteria, identification
of, 25
Acidity, human body and, 6–7
Acidosis, 7–8
Acids, digestion and, 5–6
Acne, 83–84
Acquired immune deficiency syn-
drome (AIDS), 453
Acquired immunity, 44
ACTH. *See* adrenocorticotropic
hormone.
Acute glaucoma, 243
Acute lumbosacral strain, 157
Adenine, deoxyribonucleic acid
(DNA) and, 60
Adenohypophysis, 460–61
Adenosine triphosphate (ATP), 5,
123, 420
Adipose tissue, 68, 74
Adrenal glands, 465–67
adrenal cortex and, 465
adrenal medulla, 467
glucocorticoids and, 465–66
mineralocorticoids and, 466–67
sex hormones and, 467
Adrenocorticotropic hormone, 461
Adult respiratory distress syn-
drome (ARDS), 343–44
Age, stress and, 471

AICD. *See* automatic implantable
cardioverter defibrillator
(AICD).
Albinism, 430
Albumin, 358
Alcoholic hepatitis, 382
Aldosterone, 466
urine formation and, 391–92
Algae, 18
Alimentary canal, 353–62
mouth and, 353–54
Alkaline phosphatase, bone and,
93
Alkalinity, human body and, 6–7
Alkalosis, 6
Allergic asthma, 340
Allergy, described, 33
Alveoli, 58
described, 314–16
oxygen/carbon dioxide ex-
change in, *315*
Amenorrhea, 443
Amino acids, glucocorticoids and,
466
Amphiarthrotic joints, 116
Amylase, proteins and, 360
Anabolism
fat, 364
immobility and, 52
protein, 364
Analgesics, pain and, 49–50
Anemia, 307
Anesthesia, pain and, 49–50
Aneurysms, atrial, 306
Angina pectoris, 294
location of, *294*
Angiography
cerebral, 205–6
pulmonary, 329
Angioplasty, 295
Anions, 3
Ankle, bones of, *112*
Anorexia, immobility and, 52
Anoxia, defined, 33
Antagonist muscles, 127
Anterior chamber, eyeball and,
231

Anticoagulation
cold trauma and, 36
therapy, colon/rectum cancer
and, 379
Antidiuretic hormone (ADH),
hypothalamus and, 463
Antigens, 281
described, 44
Antihistamine, allergies and, 33
Antimicrobial methods, 22–24
Antipyretic, fever and, 45
Antiseptics, 22–23
Anvil of the ear, 227
Aorta, coarctation, 301
Aortic stenosis, 300–301
Aplasia, left hemisphere and, 183
Apneustic center, 179
Appendicitis, 378
Appendicular skeleton, 99–104
arm, 99, 102
extremities, lower, 103–4
hand, 99, 102
pelvic girdle, 102
shoulder girdle, 99
Aqueduct of Sylvius, 188
Arachnoid, spinal cord and, 171
ARDS. *See* adult respiratory dis-
tress syndrome (ARDS).
Areolar connective tissues, 67–68,
74
Arm
bones of, 99, 102
muscles of, *132–33, 137*
Arterial
blood pressure, 258
disease, peripheral, 304, 306
Arteries
illustration of, *262*
lower extremity, *267*
Arteriography, 289
Arteriosclerosis, eye blood vessels
and, 239
Arthritis
gonorrhea and, 452
rheumatoid, 153–55
Articulations. *See* joints.
Asbestosis, 341–42

Note: Italic page numbers indicate non-text materials.

Aschheim-Zondek tests, 437
Ascites, cirrhosis and, 382
Aspirin, fever and, 45
Asthma, bronchial, 339–40
Astigmatism, 240
Atherosclerosis, 291–93
Athlete's foot, 87
Atoms, structures of, 2–3
ATP. See adenosine triphosphate
    (ATP).
Atrial
    aneurysms, 306
    fibrillation, 298
    septal defect, 301
Atrioventricular (A-V)
    block, 298–99
    node, 254–55
Atrophy, defined, 30
Autoclave, described, 23
Autodigestion, pancreatic en-
    zymes and, 380
Autoimmune diseases, described,
    34
Automatic implantable cardio-
    verter defibrillator (AICD),
    299
Autonomic nervous system, 190,
    192–94
    parasympathetic division of,
    193–94
    sympathetic division of, 193
Autosomal
    dominant mutations, 455
    recessive mutations, 454–55
Axial skeleton, 104–15
    skull, 104–11, 113–15
        cranium, 104–6, 114
        face, 106–8
        fontanels, 110–11
        sinuses, 108, 116
        sutures, 108, 110
    thorax, 114–15, 120
    vertebral column, 111–12, 114,
        118–19
Axons, 163

Babinski reflex, 169
Bacilli, 19
Back
    deformities of, 158
    pain in, 157–58
Bacteria, 19
    acid-fast, identification of, 25
    disease etiology and, 35–36
    distribution of, 20–21
    infections from, septic shock
        and, 47
    large intestine and, 361
    needs of, 21–22
Bacteriostatic, defined, 43–44

Barium
    enema, 369–70
    swallow, 369
Baroreceptors, 256
Bartholin's glands, 417
Basal ganglia
    described, 185, 187
    Parkinson's disease and, 218
Bases, digestion and, 6
Bed sores, immobility and, 51
Behavior, changes in, immobility
    and, 52
Benign
    prostatic hypertrophy, 449–50
    tumors, 34
Beta-lipotropin, 462
Binocular vision, 234
Biochemical alterations, disease
    etiology and, 32–33
Biofeedback, pain and, 50–51
Biopsy
    cervical, gynecological exami-
        nation and, 439
    skin, 81
Birth
    complications of, 445–46
    process of, 424, 426
Bladder
    cancer of, 404
    tumors of, 403–4
Blood
    cells,
        illustrated, 275
        radiation damage to, 13
    chemistry findings, 277–80
    circulation,
        arterial, 261–63, 265
        blood pressure and, 258–60
        capillaries, 266
        cardiac cycle and, 254
        cardiac reflexes and, 256–57
        electrical charges and, 254–55
        fetal, 270, 272–74
        flow, 257–58
        flow resistance and, 258
        heart and, 254–60
        illustrated, 261
        liver, 358
        stroke volume and, 256
        velocity of, 258
        venous return and, 266–67
    clot,
        described, 275
        immobility and, 52
    clotting, 275
    composition of, 274–80
    fecal occult, 368–69
    groups, 282–83
    hematology findings and, 276
    pH, 6
        regulation, 392

    pressure,
        blood circulation and,
            258–60
        shock and, 47
        stress and, 472
    proteins, liver and, 269
    sugar, stress and, 472
    supply, to bone, 98
    transfusion, reactions, 283
    typing, 282–83
    vessels, glucocorticoids and, 466
Body
    acidity and, 6–7
    alkalinity, 6–7
    buffers, 7
    cavities, 57–58
    cells, 60–67
        nucleus, 60–64
        See also cells.
    chemical substances in, 507
    cytoplasm and, 64–65
    defenses,
        fever and, 45–46
        gastric juices and, 43–44
        immobility and, 51–52
        immunity and, 44–45
        interferon and, 44
        lymphocytes and, 44
        mucous membranes and, 43
        nasal hairs and, 43
        pain and, 48–49
        saliva and, 43
        shock and, 46–48
        tears, 43
        temperature and, 45–46
        urine and, 43
    fluids, pH of, 6
    membranes of, 65–67, 68,
        75–76
    organelles and, 64–65
    planes of, 56, 57
    regions of, 56, 58, 59
    superficial muscles of,
        anterior view, 129
        posterior view, 130
    systems, 58–60
    tissues. See tissues.
Bones
    blood supply and, 98
    classification of, 93, 95–97
    composition of, 92–93
    dislocations of, 153
    formation of, 98–99
    fractures of, 144–52
        first aid for, 146–47
        treatment of, 147–51
        types of, 144–46
    immobility and, 51
    long, transverse section of, 96
    markings, 97
    marrow, 97–98

leukemia and, 35
  transplant, 35
osteoarthritis, 155–56
rheumatoid arthritis, 153–55
subluxations, 153
wounds to, 40, 42
  See also skeleton.
Botulism, 383
Bowel, loop, strangulation of, 159
Bowman's capsule, urine formation and, 391
Boyle's law, 321
BPH. *See* benign prostatic hypertrophy.
Brachial plexus, 173
Bradycardia, 298
Bradykinesia, Parkinson's disease
  and, 218
Brain
  blood flow and, 257–58
  blood vessels of, *264*
  cerebellum, 181
  cerebrospinal fluid and, 187–89
  cerebrum, 183, 185, 187
  cortex,
    motor, *184*
    sensory, *184*
  cranial nerves and, 190
  interbrain, 181
  left hemisphere and,
    aplasia and, 183
    lesions and, 185
  medulla oblongata, 179
  meninges, 187
  midbrain, 179
  pons, 179
  rectangular formation of,
    182–83
  spinal cord, connections with,
    177–78
  stem, 179, 181
  views of, *180*
Breasts
  abscesses of, 449
  cystic mastitis of, 448
  female, 417–18
    cross section of, *419*
  lactogenic hormone and, 461
  malignancies of, 448–49
  tumors,
    benign, 448
    diagnosis of, 439–40
    malignant, 448–49
Breathing. *See* respiration.
Broca's area of the brain, 183
Bronchi, described, 313–14
Bronchial asthma, 339–40
Bronchiectasis, 338–39
Bronchioles, described, 313–14
Bronchodilators
  asthma and, 340

chronic obstructive pulmonary
    disease and, 341
Bronchopneumonia, 334
Bronchoscopy, respiratory system,
    329
Bruise, described, 42
Buffers, human body and, 7
Bulbourethral glands, 422
Bullae, described, 81
Burns, disease etiology and, 37–39
Bursae, 117–18

Calcaneus, 103
Calcitonin, 463–64
Calcium, immobility and, 51
Calculi
  defined, 43
  renal, 403
Calluses, 87
Canal of Schlemm, 231
Cancer
  bladder, 404
  bone, 159
  colon, 378–79
  genetics and, 454
  immunotherapy and, 34–35
  larynx, 333
  lungs, 342–43
  musculoskeletal system and, 159
  prostate, 450
  rectum, 378–79
  testicular, 450
  urinary system and, 404
  uterine, 447
  See also specific type of cancer.
Canthus, tears and, 230
Capillaries, blood circulation and,
    266
Carbaminohemoglobin, respira-
    tion and, 318
Carbohydrates
  described, 5
  metabolism of, 362–64
Carbuncles, 86
Carcinoembryonic antigen (CEA),
    379
Cardiac
  catheterization, 289
  cycle, 254
  dysrhythmias, 298–99
  muscles, 68, 121, 123
    described, 60
  pacemaker, 299
  reflexes, 256–57
  sphincter, 354
Cardiogenic shock, 47
Cardiopulmonary system, immo-
    bility and, 51–52
Cardiovascular system
  anemia, 307
  atherosclerosis of, 291, 293

blood,
  composition and, 274–80
  groups and, 282–83
capillaries of, 266
circulation and, 254–60
  arterial, 261–63, 265
  fetal, 270, 272–74
diagnostic procedures and,
    288–90
  arteriography, 289
  cardiac catheterization, 289
  doppler ultrasound studies,
    289
  echocardiogram, 289
  electrocardiogram (ECG),
    288–89
  phonocardiogram, 289
  radionuclide studies, 289–90
heart, 250–54, 293–304
  cardiac dysrhythmias, 298–99
  congenital heart disease,
    301–2
  congestive heart failure,
    302–4
  infective endocarditis, 300
  ischemic heart disease,
    293–96
  valvular heart disease,
    300–301
hemorrhagic disorders of, 307
hypertension and, 293
immunity and, 281–82
lymphatic system and, 283–84
polycythemia vera and, 307
vascular diseases of, 304–7
  atrial aneurysms, 306
  peripheral arterial disease,
    304, 306
  varicose veins, 306–7
venous return, 266–70
  See also circulation and heart.
Cardioversion, 299
Carpal bones, 102, *105*
Cartilage, 68, 74–75
Cartilaginous connective tissue, 68
Casting, bone fractures, 149–51
Casts, bone fractures and,
    149–51
Catabolism, immobility and, 52
Catalysis, chemical reactions and,
    8
Cataracts, 243
Catheters, urine specimens and,
    396
Cations, 3
CEA. *See* carcinoembryonic anti-
    gen (CEA).
Cells, 60–67
  blood, illustrated, 275
  membranes of, 65–67
    diffusion and, 65–66

Cells, (*Cont.*)
    filtration and, 66
    osmosis, 66–67
    nucleus, 60–64
        deoxyribonucleic acid (DNA)
          and, 60–61, *62*
        meiosis and, 64
        mitosis and, 61, *63*, 64
    See also body and cells.
Cellular immunity, 281–82
Cerebellum, 181
  equilibrium and, 229
  testing, 201
Cerebral
  angiogram, 205–6
  cortex,
    described, 183
    stimulation of, 182
Cerebrospinal fluid
  brain and, 187–89
  circulation of, *189*
  composition of, *204*
  hydrocephalus and, 217
  lumbar puncture and, 203
Cerebrovascular accident, nervous
    system and, 211–12
Cerebrum, 183, 185, 187
Cerumen, 77, 227
  impacted, 245
  microorganisms and, 43
Ceruminous glands, 77
Cervix, biopsy of, gynecological
    examination and, 439
Chalazion, 230, 244
Chancre, syphilis and, 452
Chemical
  antimicrobial methods and,
    22–24
  burns, 38
  reactions,
    electrons and, 3
    speed of, 7–8
  transmission, nerve impulses,
    168–69
Chemoreceptors, 256–57
Chemotherapy
  breast cancer and, 449
  colon/rectum cancer and, 379
  leukemia and, 35
  testes cancer and, 450
Chest, trauma to, 344
Chlorofluorocarbons, disease
    etiology and, 31
Cholecystitis, 380
Cholecystokinin, 463
  pancreozymin, 356
Cholelithiasis, 380
Cholesterol
  liver use of, 357
  types of, 357–58
Cholinesterase, 168–69

Chondrosarcoma, 159
Choroid, 231
  plexus, cerebrospinal fluid and,
    187
Chronic
  asthma, 340
  cholecystitis, 380
  gastritis, 375
  glaucoma, 243–44
  hepatitis, 382
  obstructive pulmonary disease,
    treatment of, 341
  pancreatitis, 380
  renal failure, 405
Ciliary muscle, vision and, 231
Circle of Willis, 261
Circulation
  blood,
    arterial, 261–63, 265
    blood pressure and, 258–60
    capillaries and, 266
    cardiac cycle, 254
    cardiac reflexes and, 256–57
    electrical charges and,
      254–55
    fetal, 270, 272–74
    flow and, 257–58
    flow resistance and, 258
    illustrated, *261*
    stroke volume and, 256
    velocity of, 258
    venous return and, 266–67
  heart and, 254–60
  See also cardiovascular system.
Circulatory system, described, 59
Cirrhosis, liver, 382–83
Cisternal puncture, 203–4
Clavicle, 99, *102*
Clearance tests, renal, 397
Clitoris, 417
Coarctation, aorta, 301
Cocci, 19
Coccyx, 102, *106–9*
Cochlea
  cross section of, *229*
  implants of, 246–47
  of inner ear, 227
Codominance, 429
Cold
  common, 333
  sense of, 234
  sores, 86
  trauma, 36–37
Collagen, 92
Colon, 360
  cancer of, 378–79
  sigmoid, 361–62
Colostomy, colon/rectum cancer
    and, 379
Colposcopy, gynecological exami-
    nation and, 439

Columnar
  epithelial tissue, 67
  epithelium, 74
Common cold, 333
Compartment syndrome, bone
    fractures and, 152
Compounds
  defined, 3
  illustrated, *4*
  See also organic compounds.
Computer tomography (CT)
  bone fractures, 147
  gastrointestinal system and,
    372–73
  hydrocephalus and, 218
  myelogram, 207–8
  nervous system and, 204–5
  respiratory system and, 329
Concentrations, chemical reac-
    tions and, 8
Concussion, described, 213
Conductive hearing loss, 246
Cones, vision and, 232, 233
Congenital heart disease, 301–2
Congestive heart failure, 302–4
Conjunctiva, vision and, 230
Conjunctivitis, 244
Connective tissues, 67–68, 74–75
Consciousness, determination of,
    199
Constipation, 361
Contact dermatitis, 84–85
Continuous ambulatory perito-
    neal dialysis, 406–7
Contraception, reproduction and,
    427–28
Contraction physiology, muscles,
    123–26
Contusion, head, 213
Cornea
  described, 230
  problems of, 245–46
Corns, 87
Coronary artery, bypass graft sur-
    gery, 295, *296*
Corpus callosum, 183
Corpus luteum, 414
Corticospinal
  fibers, 178
  tracts, 178
Cowper's glands, 422
Cranial nerves, 190
  examination of, 199–200
    functions and, *200–201*
Cranium, bones of, 104–6, *114*
Creatinine, urine formation and,
    392–93
Crohn's disease, 378
Croup, 333–34
Crutches, walking with, bone
    fractures and, 152

Cryosurgery, skin, 82–83
Cryptorchidism, 420
Crystal violet, 25
CT. *See* computer tomography (CT).
Cuboidal epithelium, 67, 74
Culdoscopy, gynecological examination and, 439
Cutaneous
   membrane. *See* skin.
   pain, 48
     areas of, *49*
   senses, 234–35
CVA. *See* cerebrovascular accident.
Cyanosis, 302
Cystic
   fibrosis, 340–41
   mastitis, 448
Cystoscopy, urine tests and, 401
Cysts, sebaceous, 86–87
Cytology, defined, 30
Cytoplasm, 64–65
Cytosine, deoxyribonucleic acid (DNA) and, 60

D and C, 439
Da Nang Lung, 343
Dalton's law, 321
Dandruff, 84
Deafness, vestibular disease and, 247
Decubital ulcers, immobility and, 51
Deep tendon reflex, 169
Delirium, nervous system and, 209
Delivery. *See* birth.
Dendrites, 163
   described, 164
Dense fibrous connective tissue, 68, 74
Dental, caries, 374
Deoxyribonucleic acid (DNA), described, 60–61, *62*
Dermatitis, contact, 84–85
Dermatophytosis, 87
Dermis, described, 76
Desquamation, described, 81
Detached retina, 244
Dialysis, 405–8
Diaper rash, 87
Diaphragmatic hernia, 159
Diaphysis, 93
Diarrhea, gastrointestinal disorders and, 374
Diarthrotic joints, 116
   motion in, *118*
Diastole contraction, 254
Diastolic blood pressure, 260
Diencephalon, 181

Diet, disease etiology and, 31
Diffusion
   cells and, 65–66
   defined, 65
Digestive processes
   acids and, 5–6
   bases and, 6
   chemicals of, *361*
   esophagus and, 354
   gallbladder and, 359
   intestines,
     large, 360–62
     small and, 356–60
   liver and, 356–57
   pancreas and, 359–60
   pharynx and, 354
   stomach and, 354–55
Dilation and curettage (D and C), 439
Diplococci, 19
Disc, herniated intervertebral, 157
Disease
   body defenses to, 42–45
   etiology of, 31–42
     bacterial invasion and, 35–36
     biochemical alterations, 32–33
     direct causes, 32–42
     immunity disturbances, 33–34
     neoplasms, 34–35
     oxygen lack, 33
     poisons and, 32
     predisposing causes, 31–32
     trauma, 36–42
     viral invasion and, 35–36
Disinfectants, 22–23
Dislocations, 153
Diverticular disease, 376–77
Diverticulum, described, 376–77
DNA. *See* deoxyribonucleic acid (DNA).
Dominant
   inheritance, 428
   mutations, autosomal, 455
Dopamine, Parkinson's disease and, 218–19
Doppler ultrasound studies, cardiovascular system and, 289
Dorsal cavity, described, 58
Down syndrome, 454
Dressings, wet, skin, 82
Dropped kidney, 403
Drowning, 36
Dry heat, microbes and, 23
Duodenum, 356
   disorders of,
     gastritis, 375
     peptic ulcer disease, 375–76
Dura mater, 76
   spinal cord and, 171

Dysmenorrhea, 443
   uterine displacement and, 447
Dyspepsia, chronic gastritis and, 375
Dyspnea, defined, 33
Dysreflexia, 215
   treatment of, 215–16

Ear
   cerumen and, 77, 227
     impacted, 245
     organisms and, 43
   cross section of, *228*
   foreign bodies in, 245–46
   hearing and, 227–28
   mastoiditis and, 245
   otitis media and, 245
   See also hearing.
Ecchymosis, described, 42
ECG. *See* electrocardiogram (ECG).
Echocardiogram, 289
Ecogenetics, described, 431
Eczema, 84
Edema, defined, 36
EEG. *See* electroencephalogram (EEG).
Ejaculatory ducts, 421
Elastic cartilage, 68, 74
Electrical
   burns, 38
   stimulators, pain and, 50
   transmission, nerve impulses, 166–68
Electrocardiogram (ECG), 288–89
Electroencephalogram (EEG), 206
   described, 167
Electrolytes, described, 3
Electromyogram (EMG), 207
Electrons, 2
   chemical reactions and, 3
Electronystagmography, vestibular disease and, 247
Element, defined, 3
Embolus
   described, 275
   immobility and, 52
EMG. *See* electromyogram (EMG).
Emphysema, 338
Encephalitis, central nervous system and, 217
Encephalon. *See* brain.
Endocarditis
   gonorrhea and, 452
   infective, 300
Endocardium, 250
Endocrine system
   adrenal glands and, 465–67
   described, 60
   glands of, *459*
   gonads and, 469
   hypothalamus, 463

Endocrine system, (*Cont.*)
  kidney and, 468–69
  local hormones and, 469
  pancreas and, 467–68
  parathyroid glands and, 464
  pineal gland and, 463
  pituitary gland, 458, 460–63
    adenohypophysis and, 460–61
    adrenocorticotropic hormone
      and, 461
    antidiuretic hormone (ADH)
      and, 462
    beta-lipotropin and, 462
    gonadotropic hormones and,
      461
    melanocyte-stimulating hor-
      mone (MSH), 462
    neurohypophysis and, 462–63
    oxytocin and, 462–63
    somatotropic hormone and,
      461–62
    thyrotropic hormone and,
      461
    vasopressin and, 462
  placenta and, 469
  prostaglandins and, 469–70
  stress and, 470–73
  thymus and, 464–65
  thyroid and, 463–64
Endometrium, 415
Endoplasmic reticulum, 64
Endorphins, 50
Endoscopy, gastrointestinal sys-
  tem and, 371
Endothelium tissues, 67
Enema, barium, 369–70
Enteritis, regional, 378
Enzymes, described, 5
Epicardium, 250
Epicondylitis, 153
Epidermis, described, 76
Epididymis, 421
Epididymitis, 451
Epiglottis, taste buds and, 225
Epiglottitis, 334
Epilepsy, nervous system and,
  212–13
Epinephrine, 45
Epiphyses, 93
Epistaxis, 332
Epithelial tissues, 67, 73–74
Epithelium, simple squamous,
  73–74
Equilibrium, 228–29
Esophagus
  digestive processes and, 354
  varicose veins of, cirrhosis and,
    382–83
Estrogen
  function of, 414
  immobility and, 51

Eustachian tube, 227
  function of, 312
Evoked
  potentials, nervous system and,
    206–7
  responses, nervous system and,
    206–7
Ewing's sarcoma, 159
Excoriation, described, 82
Exocytosis, defined, 67
External
  fixation, bone fractures and, 149
  respirations, 317–19
Extracellular fluids, glucocorti-
    coids and, 466
Extrapyramidal tracts, 178
Extravascular clotting, 275
Extremities
  lower,
    bones of, 103–4
    venous blood return and,
      267, *271*
  upper, venous blood return
    and, 267
Extrinsic asthma, 340
Exudate, described, 82
Eye
  astigmatism and, 240
  cataracts and, 243
  detached retina and, 244
  examinations of, 239
  glaucoma and, 243–44
  hyperopia and, 240
  muscles of, *131*
  myopia and, 240
  presbyopia and, 241–42
  strabismus and, 242–43
  visual field defects and, 240
  See also vision.
Eyeball
  cross section of, *231*
  focusing and, 232–33
  layers of, 230–32
  protection of, 230
Eyelids, 230

Face
  bones of, 106–8
  muscles of, *131*
Failed union, bone fractures and,
  151
Fallopian tubes, 414
Falx cerebri, 187
Far-sightedness, 240
Fat
  anabolism, 364
  glucocorticoids and, 466
  metabolism, 364
Fat emboli, bone fractures and,
  151–52
Fecal occult blood, 368–69

Femur, 103, *110*
Fertility
  defined, 424
  reproduction and, 424, 427
Fertilization, pregnancy and,
  422–24
Fetal, heart monitoring of, direct,
  442
Fetus
  blood circulation in, 270,
    272–74
  body size, changes in, *423*
  development of, 422–24
Fever
  body defenses and, 45–46
  chemical reactions and, 7–8
Fibrinogen, 358
Fibroadenoma, 448
Fibroblasts, lymphocytes and, 44
Fibrosarcoma, 159
Fibrous
  connective tissues, 68, 74–75
  membranes, 76
Fibula, 103, 104, *111*
Fingernails, 77
First degree burns, 37
First-level reflexes, 169–70
Fissures
  described, 82
  of Rolando, 183
  of Sylvius, 183
Flail chest, 344
Floating kidney, 403
Follicle-stimulating hormone
    (FSH), 414, 461
  spermatogenesis and, 420
Fontanels, 110–11
Food poisoning, 383
Foot, bones of, *112*
Foramen
  of Luschka, 188
  of Magendie, 188
  of Monroe, 188
Foreign bodies, ear and, 245–46
Fornix, 417
Fractures, 144–52
  casting/cast care and, 149–51
  complications of,
    compartment syndrome, 152
    failed union, 151
    fat emboli, 151–52
    infection, 152
  crutch walking and, 152
  first aid for, 146–47
  reduction of, 147–49
  traction for, 151
  treatment of, 147–51
  types of, 144, 146
    illustrated, *145*
Freckles, 76
Friedman test, 437

Frostbite, 36
FSH. *See* follicle-stimulating hormone (FSH).
Fungi, 19
Furunculus, 86

Gag reflex, 169
Gallbladder
  digestive processes and, 359
  disorders of,
    cholecystitis, 380
    cholelithiasis, 380
Ganglia, described, 164
Gastric
  acidity, glucocorticoids and,
    466
  juices, body defenses and,
    43–44
Gastrin, 463
Gastritis, 375
Gastrointestinal system
  alimentary canal and, 353–62
  computerized tomography
    (CT) and, 372–73
  described, 60
  diagnostic procedures of,
    barium enema, 369–70
    barium swallow, 369
    colonoscopy, 372
    computer tomography (CT)
      and, 372–73
    endoscopy, 371
    fecal occult blood, 368–69
    nuclear medicine, 373
    oral cholecystogram, 370–71
    small bowel series, 369
    ultrasonography, 371–72
    upper gastrointestinal series,
      369
  diseases of,
    appendicitis and, 378
    cirrhosis, 382–83
    colon/rectum cancer, 378–79
    Crohn's disease, 378
    diverticular disease, 376–77
    hemorrhoids and, 379
    hepatitis, 381–82
    inflammatory bowel disease,
      377–78
    intestinal obstruction and, 379
    pancreatitis, 380
    peritonitis, 377
  disorders of,
    abdominal pain, 373
    cholecystitis, 380
    cholelithiasis, 380
    dental caries and, 374
    diarrhea, 374
    gastritis, 375
    mouth tumors and, 374–75
    nausea/vomiting, 374

  peptic ulcer disease and,
    375–76
  stomatitis, 374
  metabolism of,
    carbohydrate, 362–64
    fat, 364
    protein, 364
  nuclear medicine and, 373
  poison and,
    food, 383
    ingested, 383–84
    treatment of, 384–85
Genetics, reproduction and,
  428–31
Genital herpes, 452–53
Germ cells, mutation of, radioactivity and, 14
GI series, 369
Glandular epithelium, 67, 74
Glaucoma, 243–44
  test for, 239
Glisson's capsule, 357
Globulin, 358
Glomerulotropin, 463
Glucagon, 467
  insulin and, 360
Glucocorticoids, 465–66
  insulin and, 360
Gluconeogenesis, 357
Glucose
  glomerular filtrate and, 391
  glucocorticoids and, 466
Glycogen, 5
Glycolysis, 363
Glycosuria, described, 391
Golgi complex, described, 65
Gonadotropic hormone, 461
Gonads, 469
Gonorrhea, 40, 451–52
Gram-negative organisms, identification of, 25
Gram-positive organisms, identification of, 25
Gram's iodine, 25
Grand mal seizures, 212
Guanine, deoxyribonucleic acid
  (DNA) and, 60

Hair
  loss of, radiation and, 13
  nasal, body defenses and, 43
Hammer of the ear, 227
Haversian systems, bone and, 93, 95
HDL. *See* high density lipoprotein
  (HDL).
Head
  blood circulation to, 261
  hematoma of, 213–14
  injury,
    nervous system and, 213–14
    symptoms of, *214*

  venous blood return and, 267,
    268
Hearing, 227–28
  cochlear implants and, 246–47
  impaired, 246
  labyrinthitis and, 247
  loss,
    conductive, 246
    sensorineural, 246
  presbycusis and, 246
  tests of, 239–40
  vestibular disease and, 247
  See also ear.
Heart, 250–54
  attack early warnings of, *297*
  blood,
    circulation, 254–60
    supply to, 251
  cardiac dysrhythmias and,
    298–99
  chambers of, 250–51
  conduction system, 253–54
  congenital disease of, 301–302
  congestive failure of, 302–4
  cross section of, *252*
  disease, 293–304, 392–94
  ischemic heart disease, 393–96
  nerve, supply to, 251, 253
  transplantation, illustrated, *305*
  valves, 251
  valvular heart disease, 300–301
  See also cardiovascular system.
Heartburn, chronic gastritis and,
  375
Heat
  exhaustion, 37
  microbes and, 23
  sense of, 234–35
  stroke, 37
Hematemesis, chronic gastritis
  and, 375
Hematocrit, defined, 274
Hematoma, 42
  head, 213–14
Hematuria
  blood transfusions and, 283
  kidney stones and, 403
Hemodialysis, 407–8
Hemoglobin
  described, 274
  oxygen combining with, 318
Hemophilia, 307, 430, 455
Hemopoietic, bone marrow and, 97
Hemorrhage, subarachnoid, 214
Hemorrhagic disorders, 307
Hemorrhoids, 379
Hepatitis, 381–82
  A, 381
    clinical course of, 382
  B, 381–82
    clinical course of, 382

Hepatitis, (*Cont.*)
    C, 382
        viral, comparison types of, *381*
Heredity
    expressions of, 430–31
    modes of, 428–30
Hernias, 158–59
Herniated intervertebral disc, 157
Herpes
    genital, 452–53
    simplex, 86
    zoster, 86
Hiatus hernia, 159
High density lipoprotein (HDL),
        357–58
Histocytes, body defenses and, 44
Histology, defined, 30
Hives, 84
Hodgkin's disease, pruritus and, 82
Hordeolum, 244
Hormonal therapy, breast cancer
        and, 449
Hormones
    local, 469
    releasing factors of, 460–61
    See also specific type of hor-
        mone.
Humerus, 99, *103*
Humoral immunity, 281
Hyaline cartilage, 68, 75
Hydrocele, 461
Hydrocephalus, nervous system
        and, 217–18
Hydrochloric acid, 5
Hydronephrosis, 403
Hymen, 417
Hyperopia, 240
Hypersensitivity, described, 33
Hypertension, 293
    renal, 405
Hypertonic, defined, 66
Hypertrophy, defined, 30
Hypothalamus, 463
    described, 181
    temperature control and, 45
Hypothermia, 36–37
Hypotonic, defined, 66
Hypovolemic shock, 46
Hysterosalpingogram, 435, 437

ICSH. *See* interstitial cell-stimu-
        lating hormone (ICSH).
Ileocecal, 360
Ileum, 356
Ileus, paralytic, 379
Ilisarov external fixation, bone
        fractures and, 149, *150*
Ilium, 102
Imaging, bone fractures, 147–49
Immobility, body defenses and,
        51–52

Immunity
    acquired, 44
    body defenses and, 44–45
    cardiovascular system and,
        281–82
    cellular, 281–82
    disease etiology and, 33–34
    humoral, 281
Immunization, schedule, *281*
Immunologic depression, de-
        scribed, 33–34
Immunotherapy
    cancer and, 34–35
    colon/rectum cancer and, 379
Impetigo, 85
Incisional hernia, 159
Incomplete abortion, 444
Incus, 227
Induced abortion, 444
Infant respiratory distress syn-
        drome (IRDS), 343
Infections
    bacterial, septic shock and, 47
    bone fractures and, 152
    cystitis, 404
    glomerulonephritis, 404–5
    nervous system,
        encephalitis, 217
        meningitis, 216–17
    pelvic inflammatory disease, 447
    pregnancy and, 445
    puerperal, 446
    pyelonephritis, 404
    renal,
        failure, 405
        hypertension, 405
        uremia, 405
    transmission of, 22
    upper respiratory, eustachian
        tube and, 312
    vaginitis, 447
    vision and, 244
Infectious hepatitis, 381
Infective endocarditis, 300
Infertility, tests, 435, 437
Inflammatory bowel disease,
        377–78
Influenza, 333
Inheritance
    expressions of, 430–31
    modes of, 428–30
    polygenic, 455
Inner ear, 227
Innominate bone, 102
Insulin, 467–68
    glucagon and, 360
    glucocorticoids and, 360
    production of, 360
Integument. *See* skin.
Interbrain, 181
Interferon, body defenses and, 44

Intermediate inheritance, 430
Internal capsule, neural pathways
        and, 185
Internal respirations, 317–19
Interstitial cell-stimulating hor-
        mone (ICSH), 461
Intestinal obstructions, 379
Intestines
    large,
        bacteria and, 361
        digestive processes and,
            360–62
    small,
        chemicals of, *361*
        digestive processes and,
            356–60
Intracranial pressure, nervous
        system and, 210
Intradermal tests, 81
Intraocular pressure, measuring,
        239, *240*
Intravascular blood clots, 275
Ionization, defined, 3
IRDS. *See* infant respiratory dis-
        tress syndrome (IRDS).
Iris, described, 231
Ischemia
    defined, 33
    visceral pain and, 48
Ischemic heart disease, 393–96
Ischium, 102
Isotonic, defined, 66
Isotopes
    defined, 9
    radioactive, nuclear chemistry
        and, 9–11
    See also radioisotopes.

Jacksonian seizures, 212
Jejunum, 356
Joints, 116

Keratolytic agents, corns/calluses
        and, 87
Ketosis, defined, 364
Kidneys
    blood flow and, 257–58
    cross section of, *389*
    dialysis of, 405–8
    endocrine function of, 468–69
    insulin and, 360
    renal medulla, 390
    renal pelvis, 390
    shock and, 47
    stones of, 403
    transplant of, 408
    tumors of, 403–4
    urinary system and, 388–90
Klinefelter's syndrome, 453
Kupffer's cells, 43
Kyphosis, 158

Labia, 417
Labor
   complications of, 445–46
   prolonged, 445
Labyrinth of the ear, 227
Labyrinthitis, 247
Laceration, described, 40
Lacrimal
   apparatus, vision and, 230
   glands, vision and, 230
Lactase, 360
Lactogenic hormone, 461
Laparoscopic examination, 437
Large intestines
   bacteria and, 361
   digestive processes and, 360–62
Laryngopharynx, respiration and,
      313
Larynx
   cancer of, 333
   described, 313
Lateral
   corticospinal fibers, 178
   spinothalamic cord, 177
Latissimus dorsi muscle, *136*
Law of Specific Nerve Endings, 181
LDL. *See* low density lipoprotein
      (LDL).
Leg, muscles, *139–40*
Leiomyosarcoma, 159
Lesions
   left hemisphere and, 185
   skin, 81–82
Leukemia
   described, 35
   pruritus and, 82
Leukocytes, described, 274
LH. *See* luteinizing hormone (LH).
Lice, pediculosis and, 87
Ligaments, 68
Limbic system, hypothalamus
      and, 181
Linea aspera, 103
Lingual tonsils, 313
Lipids, described, 5
Liquid connective tissue, 68, 75
Liver
   blood,
      circulation and, 257–58, *358*
      proteins and, 269
   chemicals of, *361*
   cholesterol and, 357
   digestive processes and,
         356–57
   diseases of,
      cirrhosis, 382–83
      hepatitis, 381–82
   insulin and, 360
   Kupffer's cells and, 43
   transplant, cirrhosis and,
         382–83

Lobar pneumonia, 334
Longitudinal fissure, 183
Low density lipoprotein (LDL),
      357–58
Lower extremities, venous blood
      return and, 267, *271*
LTH. *See* luteotropic hormone
      (LTH).
Lumbar
   plexus, 173
   puncture, *188*
      described, 203
Lumbosacral strain, acute, 157
Lumpectomy, 449
Lungs
   air volumes, 319–20
   cancer of, 342–43
   described, 316
   diseases of,
      asbestosis, 341–42
      bronchial asthma, 339–40
      bronchiectasis, 338–39
      cancer, 342–43
      chronic bronchitis, 338
      chronic obstructive pulmo-
            nary disease, 336, 338
         treatment of, 341
      cystic fibrosis, 340–41
      pleurisy, 334
      pneumoconiosis, 341
      pneumonia, 334
      pulmonary embolism, 336,
            337
      pulmonary infarction, 336
      silicosis, 341–42
      tuberculosis, 334–36
   emphysema and, 338
   scans of, 326, 329
   secretions of, eliminating, *339*
Lupus erythematosus, 88
Luteinizing hormone (LH), 414,
      461
Lymphatic systems, 283–84
Lymphocytes, circulating, body
      defenses and, 44
Lysosomes, described, 64
Lysozyme
   described, 43
   tears and, 230

Macule, described, 82
Magnetic resonance imaging
      (MRI), 208
   bone fractures and, 147–48
   hydrocephalus and, 218
Malignant hypertension, 293
Malleus, 227
Maltase sucrase, 360
Mammary glands. *See* breasts.
Mastectomy, 449
Mastoiditis, 245

Medial malleolus, 103
Mediastinum, heart and, 250
Medulla, 178
   oblongata, 179
Meibomian glands, 230
Meiosis, described, 64
Melanin, 76
Melanocyte-stimulating hormone
      (MSH), 462
Melatonin, 463
Membranes, 68, 75–76
   active transport and, 66–67
   cell,
      active transport and, 66–67
      diffusion and, 65–66
      exocytosis and, 67
      osmosis and, 66–67
      phagocytosis and, 67
      pinocytosis and, 67
   filtration and, 66
Menarche, 416–17
Menieres disease, 247
Meninges, 187
   spinal cord and, 171
Meningitis, central nervous sys-
      tem and, 216–17
Menopause, 416–17
Menorrhagia, 443
Menstrual cycle, *415*, 416
Metabolism
   carbohydrate, 362–64
   fat, 364
   protein, 364
Metacarpal bones, 102, *105*
Metrorrhagia, 443
Microbes
   algae, 18
   bacteria, 19
   control of, 22–24
   fungi, 19
   handling of, 24–25
   identification of, 24–25
   protozoa, 19
   rickettsiae, 19
   shape of, 19–20
   viruses, 19
Microfilaments, described, 65
Microscopes, use of, 25–27
Microtubules, described, 65
Midbrain, 179
Middle ear, hearing and, 227
Miliaria, 87
Mineralocorticoids, 466–67
Minerals, in human body, 5
Missed abortion, 444
Mitochondria, described, 64
Mitosis, described, 61, *63*, 64
Mitral
   insufficiency, 300
   stenosis, 300
Mixture, described, 5

Molecule, defined, 3
Monocytes, 274
Mons pubis, 417
Morphine, health and, 32
Motor system, examination of, 200–201
Mouth
  chemicals of, *361*
  digestive processes and, 353–54
  tumors, 374–75
MRI. *See* magnetic resonance imaging (MRI).
MSH. *See* melanocyte-stimulating hormone (MSH).
Mucous membranes, 68, 75
  body defenses and, 43
Muscles
  abdominal,
    deep, *138*
    wall, *138*
  antagonists, 127
  arm, *137*
  cardiac, described, 60
  contraction physiology, 123–26
  eye, *131*
  facial expression, *131*
  hernias and, 158–59
  immobility and, 51
  latissimus dorsi, *136*
  leg, *139–40*
  naming, 126
  neck/arm/trunk, *132*
  pectoralis major, *136*
  prime mover, 127
  semispinalis capitis, *134*
  skeletal, *127–28*
    described, 60
  sternocleidomastoid, *134*
  superficial body,
    anterior view, *129*
    posterior view, *130*
  tissues, 68, 75
  tone of, 125–26
  trapezius, *135*
  types of, 120–21, 123
  visceral, described, 60
Muscular dystrophy, 430, 455
  nervous system and, 218
Musculoskeletal system
  bone,
    composition of, 92–93
    formation of, 98–99
    structure of, 93–98
  bursae, 117–18
  cartilage, 115–16
  disorders of,
    arthritis, 153–56
    back deformities, 158
    cancer, 159
    dislocations, 153
    epicondylitis, 153

  fractures, 144–52
  hernias, 158–59
  lower back pain, 157–58
  osteomyelitis, 158
  osteoporosis, 156–57
  sprains/strains, 153
  subluxations, 153
  joints, 116, *122*
  muscles of, 120–40
    abdominal, *136*
    antagonists, 127
    contraction physiology of, 123–26
    of facial expressions, *131*
    latissimus dorsi, *136*
    left eye, *131*
    leg, *139–40*
    list of, *127–28*
    naming, 126
    neck/arm/trunk, *132–33*
    pectoralis major, *136*
    prime movers, 127
    right arm, *137*
    Semispinalis capitis, *134*
    sternocleidomastoid, *134*
    superficial, *129–30*
    trapezius, *135*
    types of, 120–21, 123
  skeleton,
    appendicular, 99–104
    axial, 104–15
Mushroom poisoning, 383
Mutations
  autosomal recessive, 454
  diseases due to, 454
  dominant, autosomal, 455
  germ cells, radioactivity and, 14
  sex linked, 455
Myasthenia gravis, nervous system and, 219–20
Mycobacterium tuberculosis, 334
Myelin, described, 164
Myelogram, computerized tomography (CT) and, 207–8
Myocardial infarction, 294
Myocardium, 250
  blood, supply to, 251
Myometrium, 415
Myopia, 240
Myositis ossificans, 51

Narcotics, pain and, 49
Nasal cavities
  described, 310–12
  hairs, body defenses and, 43
Nasolacrimal ducts, described, 311
Nausea, gastrointestinal disorders and, 374
Nearsightedness, 240

Neck
  blood circulation to, 261
  muscles of, *132–33*
Neoplasms, described, 34–35
Nephroptosis, 403
  described, 388
Nephrostomy, 403
Nerves
  conduction and, 165–69
    chemical transmission, 168–69
    electrical transmission, 166–68
  cranial, 189
    examination of, 199–200
    testing function of, *200–201*
  plexuses of, 173
  reaction time and, 171
  reflexes and, 169–71
  spinal cord and, 171, 173
    brain connections with, 177–78
    origins and distribution of, 173–77
  tissue of, 68, 75, 162–65
Nervous system
  autonomic, 190, 192–94
  behavioral responses and, 208–9
  brain and, 179–87
  cerebrospinal fluid and, 187–89
  cerebrovascular accident and, 211–12
  coma and, 210–11
  cranial nerves and, 190, *191*
  delirium and, 209
  described, 60
  diagnostic tests of,
    cerebral angiogram, 205–206
    cisternal puncture, 203–204
    computerized tomography (CT) and, 204–205
    CT myelogram, 207–208
    electroencephalogram (EEG), 206
    electromyogram (EMG), 207
    evoked responses, 206–207
    lumbar puncture, 203
    magnetic resonance imaging (MRI), 208
  divisions of, 162
  encephalitis and, 217
  epilepsy and, 212–13
  evaluation of, 199–203
    history, 198–99
  head injury and, 213–14
    symptoms of, *214*
  hydrocephalus and, 217–18
  intracranial pressure and, 210

meninges and, 187
meningitis and, 216–17
muscular dystrophy and, 218
myasthenia gravis and, 219–20
nerve conduction and, 165–69
neurons and, 165
Parkinson's disease and, 218–19
poliomyelitis and, 217
reaction time and, 171
reflexes and, 169–71
seizures and, 209–10
spinal cord and, 171, 173
  brain connections with,
    177–78
  trauma and, 214–16
spinal nerves,
  cross section of, *164*
  origins/distribution of,
    173–77
tissue of, 162–65
Neurilemma, described, 164
Neurofibrils, 163
Neurogenic shock, 47
Neurohypophysis, 462–63
Neurons, *163*
  cell bodies of, 164
  classification of, 165
  hypothalamus and, 181
Neurosurgery, pain and, 50
Neutrons, 2
Nissl bodies, 163
NMR. *See* nuclear magnetic reso-
    nance (NMR).
Nodes of Ranvier, 164
Nodules, described, 82
Noncardiogenic pulmonary
    edema, 343
Nosebleed, 332
Nuclear chemistry, 8–14
  radiation damage and, 12–14
  radioactivity and, 9
    isotopes and, 9–11
Nuclear magnetic resonance
    (NMR), bone fractures
    and, 147-48
Nuclear medicine, gastrointes-
    tinal system and, 373
Nucleic acids, described, 5
Nucleus, 2
Nystagmus, labyrinthitis and, 247

Obstructions
  intestinal, 379
  urinary, 403
Obturator foramen, 102
Occult blood, fecal, 368–69
Oocyte, described, 414
Oogenesis, spermatogenesis and,
    429
Open reduction, bone fractures
    and, 149

Ophthalmoscope, 239
  neurological examination and,
    199
Optic chiasma, 233
Optic disc, vision and, 232
Optic nerves, 233
Oral cavity
  disorders of,
    dental caries and, 374
    mouth tumors and, 374–75
    stomatitis and, 374
Oral cholecystogram, 370–71
Orchitis, 450–51
Organelles, 64–65
Organic
  compounds,
    in human body, 5
    See also compounds.
  sensations, 235
Organisms, identification of,
    24–25
Organs of Corti, 227
Oropharynx, described, 313
Orthostatic hypotension, immo-
    bility and, 52
Osmosis, cells and, 66–67
Osseous connective tissue, 68, 75
Ossification, bone, 95
Osteoarthritis, 155–56
Osteoarthropathy, 51
Osteoarthrosis, 155–56
Osteoblasts, 93
Osteoclasts, 93–94
Osteocytes, 93
Osteomyelitis, 158
Osteoporosis, 156–57
Otitis media, 227, 245
Otosclerosis, hearing loss and, 246
Ovaries, 412, 414
Oviducts, 414
Ovulation, described, 414
Oxygen
  disease etiology and, 33
  hemoglobin combining with,
    318
Oxyhemoglobin, respiration and,
    318
Oxytocin, 462–63

P wave, 254
Pacemaker, cardiac, 299
Pain
  abdominal, gastrointestinal
    disorders and, 373
  anesthesia/analgesics and,
    49–50
  anginal, location of, *294*
  biofeedback and, 50–51
  body defenses and, 48–49
  cutaneous, 48
    areas of, *49*

electrical stimulators and, 50
low back, 157–58
neurosurgery for, 50
sense of, 235
threshold, 48
tolerance, 48
visceral, receptors, 48
Palatine tonsils, 313
Palpebrae. *See* eyelids.
Pancreas, 467–68
  chemicals of, *361*
  digestive processes and,
    359–60
  diseases of, pancreatitis, 380
  sodium bicarbonate and, 360
Pancreatitis, 380
Pap test, 438
Papanicolaou test, 438
Papillae, 76
Papules, described, 82
Paralytic ileus, 379
Paranasal sinuses, described,
    310–11
Parathormone, 464
  bone and, 93
Parathyroid
  bone and, 93
  glands, 464
  hormone, calcium ion reab-
    sorption and, 391
Parietal membranes, bone, 48
Parkinson's disease, nervous sys-
    tem and, 218–19
Paronychia, 86
Parotid gland, 353
Parturition, 424, *426*
Passive immunity, 45
Pasteurization, described, 23
Patch test, 81
Pathogens, boiling and, 23
Pathology, defined, 30
Pectoralis major muscle, *136*
Pediculosis, 87
Pelvic
  cavity, described, 57–58
  examination, ultrasound, 437
  girdle, 102
  inflammatory disease, 447
Pelvis, venous blood return and,
    267–68
Penetrating wounds, 42
Penicillin, gonorrhea and, 452
Penis, 422
Pepsin, described, 355
Pepsinogen, described, 355
Peptic ulcer disease, 375–76
Percutaneous transluminal coro-
    nary angioplasty (PTCA),
    295
Pericardium, 250
Perineum, 417

Periosteum, 76
  bone, pain and, 48
Peripheral arterial disease, 304, 306
Peristalsis, described, 354
Peritoneal, dialysis, 406–7
Peritoneum, 68, 75
Peritonitis, 377
Petit mal seizures, 212
Phagocytosis, defined, 67
Phalanges, 102, *105*
Pharyngeal tonsil, described, 312–13
Pharynx
  described, 312–13
  digestive processes and, 354
  taste buds and, 225
Phonocardiogram, 289
Pia mater, spinal cord and, 171
Pilonidal sinus, 88
Pineal gland, 463
Pinocytosis, defined, 67
Pituitary gland, 181, 458, 460–63
  adenohypophysis and, 460–61
  adrenocorticotropic hormone and, 461
  antidiuretic hormone (ADH) and, 462
  beta-lipotropin and, 462
  gonadotropic hormones and, 461
  melanocyte-stimulating hormone (MSH) and, 462
  neurohypophysis and, 462–63
  oxytocin and, 462–63
  somatotropic hormone and, 461–62
  thyrotropic hormone and, 461
  vasopressin and, 462
Placenta
  abruption of, 445
  blood circulation, *273*
  endocrine function of, 469
  previa, 445–46
Plantar reflex, 169
Plasma, blood, described, 274
Pleura, 68, 75
  described, 316
Pleurisy, 334
Plexus, spinal cord and, 173–74
Pneumoconiosis, 341
Pneumonia, 334
Pneumotaxic center, 179
Poisons
  disease etiology and, 32
  food, 383
  ingested, 383–84
  treatment of, 383–84
Poliomyelitis, nervous system and, 217
Pollution, disease etiology and, 31

Polycythemia vera, 307
Polygenetic inheritance, 430, 455
Pons, 179
Portal system, venous blood return and, 269
Posterior chamber, eyeball and, 231
Postpartum hemorrhage, 446
Posttraumatic pulmonary insufficiency, 343
Pregnancy
  confirmation tests, 437
  ectopic, 444
  fertilization and, 422–24
  infections and, 445
  radiation and, 14
  thrombophlebitis and, 445
  toxemia and, 444–45
Presbycusis, 246
Presbyopia, 241–42
Pressure, sense of, 234
Pressure points, illustrated, *41*
Prickly heat, 87
Prime movers, 127
Probenecid, gonorrhea and, 452
Progesterone, function of, 414
Prolapsed uterus, 447
Prostaglandins, 469–70
Prostate, 422
  benign hypertrophy of, 449–50
  cancer of, 450
  infections of, 451
Prostatitis, 451
Proteins
  amylase and, 360
  described, 5
  metabolism, 364
  pancreatic trypsin and, 360
Prothrombin, 358
  time, defined, 275
Protons, 2
Protozoa, 19
Pruritus, skin and, 82
Psoriasis, 85
PTCA. *See* percutaneous transluminal coronary angioplasty (PTCA).
Pubis, 102
Pudendal plexus, 174, 177
Puerperal infection, 446
Pulmonary
  angiography, 329
  circulation,
  described, 261
  pressure, Swan-Ganz catheter and, 260
  function tests, respiratory system and, 332
Pupils
  brain damage and, *211*
  reflexes and, 169

Purpura, 307
Pustules, described, 82
Pyelogram
  intravenous, urine tests and, 400–401
  retrograde, urine tests and, 401
Pyelonephritis, 404
Pyramidal tracts, 178

QRS complex, 254

Radiation
  breast cancer and, 449
  colon/rectum cancer and, 379
  damage, nuclear chemistry and, 12–14
  injuries by, 39–40
  lethal dose, symptoms of, 13–14
  pregnant women and, 14
  protection from, 14
  testes cancer and, 450
Radioactive, isotopes, nuclear chemistry and, 9–11
Radiographic studies
  barium,
    enema, 369–70
    swallow, 369
  endoscopy, 371
  oral cholecystogram, 370–71
  small bowel series, 369
  ultrasonography, 371–72
  upper gastrointestinal series, 369
Radioisotopes
  commonly used, *10*
  uses of, 10–11
  See also isotopes.
Radionuclide studies, cardiovascular system and, 289–90
Recessive
  autosomal mutations, 455
  inheritance, 428
Rectum
  cancer of, 378–79
  varicose veins of, cirrhosis and, 382–83
Red bone marrow, 97
Reduction
  bone fractures and, 147–51
  division. *See* meiosis.
Reflexes
  Babinski, 169
  cardiac, 256–57
  deep tendon, 169
  first-level, 169–70
  gag, 169
  midbrain and, 179
  nerves and, 169–71
  plantar, 169
  testing, 201–2

Regional enteritis, 378
Relaxin, 414
Renal
  cortex, kidney, 388–90
  failure, 405
  hypertension, 405
  medulla, kidneys and, 390
  pelvis, kidneys and, 390
Reproduction
  contraception and, 427–28
  fertility and, 424, 427
  genetics and, 428–31
  physiology of, 422–24
Reproductive system
  abortions and, 443–44
  acquired immune deficiency
    syndrome (AIDS) and, 453
  amenorrhea, 443
  autosomal,
    dominant mutations, 455
    recessive mutations and,
      454–55
  breast, 417–18
    abscess of, 449
    benign tumors of, 448
    cystic mastitis and, 448
    malignancies of, 448–49
    tumors of, 439–40
  diagnostic procedures, infertil-
    ity tests, 435, 437
  diseases of,
    benign prostatic hypertro-
      phy, 449–50
    endometriosis, 446
    epididymitis, 451
    genital herpes and, 452–53
    gonorrhea and, 451–52
    inherited, 453–54
    mutations and, 454
    orchitis, 450–51
    ovarian tumors, 446
    pelvic inflammatory disease,
      447
    prostate cancer, 450
    prostatitis, 451
    testicular cancer, 450
    toxemia and, 444–45
    uterine cancer, 447
    uterine tumors, 446
    vaginal fistulas, 448
    vaginitis, 447
    venereal, 452–53
    vesicovaginal fistula and, 448
  dysmenorrhea, 443
  female, 412–18
    cross section of, 413
    external organs of, 417
    mammary glands, 417–18
    menstruation disorders, 443
    ovaries, 412, 414
    oviducts, 414

  uterus, 414–17
  vagina, 417
  gynecological examination,
    438–39
  infections,
    epididymitis, 451
    orchitis, 450–51
    pelvic inflammatory disease,
      447
    prostatitis, 451
    vaginitis, 447
  inheritance, polygenic, 455
  labor/delivery problems,
    placenta previa, 445–46
    placental abruption, 445
    postpartum hemorrhage, 446
    prolonged labor, 445
    puerperal infection, 446
  male,
    accessory structures of,
      421–22
    cross section of, 420
    excretory ducts of, 421
    penis, 422
    semen, 422
    testes, 418, 420–21
  menorrhagia, 443
  metrorrhagia, 443
  pregnancy,
    confirmation tests, 437
    ectopic, 444
    infections and, 445
    thrombophlebitis and, 445
    toxemia and, 444–45
  sex-linked mutants and, 455
  syphilis and, 452
  tumors of,
    endometriosis, 446
    ovarian, 446
    uterine, 446
    uterine cancer, 447
  uterine displacements, 447–48
  vaginal fistulas of, 448
  venereal disease, 451–52
    examination for, 440–41
  vesicovaginal fistula and, 448
Residual air, described, 319–20
Respiration
  acid-base balance regulation
    and, 321–22
  external/internal, 317–19
  gas transport and, 318
  hemoglobin-oxygen combining
    in, 318
  physiology of, 316–19
    pressure involved in, 316
  regulation of, 319
Respiratory system
  acid-base balance regulation
    and, 321–22
  air volumes and, 319–20

  alveoli and, 314–16
  bronchi and, 313–14
  bronchioles and, 313–14
  described, 58–59
  diagnostic procedures of,
    327–32
    bronchoscopy and, 329
    computerized tomography
      (CT), 329
    pulmonary angiography, 329
    pulmonary function tests
      and, 332
    roentgenography, 327,
      329–30
    sputum specimens and, 329
    tuberculin tests and, 331
  diseases of,
    adult respiratory distress
      syndrome (ARDS), 343–44
    asbestosis, 341–42
    bronchial asthma, 339–40
    bronchiectasis, 338–39
    chest trauma, 344
    chronic bronchitis, 338
    chronic obstructive pulmo-
      nary disease, 336, 338
      treatment, 341
    common cold, 333
    croup, 333–34
    cystic fibrosis, 340–41
    emphysema and, 338
    epiglottitis, 334
    epistaxis, 332
    infant respiratory distress
      syndrome (IRDS), 343
    influenza, 333
    larynx cancer, 333
    lung cancer, 342–43
    pleurisy, 334
    pneumoconiosis, 341
    pneumonia, 334
    pneumothorax, 344–45
    pulmonary embolism, 336,
      337
    pulmonary infarction, 336
    silicosis, 341–42
    sinusitis, 332
    tonsillitis, 332–33
    tuberculosis, 334–36
  gas laws and, 321
  larynx and, 313
  lungs and, 316
  nasal cavities and, 310–12
  pharynx and, 312–13
  pleura and, 316
  respiration physiology and,
    316–19
  secretions of, eliminating, 339
  tonsils and, 312–13
  trachea and, 313
  voice production and, 313

Reticuloendothelial system, 44
    blood cells and, 274
Retina
    described, 232
    detached, 244
Rhabdomyosarcoma, 159
Rheumatic
    fever, valvular heart disease
        and, 300
    heart disease, 300
Rheumatoid arthritis, 153–55
Ribosomes, 64
Ribs, broken, 344
Rickettsiae, 19
Rods, vision and, 232, 233
Roentgenography, 327, 330
Rubin test, 435
Rubrospinal tracts, 178
Rugae, described, 354
Rule of Nines, burns and, 37–38,
        38, 39

Saccule, equilibrium and, 229
Sacral plexus, 173–74
Sacrum, 102, *106–9*
Safranine, 25
Saliva, body defenses and, 43
Salivary glands, 353
Salmonella, 383
Salts, described, 6
Saphenous vein revascularization
        procedure, *296*
Scabies, 87–88
Scapula, 99, *102*
Schiotz tonometer, *240*
Sclera, 68, 76
    described, 230
Scleroderma, 88
Scoliosis, 158
Scrotum, 421
Sebaceous
    cysts, 86–87
    glands, 76
    secretions, microorganisms
        and, 43
Seborrheic dermatitis, 84
Sebum, 76
Second degree burns, 37
Second-level reflexes, 170
Secondary hypertension, 293
Secretin, 356
Sedatives, pain and, 49
Seizures, nervous system and,
        209–10
Semen, 422
Semicircular canals
    equilibrium and, 228–29
    inner ear, 227
Seminal vesicles, 421–22
Semispinalis capitis muscle, *134*

Sensation
    characteristics of, 224–25
    mechanisms of, 224–25
Senses
    cutaneous, 234–35
    equilibrium and, 228–29
    hearing, 227–28
        tests for, 239–40
    organic, 235
    sight, 230–33
        examinations, 239
    smell, 226–27
    taste, 225–26
    vision, 229–34
        impaired, 240–45
Sensitivity tests, skin, 81
Sensorineural hearing loss, 246
Septal defect, 301
Septic shock, 47
Septicemia, gonorrhea and,
        451–52
Serotonin, 463
Serous membranes, 68, 75–76
Sex
    hormones, adrenal glands, 467
    linked inheritance, 429–30
    linked mutants, 455
Shingles, 86
Shock, body defenses and, 46–48
Shock lung, 343
Shoulder girdle, 99
Sigmoid colon, 361–62
    diverticular disease and, 377
Silicosis, 341
Simple squamous epithelium,
        73–74
Sinoatrial node, 253–54
Sinus tachycardia, 298
Sinuses, 108, *116*
Sinusitis, 332
Skeletal
    muscles, 68, 120, 121, 123
        described, 60
    system, described, 59–60
Skeleton
    anterior view of, *100*
    appendicular, 99–104
    axial, 104–15
    posterior view of, *101*
    See also bone.
Skin, 68, 76–78
    biopsy of, 81
    body defenses and, 42–43
    crusts and, 82
    cryosurgery and, 82–83
    disorders of,
        acne, 83–84
        athlete's foot, 87
        bites, 87
        calluses, 87
        carbuncles, 86

cold sores, 86
contact dermatitis, 84–85
corns, 87
dermatophytosis, 87
diaper rash, 87
eczema, 84
furuncles, 86
herpes simplex, 86
herpes zoster, 86
hives, 84
impetigo, 85
infestations, 87
lupus erythematosus, 88
miliaria, 87
paronychia, 86
pediculosis, 87
pilonidal sinus, 88
prickly heat, 87
psoriasis, 85
scabies, 87–88
scleroderma, 88
sebaceous cysts, 86–87
seborrheic dermatitis, 84
shingles, 86
warts, 85
    examination of, 80–81
    lesions, 81–82
    scales and, 82
    sensitivity tests, 81
    therapeutic measures for,
        82–83
Skull, bones of, 104–11, *113–15*
Slipped disc, 157
Small
    bowel series, 369
    intestines,
        chemicals of, *361*
        digestive processes and,
            356–60
Smell, sense of, 226–27
Smooth muscles, 68
Snellen eye chart
    eye examinations and, 239
    neurological examination and,
        199
Sodium, stress and, 472
Sodium bicarbonate, pancreas
        and, 360
Soft
    palate, taste buds and, 225
    tissue, wounds to, 40, 42
Somatic damage, radioactivity
        and, 12–14
Somatostatin, 463, 468
Somatotropic hormone, 461–62
Sordes, defined, 226
Specimens, microbes, collecting,
        24
Spermatic cords, 421
Spermatogenesis, oogenesis and,
        429

Spinal cord
  brain, connections with,
    177–78
  nerves and, 171, 173
    origins and distribution of,
      173–77
  trauma to, 214–16
  guide of, 216
Spinal tap. See lumbar puncture.
Spine, pain in, 157–58
Spinocerebellar tracts, 177
Spinothalamic cord, 177
Spinous process, 112
Spirochete, 19
Spleen, lymphatic system and,
  283
Spontaneous abortion, 444
Sprains, 153
Sputum, specimens, respiratory
  system and, 329
Squamous
  epithelial tissue, 67
  epithelium, 73–74
Stapes, 227
Staphylococci, 19
Starling's Law of the Heart, 256
Stasis, urine, immobility and, 52
Status asthmaticus, 340
Sterilization, microbes and, 23
Sternocleidomastoid muscles, 134
Steroid creams, acne and, 84
Stimulators, electrical, pain and,
  50
Stirrup of the ear, 227
Stomach
  chemicals of, 361
  cross section of, 355, 356
  digestive processes and,
    354–55
  disorders of,
    gastritis, 375
    peptic ulcer disease and,
      375–76
Stomatitis, 374
Strabismus, 242–43
Strains, 153
Strangulation, loop of bowel, 159
Stratified
  epithelium, 74
    squamous, 67
Streptococci, 19
Stress
  alarm/resistance and, 472–73
  endocrine system and, 470–73
  response to, 470
    factors determining, 471–72
  sodium and, 472
Striated muscles, 68
Strictures, renal, 403
Stroke
  nervous system and, 211–12

volume, blood circulation and,
  256
Subarachnoid hemorrhage, 214
Subluxations, 153
Succus entericus, 360
Sunlight, microbes and, 23
Sunstroke. See heat stroke.
Sutures, 108, 110
Swan-Ganz catheter, pulmonary
  circuit pressure and, 260
Sweat
  glands, 76–77
  microorganisms and, 43
Symphysis pubis, 102
Synapse, described, 165
Synarthrotic joints, 116
Syndrome, defined, 31
Synovial membranes, 68, 76
Syphilis, 452
Systemic circulation, described,
  261
Systole contraction, 254

T cells
  cellular immunity and, 281
  thymosin and, 281
T wave, 254–55
Tachycardia, 298
Talus, 103–4
Tarsal bones, 103
Taste, 225–26
  buds, 353
Tears
  body defenses and, 43
  vision and, 230
Teeth, 353, 354
  brushing of, 375
Temperature
  chemical reactions and, 7–8
  control of, body defenses and,
    45–46
Tendons, 68
Tennis elbow, 153
Tentorium cerebelli, 187
Testes
  cancer of, 450
  inflammation of, 450–51
Tetracycline, gonorrhea and, 452
Tetralogy of Fallot, 302
Thalamus
  described, 181
  nerve impulses and, 177
Thermal burns, 37–38
Thermography, breast examina-
  tions and, 440
Third degree burns, 37
Third-level reflexes, 170
Thoracentesis, 334, 335
Thoracic cavity, 57
Thorax, 114–15, 120
  venous blood return and, 267

Threatened abortion, 444
Thrombocytes, 275
Thrombophlebitis, pregnancy
  and, 445
Thrombus
  described, 275
  immobility and, 52
Thymine, deoxyribonucleic acid
  (DNA) and, 61
Thymosin, 464–65
  T cells and, 281
Thymus, 464–65
  lymphatic system and, 283
Thyrocalcitonin, bone and, 93
Thyroid, 463–64
  bone and, 93
Thyrotropic hormone, 461
Thyroxin, 463
Tibia, 103, 104, 111
Tidal air, described, 319
Tincture of benzoin, lacerations
  and, 40
Tinnitus
  labyrinthitis and, 247
  vestibular disease and, 247
Tissues, 72–75
  connective, 67–68, 74–75
  cultures, gene study and, 430
  endothelium, 68
  epithelial, 67, 73–74
  illustrated, 73
  muscle, 68, 75
  nerve, 68, 75
Toenails, 77
Tonic clonic seizures, 212
Tonometer, 239
Tonsillitis, 332–33
Tonsils
  described, 312–13
  lymphatic system and, 283
Touch, sense of, 234
Toxemia, pregnancy and, 444–45
Toxic shock, 47
Trachea, described, 313
Tracheostomy, larynx cancer and,
  333
Traction, bone fractures and, 151
Tranquilizers, pain and, 49
Transient ischemic attack (TIA),
  stroke and, 211
Transverse fissure, 183
Trapezius muscle, 135
Trauma
  cold, 36–37
  disease etiology and, 36–42
Triiodothyronine, 463
Trisomy 21, 454
Trisomy, sex chromosomes and,
  454
Trochanters, 103
Trunk, muscles of, 132–33

Trypsin, proteins and, 360
Tubal ligation, 427
Tuberculin tests, respiratory system, 331
Tuberculosis, 334–36
Tuberosity, 103
Tumors
  benign, 34
  breast,
    benign, 448
    diagnosis of, 439–40
    malignant, 448–49
  described, 82
  endometriosis, 446
  malignant, 34
  mouth, 374–75
  ovarian, 446
  urinary system, 404
  uterine, 446
    cancerous, 447
Tuning forks, hearing tests and, 238
Turner's syndrome, 453–54
Tympanic membrane, 227

Ulcers, peptic, 375–76
Ulna, 99, *104*
Ultrasonography, gastrointestinal system and, 371–72
Ultrasound, urinary system and, 401–402
Universal precautions, microbes and, 23–24
Upper extremity, venous blood return and, 267, *269*
Upper gastrointestinal series, 369
Upper respiratory tract
  diseases of,
    common cold, 333
    croup, 333–34
    epiglottitis, 334
    epistaxis, 332
    influenza, 333
    larynx cancer, 333
    sinusitis, 332
    tonsillitis, 332–33
Urea, described, 391
Uremia, 405
Uremic frost, 405
Ureters, 390
Urethra, 390–91
  male reproductive system and, 421
Urinary, obstructions, 403
Urinary system
  cancer of, 404
  cystoscopy and, 401
  described, 60
  diagnostic measures and,
    blood tests, 397
    urine tests, 396–97

X-rays, 397, 400–401
diseases of,
  calculi, 403
  cystitis, 404
  glomerulonephritis, 404–5
  nephroptosis, 403
  pyelonephritis, 404
  renal failure, 405
  renal hypertension, 405
  strictures, 403
  tumors, 403–4
  uremia, 405
  urinary obstructions, 402–3
kidneys, 388–90
micturition and, 393
ultrasound and, 401–2
ureters and, 390
urethra, 390–91
urine formation and, 391–93
Urine
  acidification of, 392
  appearance of, 397
  body defenses and, 43
  composition of, 397, *398–99*
    abnormal, *399*
  formation of, 391–93
  pregnancy testing and, 437
  specimens,
    catheterized, 396
    clean-caught midstream, 396–97
  stasis, immobility and, 52
  tests of, 396–97
  volume/concentration of, 393
Urticaria, 84
Uterus, 414–17
  displacements of, 447–48
Utricle, equilibrium and, 228–29

Vagina, 417
  mucous membranes, body defenses and, 43
Vaginal fistulas, 448
Vaginitis, 447
Vagus nerve, heart rate and, 252–53
Valves, heart, 251
Valvular heart disease, 300–301
Varicose veins, 306–7
  cirrhosis and, 382–83
Varicosities, 379
Vas deferens, 421
Vasoconstriction, fever and, 45
Vasodilation, cold trauma and, 36
Vasogenic shock, 47
Vasopressin, 462
Vasospasms, cold trauma and, 36
Veins, illustration of, *262*
Venereal diseases, 450–53
  examination for, 440–41

Venous blood pressure, 260
Ventral spinothalamic tract, 177
Ventricular
  fibrillation, 298
  septal defect, 301
Vertebral column, 111–12, 114, *118–19*
Vertigo
  described, 247
  vestibular disease and, 247
Vesicles, described, 82
Vesicovaginal fistula, 448
Vestibule, 417
  of inner ear, 227
    disease of, 247
Villi, described, 356
Viral hepatitis, comparison types of, *381*
Viruses, 19
  disease etiology and, 35–36
Visceral
  muscles, 68, 120–21, 123
    described, 60
  pain, receptors, 48
Vision, 229–34
  astigmatism and, 240
  binocular, 234
  cataracts and, 243
  corneal problems and, 245–46
  detached retina and, 244
  focusing and, 232–33
  glaucoma and, 243–44
  hyperopia and, 240
  infections and, 244
  myopia and, 240
  pathways of, 233–34, *241*
  presbyopia and, 241–42
  strabismus and, 242–43
  visual field defects and, 240
  See also eye.
Vital capacity, respiration and, 320
Voice box. *See* larynx.
Voice production, described, 313
Vomiting, gastrointestinal disorders and, 374

Warts, 85
Water, stress and, 472
Wet dressings, skin, 82
Wheals, described, 82
White blood cells, described, 274
White fibrous connective tissue, 68
Wilm's tumor, 404
Wounds, 40, 42
  healing of, 42

X-rays, bone fractures and, 147–48

Yellow bone marrow, 97